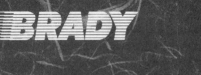

BRADY

Intermediate Emergency Care
Principles & Practice

Workbook

Robert S. Porter

BRYAN E. BLEDSOE, DO, FACEP, EMT-P
Clinical Associate Professor of Emergency Medicine
University of North Texas Health Sciences Center
Fort Worth, Texas

ROBERT S. PORTER, MA, NREMT-P
Senior Advanced Life Support Educator
Madison County Emergency Medical Services
Canastota, New York
and
Flight Paramedic
AirOne, Onondaga County Sheriff's Department
Syracuse, New York

RICHARD A. CHERRY, MS, NREMT-P
Clinical Assistant Professor of Emergency Medicine
Assistant Residency Director
SUNY Upstate Medical University
Syracuse, New York

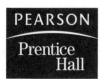

PEARSON

Prentice
Hall

Upper Saddle River, New Jersey 07458

NOTICE ON CARE PROCEDURES

It is the intent of the authors and publisher that this workbook be used as part of a formal EMT-Intermediate program taught by qualified instructors and supervised by a licensed physician. The procedures described in this workbook are based upon consultation with EMT and medical authorities. The authors and publisher have taken care to make certain that these procedures reflect currently accepted clinical practice; however, they cannot be considered absolute recommendations.

The material in this workbook contains the most current information available at the time of publication. However, federal, state, and local guidelines concerning clinical practices, including, without limitation, those governing infection control and universal precautions, change rapidly. The reader should note, therefore, that the new regulations may require changes in some procedures.

It is the responsibility of the reader to familiarize himself or herself with the policies and procedures set by federal, state, and local agencies as well as the institution or agency where the reader is employed. The authors and the publisher of this workbook disclaim any liability, loss, or risk resulting directly or indirectly from the suggested procedures and theory, from any undetected errors, or from the reader's misunderstanding of the text. It is the reader's responsibility to stay informed of any new changes or recommendations made by any federal, state, and local agency as well as by his or her employing institution or agency.

Publisher: Julie Levin Alexander
Assistant to Publisher: Regina Bruno
Executive Editor: Marlene McHugh Pratt
Managing Development Editor: Lois Berlowitz
Development Editor: Susan Simpfenderfer, Triple SSS Press Media Development
Senior Marketing Manager: Katrin Beacom
Director of Manufacturing & Production: Bruce Johnson
Senior Manufacturing Manager: Ilene Sanford
Manufacturing Buyer: Pat Brown
Managing Production Editor: Patrick Walsh
Production Editor: Jeanne Molenaar
Channel Marketing Manager: Rachele Strober
Cover Design: Blair Brown
Cover Photography: Eddie Sperling
Production Supervision: Navta Associates, Inc.
Composition: Barbara J. Barg
Cover Printer: Coral Graphics
Printing/Binding: Banta Company, Harrisonburg, Virginia

Pearson Prentice Hall™ is a trademark of Pearson Education, Inc.
Pearson® is a registered trademark of Pearson plc
Prentice Hall® is a registered trademark of Pearson Education, Inc.

Pearson Education LTD.
Pearson Education Australia PTY, Limited
Pearson Education Singapore, Pte. Ltd
Pearson Education North Asia Ltd
Pearson Education Canada, Ltd
Pearson Educación de Mexico, S.A. de C.V.
Pearson Education—Japan
Pearson Education Malaysia, Pte. Ltd
Pearson Education, Upper Saddle River, NJ

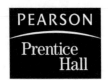

10 9 8 7 6 5 4 3 2 1
ISBN 0-13-113639-9

Dedication

This book is respectfully dedicated to the EMT professionals who toil each day in an environment that is unpredictable, often dangerous, and constantly changing. They risk their lives to aid the sick and the injured, driven only by their love of humanity and their devotion to this profession we call emergency medical services.

We remember the EMS, fire, and law enforcement personnel who have made the ultimate sacrifice for their communities and our nation. May they never be forgotten.

Contents

Self-Instructional Workbook

Intermediate Emergency Care: Principles & Practice

Introduction
To the Self-Instructional Workbook
Intermediate Emergency Care: Principles & Practice

Welcome to the self-instructional workbook for *Intermediate Emergency Care: Principles & Practice*. This workbook is designed to help guide you through an educational program for Intermediate-level training that follows the guidelines of the 1999 U.S. Department of Transportation EMT-Intermediate National Standard Curriculum. The workbook is designed to be used either in conjunction with your instructor or as a self-study guide you use on your own.

This workbook features many different ways to help you learn the material necessary to become an EMT-I, including those listed below.

FEATURES

Review of Chapter Objectives
Each chapter of *Intermediate Emergency Care: Principles & Practice* begins with objectives that identify the important information and principles addressed in the chapter reading. To help you identify and learn this material, each workbook chapter reviews the important content elements addressed by these objectives as presented in the text.

Case Study Review
Each chapter of *Intermediate Emergency Care: Principles & Practice* includes a case study, introducing and highlighting important principles presented in the chapter. The workbook reviews these case studies and points out much of the essential information and many of the applied principles they describe.

Content Self-Evaluation
Each chapter of *Intermediate Emergency Care: Principles & Practice* presents an extensive narrative explanation of the principles of EMT-I practice. The workbook chapter (or chapter part) contains between 10 and 90 multiple-choice questions to test your reading comprehension of the textbook material and to give you experience taking typical emergency medical service examinations.

Chapter Parts
Several chapters in *Intermediate Emergency Care: Principles & Practice* are long and contain a great deal of subject matter. To help you grasp this material more efficiently, the workbook breaks these chapters into parts with their own objectives and content review.

Special Projects
The workbook contains several projects that are special learning experiences designed to help you remember the information and principles necessary to perform as an EMT-I. Special projects include crossword puzzles, personal benchmarking activities, and a variety of other exercises.

Personal Benchmarking
The workbook provides exercises that direct you to learn sites for drug administration on yourself. These exercises help you develop your medication administration skills and to use normal findings as benchmarks for reference when you begin your career as an EMT-I.

National Registry Practical Evaluation Forms

Supplemental materials found at the back of the workbook include the National Registry Practical Evaluation Forms. These or similar forms will be used to test your practical skills throughout your training and, usually, for state certification exams. By reviewing them, you have a clearer picture of what is expected of you during your practical exam and a better understanding of the type of evaluation tool that is used to measure your performance.

Emergency Drug Cards

This workbook contains alphabetized 3″ × 5″ cards that present the names/classes, descriptions, indications, contraindications, precautions, and routes and dosages of drugs you are most likely to encounter in prehospital care. Detach the cards and use them in flash card fashion. Practice until you can give the correct route, dosage, indications, and contraindications for each drug.

ACKNOWLEDGMENTS

Contributors

We wish to acknowledge the extraordinary talents and efforts of the following people who contributed chapters to this workbook. In developing study guides, questions, and activities, they have upheld the highest standards of EMS instruction.

Beth Lothrop Adams, MA, RN, NREMT-P
EMS Quality Manager
Fairfax County Fire Department
Fairfax County, Virginia

Elizabeth Coolidge-Stolz, MD
Medical Writer; Health Educator
North Reading, Massachusetts

Special thanks to Tony Crystal and Bob Elling, whose tireless efforts in writing, checking, and coordinating workbook content made it possible to deliver this workbook to students in a timely manner. We are grateful for their assistance.

Tony Crystal
EMS Director
Lake Land College
Mattoon, Illinois

Bob Elling, MPA, REMT-P
Professor of Management
American College of Prehospital Medicine
Faculty Member
Hudson Valley Community College of Prehospital
    Emergency Medicine
Schenectady, New York

Reviewers

The reviewers listed below provided many excellent suggestions for improving this workbook. Their assistance is greatly appreciated.

Blaine Griffiths, BSAS, RN, NREMT-P
Youngstown State University
Youngstown, Ohio

David M. Habben, NREMT-P
EMS Consultant
Boise, Idaho

Edward B. Kuvlesky, NREMT-P
Battalion Chief
Indian River County EMS
Indian River County, Florida

Matthew R. Streger, MPA, NREMT-P
former Deputy Commissioner
Cleveland Emergency Medical Services
Cleveland, Ohio

Scott Vahradian, EMT-P
Santa Cruz, California

K. Lee Watson, NREMT-P
Martinsville-Henry County Rescue Squad
Martinsville, Virginia

HOW TO USE

The Self-Instructional Workbook

Intermediate Emergency Care: Principles & Practice

The self-instructional workbook accompanying *Intermediate Emergency Care: Principles & Practice* may be used as directed by your instructor or independently by you during your course of instruction. The recommendations listed below are intended to guide you in using the workbook independently.

- Examine your course schedule and identify the appropriate text chapter or other assigned reading.

- Read the assigned chapter in *Intermediate Emergency Care: Principles & Practice* carefully. Do this in a relaxed environment, free of distractions, and give yourself adequate time to read and digest the material. The information presented in *Intermediate Emergency Care: Principles & Practice* is often technically complex and demanding, but it is very important that you comprehend it. Be sure that you read the chapter carefully enough to understand and remember what you have read.

- Carefully read the Review of Chapter Objectives at the beginning of each workbook chapter (or part). This material includes both the objectives listed in *Intermediate Emergency Care: Principles & Practice* and narrative descriptions of their content. If you do not understand or remember what is discussed from your reading, refer to the referenced pages and reread them carefully. If you still do not feel comfortable with your understanding of any objective, consider asking your instructor about it.

- Take the Content Self-Evaluation at the end of each workbook chapter (or part), answering each question carefully. Do this in a quiet environment, free from distractions, and allow yourself adequate time to complete the exercise. Correct your self-evaluation by consulting the answers at the back of the workbook, and determine the percentage you have answered correctly (the number you got right divided by the total number of questions). If you have answered most of the questions correctly (85 to 90 percent), review those that you missed by rereading the material on the pages listed in the answer key and be sure you understand which answer is correct and why. If you have more than a few questions wrong (less than 85 percent correct), look for incorrect answers that are grouped together. This suggests that you did not understand a particular topic in the reading. Reread the text dealing with that topic carefully, and then retest yourself on the questions you got wrong. If incorrect answers are spread throughout the chapter content, reread the chapter and re-take the Content Self-Evaluation to assure that you understand the material. If you don't understand why your answer to a question is incorrect after reviewing the text, consult with your instructor.

- When you have completed *Intermediate Emergency Care: Principles & Practice* and its accompanying workbook, prepare for a course test by reviewing both the text in its entirety and your class notes.

If, during your completion of the workbook exercises, you have any questions that either the textbook or workbook doesn't answer, write them down and ask your instructor about them. Prehospital emergency medicine is a complex and complicated subject, and answers are not always black-and-white. It is also common for different EMS systems to use differing methods of care. The questions you bring up in class, and your instructor's answers to them, will help you expand and complete your knowledge of prehospital emergency medical care.

The authors and Brady Publishing continuously seek to assure the creation of the best materials to support your educational experience. We are interested in your comments. If, during your reading and study of material in *Intermediate Emergency Care: Principles & Practice*, you notice any error or have any suggestions to improve either the textbook or workbook, please direct your comments via the Internet at: harrier@localnet.com. You can also visit the Brady website at: www.prenhall.com/bledsoe.

GUIDELINES TO BETTER TEST-TAKING

The knowledge you will gain from reading the textbook, completing the exercises in the workbook, listening in your EMT-I class, and participating in your clinical and field experience will prepare you to care for patients who are seriously ill or injured. However, before you can practice these skills, you will have to pass several classroom written exams and your state's certification exam successfully. Your performance on these exams will depend not only on your knowledge but also on your ability to answer test questions correctly. The following guidelines are designed to help your performance on tests and to better demonstrate your knowledge of prehospital emergency care.

1. Relax and be calm during the test.

A test is designed to measure what you have learned and to tell you and your instructor how well you are doing. An exam is not designed to intimidate or punish you. Consider it a challenge, and just try to do your best. Get plenty of sleep prior to the examination. Avoid coffee or other stimulants for a few hours before the exam, and be prepared.

Reread the text chapters, review the objectives in the workbook, and review your class notes. It might be helpful to work with one or two other students and ask each other questions. This type of practice helps everyone better understand the knowledge presented in your course of study.

2. Read the questions carefully.

Read each word of the question and all the answers slowly. Words such as "except" or "not" may change the entire meaning of the question. If you miss such words, you may answer the question incorrectly even though you know the right answer.

EXAMPLE:
The art and science of Emergency Medical Services involves all of the following EXCEPT:

    A. sincerity and compassion.
    B. respect for human dignity.
    C. placing patient care before personal safety.
    D. delivery of sophisticated emergency medical care.
    E. none of the above

The correct answer is C, unless you miss the "EXCEPT."

3. Read each answer carefully.

Read each and every answer carefully. While the first answer may be absolutely correct, so may the rest, and thus the best answer might be "all of the above."

EXAMPLE:
Indirect medical direction is considered to be:

    A. treatment protocols.
    B. training and education.
    C. quality assurance.
    D. chart review.
    E. all of the above

While answers A, B, C, and D are correct, the best and only acceptable answer is "all of the above," E.

4. Delay answering questions you don't understand and look for clues.

When a question seems confusing or you don't know the answer, note it on your answer sheet and come back to it later. This will ensure that you have time to complete the test. You will also find that other questions in the test may give you hints to answer the one you've skipped over. It will also prevent you from being frustrated with an early question and letting it affect your performance.

EXAMPLE:
Upon successful completion of a course of training as an EMT-I, most states will

    A. certify you. (correct)
    B. license you.
    C. register you.
    D. recognize you as an EMT-I.
    E. issue you a permit.

Another question, later in the exam, may suggest the right answer:

The action of one state in recognizing the certification of another is called:

    A. reciprocity. (correct)
    B. national registration.
    C. licensure.
    D. registration.
    E. extended practice.

5. Answer all questions.

Even if you do not know the right answer, do not leave a question blank. A blank question is always wrong, while a guess might be correct. If you can eliminate some of the answers as wrong, do so. It will increase the chances of a correct guess.

EXAMPLE:
When an EMT-I is called by the patient (through the dispatcher) to the scene of a medical emergency, the medical direction physician has established a physician/patient relationship.

    A. True
    B. False

    A true/false question gives you a 50 percent chance of a correct guess.

The hospital health professional responsible for sorting patients as they arrive at the emergency department is usually the:

    A. emergency physician.
    B. ward clerk.
    C. emergency nurse.
    D. trauma surgeon.
    E. both A and C (correct)

    A multiple-choice question with five answers gives a 20 percent chance of a correct guess. If you can eliminate one or more incorrect answers, you increase your odds of a correct guess to 25 percent, 33 percent, and so on. An unanswered question has a 0 percent chance of being correct.
    Just before turning in your answer sheet, check to be sure that you have not left any items blank.

Intermediate Emergency Care: Principles & Practice

Division 1

Preparatory Information

CHAPTER 1

*

Foundations
of the EMT-Intermediate

Part 1: Introduction to Advanced Prehospital Care

Review of Chapter Objectives

With each chapter of the Workbook, we identify the objectives and the important elements of the textbook content. Because Chapter 1 is lengthy, it has been divided into parts. You should review items in these parts and refer to the pages listed if any points are not clear.

After reading this part of the chapter, you should be able to:

1. **Describe the relationship between the EMT-Intermediate and the other members of the allied health professions.** pp. 5–7

   The EMT-I is the second highest-level prehospital care provider and leader of the prehospital care team. He or she is a member of the allied health-care professions and specifically a member of the ancillary health-care professions, which include health-care professionals other than physicians and nurses. EMT-Is are credentialed or licensed by an appropriate state or provincial agency and approved by their system's medical directors.

2. **Identify the attributes and characteristics of an EMT-Intermediate.** pp. 6–7

   EMT-Is must possess the knowledge, skills, and attitudes consistent with the expectations of the public and the profession. This includes recognizing that you are an essential component in the continuum of care and an advocate for the patient. As an EMT-I, you must be flexible enough to work within the various types of EMS systems and adjust to the ever-changing emergency environment. You must be a confident leader, accept the challenges of your profession, have excellent judgement, communicate effectively, develop a rapport with a great diversity of patients, and function independently in a very unstructured environment.

3. **Explain the elements of EMT-Intermediate education and practice that support its stature as a profession.** pp. 6–7

   The 1998 U.S. Department of Transportation's EMT-I: National Standard Curriculum describes an intensive course of education with a great emphasis on anatomy, physiology, and pathophysiology. This material provides a broad foundation for your understanding of the human body and its injury and illness. Once you complete initial training, you are expected to continue your education, both to expand your knowledge of prehospital care and to ensure that you remain practiced and ready to employ those skills used less frequently. Further, you and other members of the profession must commit to supporting research both to define and improve skills and care procedures that benefit patients and to identify those that do not. Only through research can the EMT-I profession continue to grow and earn respect for the work of its members. Despite its relative youth, the field of emergency medical services enjoys growing public recognition as an important segment of the health-care professions. However, this status must not be taken for granted.

CASE STUDY REVIEW

This case study demonstrates the coming together of personnel from many agencies to meet the prehospital needs of a patient, an EMS system.

The case study highlights the different facets of EMS response. Observing the crash, you recognize the need for a response and access the system by using a cell phone to dial the universal entry number 911. The initial dispatcher quickly directs your call to the EMS area dispatcher, and the dispatcher starts numerous agencies en route to the scene—the fire department (BLS), the rescue service, and an ALS ambulance. The police are also notified and begin their response. The dispatcher gathers further information about the crash to update the responding personnel and possibly modify the response. Once on the scene, the BLS providers assume patient care responsibilities by assuring that the scene is safe, analyzing the mechanism of injury, and taking information from you. From this information and the results of a quick physical assessment (the initial assessment) of the patients, they triage the patients and call the dispatcher for an additional ALS ambulance and air medical transport.

An additional arriving fire unit further assures traffic control and scene safety and establishes a landing zone. The highest-trained EMS care provider assumes overall patient care coordination responsibilities. He calls for the patients to be distributed to the most appropriate facilities, assuring that the patients receive the best of care and that no single facility is overloaded by the arrival of patients. This process, as established by the medical direction system and supervised by a resource hospital, also assures that the most appropriate hospital resources are used for the most seriously injured patients. Patients are moved quickly to the appropriate facilities. The child is rushed by air to the pediatric trauma center, while the adults are rushed to other appropriate trauma centers. In this case study, various providers from various services work together efficiently to assure that patients are removed from the crash scene quickly. This study is thus an excellent example of an EMS system operating as it should.

What is not mentioned here is that the care given by the providers is well coordinated because the various services practice working together in disaster drills and because continuous quality improvement programs have identified system weaknesses and have taken corrective action before these patients were placed in need. Ongoing education and skills maintenance exercises keep the providers current in skills and knowledge. Finally, the system's CQI committee will review this response, identify strengths it highlights, and correct any weaknesses it reveals through education and revised protocols. Again, these are signs of a healthy EMS system.

CONTENT SELF-EVALUATION

Each of the chapters in this Workbook includes a short content review. The questions are designed to test your ability to remember what you read. At the end of this Workbook, you can find the answers to the questions as well as the pages where the topic of each question was discussed in the text. If you answered a question incorrectly or are unsure of the answer, review the pages listed.

©2004 Pearson Education, Inc.
Intermediate Emergency Care: Principles & Practice

MULTIPLE CHOICE

_____ 1. The modern ambulance is best described as a(n):
   A. rapid patient transport vehicle.
   B. vehicle for horizontal transport.
   C. mobile emergency room.
   D. mobile intensive care unit.
   E. automated care delivery center.

_____ 2. While required to be licensed, registered, or credentialed, EMT-Is still may only function as approved by and under the direct supervision of the system's medical director.
   A. True
   B. False

_____ 3. The expanding role of the EMT-I may place him in the role of:
   A. public educator.
   B. health promoter.
   C. injury and illness prevention advocate.
   D. facilitator of access to care.
   E. all of the above

_____ 4. The EMT-I is held accountable to which of the following?
   A. the public
   B. the system medical director
   C. the employer
   D. his or her peers
   E. all of the above

_____ 5. The best way to ensure that you meet the expectations of the public, peers, and the system medical director is to:
   A. know your protocols.
   B. attend all ongoing education sessions.
   C. record everything well on the prehospital care report.
   D. always act in the best interest of the patient.
   E. act confident and in control while you provide care.

_____ 6. Which of the following is NOT a characteristic of a professional EMT-I?
   A. confident leadership
   B. excellent judgement
   C. strong opinions about ethnic groups
   D. ability to develop a rapport with a wide variety of patients
   E. ability to function independently

_____ 7. Which characteristic best describes the changes made in the profession by the 1998 DOT National Standard Curriculum?
   A. It provided algorithms for most situations EMT-Is face.
   B. It raised the standards of education for the EMT-I.
   C. It allowed the EMT-I to prescribe more drugs.
   D. It required stronger math, English, and communication skills.
   E. all of the above

_____ 8. For years, EMT-I practice was based on anecdotal data and tradition.
   A. True
   B. False

_____ 9. Which of the following is a guideline for this text?
   A. AHA-CPR Standards
   B. DOH-Critical Paramedic Standards
   C. 1998 DOT Curriculum
   D. AMA EMT-I Standards
   E. all of the above

_____ 10. As a result of research, many traditional EMS treatments have been abandoned or modified.
   A. True
   B. False

CHAPTER 1

Foundations
of the EMT-Intermediate

Part 2: EMS Systems

Review of Chapter Objectives

After reading this part of the chapter, you should be able to:

1. **Describe key historical events that influenced the national development of Emergency Medical Services (EMS) systems.** **pp. 7–10**

   There is a long history of individuals providing care in the out-of-hospital setting, beginning in ancient times. The cardinal events in the history of EMS include the first organized use of patient transport (and the ambulance) by Jean Larrey, chief surgeon for Napoleon. While simply a horse-drawn cart called an ambulance volante (flying ambulance), it represented the first recognized attempt to bring the injured from the field to medical care. Wars continued to be the impetus to improve out-of-hospital care. The American Civil War, World Wars I and II, and the Korean and Vietnamese conflicts all brought substantial changes to field care and transport. The war in Vietnam saw a greater reduction in mortality associated with immediate care in the field and rapid access to surgery than was the case in any previous conflict. However, the single greatest event in the development of modern-day EMS was the National Highway Safety Act of 1966. This act, for the first time and on a national level, recognized emergency medical services and financially supported their development. Under that act, and its establishment of the Department of Transportation (DOT) as overseeing agency, the nation soon had the first national EMS training curriculum, new criteria for ambulance design (the KKK specifications), and the creation of state-led agencies to coordinate EMS development. Later federal legislation created EMS systems through the guidance of the Department of Health, Education, and Welfare, and since then several federal initiatives have continued to improve the nation's EMS system, mostly under the leadership of the DOT.

2. **Define the following terms:**

   EMS systems **p. 7**
   An emergency medical services system is a comprehensive network of personnel, equipment, and resources established to deliver aid and emergency medical care to the community.

   Licensure **p. 14**
   Licensure is a process by which a governmental agency grants permission to engage in an occupation based on an applicant's attaining a required competency sufficient to ensure the public's protection.

©2004 Pearson Education, Inc.
Intermediate Emergency Care: Principles & Practice

Certification
p. 14

Certification is a process by which an agency or association grants recognition to an individual who meets its qualifications.

Registration
p. 14

Registration is the listing of your name and essential information within a particular record of a certifying organization.

Reciprocity
p. 14

Reciprocity is the process by which an agency grants automatic certification or licensure to an individual who has comparable certification or licensure.

Profession
p. 15

A profession is a vocation requiring advanced education or training in a specialized body of knowledge and/or skills.

Professionalism
p. 15

Professionalism is the conduct or qualities that characterize a practitioner in a particular field or profession.

Health-care professional
p. 15

Health-care professionals are properly trained and licensed or certified providers of health care.

Ethics
p. 19

Ethics are rules or standards for conduct of a particular group or profession.

Peer review
p. 19

Peer review is a process of evaluation of the quality of conduct or actions performed by members of a group or profession that is undertaken by other members of that group or profession.

Medical direction
p. 11

Medical direction is the guidance of the actions of prehospital care providers by a physician associated with the emergency medical services system. Medical direction may be on-line or off-line medical direction and includes the physician's involvement in and supervision of personnel education, personnel and equipment selection, protocol development, quality improvement, and advocacy for the EMS system and the patient.

Protocols
p. 11

Protocols are policies and procedures addressing primarily triage, treatment, transport, and transfer of patients as well as special circumstances and events within the EMS system.

3. Identify national groups important to the development, education, and implementation of EMS as well as the role of national associations, the National Registry of EMTs, and the roles of various EMS standard-setting agencies. pp. 15–16

The National Association of EMTs, the National Registry of EMTs, the National Association of State EMS Directors, the National Association of Emergency Physicians, the National Council of State EMS Training Coordinators, and other like associations provide leadership, advise national regulatory bodies, and establish standards for performance related to the provision of emergency medical care. These organizations serve to guide the continuing development, initial and ongoing EMS education, and implementation and coordination of EMS systems nationally.

National associations identify standards for performance in EMS and advocate for patient care and the professional stature of their members. The National Registry of EMTs maintains a national standard, through testing, at the Basic, Intermediate, and Paramedic levels of EMT training. Other standard-setting agencies establish the criteria and standards for system performance. For example, the Joint Committee on Educational Programs for the EMT-Paramedic sets standards for institutions educating paramedics. The American Heart Association sets standards for

©2004 Pearson Education, Inc.
Intermediate Emergency Care: Principles & Practice

basic and advanced cardiac life support. The American College of Emergency Physicians recommends a list of ALS equipment for ambulances. The American College of Surgeons establishes a listing of essential BLS ambulance equipment.

4. Identify the standards (components) of an EMS system as defined by the National Highway Traffic Safety Administration. pp. 9–10

NHTSA has defined the following components for EMS systems:
- **Regulation and policy.** Each state must have laws, regulations, policies, and procedures that govern its EMS system.
- **Resources management.** Each state must have central control of health-care resources to ensure that all patients have equal access to emergency care.
- **Human resources and training.** Each state must require that all EMS providers are taught by qualified instructors using a standardized curriculum.
- **Transportation.** Each state must ensure that patients are safely and reliably transported by ground or air ambulance.
- **Facilities.** Each state must ensure that every seriously ill or injured patient is delivered to an appropriate medical facility in a timely manner.
- **Communications.** Each state must have a system for public access to EMS along with communications among dispatchers, ambulance crews, and hospital personnel.
- **Trauma systems.** Each state should develop a system of specialized care for trauma patients including the designation of trauma centers and systems to ensure that patients arrive at the appropriate facility in a timely manner.
- **Public information and education.** EMS personnel should participate in programs designed to educate the public in injury prevention, emergency recognition, system access, and first aid.
- **Medical direction.** Each EMS system must have a physician medical director responsible for delegating medical practice to prehospital care providers and overseeing patient care.
- **Evaluation.** Each state must have a quality improvement system for continuing evaluation and upgrading of the EMS system.

5. Differentiate among EMS provider levels: First Responder, Emergency Medical Technician-Basic, Emergency Medical Technician-Intermediate, and Emergency Medical Technician-Paramedic. pp. 14–15

- **First Responder.** The first responder is usually the first EMS-trained provider on the scene and is prepared to initially care for and stabilize the patient until personnel with higher levels of training arrive.
- **EMT-Basic.** The EMT-B is an EMS responder who meets the criteria of the U.S. DOT National Standard Curriculum for EMT-Basics and is prepared to assess, care for, and transport the patient at the basic life support level.
- **EMT-Intermediate.** The EMT-I is an EMS responder who meets the criteria of the U.S. DOT National Standard Curriculum for EMT-Is and is prepared to assess, care for, and transport the patient using all EMT-Basic skills plus some advanced life support level skills such as advanced airway management, IV therapy, and administration of certain medications.
- **EMT-Paramedic.** The EMT-P is an EMS responder who meets the criteria of the U.S. DOT National Standard Curriculum for EMT-Paramedics and is prepared to assess, care for, and transport the patient using advanced patient assessment, trauma management, pharmacology, cardiology, and other medical skills. The paramedic should complete advanced cardiac life support and pediatric life support courses.

6. Describe what is meant by "citizen involvement in the EMS system." p. 12

Citizen involvement in the EMS system means that average members of the public can recognize a medical or trauma emergency, know how to access the EMS system, and know how to provide basic life support assistance such as hemorrhage control, CPR, and, possibly, early defibrillation prior to the arrival of EMS personnel.

7. Discuss the role of the EMS physician in providing medical direction, prehospital and out-of-hospital care as an extension of the physician, the benefits of both on-line and off-line medical direction, and the process for the development of local policies and protocols.
pp. 10–11

An EMT-I functions only under the supervision and direction of a medical direction physician. That oversight is provided as either on-line medical direction or off-line medical direction. Off-line medical direction involves the physician's participation in personnel and equipment selection, training, protocol development, quality improvement, and acting as an EMS and patient advocate within the health profession. On-line medical direction consists of direct radio or phone consultation and oversight of EMT-Is and other prehospital care providers while they are caring for a patient. The ultimate responsibility for all care offered by the EMT-I rests with the medical direction physician.

The medical director is a physician who is legally responsible for all clinical and patient care aspects of an EMS system. Prehospital care provided by the EMT-I or other EMS personnel is provided under the license of the medical director, regardless of who his or her employer is.

The benefits of both on-line and off-line medical direction include the medical supervision of the EMS system and prehospital and out-of-hospital patient care. Among these benefits are the opportunity to practice "prehospital medicine" under the license and supervision of the medical director including use of protocols, standing orders, and algorithms developed by the medical director. Additionally, on-line medical direction provides access to direct medical consultation for EMS personnel during the care of the emergency patient.

Protocols are developed by the medical director (in cooperation with expert EMS personnel) to address the assessment and care offered during triage, treatment, transport, and transfer of the patient. The protocols and other system policies are developed to address not only commonly encountered circumstances but also special situations such as intervener physicians, child, spouse, or elderly abuse, DNR orders, patient refusals, and the like. The protocols and policies set the standards for accountability of EMS personnel and ensure uniform, medically approved care for each and every patient.

8. Describe the relationship between a physician on the scene, the EMT-Intermediate on the scene, and the EMS physician providing on-line medical direction.
pp. 11–12

At the scene of a medical or trauma emergency, the health-care professional with the highest training specific to emergency care should be responsible for patient care. When a nonsystem-affiliated physician is at the scene (an intervener physician), the on-line medical direction physician is ultimately responsible for the patient. When on-line medical direction is not available, the EMT-I may relinquish patient care responsibility to the intervener physician as long as that individual identifies him- or herself, demonstrates a willingness to assume patient care responsibilities, and agrees to provide the documentation required by the system. If treatment differs from system protocols, the intervener physician must agree to ride with the patient to the hospital.

9. Describe the components of continuous quality improvement and analyze its contribution to system improvement, continuing medical education, and research.
pp. 18–19

Continuous quality improvement (CQI) is an ongoing effort to refine and improve the system to ensure the highest level of service possible. It involves six basic components: identifying system-wide problems, elaborating on the probable causes, listing solutions, outlining a plan of corrective action, providing resources and support to ensure success, and re-evaluating the results and system performance continuously. CQI system review uses positive reinforcement and support to identify and improve patient care. It can identify areas for improvement and ways to allocate resources to make those improvements, frequently through continuing medical education. When questions arise about the benefits of care offered by a system, a CQI program can suggest research projects to investigate the real value of procedures, equipment, and protocols. The real key to effective CQI is the positive and reinforcing nature of its approach to system improvement.

10. **Describe the importance, basic principles, process of evaluating and interpreting, and benefits of research.** pp. 19–20

Research is essential to ensuring that the equipment and procedures used in the out-of-hospital setting are safe, benefit the patient, and are worth any potential risks of employing them. Research attempts to objectively evaluate the performance of interventions in an unbiased way. Research begins by asking a question (stating a hypothesis), investigating any existing research, designing a study that is unbiased and fairly measures performance, collects and analyzes data, assesses and evaluates results against the hypothesis, and reports the findings. Research is ultimately needed to determine what is in the best interest of the prehospital patient and what is the value of prehospital care in general. Research is essential to the existence of EMS and the profession's evolution.

CONTENT SELF-EVALUATION

MULTIPLE CHOICE

_____ 1. An Emergency Medical Services system is a network of personnel, equipment, and resources established to deliver aid and emergency care to the community.
   A. True
   B. False

_____ 2. The date of the earliest recorded medical care procedures is:
   A. about 5,000 years ago.
   B. about 2,000 years ago.
   C. 1497.
   D. 1562.
   E. 1666.

_____ 3. In a well-developed EMS system, trained First Responders are likely to be:
   A. police officers.
   B. firefighters.
   C. life guards.
   D. teachers.
   E. all of the above

_____ 4. Which of the following was NOT a component of the Emergency Medical Services Systems Act of 1973?
   A. communications
   B. system financing
   C. training
   D. access to care
   E. system evaluation

_____ 5. The medical director is a physician who is legally responsible for all patient care offered by the system he oversees.
   A. True
   B. False

_____ 6. The intervener physician is a physician who is:
   A. not affiliated with the system of medical direction.
   B. at the scene of an emergency.
   C. a trained emergency physician.
   D. both A and B
   E. none of the above

_____ 7. When on-line medical direction does not exist and an intervener physician is present, is willing to accept patient care responsibility, performs interventions consistent with the system protocols, and agrees to document the interventions as required by the system, the EMT-I should:
   A. relinquish patient care responsibilities.
   B. retain patient care authority.
   C. relinquish patient care responsibilities only if the physician agrees to ride to the hospital.
   D. retain patient care responsibilities in cases of physician disagreement.
   E. none of the above

©2004 Pearson Education, Inc.
Intermediate Emergency Care: Principles & Practice

_____ 8. Off-line medical direction includes which of the following?
A. protocols
B. training guidelines
C. personnel selection policies
D. quality assurance
E. all of the above

_____ 9. Which of the following is NOT one of the four "Ts" of emergency care?
A. triage
B. transfer
C. termination of care
D. transport
E. treatment

_____ 10. Which of the following statements is NOT true?
A. The ability to recognize cardiac emergencies can save lives.
B. Over 300,000 cardiac arrests per year occur before the patient reaches the hospital.
C. Most cardiac arrests happen immediately upon onset of symptoms.
D. If bystanders or the patient call in time, many cardiac arrests can be prevented.
E. all of the above

_____ 11. There are great disadvantages to dispatching EMS, fire, and police from a single control center.
A. True
B. False

_____ 12. The dispatch system that provides caller interrogation, predetermined response configurations, and pre-arrival instructions is:
A. system status management.
B. enhanced 911.
C. priority dispatch.
D. caller interrogation.
E. none of the above

_____ 13. There may be some increased liability for a system providing pre-arrival instructions.
A. True
B. False

_____ 14. The goal of dispatch and response in an effective EMS is to have:
A. BLS units on the scene within 4 minutes.
B. ALS units on the scene within 8 minutes.
C. at least 90 percent of all responses within system time limits.
D. all of the above
E. none of the above

_____ 15. The learning domain associated with skills is:
A. cognitive.
B. psychomotor.
C. affective.
D. didactic.
E. dexterous.

_____ 16. The process by which a state or other governmental agency grants permission to engage in a given occupation is:
A. licensure.
B. certification.
C. registration.
D. reciprocity.
E. tenure.

_____ 17. Granting someone recognition for meeting the qualifications of another agency is called:
A. licensure.
B. certification.
C. registration.
D. reciprocity.
E. tenure.

_____ 18. The U.S. DOT has developed curricula for how many levels of EMS providers?
A. 1
B. 2
C. 3
D. 4
E. 5

19. The EMS provider responsible for general patient assessment, CPR, hemorrhage control, and spinal immobilization is the:
    A. First Responder.
    B. EMT-Basic.
    C. EMT-Intermediate.
    D. EMT-Paramedic.
    E. all of the above

20. It is desirable for the EMT-I to complete which of the following courses?
    A. BTLS
    B. PHTLS
    C. PALS
    D. ACLS
    E. all of the above

21. The organization that administers practical and written exams and establishes qualifications for registration of EMT-Bs, EMT-Is, and EMT-Ps on a national level is the:
    A. National Association of EMTs.
    B. National Registry of EMTs.
    C. National Council of State EMS Training Coordinators.
    D. Joint Review Committee on Educational Programs for the EMT-Paramedic.
    E. American College of Emergency Physicians.

22. The body that sets standards for EMT-I education programs is the:
    A. Joint Review Committee on Educational Programs for the EMT-Paramedic.
    B. National Association of EMTs.
    C. National Registry of EMTs.
    D. National Council of State EMS Training Coordinators.
    E. American College of Emergency Physicians.

23. Fixed-wing aircraft are usually used for patient transports exceeding:
    A. 25 miles.
    B. 50 miles.
    C. 150 miles.
    D. 200 miles.
    E. none of the above

24. The agency responsible for establishing criteria for the design of ambulances is the:
    A. American College of Surgeons.
    B. American College of Emergency Physicians.
    C. U.S. General Services Administration.
    D. U.S. Military Assistance to Traffic and Safety Group.
    E. National Association of EMTs.

25. A standard van with a raised roof that is configured as an ambulance is categorized as which type of ambulance?
    A. Type I
    B. Type II
    C. Type III
    D. Type A
    E. Type B

26. A resource hospital is one that:
    A. accepts most patients for care.
    B. fulfills the role of the major trauma center.
    C. coordinates specialty services and ensures appropriate patient distribution.
    D. has the largest emergency department.
    E. provides restocking services for the system's ambulances.

27. A hospital designated as a receiving facility for the EMS system should have which of the following?
    A. an emergency department
    B. 24-hour emergency physician coverage
    C. surgical facilities and coverage
    D. critical and intensive care units
    E. all of the above

©2004 Pearson Education, Inc.
Intermediate Emergency Care: Principles & Practice

_____ 28. Which of the following is NOT a part of a well-designed disaster plan?
A. mutual aid agreements among neighboring municipalities, services, and systems
B. a rigid communications system
C. frequent disaster plan tests and drills
D. integration of all system components
E. a coordinated central management agency

_____ 29. A major complaint regarding quality assurance programs is that they tend to:
A. be one-time efforts.
B. address only procedural issues.
C. be punitive in nature.
D. not examine protocol issues.
E. create divisions among care workers on staff.

_____ 30. Continuous quality improvement differs from quality assurance in that it:
A. emphasizes customer satisfaction.
B. rewards or reinforces good behavior.
C. examines billing practices.
D. evaluates maintenance activities.
E. all the above

_____ 31. Which of the following is NOT one of the standard rules of evidence used to evaluate a proposed change in the EMS system?
A. There must be a basis for change.
B. The old procedure must be deemed no longer medically acceptable.
C. The change must be clinically important.
D. The change must be affordable, practical, and teachable.
E. none of the above

_____ 32. Ethics are best defined as:
A. protocols and policies for conduct.
B. rules or standards governing the performance of a profession.
C. legal principles governing potential law suits.
D. the four elements needed to determine negligence.
E. justifications for actions.

_____ 33. To the patient, it may be more important to receive care from a provider who seems to be interested in him or her and empathetic than to receive the most technically correct care.
A. True
B. False

_____ 34. The most common source of EMS funding is:
A. voluntary donations.
B. direct patient payments.
C. third-party payers.
D. tax subsidies.
E. residual payments.

_____ 35. The model for EMS operations that is becoming more and more popular for municipalities is the:
A. public utility model.
B. third service model.
C. fire service model.
D. volunteer model.
E. proprietary model.

LISTING

Identify the agency or association most closely linked with the following guidelines for EMS.

36. National standard curricula for EMS providers

_____

37. Criteria for ambulance design

_____

38. Listing of standard equipment for Basic Life Support ambulances

_____

39. Listing of equipment and supplies for Advanced Life Support ambulances

_____

40. Criteria for EMT-I education programs

_____

©2004 Pearson Education, Inc.
Intermediate Emergency Care: Principles & Practice

CHAPTER 1

*

Foundations
of the EMT-Intermediate

Part 3: Roles and Responsibilities
of the EMT-Intermediate

Review of Chapter Objectives

After reading this part of the chapter, you should be able to:

1. Describe the attributes of an EMT-Intermediate as a health-care professional.   **pp. 24–28**

The attributes of an EMT-I are related to his or her stature as a health-care professional and include leadership, integrity, empathy, self-motivation, appearance and personal hygiene, self-confidence, communication, time management, teamwork and diplomacy, respect, and patient advocacy.

As an EMT-I, you must demonstrate leadership in order to coordinate and direct other care providers in attending to the patient. You must know the abilities of your team and ask its members to do only what they are able to do. You must demonstrate integrity to earn the respect of your peers and the medical community. You must appreciate the plight of the patient and demonstrate an understanding of his or her situation. You must be both self-confident and self-motivated to employ life-saving procedures in the worst of conditions. You must strive for excellence in knowledge and skills and have and display confidence as you employ patient care skills. Your appearance must demonstrate a respect for both yourself and your patient. Remember that good grooming and personal hygiene both are important in presenting a professional image. You must be able to communicate effectively both orally and in writing to patients, other care providers, and physicians. You must be able to coordinate your efforts and those of others to quickly address the needs of the patient and to fulfill your responsibilities as an EMT-I. You must respect others and, through demonstrating that respect, earn respect for yourself. One way of demonstrating that respect is showing a heightened sensitivity to your patient's rights as a person, including the right to confidentiality. You must become a patient advocate, promoting and ensuring that patients receive the care and attention their illness or injury requires. And finally, you must ensure that you maintain the attributes of a professional through careful delivery of your service, including mastering and refreshing skills; following protocols, policies, and procedures; checking your equipment before its use; and operating the ambulance and equipment safely.

2. Describe the benefits of EMT-Intermediate continuing education and the importance of maintaining one's EMT-Intermediate license/certification. p. 28

Continuing education helps you maintain the knowledge you acquired through your initial EMT-I education and expands your own personal knowledge and skills. It helps you keep up with changes in prehospital care and is essential to maintaining your certification and ability to practice.

3. List the primary and additional responsibilities of EMT-Intermediates. pp. 21–28

The primary responsibilities of the EMT-I include:
- **Preparation:** You must be mentally, physically, and emotionally ready to respond to the call; know your protocols, geography, and equipment; and ensure that your vehicle and equipment are all in proper working order.
- **Response:** You must drive responsibly, ensuring a timely, yet safe, response.
- **Scene size-up:** You must assess the scene to determine: the safety of the scene (including identification of any hazards and the need for BSI; the number of ill or injured; the need for any additional resources; and the mechanism of injury or the nature of the illness.
- **Patient assessment:** Once at the patient's side, you must determine whether or not the patient needs cervical immobilization as well as his or her level of consciousness (or responsiveness) and the stability of the airway, breathing, and circulation. You will then assess for specific injury or illness signs through a focused or rapid trauma assessment. You will also evaluate the patient's medical history and perform ongoing assessments.
- **Recognition of injury or illness:** As a result of the scene size-up and patient assessment, you will identify the illness or injury and the patient's priority for care and transport.
- **Patient management:** You will employ appropriate care procedures, guided by protocols, with your patient and, at times, consult with medical direction to further guide your care.
- **Appropriate disposition:** Based upon the results of your assessment, the effects of the care measures you have employed, and your system's protocols, you will determine the disposition of your patient. That disposition may be transport to a level I, II, or III trauma center or to another specialized hospital, the closest hospital, or an alternative care facility. An additional possible disposition is to treat and release the patient with instructions to seek the advice of a personal physician.
- **Patient transfer:** As the health-care system becomes more complex and facilities become more specialized, you may be charged with the safe and efficient transfer of patients from one facility to another.
- **Documentation:** At the conclusion of your patient care, you will be required to document the results of your assessment and care to ensure the continuity of patient care.
- **Return to service:** At the end of your response, you must ensure that you, your crew, and your ambulance are ready to return to service. This includes cleaning and refueling the vehicle, maintaining equipment, and replacing supplies used during the call.

Additional responsibilities include:
- **Community involvement:** You should promote and participate in programs to help the community recognize when EMS is needed, how to access the system, and what to do until the ambulance arrives. Community involvement also includes participation in the development and presentation of programs to improve health—stressing a healthy diet, for example—and to reduce injury—such as promoting seat belt use.
- **Support for primary care:** Modern health care is evolving in ways aimed at ensuring that costly resources are best directed to serve the patient. In support of this aim, you may be responsible for transporting or directing patients with minor injury or illness to alternate facilities like urgent care centers or physicians' offices.
- **Citizen involvement in EMS:** Ordinary citizens can be highly important evaluators of the EMS system, as they are its consumers and can best say what elements of it are important to them. Pay attention to the comments, suggestions, and criticisms of the patients/citizens you contact and pass what you learn along to the appropriate personnel in your system.
- **Personal and professional development:** To maintain and improve your ability to provide prehospital (and out-of-hospital) care, you must participate in professional development. This

©2004 Pearson Education, Inc.
Intermediate Emergency Care: Principles & Practice

may include taking refresher and continuing education courses, engaging in skill maintenance exercises, and other activities.

4. Define the role of the EMT-Intermediate relative to the safety of the crew, the patient, and the bystanders. pp. 21–23

You must evaluate information obtained from the dispatcher and gathered during your scene size-up to identify any potential scene hazards. Then you must take action to ensure your safety and the safety of the patient, other crew members and rescue personnel, and bystanders. You must also monitor the scene during your care to ensure that no hazards develop to threaten you, your patient, fellow rescuers, or bystanders.

5. Describe the role of the EMT-Intermediate in health education activities related to illness and injury prevention. p. 24

As EMS matures, its members will be expected to become more involved in both injury and illness prevention programs for the public. Such programs provide the most effective ways of increasing overall public health and reducing both death and disability from accidents and injuries.

6. Describe examples of professional behaviors in the following areas: pp. 25–28

- **Integrity:** Be honest and trustworthy in your contacts with patients, crew members, and other health-care professionals. Doing this is essential to maintaining personal integrity.
- **Empathy:** You can convey empathy by attempting to understand and appreciate a patient's situation.
- **Self-motivation:** Doing your job well without direct supervision represents self-motivation.
- **Appearance and personal hygiene:** A clean, pressed shirt and trousers and well-kept hair demonstrate a good appearance and appropriate personal hygiene.
- **Self-confidence:** Displaying comfort with the application of emergency skills demonstrates self-confidence.
- **Communications:** In emergency medical services, it is essential to communicate quickly, concisely, accurately, and effectively.
- **Time management:** An emergency scene is often a chaotic place. It is imperative that you be able to organize and direct your actions and those of others quickly and efficiently to ensure that your patient receives appropriate emergency care and transport to definitive care as rapidly as possible.
- **Teamwork and diplomacy:** The emergency response is a team event, and the EMT-I, as team leader, must direct many individuals to work together in the patient's best interest.
- **Respect:** Respect is demonstrated by showing regard and consideration for patients, care providers, and others. Listening to these people and indicating that you really hear what they say shows your respect for them and earns you their respect.
- **Patient advocacy:** Ensuring that the needs of your patient remain the first priority of your prehospital emergency care will help you meet your responsibility as patient advocate.
- **Careful delivery of service:** Demonstrate professional behavior by performing your job to the highest level of excellence, by mastering and maintaining your skills and knowledge, and by conscientiously carrying out equipment checks, driving safely, and following protocols, policies, and procedures.

7. Identify the benefits of EMT-Intermediates teaching in their community. p. 24

Teaching in your community places you before your "consumers" before they call for help. This gives you an opportunity to develop a positive public image and explain the workings of the system. It will also help you integrate with the other members of the health-care system.

8. Analyze how the EMT-Intermediate can benefit the health-care system by supporting primary care for patients in the out-of-hospital setting. p. 23

With the increasing costs of health care, it has become necessary to ensure that the patient's needs are best matched to the available resources. This may mean that the EMT-I, through assessment and consultation with the medical direction physician, may direct patients to facilities other than the emergency department.

9. **Describe how professionalism applies to the EMT-Intermediate while on and off duty.** pp. 24–25

It is essential that the EMT-I display a professional attitude toward his or her patient and the profession as a whole. This applies while both on and off duty since the public often judges a profession by the actions of its members.

CONTENT SELF-EVALUATION

MULTIPLE CHOICE

_____ 1. In the past 10 years, the health-care and EMS systems have seen dramatic changes in care delivery.
   A. True
   B. False

_____ 2. Prior to responding to a call, you must be:
   A. emotionally able to meet the demands of patient care.
   B. physically able to meet the demands of patient care.
   C. mentally able to meet the demands of patient care.
   D. sure the ambulance and equipment are ready for the response.
   E. all of the above

_____ 3. Prior to responding to a call, you must be familiar with:
   A. local EMS protocols.   D. neighboring EMS agencies.
   B. the local communications system.   E. all of the above
   C. local geography.

_____ 4. A call involving which of the following is least likely to require additional assistance?
   A. a single ill patient   D. hazardous materials
   B. reported use of a weapon   E. a rescue situation
   C. knowledge of previous violence

_____ 5. When a patient receives a minor injury and is transported to an alternate care facility like an outpatient clinic, this care is best described as:
   A. basic care.   D. diversion of care.
   B. primary care.   E. health maintenance.
   C. treat and release.

_____ 6. Which of the following items is NOT an essential part of the transfer of a patient between health-care facilities?
   A. a verbal patient report from the transferring primary care provider
   B. a copy of the essential parts of the patient's chart
   C. the results of all diagnostic tests
   D. a summary of the patient's past medical history
   E. a summary of the patient's present medical history

_____ 7. The patient care report should normally be completed:
   A. before arrival at the emergency department.
   B. upon arrival at the emergency department.
   C. as soon as care is completed.
   D. upon arrival at your base station.
   E. either C or D

©2004 Pearson Education, Inc.
Intermediate Emergency Care: Principles & Practice

8. Which of the following is a component of returning to service after a call?
   A. refueling the ambulance
   B. restocking supplies
   C. stowing equipment
   D. reviewing the call with the crew
   E. all of the above

9. Which of the following is NOT a part of community involvement for the EMT-I?
   A. teaching CPR
   B. transporting patients to alternate care facilities
   C. conducting EMS demonstrations
   D. providing prevention programs
   E. sponsoring programs that help the public recognize when to access EMS

10. What is the unique benefit of having citizen consumers involved in the development, evaluation, and regulation of the EMS system?
   A. They can help seek out alternative funding.
   B. They provide an outside objective view of the EMS system.
   C. They do not have the prejudices of most EMS providers.
   D. They can provide insight into new care procedures.
   E. all of the above

11. Which of the following is NOT an attribute of a professional?
   A. leadership
   B. excited demeanor
   C. empathy
   D. self-motivation
   E. diplomacy

12. When presented with a complex situation, a self-confident EMT-I will ask for assistance.
   A. True
   B. False

13. Which of the following is NOT a method of displaying empathy?
   A. being supportive and reassuring
   B. demonstrating respect for others
   C. having a calm and helpful demeanor
   D. accepting constructive feedback
   E. understanding a patient's feelings

14. In general, the more patches you wear, the more respect you gain from patients.
   A. True
   B. False

15. Placing the patient's needs above your own represents which professional attribute?
   A. empathy
   B. diplomacy
   C. patient advocacy
   D. initiative
   E. self-confidence

MATCHING

Write the letter of the EMT-I responsibility in the space provided next to the action to which it applies.

Responsibility
- A. Preparation
- B. Response
- C. Patient assessment and management
- D. Appropriate disposition
- E. Patient transfer
- F. Documentation
- G. Return to service

Action

_____ 16. Refuel the vehicle.

_____ 17. Follow patient care protocols.

_____ 18. Transport a patient to an outpatient center.

_____ 19. Determine the mechanism of injury.

_____ 20. Record the care you provided.

_____ 21. Be familiar with local protocols.

_____ 22. Determine the patient's medical history.

_____ 23. Categorize the patient's priority for transport.

_____ 24. Take a report from the sending facility.

_____ 25. Drive responsibly and safely.

_____ 26. Deliver a patient to a Level II trauma center.

_____ 27. Be mentally fit to respond to a call.

_____ 28. Check crew members for signs of stress.

_____ 29. Identify the nature of the illness.

_____ 30. Determine the seriousness of the injury.

©2004 Pearson Education, Inc.
Intermediate Emergency Care: Principles & Practice

CHAPTER 1

Foundations
of the EMT-Intermediate

Part 4: The Well-Being of the EMT-Intermediate

Review of Chapter Objectives

After reading this part of the chapter, you should be able to:

1. Discuss the concept of wellness and its benefits, components of wellness, and the role of the EMT-Intermediate in promoting wellness.   p. 28

Wellness, or personal physical, mental, and emotional well-being, is the result of proper nutrition, basic physical fitness, safe practices to protect you from disease and injury, and the development of effective mechanisms to deal with the stress of the profession. The results of observing practices that promote wellness in your own life are a reduced incidence of work-related injury and illness, a good attitude toward the profession, and a long fruitful career in emergency medical services.

Basic physical fitness is the muscular strength, cardiovascular endurance (aerobic capacity), and flexibility that permit you to perform the tasks associated with prehospital emergency care without risk to the musculoskeletal system.

Good nutrition is the controlled and balanced consumption of carbohydrates, fats, proteins, vitamins, and minerals that meet the body's needs yet is not consumption in excess.

Personal protection from disease includes application of body substance isolation procedures and acquisition of proper immunizations for protection from contagious disease.

Stress and stress management involve the recognition that prehospital emergency care is a stressful profession and that stress management techniques, including critical incident stress management, are essential to a long career in EMS.

General safety considerations include such principles as safe lifting, ensuring a safe environment for EMS operations, safe driving practices, appropriate interpersonal relationships, and the proper dealing with habits and addictions.

The EMT-I should, by example, promote basic physical fitness, proper nutrition, the following of safe practices, and the use of appropriate mechanisms to deal with job-related stress. He or she can be a model to peers, patients, and the community in general.

2. Discuss how cardiovascular endurance, weight control, muscle strength, and flexibility contribute to physical fitness.   pp. 28–32

Cardiovascular endurance, weight control, muscular strength, and flexibility are all essential to the physical fitness required of the EMT-I. Cardiovascular endurance is the measure of the heart's and blood vessels' ability to support physical exercise. Increased cardiovascular endurance improves the body's ability to accommodate the physical stress associated with patient lifting and movement and the carrying of equipment. Weight control is essential to limit cardiovascular and musculoskeletal stresses on the body. Muscular strength is achieved by regular exercise and helps keep the body ready for the stresses of lifting and moving the patient and EMS equipment. Flexibility is the strength and ease of motion through the normal range of motion of the body's major joints. Good flexibility will reduce back pain and the potential for joint and muscle injury during your EMS career.

3. **Describe the impact of shift work on circadian rhythms.** p. 41

Shift work disturbs the normal biorhythms of the body, called circadian rhythms. Dramatic changes in a person's daily time schedule disturb the normal sleep/awake, appetite, hormonal, and temperature fluctuation cycles of the body and may result in drowsiness and fatigue. To diminish the negative effects of shift work, it is best to maintain a regular 24-hour sleep/awake cycle (sleeping at about the same time), even on days when you do not work.

4. **Discuss the contributions that periodic risk assessments and warning sign recognition make to cancer and cardiovascular disease prevention.** p. 30

Periodic assessment of your risk for disease is important. Have frequent physical exams and examine your family history to determine the risk for cancer and cardiovascular disease. Know your cholesterol and triglyceride levels and keep them in check. Women past menopause might consider the use of hormonal therapy and have frequent mammograms and Pap smears with advancing age. Males should have periodic prostate exams with advancing age. Also watch for blood in the stool, changes in moles, unexplained weight loss, unexplained chronic fatigue, and unusual lumps.

5. **Differentiate proper from improper body mechanics for lifting and moving patients in emergency and non-emergency situations.** pp. 30, 32

Proper lifting and moving techniques, especially when coupled with good physical fitness and good nutrition, help protect the musculoskeletal system from the high risks for injury associated with prehospital emergency care. Good posture, lifting with the leg muscles, and keeping the back straight, the palms up, and the body close to the object being lifted will reduce the potential for injury. Exhale during a lift, keep your feet apart with one foot ahead of the other, take your time, and ask for help when you think you will need it. These principles will make lifting easier and help keep you from back injury during your years of service.

6. **Describe the problems that an EMT-Intermediate might encounter in a hostile situation and the techniques used to manage the situation.** pp. 44–45

Emergency responses occasionally put the caregiver into contact with hostile patients, family members, and bystanders. These individuals may affect your ability to provide care and, at the extreme, threaten you or your patient with physical harm. If there is a significant threat, remove yourself from the scene immediately. Often, however, the hostility of people at the scene can be overcome by appreciating the cultural diversity of those you treat and helping them understand that your reason for being there is to offer help. Treating everyone you attend with dignity and respect will go a long way toward establishing trust in you and in EMS providers in general.

7. **Describe the special considerations that should be given to using escorts, dealing with adverse environmental conditions, using lights and siren, proceeding through intersections, and parking at an emergency scene.** pp. 44–45

Driving an emergency vehicle provides you with some privileges, but with them come some very important added responsibilities. In general, you must remain especially aware of others on the roadway and remember that they may react unexpectedly to your approach and passage. Also consider the following steps when dealing with these specific situations:

©2004 Pearson Education, Inc.
Intermediate Emergency Care: Principles & Practice

- When following an escort, be aware that some drivers may not realize that you are following from behind and may pull out in front of you.
- Adverse driving conditions (rain, snow, ice, fog) reduce visibility and traction. Give other drivers more time to see you and stop, and respect the increased stopping time and reduced maneuverability of your ambulance in these conditions.
- Lights and sirens are used to alert others of your approach and ask them to yield the right of way. However, some drivers may neither see nor hear them or may react in an unexpected manner. Be alert while using lights and sirens and anticipate the actions of others.
- Intersections pose special problems for emergency vehicles. Driving through a red light or a stop sign is dangerous because other drivers may presume they have the right of way. The situation becomes more complicated and dangerous when multiple emergency vehicles are responding. When proceeding through an intersection, and especially when passing through a red light, slow to almost a stop and keep a good lookout for other vehicles not yielding the right of way.
- Once at the scene, park so as to protect you and your crew, the patient, and other drivers. Place your emergency vehicle between traffic and the crash/care scene and be sure the lights can be seen by all oncoming traffic.

8. Discuss the concept of "due regard for the safety of all others" while operating an emergency vehicle. p. 45

The concept of exercising due regard for the safety of others recognizes that different drivers will react differently to the approach of emergency vehicles. This means that you must maintain an intense lookout for hazards while driving the emergency vehicle. You must anticipate the actions of other drivers on the highway, including those that are unexpected and not in keeping with the right of way given you under the law. Otherwise you may find yourself responsible for injury when your intent was to provide care or, worse, injure yourself.

9. Describe the equipment available in a variety of adverse situations for self-protection, including body substance isolation steps for protection from airborne and bloodborne pathogens. pp. 33–35, 44–45

Equipment available to help protect you from the more common hazards of emergency medical service include helmets, footwear with toe and ankle support, body armor, reflective tape for night visibility, seatbelts, and personal protective equipment used for body substance isolation (gloves, masks, eyewear, respirators, gowns, resuscitation equipment).

Body substance isolation (BSI) practices include the use of personal protective equipment (PPE) to isolate the body from contaminants found in the air and body fluids while caring for a patient. These practices involve using protective latex or plastic gloves to protect yourself when touching a patient if there is reasonable expectation of contact with body fluids, including tears, vomit, saliva, blood, urine, fecal material, cerebrospinal fluid, or any other body fluid or substance. Masks and protective eyewear should be used whenever there is a reasonable expectation that fluid or droplets will be splattered, as is the case with arterial hemorrhage, endotracheal intubation, intensive airway care, childbirths, and the cleaning of contaminated equipment. When a patient has or is suspected of having tuberculosis or another highly contagious airborne disease, use of a special type of mask, either the high-efficiency particulate air (HEPA) or N-95 respirator, offers protection by removing small infectious particles from the air. Gowns are worn to protect clothing and the body from contamination by splashing of body fluids in extreme circumstances (like childbirth). A gown impervious to fluid movement is recommended. When possible, use disposable equipment for patient ventilation and other invasive procedures.

10. Given a scenario in which equipment and supplies have been exposed to body substances, plan for the proper cleaning, disinfection, and disposal of the items. p. 35

When EMS equipment becomes contaminated (or possibly contaminated), it should be disposed of or properly cleaned and disinfected. Single-use devices, bandaging materials, and other disposable EMS equipment and materials should be placed in a sealed biohazard waste container and disposed of properly. Needles and other sharp contaminated items should be placed in a puncture-proof "sharps" container and disposed of properly. Equipment that has been in contact with a patient or otherwise becomes contaminated should be cleaned with soap and water, disinfected with an appropriate agent (commercial or a bleach solution), or sterilized (by heat, steam, or radiation) as per your service's policies and procedures. Any contaminated cleaning or disinfecting supplies should be disposed of properly.

11. Describe the benefits and methods of smoking cessation.   p. 30

Smoking and the effects of nicotine are well known to be detrimental to respiratory and cardiovascular health and well linked to lung cancer. Smoking cessation programs using replacement therapy (nicotine patches), behavior modification, aversion therapy, hypnotism, and "cold turkey" approaches represent structured programs of controlled withdrawal from sociocultural, psychological, and physiological dependency on the drug. The result of a successful smoking cessation program is better respiratory and cardiovascular health and a reduced risk of respiratory infection and cancer.

12. Identify and describe the three phases of the stress response, factors that trigger the stress response, and causes of stress in EMS.   p. 40

There are three stages to the human response to stress: alarm, resistance, and exhaustion. Alarm is the initial response, more commonly known as the "fight-or-flight" response. The autonomic nervous system prepares the body to deal with a threat to its well-being by releasing hormones that increase cardiac output (increase heart rate, the strength of contraction, and preload) and blood pressure, induce pupil dilation, increase blood sugar, and relax the respiratory tree. Resistance begins as the body starts to adjust and cope with the stress. During this phase, the blood pressure and pulse rate may return to normal. The final stress response phase is exhaustion. If the exposure to stress is prolonged, the body may become exhausted and lose its ability to resist and adapt to the stressors. The individual becomes more susceptible to physical and psychological ailments.

Stress is a stimulus from the environment that affects the body. Stress can have positive effects (eustress), or it can generate negative effects (distress). Factors that induce the stress response are anything that threatens (or is perceived to threaten) the well-being of the individual. These factors include physical ones, like the threat of violence; emotional ones, like the loss of a loved one; and physiological ones, like physical fatigue or extreme hunger. Each person reacts differently to stressors, bringing his or her previous experiences into the equation.

13. Differentiate between normal/healthy and detrimental physiological and psychological reactions to anxiety and stress.   pp. 39–40

The human stress response is the body's way of dealing with stress, and the outcome is either healthy or unhealthy. Healthy responses result in the individual's quickly adjusting to the stressor and physiologically and psychologically returning to normal. Unhealthy responses result in behavioral and physiologic manifestations like gastrointestinal disturbances, sleep disturbances, headaches, vision problems, fatigue, chest pains, confusion, a reduced attention span, poor concentration, disorientation, memory problems, inappropriate fear, panic, grief, depression, anxiety, and feelings of being overwhelmed, abandoned, or numb to emotion. A person with an unhealthy response may also experience withdrawal from normal social activities, increased use of drugs or alcohol, or inappropriate humor, silence, crying, suspiciousness, or activity levels.

EMS provides an abundant amount of stressors because of the nature of the profession. These stressors include shift work; loud pagers and sounds; poor pay; long hours; periods of boredom followed by short periods of extreme excitement; scene violence; abusive patients; vomit; blood; gory scenes; chaotic scenes; personal fears; frustration; exhaustion; demands of family members, friends, or bystanders; inclement weather; conflicts with co-workers or supervisors; hunger and thirst; and physical demands on the body, like heavy lifting. The personality traits commonly found in EMS members, a strong need to be liked and often unrealistically high self-expectations, also leave these individuals more likely to develop adverse responses to stress.

©2004 Pearson Education, Inc.
Intermediate Emergency Care: Principles & Practice

14. **Describe behavior that is a manifestation of stress in patients and those close to them, and describe how that behavior relates to EMT-Intermediate stress.** pp. 39–44

Stress may become evident through almost any unusual behavior exhibited by the patient, family, or bystanders. It may manifest with hyper- or hypoactivity, withdrawal, suspiciousness, increased smoking, increased alcohol or drug intake, excessive humor or silence, crying spells, or any changes in behavior, communications, interactions with others, or eating habits. These behaviors can confound the assessment of the patient's mental status and place additional stress on the EMT-I.

15. **Identify and describe the defense mechanisms and management techniques commonly used to deal with stress and the role of a personal support system in dealing with EMS stress.** pp. 41, 44

Constructive mechanisms and management techniques used to deal with stress can be divided into two categories—immediate and long term. Immediate coping mechanisms include controlling breathing to reduce adrenaline levels and heart rate, reframing thoughts to encourage or support any needed behavior on your behalf (like saying to yourself "I can do this!"), and focusing your concentration on the responsibilities at hand (i.e., the needs of the patient), not the stressful problem. For long-term well-being, ensure your physical, mental, and emotional health. Exercise, watch your diet, and work toward supportive and pleasant distractions from the stress, like a non-EMS circle of friends or a vacation away from the job.

Critical incident stress management recognizes that EMS personnel experience events with powerful emotional impacts that may cause acute stress reactions. Such events include the injury or death of an infant, an EMS co-worker, or someone known to EMS personnel; an injury or death of someone due to EMS operations; threats of personal harm; extreme media attention; or prolonged or especially gruesome events. CISM supports EMS personnel by providing pre-incident stress training, on-scene support, advice to command staff during large incidents, follow-up services, and special debriefings to spouses and families. The major components of CISM include initial discussion, defusing, demobilization, and critical incident stress debriefing services. Initial discussion permits those involved to discuss and air their feelings immediately after the incident. Defusing is a more formal gathering within 2 to 12 hours after an incident in which personnel can vent their feelings at a session monitored by a CISM-trained peer. Demobilization is performed at a staging sector at a large incident to help caregivers transition to everyday life. The critical incident stress debriefing is a formal session, proctored by a mental health provider, 24 to 72 hours after an incident.

16. **Given a scenario involving a stressful situation, formulate a strategy to help adapt to the stress.** pp. 39–44

When you are called to a situation that places you under stress, make a conscious decision to deal with it in an appropriate manner. Immediately control your breathing by taking deep breaths and letting the air out slowly through your mouth. Repeat this as needed, and then focus your energy on the essential tasks at hand. Tell yourself "I can do it" or "I can make it through this" and attend to the immediate needs of your patient. Once the immediate stressor is removed, make sure that you take care of yourself physically, emotionally, and mentally. Talk with members of your team about the event, and identify what you have done well and areas in which you can improve. Exercise regularly, eat properly, and take a vacation or a few days off. Examine the situation and your options, decide how best to handle the situation in the long term, and go on with your life. If a situation is extremely stressful, take advantage of your system's CISM services.

17. **Describe the stages of the grieving process (Kübler-Ross) and the unique challenges for EMT-Intermediates in dealing with themselves, adults, children, and other special populations related to their understanding or experience of death and dying.** pp. 36–37

The grieving patient is likely to progress through five stages of the grieving process as described by Elisabeth Kübler-Ross. Those stages include anger, denial, bargaining, depression, and acceptance. A grieving person usually progresses though these stages in order, though he or she may skip around or move back and forth between stages. In the anger stage, the person vents the frustration over the inability to control the situation or control the outcome. Denial represents the inability or refusal to accept the reality of the event or situation. Bargaining is an unrealistic attempt to change or put off the outcome. Depression represents despair over the inevitable and withdrawal into a private world. Acceptance is realization and acceptance of the event or the patient's fate.

Even though EMT-Is are exposed to death and dying, they don't necessarily handle these events better than other people. All people tend to move through the same stages of the grieving process, although age and the patient's special circumstances may alter the presentation of those stages. Children may not recognize the significance and finality of the event or may fear that death may soon happen to themselves or others. Adults react differently, usually experiencing a "paralyzing" feeling followed by intense grief for weeks. The intensity gradually subsides with later peaks of feeling associated with anniversaries, birthdays, and the like. The elderly usually are concerned about the effects of their death on others and their loss of independence.

18. Given photos of various motor-vehicle collisions, assess scene safety and propose ways to make the scene safer. pp. 44–45

The scene of an emergency is inherently dangerous, especially when it involves an auto crash. The roadway becomes a hazard as oncoming traffic may collide with your ambulance, personnel on the scene, and the wrecked auto(s). The crash produces broken glass, jagged metal, and spilled fluids that may be slippery, hot, caustic (battery acid), or flammable. If the patient involved in the crash is hostile, he or she may pose a threat to care providers as may the patient's friends and family members or other bystanders. The incident may also affect utility poles, breaking their wires to create electrical hazards. The EMT-I must use caution when approaching the scene and carefully rule out hazards. If any exist, you must eliminate them or not approach the scene. Do not attempt to correct a scene hazard unless you are specifically and properly trained and equipped to handle it. Place your vehicle to caution oncoming traffic and create a barrier between you and that traffic. At all scenes with jagged metal and broken glass, wear protective clothing, including gloves, boots, helmet, and a protective coat (turnout gear). If need be, "blind" the occupants of a stopped vehicle with a spotlight until you are sure it is safe to enter the scene. If there is any possibility of blood or body fluid exposure, observe body substance isolation procedures.

CONTENT SELF-EVALUATION

MULTIPLE CHOICE

_____ 1. All of the following are benefits of physical fitness EXCEPT:
- A. decreased resting heart rate.
- B. decreased resting blood pressure.
- C. increased anxiety levels.
- D. enhanced quality of life.
- E. increased resistance to disease.

_____ 2. The basic elements of physical fitness include all of the following EXCEPT:
- A. disease resistance.
- B. muscular strength.
- C. flexibility.
- D. cardiovascular endurance.
- E. aerobic capacity.

_____ 3. Exercise performed against stable resistance, where muscles are exercised in a motionless manner, is called:
- A. isometric.
- B. polymeric.
- C. aerobic.
- D. isotonic.
- E. polytonic.

_____ 4. The target heart rate for a 50-year-old female with a resting heart rate of 65 is:
- A. 103.
- B. 139.
- C. 152.
- D. 170.
- E. 220.

_____ 5. Flexibility is obtained by:
   A. isometric exercise.
   B. isotonic exercise.
   C. stretching.
   D. bouncing at the end of a range-of-motion exercise.
   E. weight lifting.

_____ 6. Which of the following is NOT a major food group?
   A. grains and breads   D. meat and fish
   B. dairy products   E. simple sugars
   C. fruits

_____ 7. A proper and healthy diet minimizes intake of which of the following?
   A. carbohydrates   D. protein
   B. vitamins   E. grains
   C. salt

_____ 8. Which of the following does NOT increase your risk for cancer?
   A. prolonged, chronic, and unprotected sun exposure
   B. consumption of charcoal-grilled foods
   C. eating broccoli
   D. being a postmenopausal woman
   E. elevated cholesterol levels

_____ 9. Which of the following can reduce the risk of back injury?
   A. doing abdominal crunches
   B. stopping smoking
   C. following good nutritional practices
   D. getting adequate rest
   E. all of the above

_____ 10. Which of the following is NOT part of proper lifting?
   A. positioning the load as close to the body as possible
   B. locking your back in a slightly extended position
   C. reaching while twisting to distribute weight
   D. bending your knees
   E. keeping your palms up

_____ 11. Because a person carrying a contagious disease may present without signs, you must consider the blood and body fluids of every patient you treat as infectious.
   A. True
   B. False

_____ 12. Which of the following infectious diseases is NOT transmitted via airborne pathogens?
   A. hepatitis C   D. varicella
   B. pertussis   E. rubella
   C. tuberculosis

_____ 13. Which of the following items of personal protective equipment is/are recommended when suctioning a patient?
   A. gloves   D. both A and B
   B. eyewear and mask   E. A, B, and C
   C. gown

_____ 14. Which of the following items of personal protective equipment is/are recommended when assisting a mother with childbirth?
   A. gloves   D. both A and B
   B. eyewear and mask   E. A, B, and C
   C. gown

_____ 15. HEPA and N-95 respirators are intended to protect against:
A. HIV/AIDS.   D. hepatitis C.
B. tuberculosis.   E. bacterial meningitis.
C. hepatitis B.

_____ 16. Proper handwashing requires:
A. removing rings.
B. lathering hands vigorously.
C. scrubbing vigorously for at least 15 seconds.
D. scrubbing under fingernails and in creases of the knuckles.
E. all of the above

_____ 17. Which of the following is a recommended immunization for the EMT-I?
A. tetanus/diphtheria   D. rubella
B. polio   E. all of the above
C. hepatitis B and C

_____ 18. Used needles are to be disposed by:
A. placing them in a properly labeled puncture-proof container.
B. recapping them and placing them in a biohazard bag.
C. returning them to the pharmacy for disposal.
D. driving them deeply into the ground.
E. breaking them and taping them together with the tips covered.

_____ 19. Sterilization uses which of the following to kill pathogens?
A. bleach   D. pressurized steam
B. radiation   E. all of the above except A
C. EPA-approved chemical agents

_____ 20. Which of the following represent the standard progression through the stages of grieving?
A. anger, denial, bargaining, acceptance, depression
B. denial, bargaining, anger, depression, acceptance
C. denial, anger, bargaining, depression, acceptance
D. anger, denial, bargaining, depression, acceptance
E. depression, anger, denial, bargaining, acceptance

_____ 21. A grieving patient who is withdrawing from friends and family and is unwilling to communicate with others is most likely in which stage of loss?
A. denial   D. bargaining
B. anger   E. acceptance
C. depression

_____ 22. Because EMT-Is experience death more often than the general population, they experience less stress and are better able to cope with it.
A. True
B. False

_____ 23. At which age are children most likely to feel that death is a temporary absence from which the deceased person will return?
A. newborn to age 3   D. ages 9 to 12
B. ages 3 to 6   E. ages 12 to 18
C. ages 6 to 9

_____ 24. When informed of the death of a loved one, some family members may explode in anger, throw things, and scream.
A. True
B. False

_____ 25. When informing the family of the death of a member, use the words "dead" or "died" rather than less definitive ones such as "moved on" or "has gone to a better place."
A. True
B. False

©2004 Pearson Education, Inc.
Intermediate Emergency Care: Principles & Practice

26. The type of stress that has positive effects is:
    A. distress.   D. eustress.
    B. halcion.   E. gravitas.
    C. stimulation.

27. Which of the following is NOT a typical stressor for people working in emergency medical services?
    A. shift work   D. limited responsibilities
    B. violent people   E. thirst
    C. waiting for calls

28. The human response to stress progresses through three stages, in this order:
    A. resistance, alarm, exhaustion.   D. resistance, exhaustion, alarm.
    B. alarm, resistance, exhaustion.   E. exhaustion, alarm, resistance.
    C. alarm, exhaustion, resistance.

29. The physiological phenomena that occur at approximately 24-hour intervals and regulate body temperature, sleepiness, and appetite are called:
    A. estrorhythms.   D. fatigue/rest cycles.
    B. circadian rhythms.   E. solar epochs.
    C. lunar tidals.

30. When you work a regular night shift, a technique that may help you maintain the appropriate awake/sleep cycle is:
    A. sleeping during one "anchor time" for both on- and off-duty days.
    B. eating well before going to bed.
    C. sleeping during the day after you work a night shift and at night when off duty.
    D. sleeping in a warm place during the day.
    E. taking short naps rather than long sleep.

31. Which of the following is a warning sign of stress?
    A. withdrawal   D. aching muscles and joints
    B. feeling of being abandoned   E. all of the above
    C. difficulty making decisions

32. Which of the following is NOT a healthy behavior for dealing with or reducing stress?
    A. controlled breathing
    B. remaining distant from co-workers
    C. reframing
    D. creating a non-EMS circle of friends
    E. taking a vacation

33. An example of an event that is likely to be stressful for an EMS provider is:
    A. serious injury to a child.
    B. the death of a co-worker.
    C. an EMS operation causing a civilian death.
    D. a disaster.
    E. all of the above

34. Interpersonal safety begins with effective and positive communications.
    A. True
    B. False

35. When driving an ambulance, an EMT-I must:
    A. ignore highway regulations as necessary to reach the patient.
    B. practice due regard for the safety of others.
    C. never exceed speed limits.
    D. always use an escort vehicle.
    E. none of the above

©2004 Pearson Education, Inc.
Intermediate Emergency Care: Principles & Practice

MATCHING

Body Substance Isolation Procedures

Write the letter or letters of the appropriate personal protective equipment necessary for each of the following procedures in the space provided.

A. gloves
B. mask and eyewear
C. HEPA or N-95 respirator
D. gown

A,B   36. Suctioning

A,B,D   37. Childbirth

A,B   38. Endotracheal intubation

A,B,C   39. Patient with suspected TB

A,B,D   40. Serious arterial blood loss

©2004 Pearson Education, Inc.
Intermediate Emergency Care: Principles & Practice

CHAPTER 1

Foundations
of the EMT-Intermediate

Part 5: Illness and Injury Prevention

Review of Chapter Objectives

After reading this part of the chapter, you should be able to:

1. Describe the incidence, morbidity and mortality, and the human, environmental, and socioeconomic impact of unintentional and allegedly unintentional injuries. pp. 45–46

Injuries are the third leading cause of death in the United States overall and the leading cause of death for individuals between the ages of 1 and 44. Nearly 70,000 deaths are nonintentional, and the largest part of these are the result of vehicle collisions, fires, burns, falls, drownings, and poisonings. For every death there are approximately 19 hospitalizations and 254 emergency department visits. The lifetime cost of trauma exceeds $114 billion.

2. Identify health hazards and potential crime areas within the community. pp. 49–50

Health hazards are plentiful in a community. Homes are frequent sites of injuries to children from burns, falls, and firearm discharges. Geriatric patients also frequently fall in their homes. The home setting is also a place where EMT-Is are likely to encounter infants of low birth weight, patients discharged early from health-care facilities, and patients having problems with medication noncompliance—all groups that are at greater likelihood for needing emergency care. Recreational and workplace injuries are also common in communities. Bars and areas with previous records of high crime rates should also be considered as potential crime areas.

3. Identify local municipal and community resources available for physical, socioeconomic crises. pp. 47–48, 50–52

Establish a list of community resources in your locality that are available to assist patients in crisis. Such sites might include prenatal clinics, urgent care centers, and social services organizations that can offer food, shelter, clothing, and mental health counseling or services or referral to clinics or other forms of health-care service.

4. List the general and specific environmental parameters that should be inspected to assess a patient's need for preventative information and direction. pp. 49–52

Factors that should be considered when assessing the need for injury/illness prevention include the availability of prenatal care; level of public compliance with use of proper vehicular restraints for infants and children; awareness of proper firearm control measures; awareness of the dangers of drinking and driving; the home environments of geriatric patients (who are susceptible to falls); awareness of the need for patients to comply with directions for using medications; and local hospital/health organization policies involving the early discharge of patients with illness or injury. By surveying your community in these areas, you may identify parameters in which public education and direction may be beneficial in preventing illness and injury.

5. Identify the role of EMS in local municipal and community prevention programs.   pp. 50–52

The EMS provider can promote prevention by becoming an advocate of injury prevention. This may include teaching CPR and first aid courses for the public, teaching and supporting prevention programs, and being a role model and example by following safe practices (including BSI and ensuring scene safety) him- or herself.

6. Identify the injury and illness prevention programs that promote safety for all age populations.   pp. 49–52

Childhood and flu immunization programs; prenatal, well baby, and elder-care clinics; defensive driving programs; workplace safety courses; and health clinics sponsored by hospitals or health-care organizations are just some examples of injury and illness prevention programs available to people across a range of ages in the community.

7. Identify patient situations in which the EMT-Intermediate can intervene in a preventative manner.   pp. 49–52

The EMT-I can intervene at the scene of an illness or injury and take advantage of a teachable moment. In a nonjudgmental, nonthreatening way, the EMT-I may identify behaviors that would prevent illness or injury—for example, wearing protective equipment like seat belts in a car or helmets when biking—and instruct the patient in their use. The EMT-I may also identify community risks like improperly enclosed swimming pools, which are common sites of children drowning, or poorly designed railway crossings, which are likely sites of train-vs.-auto collisions.

8. Document primary and secondary injury prevention data.   pp. 50–52

Frequently, prehospital care reports contain or can be designed to collect information about the patient behavior regarding safe practices. Information on seatbelt use, airbag deployment, medication compliance, and the like may be helpful in identifying areas in which programs promoting safe practices could reduce illness and injury. The patient care report may also identify mechanisms that frequently result in injury and suggest areas in which preventative practices or safety equipment may help reduce mortality and morbidity.

CONTENT SELF-EVALUATION

MULTIPLE CHOICE

C   1. Injury represents the _____ leading cause of death in the United States.
    A. first
    B. second
    C. third
    D. fourth
    E. fifth

A   2. While injuries are often considered to be caused by accident, they are most likely predictable and preventable.
    A. True
    B. False

A   3. The calculation made by subtracting a person's age at death from 65 produces a result called the:
    A. years of productive life.
    B. injury risk factor.
    C. secondary span.
    D. epidemiological age.
    E. vital factor.

©2004 Pearson Education, Inc.
Intermediate Emergency Care: Principles & Practice

B 4. A systematic method to collect, analyze, and interpret information about injury data is a(n):
A. injury risk program.
B. injury surveillance program.
C. epidemiological intervention.
D. secondary prevention program.
E. risk data analysis.

A 5. EMS providers are well distributed throughout the population, are often considered to be champions of the health-care consumer, and are high-profile health-care role models.
A. True
B. False

B 6. An EMT-I should enter a hazardous scene only when the proper rescue, utility, or hazardous materials teams are not available.
A. True
B. False

A 7. What percentage of child deaths are the result of injuries?
A. one third
B. one quarter
C. one fifth
D. one sixth
E. one tenth

B 8. The most serious injuries associated with pediatric bicycle collisions are to the:
A. neck.
B. head.
C. abdomen.
D. chest.
E. extremities.

C 9. The most common cause of injury to children younger than six years old is:
A. bicycle collisions.
B. auto crashes.
C. falls.
D. abuse.
E. fire.

A 10. The term *accident* does not accurately reflect the nature of auto collisions.
A. True
B. False

C 11. The greatest cause of preventable injuries in the geriatric population is:
A. skeletal failure.
B. motor vehicle accidents.
C. falls.
D. intentional mechanisms.
E. burns.

A 12. The early release of patients from health-care facilities to help control heath care costs is likely to cause an increase in the number of EMS responses.
A. True
B. False

E 13. Which of the following is an action you should take as an EMS responder to implement injury prevention strategies?
A. Preserve response team safety.
B. Recognize scene hazards.
C. Engage in on-scene education.
D. Know your community resources.
E. all of the above

B 14. The opportunity presented by an emergency call to provide information to patients/bystanders about the future prevention of such an emergency is:
A. a prevention protocol.
B. a teachable moment.
C. EMS empowerment.
D. patient/provider prevention.
E. tertiary prevention.

E 15. Which of the following is a possible community resource for injury or illness prevention?
A. childhood and flu immunization program
B. elder-care clinic
C. workplace safety course
D. prenatal and well-baby clinic
E. all of the above

CHAPTER 1

Foundations
of the EMT-Intermediate

Part 6: Medical-Legal Considerations in Prehospital Care

Review of Chapter Objectives

After reading this part of the chapter, you should be able to:

1. **Differentiate legal, ethical, and moral responsibilities.** p. 52

An EMT-I's legal responsibility to the patient and others is defined by statute, regulation, and common law. Failure to meet this responsibility may result in criminal or civil liability. Ethical responsibilities are those actions expected of an EMT-I by the health-care profession and by the public. Moral responsibilities are personal values of right and wrong and are governed by conscience. Legal, ethical, and moral factors guide an individual in his or her actions as an EMT-I.

2. **Describe the basic structure of the legal system and differentiate between civil and criminal law.** pp. 52–53

There are four primary sources of law in the United States: constitutional, common, legislative, and administrative. Constitutional law defines governmental authority and gives the individual certain rights. Common law is based upon past judge-decided cases (case law) and is a fundamental principle of our legal system. Legislative law consists of statutes enacted at the federal, state, or local level. Administrative law consists of the regulations and rules that a governmental agency uses to implement legislative law. These four sources of law affect the legal responsibilities of the practicing EMT-I.

Civil law is non-criminal legal action between individuals for such things as matrimonial, contract, and personal injury disputes. It may also include civil wrongs such as assault, battery, medical malpractice, and negligence. Criminal law addresses actions against society (crimes) such as rape, murder, and burglary and will fine or imprison those found guilty.

3. **Differentiate licensure and certification.** p. 55

Certification is the recognition of an individual who has met predetermined qualifications to participate in a certain activity. It may be given by a governmental or other agency or by a professional association. Licensure is a process whereby a governmental agency grants permission to an individual, after meeting certain qualifications, to engage in a particular profession. A particular state may choose to require certification, licensure, or both for an EMT-I to practice.

4. List reportable problems or conditions and to whom the reports are to be made.   p. 55

Each state, through statutes and administrative regulation, may require prehospital care providers to report such matters as suspected spousal abuse, child neglect and abuse, abuse of the elderly, violent crimes, and public health threats such as animal bites and communicable diseases. Reports are made to the department of health, police, or other agencies as defined in statute or regulation.

5. Define:

a. Abandonment   p. 64

This is the termination of a patient–EMT-I relationship while the patient still desires and needs care without the EMT-I's providing for the appropriate continuation of care.

b. Advance directives   p. 66

These are documents created to express the patient's treatment choices should he or she become incapacitated or otherwise unable to express a choice of treatment.

c. Assault   p. 66

This is placing a person in apprehension of immediate bodily harm without his or her consent.

d. Battery   pp. 65

This is the unlawful touching of an individual without his or her consent.

e. Breach of duty   p. 57

This is the failure to act with the skill and judgement expected of a similarly trained EMT-I under similar circumstances.

f. Confidentiality   p. 59

This is the principle of law that prohibits the release of medical or other information about a patient without his or her permission.

g. Consent (expressed, implied, informed, involuntary)   pp. 61–62

Consent is the granting of permission to treat. Expressed consent occurs when a patient gives verbal or written permission to treat. Implied consent occurs when you presume the patient would give expressed consent if he or she were able. Informed consent is consent granted by the patient who knows the necessity, nature, and risks of treatment. Involuntary consent is consent to treat a patient given by the authority of a police agency or court.

h. Do not resuscitate (DNR) orders   p. 66

These are advance directives that define the life-sustaining equipment or procedures that may be used if the patient's heart or respirations cease.

i. Duty to act   p. 56

This is the formal or informal responsibility of the EMT-I to provide care.

j. Emancipated minor   p. 62

This is generally someone under 18 years of age who is married, pregnant, a parent, a member of the armed forces, or financially independent and living away from home. Such a person is often considered legally able to give informed consent.

k. False imprisonment   p. 65

This is the restraint or transport of a patient without consent, proper justification, or authority.

l. Immunity   p. 55

This is the exemption from legal liability.

m. Liability   p. 52

This is the legal responsibility for one's actions. Any deviation from the duty to act or the standard of care exposes the care provider to liability.

n. Libel   p. 61

This is the act of injuring a person's character, name, or reputation by false and malicious written statements.

o. Minor
                              p. 62

A minor is a person under 18 years of age for whom a parent, legal guardian, or court-appointed custodian gives informed consent.

p. Negligence
                              p. 56

This is the deviation from accepted standards of care recognized by the law for the protection of others against the unreasonable risk of harm.

q. Proximate cause
                              p. 57

This is the action or inaction of the EMT-I that caused or worsened the damage suffered by the patient.

r. Scope of practice
                              p. 54

This is the range of duties and skills EMT-Is are allowed and expected to perform.

s. Slander
                              p. 61

This is the act of injuring a person's character, name, or reputation by false and malicious spoken statements.

t. Standard of care
                              p. 57

This is the degree of skill and judgment expected of an individual when caring for a patient and is defined by training, protocols, and the expected actions of care providers with similar training and experience, working under similar conditions.

u. Tort
                              p. 53

This is a category of law dealing with civil wrongs against an individual such as negligence, medical malpractice, assault, battery, and slander.

6. Discuss the legal implications of medical direction.   **pp. 54, 59**

Medical direction, both on-line and off-line, helps define the EMT-I's scope of practice. Protocols, policies, and procedures as well as medical direction from an on-line physician define what is the acceptable standard of care. The system medical director is responsible for supervising the protocols and continuing education of the EMT-I. The on-line medical direction physician is responsible for supervising and directing the EMT-I's actions at the scene and during transport. The EMT-I is responsible for ensuring that the medical care given to the patient is appropriate and in keeping with the protocols. Any breach of duty or deviation from the standard of care that results in patient injury may result in charges of negligence.

7. Describe the four elements necessary to prove negligence.   **p. 56**

Four elements must exist before negligence can be proven. They include the duty to act, breach of duty, actual damages, and proximate cause. The duty to act is the direct or indirect responsibility to provide the patient with care. Breach of duty is the failure to meet the standard of care associated with the patient's needs. Damages are the actual physical, psychological, or financial harm suffered by the patient. Proximate cause means that the EMT-I's action or inaction directly caused or worsened the harm suffered by the patient.

8. Explain liability as it applies to emergency medical services.   **pp. 52, 56–59**

Liability in EMS is the legal responsibility to provide appropriate assessment, care, and transport of the ill or injured patient. That liability extends to the system medical director and on-line medical direction physician as well as to the EMT-I who supervises the actions of others while at the emergency scene. They must ensure that those they supervise follow the standard of care.

9. Discuss immunity, including Good Samaritan statutes and governmental immunity, as it applies to the EMT-Intermediate.   **pp. 55–56**

The Good Samaritan statute may offer some liability protection to someone who assists at the emergency scene if that person acts in good faith, is not grossly negligent, acts within his or her scope of practice, and does not receive payment for his or her services. In some states, Good Samaritan statutes have been expanded to include both paid and unpaid EMS providers.

©2004 Pearson Education, Inc.
Intermediate Emergency Care: Principles & Practice

Governmental immunity is a judicial doctrine that protects the government from liability unless it accepts that liability. However, most states have waived these rights, and courts are becoming increasingly likely to strike any remaining immunity down.

10. Explain the necessity and standards for maintaining patient confidentiality that apply to the EMT-Intermediate. pp. 59–61

The EMT-I, through his or her involvement in patient care, learns sensitive information about the patients he or she treats. To encourage patients to continue to divulge this information, EMT-Is must respect its confidential nature and only divulge it to those with a need to know. Information regarding a patient may be released to those continuing care, in accordance with the patient's consent to release information, as required by law, and as necessary for billing purposes.

11. Differentiate expressed, informed, implied, and involuntary consent and describe the process used to obtain informed or implied consent. pp. 61–62

Expressed consent is that given in writing or verbally, while implied consent is assumed consent from a patient who is unable to give expressed consent. Informed consent is the consent for treatment given by a patient when he or she understands the necessity, nature, risks, and alternatives to care. Involuntary consent is the consent given by the authority of a police agency or court to treat an individual.

When a patient summons an ambulance, that action suggests that he or she is asking for help and consenting to treatment. However, an EMT-I is obligated to explain what he or she is going to do to and for the patient and why he or she is going to do it. The EMT-I must also determine if the patient is alert, oriented, and rational enough to make a competent decision to accept or refuse care. If the patient is not able to make a rational decision regarding care, then the EMT-I may need to invoke implied consent. If the patient is a minor and the legal parent or guardian cannot be reached, consent is assumed (implied consent).

12. Discuss appropriate patient interaction and documentation techniques regarding refusal of care. pp. 62–64

When a patient refuses care, the EMT-I must assure and document the following: the patient was legally able and competent to make the decision; the need for care and potential consequences of refusing care were explained; on-line medical direction was consulted; the patient was directed to see his or her own physician; and the patient was directed to call the ambulance if the symptoms return or get worse. The refusal form should be signed by the patient and either a family member or a police officer. If the patient refuses to sign a refusal of treatment form, then have his or her refusal witnessed by a family member or police officer.

13. Identify legal issues involved in the decision not to transport a patient, or to reduce the level of care. pp. 64–65

A decision not to continue the care of a patient or to relinquish care to a lesser level of provider may expose the EMT-I to charges of abandonment or negligence if the patient suffers harm. This is especially true if the EMT-I has initiated advanced life support procedures like starting an IV or administering a medication.

14. Describe the criteria and the role of the EMT-Intermediate in selecting hospitals to receive patients. pp. 65–66

The patient's request to be transported to a particular hospital should be honored unless his or her particular care needs demonstrate otherwise. The decision to transport a patient to a facility other than the one requested must be based upon the patient's care needs, the capabilities of the requested facility, protocols, and interaction with the on-line medical direction physician.

©2004 Pearson Education, Inc.
Intermediate Emergency Care: Principles & Practice

15. Differentiate assault and battery. p. 65

Assault threatens bodily harm, while battery is unauthorized touching. These civil and criminal actions can be avoided by the EMT-I's making sure to obtain expressed consent for treatment and to explain what he or she is planning to do for the patient before doing it.

16. Describe the conditions under which the use of force, including restraint, is acceptable. p. 65

The use of force to restrain a patient may be necessary when the patient is violent or poses a danger to him- or herself or to others. Then only such force and restraint should be used as is required. In conditions where force and restraint are necessary to care for a patient, the police should be involved.

17. Explain advance directives and how they impact patient care. pp. 66–67

Advance directives permit the patient to define what care he or she would desire should they become incapacitated. Advance directives include Do Not Resuscitate (DNR) orders, which limit care actions that can be taken should the patient go into cardiac or respiratory arrest. Living wills are legal documents that also prescribe the care a patient may receive, including his or her desire to donate organs and to die at home or elsewhere. State statutes usually define the authority of DNRs, living wills, and other advance directives.

18. Discuss the EMT-Intermediate's responsibilities relative to resuscitation efforts for patients who are potential organ donors. p. 67

When presented with a patient who is a possible organ donor, it is essential for the EMT-I to maintain adequate perfusion of that organ to ensure its viability. Employ resuscitation procedures including fluid therapy, cardiac compressions, and ventilation and notify the medical direction physician that you are transporting a possible organ donor.

19. Describe how a EMT-Intermediate may preserve evidence at a crime or accident scene. pp. 67–68

Your responsibility at the crime scene is first to ensure your safety and that of your patient and then to ensure the health of the victim (your patient). If the patient is not obviously dead, initiate resuscitation and care directed at his or her injuries. Limit any movement of articles around the patient and at the scene and, if possible, document what you moved and from what location you moved it. Do not cut through clothing where objects entered the body; remove the clothing without cutting it, or cut around the openings.

20. Describe the importance of providing accurate documentation of an EMS response. pp. 68–69

Documentation establishes what was found and what was done at the emergency scene. It must be completed promptly, thoroughly, objectively, and accurately. At the same time, the confidentiality of the information obtained must be maintained. The documentation will become a part of the patient's medical record and help guide continuing patient care. It will also become a record of what you did at the emergency scene and during transport should your actions ever come into question. It may also become a legal document in a court of law when someone feels they have been injured (damaged) by someone else.

21. Describe what is required to make the patient care report an effective legal document. pp. 68–69

A patient care report must be completed in a timely manner, must be thorough, must be objective, must be accurate, and must ensure patient confidentiality to be an effective legal document.

©2004 Pearson Education, Inc.
Intermediate Emergency Care: Principles & Practice

CONTENT SELF-EVALUATION

MULTIPLE CHOICE

B   1. The term liability best refers to:
- A. an illegal act.
- B. legal responsibility.
- C. an act of negligence.
- D. civil responsibility.
- E. responsibility for damages.

C   2. Ethical responsibilities are best described as:
- A. requirements of case law.
- B. requirements of statute law.
- C. standards of a profession.
- D. personal feelings of right and wrong.
- E. legal concepts of right and wrong.

C   3. Which type of law is also called statutory law?
- A. "case" law
- B. common law
- C. legislative law
- D. administrative law
- E. regulatory law

A   4. Criminal law is best described as dealing with:
- A. wrongs committed against society.
- B. conflicts between two or more parties.
- C. contract disputes.
- D. negligence.
- E. breaches of faith.

E   5. Which of the following is a component of an EMT-I's scope of practice?
- A. protocols
- B. system policies and procedures
- C. on-line medical direction
- D. training and continuing education
- E. all of the above

D   6. Which of the following is NOT a common mandatory reporting event?
- A. rape
- B. spousal abuse
- C. child abuse
- D. a seizure episode
- E. animal bites

B   7. Governmental immunity is a likely protection for the EMT-I working for a municipality.
- A. True
- B. False

A   8. The Ryan White CARE act provides what protection to the EMT-I?
- A. It requires a notification system for contagious disease exposure.
- B. It compensates EMS providers who contract AIDS.
- C. It permits EMS review of any patient records.
- D. It grants immunity to civil litigation in cases of ordinary negligence.
- E. It defines the restraints permissible while treating a violent patient.

D   9. Which of the following is NOT one of the elements required to prove a charge of negligence against an EMT-I?
- A. duty to act
- B. proximate cause
- C. actual damages suffered by the patient
- D. payment to the EMT-I
- E. breach of duty

_E_ **10.** Which of the following is a duty expected of the EMT-I?
  A. to respond to the scene of an emergency
  B. to conform to the expected standard of care
  C. to provide care in accordance with the system's protocols
  D. to drive, or ensure the emergency vehicle is driven, appropriately
  E. all of the above

_C_ **11.** The degree of care, skill, and judgment that would be expected under like or similar circumstances by a similarly trained, reasonable EMT-I is:
  A. the duty to act.   D. a proximate cause.
  B. the scope of practice.   E. malfeasance.
  C. the standard of care.

_C_ **12.** *Res ipsa loquitur* is a legal term that refers to:
  A. contributory negligence.   D. the victim's liability.
  B. immunity from prosecution.   E. the reliability of evidence.
  C. a matter that is self-evident.

_E_ **13.** Which of the following may protect an EMT-I from charges of negligence?
  A. Good Samaritan statute   D. contributory negligence
  B. governmental immunity   E. all of the above
  C. the statute of limitations

_A_ **14.** Although many employers and agencies carry insurance coverage, it is a good idea for an EMT-I to obtain personal coverage because the agency's coverage may be inadequate.
  A. True
  B. False

_A_ **15.** In many states, an EMT-I would be guilty of practicing without a license if, while off duty, he or she performed advanced life support skills outside his or her system of medical direction.
  A. True
  B. False

_D_ **16.** Which of the following is NOT an acceptable reason for the release of confidential patient information?
  A. Medical providers need it to care for the patient.
  B. A judge has signed a court order demanding its release.
  C. It is necessary for third party billing.
  D. Other EMT-Is, not on the call, have requested it.
  E. The patient has made a written request for its release.

_E_ **17.** The act of injuring an individual's character, name, or reputation by false written statements and with malicious intent is:
  A. slander.   D. misfeasance.
  B. breach of confidentiality.   E. libel.
  C. malfeasance.

_B_ **18.** Before beginning to treat a patient, an EMT-I must obtain expressed consent.
  A. True
  B. False

_C_ **19.** The type of consent that is given by the authority of a court is:
  A. expressed.   D. informed.
  B. implied.   E. common.
  C. involuntary.

©2004 Pearson Education, Inc.
Intermediate Emergency Care: Principles & Practice

_E_ 20. For a patient's consent to be informed, the patient must be told and understand:
A. the nature of the treatment.
B. the necessity of the treatment.
C. the risks of the treatment.
D. the risks of refusing the treatment.
E. all of the above

_B_ 21. Once a patient has given consent for treatment, he or she may not withdraw that consent.
A. True
B. False

_B_ 22. A minor is <u>usually</u> considered someone under the age of:
A. 16.
B. 18.
C. 19.
D. 21.
E. 25.

_E_ 23. Conditions that may define a person as an emancipated minor include being:
A. married.
B. pregnant.
C. a parent.
D. a member of the armed forces.
E. all of the above

_B_ 24. Once a patient has withdrawn his consent to care, it may be considered assault to encourage him to go to the hospital.
A. True
B. False

_B_ 25. Which of the following is NOT an essential element in accepting a patient's refusal of care?
A. The patient is conscious, alert, and rational.
B. The patient is a minor.
C. The patient is aware of the possible consequences of his or her decision.
D. The patient has been advised that he or she may call again for help if necessary.
E. The patient and/or a disinterested witness has signed a release-from-liability form.

_A_ 26. Ideally, a police officer should respond to the scene of all problem patients and sign the patient care report as a witness or, if the patient poses a threat to the EMT-I, accompany the EMT-I and patient to the hospital.
A. True
B. False

_D_ 27. Ending a patient–care giver relationship without providing the appropriate continuing care and without the patient's approval could be found to be:
A. battery.
B. defamation.
C. nonfeasance.
D. abandonment.
E. assault.

_C_ 28. The unlawful act of touching another person without permission is:
A. assault.
B. abandonment.
C. battery.
D. slander.
E. libel.

_D_ 29. An important question to ask yourself when considering the restraint of a patient is:
A. Does the patient need immediate treatment?
B. Does the patient pose a threat to himself?
C. Does the patient pose a threat to others?
D. all of the above
E. none of the above

_A_ 30. If you need to use force to restrain a patient, it is best to involve law enforcement whenever possible.
A. True
B. False

_E_ **31.** Under what situation should an EMT-I NOT begin resuscitation of a pulseless, non-breathing patient?
  A. The patient is are obviously dead.
  B. The patient has a valid DNR order.
  C. There is obvious tissue decomposition.
  D. There is extreme dependant lividity.
  E. all of the above

_A_ **32.** Do Not Resuscitate orders usually restrict care providers from:
  A. performing CPR in case of cardiac arrest.
  B. performing a "slow code."
  C. performing a "chemical code."
  D. leaving the scene until the coroner arrives.
  E. contacting medical direction.

_A_ **33.** If there is any doubt about the authenticity or applicability of a DNR order, an EMT-I should initiate resuscitation immediately.
  A. True
  B. False

_C_ **34.** Which of the following statements is NOT true regarding an EMT-I's responsibility at the crime scene?
  A. He or she should contact law enforcement officers if they are not on the scene.
  B. He or she should not enter the scene unless it is safe.
  C. His or her primary responsibility is to preserve the evidence at the scene.
  D. He or she should not disturb the scene unless it is necessary for patient care.
  E. He or she should document the movement of any item at the scene.

_C_ **35.** Which of the following is NOT required when documenting a patient care response?
  A. Completing documentation promptly.
  B. Ensuring that documentation is accurate.
  C. Ensuring that documentation is subjective.
  D. Ensuring that patient confidentiality is maintained.
  E. Ensuring that documentation is thorough.

©2004 Pearson Education, Inc.
Intermediate Emergency Care: Principles & Practice

CHAPTER 1

*

Foundations
of the EMT-Intermediate

Part 7: Ethics in Advanced Prehospital Care

Review of Chapter Objectives

After reading this part of the chapter, you should be able to:

1. **Define ethics and morals and distinguish between ethical and moral decisions in emergency medical service.** pp. 69–71

   Morals are social, religious, or personal standards of right and wrong. Ethics are rules or standards that govern the conduct of a group or profession. Ethics and morals, along with common law, govern how we function in prehospital emergency care.

   Ethical decisions regarding patient care involve what the public and peers expect of the EMT-I. Moral decisions involve the EMT-I's own values of right and wrong.

2. **Identify the premise that should underlie the EMT-Intermediate's ethical decisions in out-of-hospital care.** pp. 70–71

   Ultimately, the decisions made by the EMT-I should be guided by the question: What is in the best interest of the patient?

3. **Analyze the relationship between the law and ethics in EMS.** p. 69

   In general, the law takes a narrower and more specific look at behavior and identifies what is wrong in the eyes of society. Ethics takes a more general view of what is right or good behavior. Laws or the results of following them may be unethical, and the law often does not resolve ethical dilemmas.

4. **Compare and contrast the criteria used in allocating scarce EMS resources.** pp. 76–77

   The most common situation regarding allocation of resources that a member of EMS is likely to face is a multiple-casualty incident (MCI). At an MCI, the triage process sorts casualties into priorities for care because patient needs outstrip the available resources. In the civilian environment, the person with the most need for care (excepting those with mortal injuries) receives care first. In the military domain, those with the least serious injuries receive care first to help maintain the fighting force (and win the battle).

5. **Identify issues surrounding advance directives in making a prehospital resuscitation decision.** pp. 73–74

Advance directives, such as living wills and Do Not Resuscitate orders, are ways that patients can indicate their desire for the type of medical care they wish to receive should they become incapacitated. Such directives often present ethical dilemmas for EMT-Is because they are trained and expected to do all that is necessary to preserve life. When an EMT-I confronts a situation involving an advance directive, he or she must weigh the patient's right to autonomy against what he or she feels is in the patient's medical best interest. Whenever you are presented with an advance directive, ensure that it is valid, current, and conforms to requirements in your state for such documents. When in doubt, resuscitate.

CONTENT SELF-EVALUATION

MULTIPLE CHOICE

 1. Although ethical problems often have a legal aspect, most ethical problems are solved in the field and not in a courtroom.
   A. True
   B. False

 2. Most codes of ethics provide specific guidance for performance of the professional.
   A. True
   B. False

 3. When faced with an ethical challenge, the best guiding question is which of the following?
   A. How would I like to be treated?
   B. What would the patient want?
   C. Which actions will account for the greatest good?
   D. What is in the best interest of the patient?
   E. What actions can I defend?

4. The term that means "desiring to do good" is:
   A. benevolence.   D. autonomy.
   B. justice.   E. euphylanthropnia.
   C. beneficence.

 5. The Latin phrase *primum non nocere* means:
   A. "Do the best you can."
   B. "Avoid mistakes."
   C. "Maintain the patient's best interests."
   D. "First, do no harm."
   E. "Treat all patients fairly."

 6. Which question best describes the impartiality test for analyzing an ethical situation?
   A. Can you justify this action to others?
   B. Would you want this procedure if you were in the patient's place?
   C. Would you want this procedure performed on you if you were in similar circumstances?
   D. Will you likely be questioned about the need for this procedure later?
   E. none of the above

©2004 Pearson Education, Inc.
Intermediate Emergency Care: Principles & Practice

_A_ 7. When in doubt about the validity of a DNR order or the patient's desire to be resuscitated, you should:
   A. begin resuscitation immediately.
   B. await arrival of the DNR to verify its validity.
   C. contact medical direction for advice before beginning resuscitation.
   D. not resuscitate.
   E. begin with CPR and delay advanced interventions.

_B_ 8. There are no circumstances in which it is appropriate to breach patient confidentiality.
   A. True
   B. False

_A_ 9. When presented with a patient who is enrolled in a health maintenance organization (HMO) whose policy states that the patient must be cared for at a member institution, you are responsible to act in the patient's best interest.
   A. True
   B. False

_E_ 10. When presented with orders from a physician that do not comply with your protocols and that you believe are not in the patient's best interest, you should:
   A. follow the physician's order and report your concerns to the medical director.
   B. ask the physician to repeat or confirm the order.
   C. ask the physician for an explanation of the order.
   D. not follow the physician's order.
   E. do all except A.

SPECIAL PROJECT

Crossword Puzzle

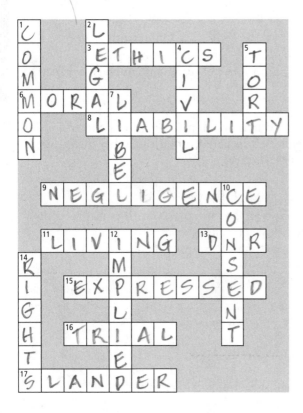

Across

3. Rules or standards of conduct that govern members of a profession
6. Right as determined by personal conscience
8. Legal responsibility
9. Deviation from the accepted standard of care
11. _____ will: document that allows a person to specify the kinds of treatment he or she would desire
13. _____ order: legal document indicating the life-sustaining measures to take during cardio-pulmonary arrest (abbr.)
15. _____ consent: communication from the patient indicating that he or she agrees to care
16. Component of a law suit in which both sides present testimony and evidence
17. Injuring a patient's character by false spoken statements

Down

1. _____ law: type of law derived from society's acceptance of customs and norms over time
2. Pertaining to the law
4. _____ law: division of the legal system that deals with non-criminal issues
5. A civil wrong committed by one individual against another
7. Injuring a patient's character by false written statements
10. A patient's permission to give care
12. _____ consent: type of permission to treat that is presumed from an otherwise incapacitated patient
14. Privileges that one is given by law and tradition

©2004 Pearson Education, Inc.
Intermediate Emergency Care: Principles & Practice

CHAPTER 2
✳
Overview of Human Systems

Part 1: The Cell and the Cellular Environment

Review of Chapter Objectives

Because Chapter 2 is lengthy, it has been divided into parts to aid your study. Read the assigned textbook pages, then progress through the objectives and self-evaluation materials as you would with other chapters. When you feel secure in your grasp of the content, proceed to the next part.

After reading this part of the chapter, you should be able to:

1. **Define the following terms: anabolism, anatomy, blood pressure, catabolism, homeostasis, metabolism, pathophysiology, physiology.** p. 87

   Anabolism is the building up of biochemical substances to produce energy. **Anatomy** is the study of the structure of the organisms. **Blood pressure** is a fraction formed by the systolic pressure over the diastolic pressure. The systolic represents the pressure in the arteries when the left ventricle contracts and the diastolic represents the pressure when the left ventricle relaxes. **Catabolism is the breaking down of biochemical substances to produce energy.** **Homeostasis** is the term for the body's natural tendency to keep the internal environment and metabolism steady and normal. **Metabolism** is the term used to refer to the building up and breaking down of biochemical substances to produce energy. **Pathophysiology** is the study of abnormal function of organisms. **Physiology** is the study of the function of organisms.

2. **Name the levels of organization of the body from simplest to most complex, and explain each.** pp. 83–100

   The body is organized from simple levels to complex in the following way:
   - The cell is the fundamental unit of the human body which contains all necessary components to turn essential nutrients into energy, remove waste products, reproduce, and carry on other essential life functions.
   - Tissues refer to a group of cells that perform a similar function. There are four basic types of tissue: epithelial, muscle, connective, and nerve.
   - Organs are a group of tissues working together to perform a specific function.
   - Organ system is a group of organs that are working together for a specific functions such as the: cardiovascular system, respiratory system, gastrointestinal system, genitourinary system, reproductive system, nervous system, endocrine system, lymphatic system, muscular system, and skeletal system.
   - The organism consists of the sum of all cells, tissues, organs, and organ systems.

©2004 Pearson Education, Inc.
Intermediate Emergency Care: Principles & Practice

3. **Describe the general characteristics of each of the four major categories of tissues.** pp. 85–86

Tissue refers to a group of cells that perform a similar function. The following are the four basic types of tissue:

- **Epithelial tissue** lines internal and external body surfaces and protects the body. In addition, certain types of epithelial tissue perform specialized functions such as secretion, absorption, diffusion, and filtration. Examples of epithelial tissue are skin, mucous membranes, and the lining of the intestinal tract.
- **Muscle tissue** has the capability of contraction when stimulated. There are three types of muscle tissue: 1) Cardiac muscle which is tissue found only within the heart. It has the unique capability of spontaneous contraction without external stimulation. 2) Smooth muscle is the muscle found within the intestines and encircling blood vessels. Smooth muscle is generally under the control of the involuntary, or autonomic, component of the nervous system. 3) Skeletal muscle is the most abundant muscle type. It allows movement and is mostly under voluntary control.
- **Connective tissue** is the most abundant tissue in the body. It provides support, connection, and insulation. Examples of connective tissue include bones, cartilage, and fat. Blood is also sometimes classified as connective tissue.
- **Nerve tissue** is tissue specialized to transmit electrical impulses throughout the body. Examples of nerve tissue include the brain, spinal cord, and peripheral nerves.

4. **Define each of the cellular transport mechanisms and give an example of the role of each in the body: diffusion, osmosis, facilitated diffusion, and active transport.** pp. 94–96

Cellular transport is conducted by various methods such as:

- **Diffusion** is the tendency of molecules to move from an area of higher concentration to an area of lower concentration. This process does not require energy. The diffusion of a solute (usually an electrolyte) across a cell membrane from the area of higher concentration to the area of lower concentration continues until the natural balance is again attained.
- **Osmosis** is the passage of any solvent, usually water, through a membrane. It occurs in the direction opposite to the direction of solute movement. For example, if a semipermeable membrane separates solutions of water and sodium, and if the concentration of sodium is two times higher on one side of the membrane than on the other, then two things will occur. Sodium will diffuse from the area of higher concentration to the area of lesser concentration. Concurrently, water will diffuse in the opposite direction. These actions will continue until the concentration of water and sodium on both sides has equalized.
- **Facilitated diffusion** requires the assistance of "helper proteins," parts of a membrane transport system, on the surface of the cell membrane for the molecule to move across a cell membrane. These proteins, once activated, bind to the glucose molecule. Following binding, the proteins change their configuration and transport the glucose molecule to the inside of the cell, where it is released. Depending on the substance being transported, facilitated diffusion may or may not require energy.
- **Active transport** is the movement of a substance across the cell membrane against the osmotic gradient toward the side that already has more of the substance. For example the body requires cells of the myocardium to be negatively charged on the inside of the cells compared to the outside. However, sodium, with its positive charge, tends to diffuse passively into the cell. This would destroy the negative charge inside the cell. In order to maintain the desired negative charge, sodium ions are actively pumped out of the cell, while potassium ions are pumped into the cell, by a mechanism known as the sodium-potassium pump.

5. **Describe the water compartments and name the fluid in each.** pp. 89–91

Water is distributed into various compartments of the body and is separated by cell membranes. The compartments are the intracellular compartment and the extracellular compartment. The intracellular compartment contains the intracellular fluid, which is all of the fluid found inside the body cells. The extracellular compartment contains intravascular fluid—the fluid found outside of

©2004 Pearson Education, Inc.
Intermediate Emergency Care: Principles & Practice

the cells and within the circulatory system—and interstitial fluid—all the fluid found outside of the cell membranes yet are not within the circulatory system.

6. Explain how water moves between compartments. pp. 94–96

Normally the total volume of water in the body, as well as the distribution of fluid remains relatively constant. However, at different ages total body water varies, being the highest in infants and the lowest in the elderly. The body also maintains fluid balance by shifting water from one body space or compartment to another.

7. Explain the regulation of the intake and output of water. pp. 91–94

To maintain homeostasis, the intake of fluid must equal the output. Several mechanisms work to maintain this balance. When the fluid volume drops, the pituitary gland secretes antidiuretic hormone (ADH), which causes the kidney tubules to reabsorb more water into the blood and to excrete less urine. This process helps to restore the fluid volume to normal values. Thirst also regulates fluid intake. When sensing thirst, the person is stimulated to take in more fluids orally. Conversely when too many fluids enter the body, the kidneys are activated and more urine is excreted.

8. Describe the three buffer systems in body fluids. pp. 97–100

The three major buffer systems are part of the process to maintain the acid-base balance, since hydrogen ions must be constantly eliminated from the body.

- **Bicarbonate Buffer System**
  In a healthy individual, for every molecule of carbonic acid, there are 20 molecules of bicarbonate ion. Any change in this 20:1 ratio is immediately corrected without significant change in the total body pH. An increase in hydrogen ion (acidosis) is corrected as the excess hydrogen ions combine with bicarbonate ions to form carbonic acid. Conversely, when there is a deficit in hydrogen ions (alkalosis), carbonic acid will dissociate into bicarbonate ions and hydrogen ions.

- **Respiratory Function**
  An increase in respirations cases increased elimination of CO_2, which results in a decrease in hydrogen ions and an increase in pH. Conversely, decreased respirations cause CO_2 to be retained, causing an increase in hydrogen ions and a decrease in pH.

- **Kidney Function**
  The kidneys also regulate the pH by altering the concentration of bicarbonate ions (HCO_3) in the blood. Increased elimination of HCO_3 results in a lowered pH. Conversely, retention of HCO_3 causes an increase in pH.

9. Explain the renal mechanisms for pH regulation of extracellular fluid. pp. 97–100

See objective 8.

10. Describe the effects of acidosis and alkalosis. pp. 97–100

The total number of hydrogen ions present in the body at any given time is very high. Because of this the pH system is used. The pH scale ranges from 1 to 14. A pH of 1 means that only hydrogen ions are present. A pH of 14 means that virtually no hydrogen ions are present. The pH of the body is normally 7.35 to 7.45. A pH below 7.35 is called acidosis. A pH above 7.45 is called alkalosis. A variation in humans of only 0.4 of a pH unit in either direction from normal can be fatal.

©2004 Pearson Education, Inc.
Intermediate Emergency Care: Principles & Practice

CASE STUDY REVIEW

This case study demonstrates the important link between understanding the disease process (pathophysiology) and the assessment and care of the patient.

EMT-I Terry Martinez and Mark Westbrook are presented with a patient who displays the signs and symptoms of a serious emergency. However, these signs and symptoms are from several body systems and seem unrelated. They include a reduced mental status (CNS), difficulty swallowing (gastrointestinal), cold, pale, diaphoretic skin and a rash (integumentary), and difficulty breathing, with wheezes and chest tightness (respiratory). These EMT-Is might treat each symptom as a separate problem if they did not recognize how they are related. The crew can recognize this relationship, however, because of their understanding of the pathophysiology of disease.

The patient presents with some signs and symptoms of inadequate tissue perfusion, also known as shock. These include the anxiousness and confusion, difficulty breathing (dyspnea), the rapid and weak pulse, the diaphoresis, and cold and clammy skin. These assessment findings are a result of the body's attempts to compensate for the migration of fluid out of the vascular system and into the lungs, skin, and other tissue and the reduced respiratory efficiency caused by the airway restrictions and fluid build-up (pulmonary edema). The lowered level of consciousness and agitation occur because the brain is not well perfused or oxygenated. The air hunger occurs as the body tries to increase the oxygen available to the blood and body cells. The rapid weak pulse is a result of the body's increasing the heart rate to compensate for a reduced blood volume and cardiac output. Finally, the cool, clammy (diaphoretic), and pale skin represents the body's directing blood away from non-critical organs to the brain, heart, and kidneys. Mark and Terry recognize these assessment findings as indications of the serious medical condition we call shock. They know something is seriously wrong with the 34-year-old female.

Their assessment reveals signs and symptoms specific to the patient's problem. They discover complaints of tightness in the chest, difficulty swallowing, and a hoarse voice and notice wheezes in the lung fields and hives on her chest and abdomen. These symptoms and signs are consistent with the body's overly aggressive response to an invading agent. The term for a mild reaction to an invading agent is "allergy," while the drastic response this patient displays is called "anaphylaxis." To prevent further absorption of the toxin, the body constricts the airways and begins the inflammatory response by allowing fluid to leak into the interstitial spaces. These responses are initiated by the body's release of a powerful hormone called histamine.

Understanding the significance of this problem and knowing that it can rapidly lead to death, Mark and Terry immediately intervene. They administer another body hormone, epinephrine, to counteract the effects of histamine and then administer fluids to replace the fluid shifting into the interstitial spaces. Providing the patient with oxygen helps increase respiratory efficiency. Once the immediate effects are addressed, the EMT-Is administer diphenhydramine (Benadryl) to negate the more long-term effects of the histamine.

Mark and Terry are only able to recognize and treat this serious emergency because they understand the pathophysiology of anaphylaxis. To be a good EMT-I, you must understand the pathologic processes at work behind the signs and symptoms of the most frequent diseases threatening life. Understanding the material in this chapter is a good beginning.

CONTENT SELF-EVALUATION

MULTIPLE CHOICE

____ 1. The fundamental unit of life is:
   A. the cell.
   B. tissue.
   C. the organ.
   D. the organism.
   E. DNA.

____ 2. One of the three main elements of a typical cell is the:
   A. cell membrane.
   B. cilia.
   C. leukocyte.
   D. eosinophil.
   E. basophil.

©2004 Pearson Education, Inc.
Intermediate Emergency Care: Principles & Practice

_C_   3. The characteristic ability of a cell membrane to selectively permit material to pass
through it is called:
A. diffusiveness.   D. cytoplasmicism.
B. imperviousness.   E. isotonicism.
C. semipermeability.

_E_   4. The thick viscous fluid that fills the cell and gives it shape is called:
A. ribosome.   D. protoplasm.
B. lysosome.   E. either C or D
C. cytoplasm.

_C_   5. The structure that contains the genetic material including the cell's DNA is the:
A. endoplasmic reticulum.   D. mitochondria.
B. Golgi apparatus.   E. cytokine.
C. nucleus.

_D_   6. The compound that provides the cell with most of its energy is:
A. DNA.   D. ATP.
B. phosgene.   E. carbohydrate.
C. carbon dioxide.

_A_   7. The tissue type that covers the internal and external body surfaces is:
A. epithelial.   D. connective.
B. smooth muscle.   E. skeletal muscle.
C. nerve.

_E_   8. The tissue type that is mostly under voluntary control is:
A. epithelial.   D. connective.
B. cardiac muscle.   E. skeletal muscle.
C. nerve.

_D_   9. The tissue type that provides support and insulation is:
A. epithelial.   D. connective.
B. cardiac muscle.   E. skeletal muscle.
C. nerve.

_A_   10. The body organ system that produces most body heat is the:
A. muscular system.   D. endocrine system.
B. gastrointestinal system.   E. lymphatic system.
C. genitourinary system.

_E_   11. The body organ system that is important in fighting disease and filtration is the:
A. muscular system.   D. endocrine system.
B. gastrointestinal system.   E. lymphatic system.
C. genitourinary system.

_E_   12. The term that is applied to the building up and tearing down of biochemical substances
to produce energy is:
A. anatomy.   D. anabolism.
B. physiology.   E. metabolism.
C. catabolism.

_A_   13. Ductless or endocrine glands secrete directly into the circulatory system.
A. True
B. False

_B_   14. The natural tendency of the body to maintain a constant internal environment is:
A. cellular equilibrium.   D. physiology.
B. homeostasis.   E. paracrine signaling.
C. metabolism.

A   15. The body's major baroreceptors are located in the:
        A. arch of the aorta.   D. inner ears.
        B. brainstem.   E. medulla oblongata.
        C. lung tissue.

B   16. Most of the input affecting body organs and homeostasis occurs via the positive
            feedback loop.
        A. True
        B. False

B   17. The feedback system that decreases stimulation as the target organ responds is the:
        A. positive feedback loop.   D. beta adrenergic system.
        B. negative feedback loop.   E. cholinergic loop.
        C. decompensation system.

C   18. Extracellular fluid accounts for what percentage of total body water?
        A. 75 percent   D. 17.5 percent
        B. 60 percent   E. 7.5 percent
        C. 25 percent

B   19. The fluid space found between the vascular and cellular compartments is the
            extracellular compartment.
        A. True
        B. False

D   20. A fluid that dissolves other substances is a(n):
        A. solute.   D. solvent.
        B. electrolyte.   E. anhydrous.
        C. hydrate.

E   21. Which of the following is a source of body fluid loss and dehydration?
        A. diarrhea   D. poor nutritional states
        B. hyperventilation   E. all of the above
        C. pancreatitis

B   22. The term *turgor* refers to:
        A. intense thirst.   D. sunken fontanelles.
        B. skin tension.   E. extreme obesity.
        C. highly concentrated urine.

A   23. Which element is most common in the human body?
        A. hydrogen   D. nitrogen
        B. oxygen   E. sodium
        C. carbon

B   24. A positively charged ion is a(n):
        A. anion.   D. dissociated element.
        B. cation.   E. reagent.
        C. electrolyte.

E   25. The most prevalent cation in the human body is:
        A. magnesium.   D. bicarbonate.
        B. chloride.   E. sodium.
        C. potassium.

D   26. Which of the following ions is responsible for buffering the acid concentrations in the
            body?
        A. magnesium   D. bicarbonate
        B. chloride   E. sodium
        C. potassium

©2004 Pearson Education, Inc.
Intermediate Emergency Care: Principles & Practice

_A_ 27. A solution that contains more solute concentration on one side of a semipermeable membrane than on the other is said to be:
A. hypertonic. D. osmotic.
B. isotonic. E. diffused.
C. hypotonic.

_B_ 28. When an isotonic solution is placed in the human bloodstream, water moves in which direction?
A. into the vascular space D. in both directions
B. does not move E. none of the above
C. out of the vascular space

_A_ 29. When a hypertonic solution is placed in the human bloodstream, water moves in which direction?
A. into the vascular space D. in both directions
B. does not move E. none of the above
C. out of the vascular space

_B_ 30. The movement of a solvent from an area of higher concentration through a semipermeable membrane to an area of lower concentration is termed:
A. diffusion. D. facilitated transport.
B. osmosis. E. oncosis.
C. active transport.

_A_ 31. The movement of water out of and then back into the capillary as it travels through the capillary is regulated by the protein concentration within the blood and the pressure as the blood is pushed through the capillary.
A. True
B. False

_D_ 32. The pressure that draws water into the blood because of the proteins there is called:
A. osmolarity. D. oncotic force.
B. osmotic pressure. E. filtration.
C. hydrostatic pressure.

_E_ 33. The movement of water out of the plasma across the capillary membrane into the interstitial space is:
A. osmolarity. D. oncotic force.
B. osmotic pressure. E. filtration.
C. hydrostatic pressure.

_A_ 34. The higher the pH value, the lower the concentration of hydrogen ions.
A. True
B. False

_B_ 35. The normal pH range in the human body is:
A. 6.9 to 7.35. D. 6.9 to 7.8.
B. 7.35 to 7.45. E. none of the above
C. 7.45 to 7.8.

_C_ 36. Which of the following would be considered alkalosis in the human?
A. 6.9 to 7.35 D. 6.4 to 6.9
B. 7.35 to 7.45 E. none of the above
C. 7.45 to 7.8

_B_ 37. A decrease in pH of 1 would reflect which change in the concentration of hydrogen ions?
A. 100 times as great D. 1/100th as great
B. 10 times as great E. a doubling
C. 1/10th as great

_B_ **38.** The cellular environment of the human body is slightly acidic.
   A. True
   B. False

_D_ **39.** The body system that responds most rapidly to a change in the pH is the:
   A. respiratory system.   **D.** buffer system.
   B. cardiovascular system.   **E.** genitourinary system.
   C. digestive system.

_B_ **40.** The addition of hydrogen ions to the bloodstream will result in an increase in carbon dioxide.
   A. True
   B. False

©2004 Pearson Education, Inc.
Intermediate Emergency Care: Principles & Practice

CHAPTER 2

*

Overview of Human Systems

Part 2: Body Systems

Review of Chapter Objectives

After reading this part of the chapter, you should be able to:

1. **Identify the anatomical terms for the parts of the body, for the anatomical planes, and for describing location of body parts with respect to one another.** **pp. 102, 115, 126, 134, 164**

The following are anatomical terms for parts of the body, anatomical planes, and for describing locations of body parts with respect to one another that the EMT-I should be familiar with:

—**Joint** is the area where the adjacent bones articulate.
—**Synovial joint** is a joint that permits the greatest degree of independent motion.
—**Flexion** is bending motion that reduces the angle between articulating elements.
—**Extension** is bending motion that increases the angle between articulating elements.
—**Adduction** is movement of a body part toward the midline.
—**Abduction** is movement of a body part away from the midline.
—**Anterior** is the front of the body.
—**Posterior** is the back of the body.
—**Superior** means above.
—**Inferior** means below.
—**Proximal** means closer to the torso of the body.
—**Distal** means further away from the torso of the body.
—**Rotation** is a turning along the axis of a bone or joint.
—**Circumduction** is movement at a synovial joint where the distal end of a bone describes a circle but the shaft does not rotate, movement through an arc of a circle.
—**Ligaments** connect tissue that connect bone to bone and hold joints together.
—**Joint capsule** are the ligaments that surround a joint.
—**Axial skeleton** is the bones of the head, thorax, and spine.
—**Appendicular skeleton** is the bones of the extremities, shoulder girdle, and pelvis.
—**Cranium** is the vault-like portion of the skull encasing the brain.
—**Meninges** are the three membranes that surround and protect the brain and spinal cord. They are the dura mater, pia mater, and arachnoid membrane.
—**Vertebrae** are the 33 bones making up the vertebral column.
—**Trachea** is a 10–12 cm long tube that connects the larynx to the main stem bronchi.
—**Bronchi** are tubes from the trachea into the lungs.
—**Alveoli** are microscopic air sacs where most oxygen and carbon dioxide gas exchange takes place.
—**Pleura** is membranous connective tissue covering the lungs.
—**Larynx** is the complex structure that joins the pharynx with the trachea.

©2004 Pearson Education, Inc.
Intermediate Emergency Care: Principles & Practice

—**Pharynx** is a muscular tube that extends vertically from the back of the soft palate to the superior aspect of the esophagus.

—**Nare** is the nostril.

2. **Review the body cavities and the major organs within each, including the abdomen and in its underlying organs.** pp. 213–216

The human body has multiple cavities which contain its major organs. The main cavities are as follows:

* **Cranium**—contains the brain consisting of the cerebrum, cerebellum, pons, thalamus, and medulla oblongata.
* **Thorax**—contains the lungs, trachea, bronchi, alveoli, diaphragm, great vessels, heart, and spine.
* **Abdomen**—contains the small intestine, large intestine, spleen, stomach, pancreas, liver, gall bladder, appendix.
* **Spinal cavity**—contains the meninges and spinal cord.
* **Pelvic cavity**—contains the reproductive organs and the urinary system.

3. **Name the three major layers of the skin.** pp. 100–102

The epidermis, dermis, and subcutaneous tissue layers comprise what is commonly known as the skin. Each of these layers performs functions essential to helping the body maintain homeostasis and each plays an important role in the wound repair process.

Epidermis
The epidermis is the most superficial layer of the skin and consists of numerous layers of dead or dying cells. The epidermis provides a flexible covering for the skin and a barrier to fluid loss, absorption, and the entrance of pathogens.

Dermis
The dermis is the true skin. It is made up of connective tissue and houses the sensory nerve endings; many of the specialized skin cells that produce sweat, oil, etc.; and the upper-level capillary beds that allow for the conduction of heat to the body's surface.

Subcutaneous Tissue
The subcutaneous layer, although not a true part of the skin, works in concert with the epidermis and dermis to insulate the body from heat loss and the effects of trauma. It consists of connective and adipose (fatty) tissues.

4. **Describe how glucose is converted to energy during cellular respiration.** pp. 180–181

The mitochondria are the energy factories, sometimes called the "powerhouses," of the cells. They convert essential nutrients, such as glucose, into energy sources, often in the form of adenosine triphosphate or ATP.

5. **Describe the functions of the skeleton, and explain how bones and joints are classified.** pp. 113–128

The skeletal system is a living body system that protects vital organs, acts as a storehouse for body salts and other materials needed for metabolism, produces erythrocytes, permits us to have an upright stature, and permits us to move with relative ease through the environment.

The skeletal system is organized into the axial and appendicular skeletons. The axial skeleton consists of the skull, thorax, and pelvis and the cervical, thoracic, lumbar, sacral, and coccygeal spine. The appendicular skeleton consists of the upper extremity (the humerus, radius and ulna, carpals, metacarpals, and phalanges) and the lower extremity (femur, tibia and fibula, tarsals, metatarsals, and phalanges).

The common long bone consists of a diaphysis, metaphysis, and epiphysis. The diaphysis is the hollow skeletal shaft of the long bone and contains the yellow bone marrow. It is covered by the periosteum, which contains sensory nerve fibers and initiates the bone repair cycle. The metaphysis is the transitional region between the diaphysis and the epiphysis. In this region, the thin

©2004 Pearson Education, Inc.
Intermediate Emergency Care: Principles & Practice

layer of compact bone of the diaphysis shaft becomes the honeycomb of the weight-bearing epiphyseal region. The epiphysis is the articular end of the bone. Through the widening of the metaphysis and the cancellous bone underneath, the weight-bearing, articular surface distributes support over a large surface area.

Bones join at an area called a joint, where they move together to permit articulation. The actual surface of movement is the articular surface and is covered with cartilage, a smooth, shock-absorbing surface that allows free movement between the two ends of the adjoining bones. It is the actual joint surface. The joint is held together with ligaments, which are bands of connective tissue attaching bones to each other. These bands encapsulate the joint and allow some stretch, while holding the articulating bones firmly together.

6. List the three types of muscles, and describe the structure and function of each. pp. 130–134

Muscles make up most of the body's mass, are the driving power behind body motion, and also provide most of the body's heat energy. They only have the ability to contract with force, hence are usually paired with one opposing the motion of the other. Muscles are usually attached by strong connective tissue called tendons. The point of attachment that remains stationary with muscle contraction is the origin, while the point of attachment that moves is the insertion.

There are three types of muscle tissue: cardiac, smooth, and skeletal. The specific structure and function of each is as follows:

- Cardiac muscle is tissue that is found only within the heart. It has the unique capability of spontaneous contraction without external stimulation. It also has a feature known as automaticity which means that each fiber has the ability, under the right circumstances, to generate an electrical impulse.
- Smooth muscle or involuntary muscle is found within the intestines and encircling the blood vessels. Smooth muscle is generally under the control of the autonomic component of the nervous system.
- Skeletal muscle, or striated or voluntary muscle, is the most abundant muscle type. It allows movement and is mostly under voluntary control, and gives the body most of its bulk and shape. Muscles help to move the bones.

7. Describe the anatomy and physiology of the nervous system, including the meninges and cerebrospinal fluid. pp. 155–174

The nervous system is the body's chief control for virtually every major function. It is divided physically into the central nervous system (CNS) and peripheral nervous system (PNS). The CNS consists of the brain and spinal cord. If the body were visualized as a computer, the CNS would be the central processing unit. Basic functions, such as continuance of heartbeat and respiration, and complex functions, such as listening to Mozart and anticipating a musical passage you particularly like, are controlled by cells in the brain. Messages within the CNS, as well as those that connect it with the rest of the body, travel as nerve impulses. The complex network of nerves outside the CNS makes up the peripheral nervous system.

The messages that carry information regarding critical body functions such as respiration pass through a part of the PNS called the autonomic nervous system; these functions do not require any conscious effort to maintain them. In contrast, messages that involve voluntary, or conscious, actions and thoughts travel through the other part of the PNS, the somatic nervous system. Both the autonomic and somatic nervous systems have two parallel tracks: one of nerves that carry messages to the brain, and another that carries messages from the brain. In terms of the computer analogy, the PNS carries the various input and output messages that run between the brain and spinal cord and the rest of the body. The autonomic nervous system is also structurally and functionally broken into two parts: the sympathetic and parasympathetic nervous systems. These two parts work together to make sure the net balance of stimulatory and inhibitory messages from the brain keep body functions such as blood pressure within normal limits.

8. **Describe the structures of neuron, types of nerves, and the roles of polarization, depolarization, and repolarization in nerve impulse transmission.** pp. 155–174

The basic structural and functional unit is the neuron, or nerve cell. Nerve cells have a body that contains the essential cell machinery of nucleus, mitochondria, etc. Nerve processes (usually there are many) that are capable of receiving impulses from other neurons or body cells are called dendrites. An impulse that is picked up by a dendrite travels toward the cell body. Another process, the axon, carries the impulse away from the cell body. Axons may have multiple tips, which means the neuron has the capacity to send the impulse onward to more than one other nerve or other cell. Dendrites associated with neurons of the major sense organs (such as the eye or ear) convert an environmental stimulus into a nerve impulse that can be forwarded via the axon to other nerves, and eventually the brain. Dendrites associated with neurons that monitor internal conditions such as PaO_2 also convert that information into an impulse and send it to the brain. Eventually all such information is analyzed by neurons in the brain, and response impulses travel back through the PNS. These impulses eventually affect a motor neuron, causing a muscle cell to contract, or affect another type of cell such as one in a gland. Messages cannot pass directly from an axon to a dendrite because there is a tiny physical gap, called a synapse, between each pair of neurons. As the wave of electrical depolarization (due to ion fluxes of potassium rapidly leaving the neuron and sodium rapidly entering) reaches the axon tip, it causes a chemical called a neurotransmitter to be released into the synapse. (There are multiple neurotransmitters within the body. Either acetylcholine or norepinephrine is found in the neurons of the PNS. Neurotransmitters within the CNS include dopamine and serotonin.) When the neurotransmitter crosses the synapse and is taken up by the dendrite on the other side, a wave of depolarization is started in that dendrite, and the nerve impulse is then carried toward the cell body.

9. **State the functions of hormones, including the hormones of the pancreas, and discuss the regulator processes of hormonal secretion.** pp. 174–183

There are eight major structures associated with the endocrine system located throughout the body: the hypothalamus, pituitary gland, thyroid gland, parathyroid glands, thymus, pancreas, adrenal glands, and gonads. The pineal gland is also part of the endocrine system.

The hypothalamus, located deep within the cerebrum of the brain, is the junction between the endocrine system and the central nervous system. About the size of a pea, the pituitary gland is located adjacent to the hypothalamus within the cerebrum. The pineal gland is also located adjacent to the hypothalamus. The double-lobed thyroid gland is located in the neck anterior to and just below the cartilage of the larynx. The parathyroid glands are very small and are found on the posterior lateral surface of the thyroid gland. The thymus is located in the mediastinum just behind the sternum. The pancreas is located in the upper abdomen behind the stomach and between the duodenum and the spleen. The adrenal glands are somewhat triangular in shape and are located on the superior surface of the kidneys. Gonads can be found in the lower pelvis in women, with each ovary resembling an almond in size and shape. In men, the gonads are located in the scrotum.

The endocrine system is closely linked to the nervous system and plays a critical role in our ability to maintain life by regulating many bodily functions through chemical substances called hormones. The endocrine system is made up of ductless glands, which manufacture and secrete hormones that act in adjacent tissues or travel via the bloodstream to target organs or other endocrine glands to produce specific or generalized effects. Hormones regulate metabolic activity, growth and development, as well as mediate chemical reactions, maintain homeostatic balance, and initiate our adaptive response to stress.

10. **State the functions of epinephrine and norepinephrine and explain their relationship to the sympathetic division of the autonomic nervous system.** pp. 166–171

The involuntary division of the PNS is called the autonomic nervous system, and it has two components: the sympathetic nervous system and the parasympathetic nervous system. The sympathetic system is associated with the primitive "fight or flight" response to sensory stimuli. Its

©2004 Pearson Education, Inc.
Intermediate Emergency Care: Principles & Practice

major nerve roots are located near the thoracic and lumbar part of the spinal cord. Stimulation causes increased heart rate and blood pressure, pupillary dilation, rise in blood sugar, as well as bronchodilation, all responses that ready the body for stress. The neurotransmitters norepinephrine and epinephrine mediate the sympathetic nervous system's actions. Sympathetic activity is also closely correlated to activity in the adrenal medulla, tissue that is of nervous system origin and that also relies on norepinephrine and epinephrine. The parasympathetic nervous system is responsible for controlling vegetative functions such as normal heart rate and blood pressure. It is associated with the cranial nerves and the sacral plexus of nerves, and it is mediated by the neurotransmitter acetylcholine. When stimulated, it causes a decrease in heart rate, an increase in digestive activity, pupillary constriction, and a reduction in blood sugar.

11. Describe the characteristics and composition of blood, as well as the function of the red and white blood cells and platelets. pp. 103–112

The components of the blood include the white blood cells, platelets, red blood cells, and plasma. White blood cells (WBCs) originate in the bone marrow from undifferentiated stem cells. Leukopoiesis is the process by which stem cells differentiate into the various immature forms of the white blood cell (leukocyte). These immature forms known as -blasts mature to become granulocytes, monocytes, or lymphocytes. While leukocytes provide protection from foreign invasion, each type of white blood cell has its own unique function. Healthy people have between 5,000 and 9,000 white blood cells per milliliter of blood, but the presence of an infection can cause that number to rise to greater than 16,000.

Granulocytic white blood cells are of three types: basophils, eosinophils, and neutrophils. The basophils' primary function is in allergic reactions as they are storage sites for all of the body's circulating histamine. When stimulated, they degranulate and release histamine. Eosinophils can inactivate the chemical mediators of acute allergic response, thus modulating the anaphylactic response. The neutrophils' primary function is to fight infection.

Monocytes, another of the specialized WBCs, serve as the body's trash collectors, moving throughout the body to engulf both foreign invaders and dead neutrophils. Some monocytes remain in circulation, while others migrate to other sites to further mature into macrophages. Monocytes and macrophages also secrete growth factors to stimulate the formation of red blood cells and granulocytes. Some macrophages become fixed within tissues of the liver, spleen, lungs, and lymphatic system, becoming part of the reticuloendothelial system and having the capability to stimulate lymphocyte production in an immune response.

Lymphocytes, the primary cells of the body's immune response, can be found in the circulating blood, as well as in the lymph fluid and nodes, bone marrow, spleen, liver, lungs, skin, and intestine. These highly specialized cells contain surface receptor sites specific to a single antigen and initiate an immune response in order to rid the body of such agents.

Platelets or thrombocytes function to form a plug at an initial bleeding site and secrete several factors important to clotting. The normal number of platelets ranges from 150,000 to 450,000 per milliliter. Derived from megakaryocytes that arise from an undifferentiated stem cell in the bone marrow, platelets survive from 7 to 10 days and are removed from circulation by the spleen.

Erythropoiesis, the process of red blood cell (RBC) production, is stimulated by erythropoietin that is secreted by the kidneys when the renal cells sense hypoxia. In turn, this stimulates the bone marrow to increase RBC production resulting in increased RBC mass and thus effectively, albeit slowly, increasing the oxygen-carrying capacity of the blood.

The life span of a red blood cell is approximately 4 months, although hemorrhage, hemolysis (RBC destruction), or sequestration by the liver or spleen may significantly reduce its life span. The spleen and liver contain macrophages (a specialized type of scavenger white blood cell) that can remove damaged or abnormal cells from circulation.

Plasma is the fluid portion of the blood and is a thick, pale yellow fluid that is 90 to 92 percent water and 6 to 7 percent proteins. It also contains electrolytes, fats, carbohydrates, gases, and chemical messengers. It transports nutrients and waste products to and from the body's cells and maintains the blood's oncotic pressure. The proteins with the plasma also assist in the clotting mechanisms and buffering the bloods pH balance.

12. State the importance of blood clotting. pp. 110–113

Hemostasis involves three mechanisms that work to prevent or control blood loss, including vascular spasms that reduce the size of a vascular tear, platelet plugs (an aggregate of platelets that adheres to collagen), and lastly the formation of stable fibrin clots (coagulation).

Damage to cells or to the tunica intima (innermost lining of the blood vessels) triggers the clotting or coagulation cascade. This sequence of events (cascade) can be activated by either an intrinsic pathway (trauma to blood cells from turbulence) or an extrinsic pathway (damage to vessels).

Following the intrinsic pathway: platelets release substances that lead to the formation of prothrombin activator, which in the presence of calcium converts prothrombin to thrombin. Thrombin converts fibrinogen to stable fibrin, again in the presence of calcium, which then traps blood cells and more platelets to form a clot.

The extrinsic pathway is triggered with the development of a tear in a blood vessel. When this occurs, the smooth muscle fibers in the tunica media (middle lining of the blood vessels) contract and the resultant vasoconstriction reduces the size of the injury. This action reduces blood flow through the area, effectively limiting blood loss and allowing platelet aggregation (formation of a platelet plug) and the subsequent conversion of prothrombin activator.

Clotting factors or proteins are primarily produced in the liver and circulate in an inactive state. Prothrombin and fibrinogen are the best known of these factors. Damaged cells send out a chemical message that activates a specific clotting factor. This activates each protein in sequence until a stable clot is formed.

An enzyme on the surface of the platelet membrane makes it sticky. It is this stickiness that allows platelet aggregation to occur.

13. Describe the anatomy and physiology of the cardiovascular system, including the pericardium, the valves, and the major vessels and chambers. pp. 183–200

The adult heart is roughly the size of a clenched fist, and it lies in the center of the mediastinum posterior to the sternum and anterior to the spine. Roughly two thirds of the heart lies to the left of midline, with roughly one-third to the right. The bottom of the heart, the apex, lies just above the diaphragm, whereas the top of the heart, or base, lies at roughly the level of the second rib. The heart's connections with the great vessels are at the base. The heart is made up of three tissue layers: The innermost is the endocardium, which has the same type of cells as the endothelial lining of blood vessels and is continuous with the linings of the vessels entering and leaving the heart. The thickest layer is the middle layer of muscle cells, the myocardium. These unique muscle cells physically resemble skeletal muscle but have electrical properties similar to smooth muscle cells. The outermost layer of the heart is the pericardium, a protective sac made of connective tissue arranged in two layers, the visceral pericardium (also called the epicardium) and the parietal pericardium. Normally, about 25 mL of pericardial fluid is contained between the two layers of pericardium, and the heart moves freely within the pericardial sac.

The heart is made up of two side-by-side pumps, the left side and the right side. Each side has an upper chamber, the atrium, which receives blood, and a lower chamber, the ventricle, which pumps blood into other blood vessels. The atria are separated by an interatrial septum, and the ventricles are separated by an interventricular septum. The atrial walls are thin in contrast with the ventricular walls, and almost all of the heart's pumping force is generated by the ventricles. The left ventricle, which pumps blood into the aorta, has a much thicker wall than the right ventricle, which pumps blood into the pulmonary artery.

The heart contains two sets of valves that help to keep blood flowing properly through the chambers and into the aorta and pulmonary artery: The atrioventricular valves lie between each atrium and ventricle. The left atrioventricular valve is called the mitral valve, and it has two characteristic leaflets. The right atrioventricular valve is called the tricuspid valve, and it has three characteristic leaflets. When the papillary muscles that connect the valves to the walls of the heart relax, the leaflets open and blood flows from the atria into the ventricles. Special fibers called the chordae tendoneae connect the leaflets of a valve to the papillary muscles, and these fibers prevent the leaflets from prolapsing back into the atrium when the valve is open. The semilunar

©2004 Pearson Education, Inc.
Intermediate Emergency Care: Principles & Practice

valves lie between the ventricles and the artery into which each empties. The left semilunar valve, or aortic valve, lies between the left ventricle and the aorta. The right semilunar valve, or pulmonic valve, lies between the right ventricle and the pulmonary artery. When these valves open, blood flows in a one-way path from the ventricles into the arteries, and backflow into the ventricles is prevented.

The superior and inferior vena cavae carry deoxygenated blood from the body to the right atrium. Blood flows through the right atrium and ventricle before entering the pulmonary artery, which carries it to the lungs. Oxygenated blood leaves the lungs through the pulmonary veins and enters the left atrium. The left ventricle pumps the blood into the aorta, which feeds the oxygenated blood into peripheral arteries to flow to the rest of the body. Pressure within the heart is markedly higher on the left than on the right because resistance to flow is higher in the peripheral circulation than it is in the pulmonary circulation. Consequently, the myocardium of the left ventricle thickens as an infant ages to the point that the adult left ventricle is markedly thicker than the right.

The circulatory system consists of two subsystems. In pulmonary circulation, blood enters the lungs via the pulmonary arteries and their smaller branches, the arterioles. It eventually flows through capillaries that form networks over alveoli, and gas exchange (movement of oxygen into the blood and carbon dioxide from the blood) takes place here. The oxygenated blood then flows into the pulmonary venules and larger pulmonary veins and enters the left atrium. The peripheral circulation begins with the aorta, which receives oxygenated blood from the left ventricle. The aorta has numerous branches. These arteries and the smaller arterioles ensure that oxygenated blood flows to all parts of the body. Oxygenated blood eventually enters capillary beds, and oxygen exchange between blood and tissues occurs. Deoxygenated blood enters smaller venules, which empty into the larger veins that return blood to the right atrium. Gas exchange occurs in capillaries because their walls are only one cell thick. This same cell layer, the endothelium, is the innermost layer of arteries and veins.

14. Describe coronary circulation, the cardiac cycle, and the parts of the cardiac conduction pathway. pp. 186–192

The coronary arteries originate in the aorta, just above the leaflets of the aortic valve. The main coronary arteries lie on the surface of the heart, and small penetrating arterioles supply the myocardial muscle. The left coronary artery supplies the left ventricle, the interventricular septum, part of the right ventricle, and the heart's conduction system. Its two major branches are the anterior descending artery and the circumflex artery.

The right coronary artery supplies a portion of the right atrium and right ventricle and part of the conduction system. Its two major branches are the posterior descending artery and the marginal artery. The coronary vessels receive blood during diastole, when the heart relaxes, because the aortic valve leaflets cover the coronary artery openings (ostia) during systole, when the heart contracts.

Blood drains from the left coronary artery system via the anterior great cardiac vein and the lateral marginal veins. These empty into the cardiac sinus. The right coronary artery empties directly into the right atrium via smaller cardiac veins.

The cardiac cycle is the sequence of events that occurs between the end of one heart contraction and the end of the next. To evaluate heart sounds and read electrocardiographs, you must thoroughly understand the pumping action of the cardiac cycle. Diastole is the relaxation phase. Systole is when the heart contracts. At this point blood flows out of the ventricles through pulmonic and aortic valves and into the arteries. The pressure closes the mitral and tricuspid valves and, if working properly, prevents backflow of blood into the atria. When pressures in the artery exceed the pressures in the ventricles, the valves close and diastole begins again.

The cardiac conductive system stimulates the ventricles to depolarize in the proper direction. This system must initiate an impulse, spread it through the atria, transmit it quickly to the apex of the heart, and then stimulate the ventricles to depolarize from inferior to superior. Important properties of the cardiac conductive system are: excitability, conductivity, automaticity, and contractility.

15. **Explain how the nervous system regulates heart rate and the force of contractions.** pp. 188–192

Perfusion is the process by which oxygen and nutrients and waste products and carbon dioxide are brought to and taken from the body cells. It is essential to life, and its breakdown is the process we call shock. To ensure adequate perfusion the body requires a pump, fluid volume, and a container. The pump is the heart and for proper cardiac output, the heart must receive an adequate supply of blood (preload) and have an adequate contractile force and a proper rate of contractions. The vascular system's fluid, blood, must be in adequate supply and fill the container, the vascular system. Additionally, the container must maintain an adequate pressure so it is able to direct blood to the tissues in need. It maintains this pressure by constricting or dilating the arterioles to maintain blood pressure. Baroreceptors monitor blood pressure and control it by changing the heart rate, strength of contraction, size of the vascular container, or the number and degree of arterioles in constriction or dilation.

When the baroreceptors, in the aortic arch and carotid sinus, sense a minute drop in pressure they send a message to the brain that there is "low pressure." This in turn sends a message down the spinal cord to the adrenal glands, located on top of the kidneys, to "dump epinephrine and norepinephrine" into the bloodstream. The intended end organ for these two substances is the heart, where the epinephrine picks up the rate and contractility or strength of the pumping and norepinephrine helps constrict the peripheral vessels so more blood can be shunted to the brain where it is needed.

16. **Explain the relationship among stroke volume, heart rate, and cardiac output.** pp. 195–199

Stroke volume (the volume of blood pumped in one heartbeat) depends on three factors: preload, cardiac contractility, and afterload. The heart can only pump out the blood it receives during diastole. The pressure in the filled ventricle at the end of diastole is termed preload, or end-diastolic volume. Starling's law states that as the stretch on cardiac muscle increases (that is, as preload increases), the greater will be the force of the subsequent contraction. When preload increases, contraction pressure increases. Because the major factor determining preload is venous return from the body (or the lungs), the greater the venous return, the greater the preload and the greater the ventricular contraction pressure. Obviously, this only applies to a range of normal return volumes. If an excessive volume flows into the atrium, the atrium will become overly stretched and eventually weaken. For the left ventricle, which pumps blood to the body (including the vital brain, myocardium, and kidneys), preload is determined by venous return from the lungs. Afterload is the pressure against which the ventricles must contract to pump blood into the aorta and pulmonary arteries. An increase in afterload (peripheral resistance) decreases stroke volume. Conversely, a decrease in afterload eases the work of the ventricles and increases stroke volume.

Cardiac output (the amount of blood pumped into the aorta per minute) depends on left ventricular end-diastolic volume, myocardial contractility, and peripheral vascular resistance as measured at the origin of the aorta. Heart failure, the inability of the left ventricle to pump a physiologically adequate supply of blood, can result from a preload (ventricular end-diastolic volume) that is too low to allow effective pumping (a clinical example is shock), a reduction in cardiac contractility such that effective pumping is impossible (a clinical example is loss of myocardium through one or more MIs), or a significant increase in systemic vascular resistance (hypertension). In many cases, more than one factor (preload, contractility, afterload) may be chronically disturbed.

17. **Describe the structure of arteries and veins, and relate their structure to function.** pp. 193–195

The arterial system, which caries oxygenated blood from the heart, functions under high pressure. The larger arterial vessels are the arteries. The arteries branch into smaller structures called arterioles, which control blood flow to various organs by their degree of resistance. The arterioles continue to divide until they become capillaries, which are the connection points between the arterial and venous systems. The walls of the arteries are thick and muscular and that is why the contraction of the left ventricle of the heart can be felt, as a pulse, when an artery which runs over a bone and close to the surface of the skin is palpated. The venous system transports blood

©2004 Pearson Education, Inc.
Intermediate Emergency Care: Principles & Practice

from the peripheral tissues back to the heart. It functions under low pressure with the aid of surrounding muscles and one-way valves within the veins. Blood enters the venous system through the capillaries, which drain into the venules. The venules, in turn, drain into the veins, the veins into the vena cava, and the vena cava into the atria. The veins must fight against gravity to get the blood back up to the heart. There is in effect a series of "elevators" or valves in the veins that help keep the blood from all pooling in the legs when we stand upright.

18. Describe the structure of capillaries, and explain the exchange processes that take place there. pp. 193–195

The vascular system and tissues are able to exchange gases, fluids, and nutrients through the very thin capillary walls. When arterial blood flows into a capillary bed, hydrostatic pressure pushes fluid across the capillary membrane into the tissue. As the blood flows through the capillary bed, this pressure diminishes. Plasma proteins in the capillaries create an oncotic pressure gradient that draws fluid back into the bloodstream. On the venous side of the capillary bed, the oncotic pressure drawing fluid in is greater than the hydrostatic pressure pushing the fluid out. The net effect is that fluid returns to the capillary for its return to the heart. In a perfect system, whatever fluid enters the tissues at one end of the capillary bed should return to the circulation at the other end. In reality, some fluid usually remains in the tissues. The lymph system acts as an auxiliary drainage system, collecting the remaining fluid from the tissues and returning it to the heart.

19. Describe the pathway and purpose of pulmonary circulation. pp. 199–200

Respiration also requires an intact circulatory system. In fact, during each cardiac cycle, the heart pumps as much blood to the lungs as it pumps to the peripheral tissues. In the capillaries, these cells take oxygen from red blood cells coming from the arterial system and give up carbon dioxide to blood returning to the venous system. The venous system carries this deoxygenated blood to the right side of the heart, and the right ventricle pumps it into the pulmonary artery.

The pulmonary artery immediately branches into the right and the left pulmonary arteries, each supplying its respective lung. In turn, both branches quickly fan into smaller arteries that end in the pulmonary capillaries. These capillaries are spread over the surfaces of the alveoli, where the red blood cells exchange carbon dioxide for oxygen. The pulmonary capillaries recombine into larger veins, eventually terminating in the pulmonary vein. The pulmonary vein empties the oxygenated blood into the left atrium of the heart. Finally, the heart transports the oxygenated blood through the left ventricle and into the systemic arterial system via the aorta and its tributaries.

The lungs themselves receive little of their blood supply from the pulmonary arteries or veins. Instead, bronchial arteries that branch from the aorta supply most of their blood. Bronchial veins return this blood from the lungs to the superior vena cava.

20. Describe the pathway and purpose of systemic circulation. pp. 199–200

The systemic circulation is the pathway that oxygenated blood travels as it exits the left ventricle, through the largest artery of the body, the aorta. The first artery to branch off of the aorta is designed to provide the heart's own circulation, the coronary arteries. Then branches come off the aorta and travel to the head as well as the aorta descends into the abdomen and splits further into arteries which serve the lower extremities. As the blood is collected and makes its way back in the direction of the heart it ends up in the venous system, ultimately in the vena cava, which is the largest vein in the body which enters the right atrium of the heart.

21. Explain the factors that maintain and regulate blood pressure. pp. 195–199

Blood pressure (BP) is the tension exerted by blood against the arterial walls and is dependent upon both cardiac output and peripheral vascular resistance. Thus the BP equals the cardiac output times the peripheral vascular resistance (PVR). The PVR is the pressure against which the heart must pump. Since the circulatory system is a closed system, increasing either cardiac output or peripheral vascular resistance will increase BP. Likewise, a decrease in cardiac output or a decrease in peripheral vascular resistance will decrease BP.

The body does its best to keep the BP relatively constant by employing compensatory mechanisms and negative feedback loops to regulate the elements of the above formula. As noted earlier, baroreceptors in the carotid sinuses and in the arch of the aorta closely monitor BP. If BP increases, the baroreceptors send signals to the brain that cause the BP to return to its normal values. This is accomplished by decreasing the heart rate, decreasing the preload, or decreasing peripheral vascular resistance.

The baroreceptors are also stimulated if the BP falls. The heart rate is increased, as is the strength of the cardiac contractions. There is also arteriolar constriction, venous constriction, and overall increased PVR. Also, the adrenal medulla is stimulated. This results in the secretion of epinephrine and norepinephrine, which further enhance the response.

22. Describe the functions of the lymphatic system. p. 195

The lymph system acts as an auxiliary drainage system, collecting the excess fluid from the tissues and returning it to the heart.

23. Describe the immune response. pp. 106–110

Foreign and invading cells or substances often have unique proteins on their surfaces called antigens. The immune system detects these antigens as being unlike those of the body's cells and initiates a response. This response uses antibodies to selectively control or destroy the foreign substance. As a result of the first contact with the foreign agent, the body develops a "memory" that produces a more rapid and effective response should the same antigen be recognized again. This response is called immunity.

Immunity can be acquired or natural. Natural immunity is not generated by the immune response but is a genetically inhospitable environment for a particular organism—for example, human resistance to canine distemper. Active acquired immunity is that immunity gained from a response to an invading antigen and is long lasting. Passive immunity is acquired from an outside source such as an immunization or from maternal blood during gestation and is temporary.

The primary immune response occurs with the first exposure to an antigen and lags from five to seven days after exposure. The secondary response occurs as the immune system is sensitized to the antigen by the first response. If it is again exposed to the antigen, it presents a more aggressive and faster response.

Humoral immunity is immunity resident in the blood and lymphatic fluid, primarily from B lymphocytes that produce antibodies. Cell-mediated immunity is immunity provided by T lymphocytes that recognize and directly attack the foreign antigen.

24. Describe the anatomy and physiology of the respiratory system, including the nervous and chemical mechanisms that regulate it. pp. 200–213

The mouth, or oral cavity, is a single cavity that serves as an auxiliary air passage. The posterior upper surface is the soft palate, which moves upward and closes off the passages from the nose to the pharynx during swallowing. The nasal cavity is a hollow two-sided chamber lined with mucous membranes that warms, filters, and humidifies air as it enters the respiratory system. Its anterior openings are the nares, or nostrils. The nasal and oral cavities empty into the pharynx, or throat. The pharynx is a muscular tube that functions as the transitional area for food and air between the nose and mouth and between the esophagus and larynx.

The larynx is the tubular structure that begins the lower airway. It consists of the thyroid and cricoid cartilages, the vocal cords, the arytenoid folds, and the upper portion of the trachea. It is the "Adam's apple" located in the anterior neck. The epiglottis is a flap-like structure covering the opening of the trachea, the glottis. It closes during swallowing to prevent food or fluids from entering the trachea and respiratory system. The vallecula is a fold formed by the epiglottis and base of the tongue. The larynx opens into the trachea, a series of cartilaginous C-shaped structures that hold the airway open. The trachea divides into two main stem bronchi at the carina. The bronchi subdivide, finally reaching the respiratory bronchioles, the alveolar ducts, and, finally, the alveoli. The alveoli are the primary exchange structures between the respiratory system and the pulmonary capillaries of the cardiovascular system for oxygen and carbon dioxide.

©2004 Pearson Education, Inc.
Intermediate Emergency Care: Principles & Practice

The gross anatomy of the pediatric airway is very similar to that of the adult but is smaller in size with smaller airway clearances and a greater proportion of soft tissue. The larynx is more superior and anterior than in the adult, and the smallest clearance of the airway is the cricoid cartilage rather than the glottis as it is in the adult. The child's tongue is proportionally larger and more easily obstructs the airway. Because of the smaller lumen size, the soft tissue of the airway may swell more quickly to cause obstruction.

25. Describe normal inhalation and exhalation. pp. 206–208

Respiration is the exchange of gases between a living organism and its environment. The volume of the thorax expands as the diaphragm contracts and displaces downward. The intercostal muscles contract, pulling the rib cage upward and outward. The muscles of the neck enhance this action as they lift the sternum. The lungs expand with the chest as the pleural seal secures the exterior of the lung to the interior of the thorax. The expansion of the lungs reduces the air pressure within them, and air flows into the alveoli. Gravity and the intrinsic elasticity of the lungs then cause the thorax to settle, the pressure within the lungs to increase, and air to be exhaled.

26. Differentiate between ventilation and respiration. pp. 206–208

The respiratory system provides a passage for oxygen, a gas necessary for energy production, to enter the body and for carbon dioxide, a waste product of the body's metabolism, to exit. This exchange is called respiration. Ventilation is the mechanical process that moves air in and out of the lungs. Ventilation is necessary for respiration to occur.

27. Explain the diffusion of gases across the alveolar-capillary junction and how oxygen and carbon dioxide are transported in the blood. pp. 209–211

The air brought into the lungs contains 21 percent oxygen and very little carbon dioxide. Oxygen diffuses through the alveolar and capillary walls and is bound to the hemoglobin, while carbon dioxide diffuses in the opposite direction. The air exhaled contains about 14 percent oxygen and 5 percent carbon dioxide. The oxygen from inspired air diffuses from the alveolar space through the alveolar wall and the pulmonary capillary membrane, where it attaches to the hemoglobin of the blood. Carbon dioxide, mostly transported as bicarbonate, diffuses from the blood plasma across the capillary membrane and through the alveolar wall.

28. Describe the functions of the digestive system and name its major divisions. pp. 216–218

The gastrointestinal (GI) tract is a long tube that extends from the mouth to the anus and is divided structurally and functionally into different parts. In general, the digestive system is divided into the upper and lower GI tracts. The upper tract includes mouth, esophagus, stomach, and duodenum, whereas the lower tract includes the remainder of the small intestine and the large intestine, rectum, and anus. In the upper GI tract, food is ingested, and preliminary physical and chemical digestion is begun. In the lower GI tract, digestion of food is completed, nutrients are absorbed into the body, and remaining fiber, intestinal bacteria, and other materials are eliminated through the anus as feces. In addition, three more organs, the liver, gallbladder, and pancreas, are intimately associated with the GI system both structurally (through connections with the duodenum) and functionally. The vermiform appendix, a blind sac found at the junction of the small and large intestines, does not have any apparent physiologic role in GI function but is important to you because of the inflammatory condition called appendicitis, which you will see in patients in the field.

29. Explain why the respiratory system has an effect on pH and describe the respiratory compensating mechanisms. p. 211

See Part 1, objective 8.

CONTENT SELF-EVALUATION

MULTIPLE CHOICE

A 1. The outermost layer of the skin is the:
A. epidermis.
B. subcutaneous tissue.
C. cutical.
D. dermis.
E. sebum.

A 2. Which of the following glands secrete sweat?
A. sudoriferous glands
B. sebaceous glands
C. subcutaneous glands
D. adrenal glands
E. none of the above

E 3. Which of the following types of cells are found in the dermis?
A. lymphocytes
B. macrophages
C. mast cells
D. fibroblasts
E. all of the above

A 4. The macrophages and lymphocytes begin the inflammation response by killing invading bodies and triggering a call for other, similar cells.
A. True
B. False

D 5. The type of hair that is short, fine, and lacks pigment is called:
A. terminal.
B. formative.
C. scalioned.
D. vellus.
E. none of the above

C 6. All of the following are components of the adult hematopoietic system EXCEPT the:
A. blood.
B. bone marrow.
C. thymus.
D. liver.
E. spleen.

B 7. The major determinants of blood volume are red blood cell mass and:
A. erythropoietin levels.
B. plasma volume.
C. total body water.
D. stem cell percentage.
E. bone marrow volume.

C 8. The component of the red blood cell that is responsible for transporting oxygen is the:
A. basophil.
B. granulocyte.
C. hemoglobin.
D. neutrophil.
E. lymphocyte.

A 9. The Bohr effect describes the relationship between pH and oxygen delivery in that the more acidic the blood, the more readily oxygen is released to the tissues.
A. True
B. False

D 10. All of the following will cause a right shift of the oxyhemoglobin dissociation curve and thus increase the rate that oxygen is released to the tissues EXCEPT:
A. increased carbon dioxide.
B. increased temperature.
C. decreased pH.
D. decreased activity.
E. increased activity.

A 11. The term for the packed cell volume of red blood cells per unit of blood volume is:
A. hematocrit.
B. hemoglobin.
C. red blood cell count.
D. blood type.
E. white blood cell count.

©2004 Pearson Education, Inc.
Intermediate Emergency Care: Principles & Practice

©2004 Pearson Education, Inc.
Intermediate Emergency Care: Principles & Practice

_E_ 12. White blood cells that primarily function in allergic reactions to release histamine are called:
- A. lymphocytes.
- B. neutrophils.
- C. eosinophils.
- D. monocytes.
- E. basophils.

_B_ 13. White blood cells that primarily function to fight infection are called:
- A. lymphocytes.
- B. neutrophils.
- C. eosinophils.
- D. monocytes.
- E. basophils.

_A_ 14. T cells and B cells, which play critical roles in immunity, are types of white blood cells called:
- A. lymphocytes.
- B. neutrophils.
- C. eosinophils.
- D. monocytes.
- E. basophils.

_B_ 15. The condition that occurs when the body develops antibodies against itself is called:
- A. acquired immunodeficiency.
- B. autoimmune disease.
- C. rejection.
- D. chemotaxis.
- E. inherited immunodeficiency.

_E_ 16. Causes of the inflammatory process include all of the following EXCEPT:
- A. infectious agents.
- B. chemical agents.
- C. trauma.
- D. immunologic agents.
- E. genetics.

_D_ 17. The formed blood cell components responsible for blood clotting are:
- A. red blood cells.
- B. white blood cells.
- C. lymphocytes.
- D. platelets.
- E. monocytes.

_B_ 18. Which of the following is NOT a function performed by the musculoskeletal system?
- A. vital organ protection
- B. a portion of the immune response
- C. storage of material necessary for metabolism
- D. hemopoietic activities
- E. efficient movement against gravity

_C_ 19. The bone cell responsible for maintaining bone tissue is the:
- A. osteoblast.
- B. osteoclast.
- C. osteocyte.
- D. osteocrit.
- E. none of the above

_B_ 20. The bone cell responsible for dissolving bone tissue is the:
- A. osteoblast.
- B. osteoclast.
- C. osteocyte.
- D. osteocrit.
- E. none of the above

_A_ 21. The central portion of a long bone is called the:
- A. diaphysis.
- B. epiphysis.
- C. metaphysis.
- D. cancellous bone.
- E. compact bone.

_C_ 22. The transitional area between the end and central portion of the long bone is called the:
- A. diaphysis.
- B. epiphysis.
- C. metaphysis.
- D. cancellous bone.
- E. compact bone.

_D_ 23. The type of bone tissue filling the end of the long bone is called the:
   A. diaphysis.
   B. epiphysis.
   C. metaphysis.
   D. cancellous bone.
   E. compact bone.

_A_ 24. The covering of the shaft of the long bones that initiates the bone repair cycle is the:
   A. periosteum.
   B. peritoneum.
   C. perforating canal.
   D. osteocyte.
   E. epiphysis.

_B_ 25. Immovable joints such as those of the skull are termed:
   A. synovial.
   B. synarthroses.
   C. amphiarthroses.
   D. diarthroses.
   E. A or D

_A_ 26. The elbow is an example of which type of joint?
   A. monaxial
   B. biaxial
   C. triaxial
   D. synarthrosis
   E. amphiarthrosis

_C_ 27. Bands of strong material that stretch and hold the joint together while permitting movement are the:
   A. bursae.
   B. tendons.
   C. ligaments.
   D. cartilage.
   E. metaphyses.

_A_ 28. The small sacs filled with synovial fluid that reduce friction and absorb shock are the:
   A. bursae.
   B. tendons.
   C. ligaments.
   D. cartilage.
   E. metaphyses.

_C_ 29. Skeletal maturity is reached by age:
   A. 6.
   B. 10.
   C. 20.
   D. 40.
   E. 45.

_E_ 30. The muscular system consists of about how many muscle groups?
   A. 100
   B. 200
   C. 300
   D. 500
   E. 600

_D_ 31. The muscle attachment to the bone that moves when the muscle mass contracts is the:
   A. flexor.
   B. extensor.
   C. origin.
   D. insertion.
   E. articulation.

_A_ 32. More than half the energy created by muscle motion is in the form of heat energy.
   A. True
   B. False

_E_ 33. Which of the following is a layer of the scalp?
   A. the skin
   B. occipitalis muscle
   C. galea aponeurotica
   D. areolar tissue
   E. all of the above

_B_ 34. Which of the following is NOT a bone of the cranium?
   A. frontal
   B. mandible
   C. parietal
   D. sphenoid
   E. ethmoid

C ___ 35. The largest opening in the cranium is the:
A. auditory canal. D. tentorium.
B. orbit of the eye. E. transverse foramen.
C. foramen magnum.

E ___ 36. Place the following layers of the meninges as they occur from the cerebrum to the skull.
A. dura mater, pia mater, arachnoid D. arachnoid, dura mater, pia mater
B. dura mater, arachnoid, pia mater E. pia mater, arachnoid, dura mater
C. arachnoid, pia mater, dura mater

D ___ 37. The layer of the meninges that is strong and lines the interior of the cranium is the:
A. pia mater. D. dura mater.
B. falx cerebri. E. tentorium.
C. arachnoid.

B ___ 38. The structure that divides the cerebrum into left and right halves is the:
A. pia mater. D. dura mater.
B. falx cerebri. E. tentorium.
C. arachnoid.

B ___ 39. The cerebellum is the center of conscious thought and perception.
A. True
B. False

A ___ 40. Which of the following is a function of the hypothalamus?
A. body temperature control
B. control of the ascending reticular activating system
C. control of respiration
D. responsibility for sleeping
E. maintaining balance

C ___ 41. Which of the following is a function of the medulla oblongata?
A. body temperature control
B. control of the ascending reticular activating system
C. control of respiration
D. responsibility for sleeping
E. maintaining balance

A ___ 42. While the brain accounts for only 2 percent of the total body weight, it requires 15 percent of the cardiac output and 20 percent of the body's oxygen supply.
A. True
B. False

A ___ 43. The capillaries serving the brain are thicker and less permeable than those in the rest of the body.
A. True
B. False

E ___ 44. The normal intracranial pressure is:
A. 120 mmHg. D. 25 mmHg.
B. 90 mmHg. E. less than 10 mmHg.
C. 50 mmHg.

C ___ 45. The reflex that increases the systemic blood pressure to maintain cerebral blood flow is called:
A. the ascending reticular activating system.
B. the descending reticular activating system.
C. autoregulation.
D. Cushing's reflex.
E. mean arterial pressure.

_E_ **46.** Which of the following nerves is responsible for voluntary movement of the tongue?
  A. CN-I
  B. CN-III
  C. CN-VIII
  D. CN-X
  E. CN-XII

_B_ **47.** Which of the following is the lower and moveable jaw bone?
  A. maxilla
  B. mandible
  C. zygoma
  D. stapes
  E. pinna

_C_ **48.** Which of the following is the bone of the cheek?
  A. the maxilla
  B. the mandible
  C. the zygoma
  D. the stapes
  E. the pinna

_C_ **49.** The structure responsible for our positional sense is the:
  A. ossicle.
  B. cochlea.
  C. semicircular canals.
  D. sinuses.
  E. vitreous humor.

_D_ **50.** Which of the following is the opening through which light travels to contact the light-sensing tissue in the eye?
  A. retina
  B. aqueous humor
  C. vitreous humor
  D. pupil
  E. iris

_A_ **51.** Which of the following is the light-sensing tissue in the eye?
  A. retina
  B. aqueous humor
  C. vitreous humor
  D. pupil
  E. iris

_A_ **52.** The white of the eye is the:
  A. sclera.
  B. conjunctiva.
  C. cornea.
  D. aqueous humor.
  E. vitreous humor.

_C_ **53.** The delicate, clear tissue covering the pupil and iris is the:
  A. sclera.
  B. conjunctiva.
  C. cornea.
  D. aqueous humor.
  E. vitreous humor.

_B_ **54.** The vertebral column is made up of how many vertebrae?
  A. 24
  B. 33
  C. 43
  D. 45
  E. 54

_C_ **55.** The major weight-bearing component of the vertebral column is the:
  A. spinous process.
  B. transverse process.
  C. vertebral body.
  D. spinal foramen.
  E. lamina.

_B_ **56.** The region of the vertebral column that has 12 vertebrae is the:
  A. cervical.
  B. thoracic.
  C. lumbar.
  D. sacral.
  E. coccygeal.

_A_ **57.** The region of the vertebral column that permits the greatest movement is the:
  A. cervical.
  B. thoracic.
  C. lumbar.
  D. sacral.
  E. coccygeal.

C _____ 58. The region of the vertebral column that has five separate vertebrae is the:
- A. cervical.
- B. thoracic.
- C. lumbar.
- D. sacral.
- E. coccygeal.

A _____ 59. The structure of the meninges of the spinal column is similar to the structure of the meninges of the cranium.
- A. True
- B. False

E _____ 60. At its distal end, the spinal cord is attached to the:
- A. foramen magnum.
- B. peripheral nerve roots.
- C. sacral ligament.
- D. lumbar process.
- E. coccygeal ligament.

B _____ 61. The region of the spine with the closest tolerance between the spinal cord and the interior of the spinal foramen is the:
- A. cervical spine.
- B. thoracic spine.
- C. lumbar spine.
- D. sacral spine.
- E. coccygeal spine.

E _____ 62. Which of the following is located within the thorax?
- A. the heart
- B. both lungs
- C. the esophagus
- D. the trachea
- E. all of the above

B _____ 63. How many rib pairs are floating ribs?
- A. 1
- B. 2
- C. 3
- D. 6
- E. 8

E _____ 64. Which of the following lines is used to describe position on the chest wall?
- A. posterior axillary line
- B. anterior axillary line
- C. medial axillary line
- D. midclavicular line
- E. all of the above

C _____ 65. How high does the diaphragm rise in the chest during a maximum inspiration?
- A. to the 2nd intercostal space posteriorly
- B. to the 4th intercostal space posteriorly
- C. to the 6th intercostal space posteriorly
- D. to the 8th intercostal space posteriorly
- E. to the manubrium anteriorly

A _____ 66. The muscle(s) of respiration responsible for reducing the distance between ribs and helping lift the thorax is(are) the:
- A. intercostal muscles.
- B. diaphragm.
- C. sternocleidomastoid muscles.
- D. scalene.
- E. rectus abdominis.

D _____ 67. The structure that separates the chest cavity from the abdominal cavity is the:
- A. mediastinum.
- B. peritoneum.
- C. perineum.
- D. diaphragm.
- E. vena cava.

B _____ 68. At the beginning of and during most of expiration, the pressure within the thorax is:
- A. less than the environmental pressure.
- B. more than the environmental pressure.
- C. equal to the environmental pressure.
- D. first lower than and then higher than the environmental pressure.
- E. first higher than and then lower than the environmental pressure.

_E_ 69. Which structures enter or exit the lungs at the pulmonary hilum?
   A. right mainstem bronchus   D. pulmonary veins
   B. thoracic duct   E. all except B
   C. pulmonary artery

_B_ 70. The right lung has only two lobes because the heart's greatest mass is on the right.
   A. True
   B. False

_A_ 71. The serous structure that ensures that the lungs expand with the thoracic cage wall and diaphragm is the:
   A. pleura.   D. lobular attachment.
   B. hilum.   E. mediastinum.
   C. ligamentum arteriosum.

_C_ 72. Which of the following structures is NOT located within the mediastinum?
   A. thoracic duct   D. vagus nerve
   B. phrenic nerve   E. esophagus
   C. pulmonary hilum

_D_ 73. The intercostal arteries and nerves run:
   A. behind the ribs.   D. under the ribs.
   B. above the ribs.   E. both A and D
   C. in front of the ribs.

_C_ 74. The somatic nervous system primarily innervates the:
   A. cardiac muscle.   D. smooth muscle.
   B. glands.   E. respiratory system.
   C. skeletal muscle.

_C_ 75. The space between the pia mater and the arachnoid membrane is the:
   A. epiarachnoid space.   D. subdural space.
   B. epidural space.   E. cerebral space.
   C. subarachnoid space.

_C_ 76. This portion of the brain connects the two hemispheres of the cerebrum:
   A. cerebellum.   D. midbrain.
   B. cerebral cortex.   E. diencephalon.
   C. corpus callosum.

_A_ 77. The area of the brain responsible for emotions, hormone production, and autonomic functions is the:
   A. hypothalamus.   D. thalamus.
   B. pituitary gland.   E. medulla oblongata.
   C. pons.

_E_ 78. This portion of the brain regulates cardiovascular, respiratory, and digestive system activities:
   A. cerebellum.   D. thalamus.
   B. hypothalamus.   E. medulla oblongata.
   C. pons.

_D_ 79. The _____ lobe of the brain is responsible for speech.
   A. frontal   D. temporal
   B. occipital   E. semiparietal
   C. parietal

_D_ 80. The _____ system is responsible for consciousness and stimuli response.
   A. carotid   D. reticular activating
   B. limbic   E. cephalic
   C. vertebrobasilar

©2004 Pearson Education, Inc.
Intermediate Emergency Care: Principles & Practice

_A_ 81. Which efferent fibers carry impulses to the skeletal muscles?
- **A.** somatic motor
- **B.** somatic sensory
- **C.** visceral motor
- **D.** visceral sensory
- **E.** visceral lymphatic

_D_ 82. The _____ nervous system is mediated by epinephrine and norepinephrine.
- **A.** afferent
- **B.** parasympathetic
- **C.** somatic
- **D.** sympathetic
- **E.** central

_C_ 83. Acetylcholine is the neurotransmitter of which nervous system?
- **A.** adrenergic
- **B.** afferent
- **C.** parasympathetic
- **D.** sympathetic
- **E.** central

_B_ 84. The gland that is the connection between the endocrine system and the central nervous system is the:
- **A.** pituitary.
- **B.** hypothalamus.
- **C.** thymus.
- **D.** pineal.
- **E.** thyroid.

_A_ 85. Antidiuretic hormone plays a role in maintaining fluid balance by increasing water reabsorption.
- **A.** True
- **B.** False

_B_ 86. All of the following are hormones secreted by the anterior pituitary gland EXCEPT:
- **A.** growth hormone.
- **B.** oxytocin.
- **C.** prolactin.
- **D.** adrenocorticotropic hormone.
- **E.** thyroid-stimulating hormone.

_B_ 87. In children, the thymus secretes a hormone that is critical to the maturation of T-lymphocytes, which play a significant role in:
- **A.** maintaining blood calcium levels.
- **B.** cell-mediated immunity.
- **C.** cellular metabolism.
- **D.** carbohydrate metabolism.
- **E.** gluconeogenesis.

_D_ 88. All of the following are pancreatic hormones EXCEPT:
- **A.** polypeptide.
- **B.** glucagon.
- **C.** somatostatin.
- **D.** cortisol.
- **E.** insulin.

_B_ 89. Homeostasis of blood glucose is controlled by insulin and:
- **A.** polypeptide.
- **B.** glucagon.
- **C.** somatostatin.
- **D.** cortisol.
- **E.** thymosin.

_B_ 90. The substance that the alpha cells of the pancreas secrete when blood glucose levels fall is:
- **A.** polypeptide.
- **B.** glucagon.
- **C.** somatostatin.
- **D.** cortisol.
- **E.** insulin.

_E_ 91. The substance secreted by the beta cells of the pancreas when blood glucose levels rise is:
- **A.** polypeptide.
- **B.** glucagon.
- **C.** somatostatin.
- **D.** cortisol.
- **E.** insulin.

_C_ 92. Insulin's primary function is to:
A. metabolize glucose at the cellular level.
B. free glucose from muscle storage sites.
C. transport glucose across the cell membrane.
D. store glucose at the cellular level.
E. enhance the function of glucagon.

_B_ 93. The production of glucose by the processes of glycogenolysis and gluconeogenesis is triggered by:
A. polypeptide.   D. cortisol.
B. glucagon.   E. insulin.
C. somatostatin.

_C_ 94. All of the following are hormones secreted by the adrenal glands EXCEPT:
A. epinephrine.   D. norepinephrine.
B. cortisol.   E. aldosterone.
C. somatostatin.

_A_ 95. Glucocorticoids play a role in maintaining blood glucose levels by promoting gluconeogenesis and:
A. decreasing glucose utilization.
B. increasing glucose utilization.
C. promoting salt and fluid retention.
D. decreasing salt and fluid retention.
E. potentiating the effects of catecholamines.

_A_ 96. Catecholamines such as epinephrine and norepinephrine are hormones secreted by the adrenal medulla.
A. True
B. False

_A_ 97. The primary function of aldosterone is to:
A. regulate sodium and potassium excretion.
B. regulate calcium and magnesium excretion.
C. promote gluconeogenesis.
D. inhibit gluconeogenesis.
E. stimulate glucocorticoid production.

_C_ 98. From innermost to outermost, the three tissue layers of the heart are:
A. the endocardium, the pericardium, and the myocardium.
B. the endocardium, the myocardium, and the syncytium.
C. the endocardium, the myocardium, and the pericardium.
D. the myocardium, the epicardium, and the pericardium.
E. the epicardium, the myocardium, and the endocardium.

_B_ 99. The small, specialized fibers that connect to the heart valve leaflets and prevent the valves from prolapsing are called:
A. atrial strictures.   D. semilunar structures.
B. chordae tendoneae.   E. none of the above
C. papillary muscles.

_E_ 100. The blood vessel that returns blood to the atria from the body is the:
A. aorta.   D. pulmonary vein.
B. inferior vena cava.   E. both B and C
C. superior vena cava.

©2004 Pearson Education, Inc.
Intermediate Emergency Care: Principles & Practice

_A_ 101. The blood supply to the left ventricle, interventricular septum, part of the right ventricle, and the heart's conduction system comes from the two branches of the left coronary artery, which are the:
   A. anterior descending artery and the circumflex artery.
   B. anterior descending artery and the posterior descending artery.
   C. circumflex artery and the posterior descending artery.
   D. circumflex artery and the marginal artery.
   E. marginal artery and the posterior descending artery.

_A_ 102. The relaxation phase of the cardiac cycle is called diastole.
   A. True
   B. False

_D_ 103. Stimulation of the heart by the sympathetic nervous system results in:
   A. negative inotropic and chronotropic effects.
   B. negative chronotropic and dromotropic effects.
   C. positive chronotropic and dromotropic effects.
   D. positive inotropic and chronotropic effects.
   E. positive inotropic and dromotropic effects.

_A_ 104. Specialized myocardial structures called intercalated discs enable the atria to act as an electrophysiologic syncytium and the ventricles to act as another one.
   A. True
   B. False

_D_ 105. The difference between the charge of the inside of a myocardial cell and its exterior before contraction is termed:
   A. action potential.   D. resting potential.
   B. depolarization.   E. none of the above
   C. sodium/potassium balance.

_D_ 106. The myocardial property that permits the heart cells to depolarize on their own is called:
   A. depolarization.   D. automaticity.
   B. conductivity.   E. conductivity.
   C. excitability.

_B_ 107. The inner layer of the blood vessels are which of the following?
   A. lumen   D. tunica adventitia
   B. tunica intima   E. Purkinje
   C. tunica media

_C_ 108. An inadequate delivery of oxygenated blood to body cells is:
   A. hypoxia.   D. ischemia.
   B. anoxia.   E. infarction.
   C. hypoperfusion.

_C_ 109. The normal cardiac stroke volume is about:
   A. 50 mL   D. 100 mL
   B. 60 mL   E. 120 mL
   C. 70 mL

_E_ 110. Which of the following affects the cardiac output?
   A. preload   D. cardiac rate
   B. afterload   E. all of the above
   C. cardiac contractile force

_D_ 111. The arteriole has the ability to change its internal diameter by as much as:
   A. twice.   D. fivefold.
   B. three times.   E. seven times.
   C. fourfold.

_D_ 112. Which of the following blood vessel(s) have (has) the greatest effect on blood pressure?
  A. aorta   D. arterioles
  B. the major arteries   E. venules
  C. the veins

_A_ 113. The sinuses help trap bacteria and can become infected.
  A. True
  B. False

_B_ 114. The nasal cavity is responsible for all of the functions listed below EXCEPT:
  A. warming the air.   D. cleansing the air.
  B. deoxygenating the air.   E. the sense of smell.
  C. humidifying the air.

_A_ 115. The space located between the base of the tongue and the epiglottis is called the:
  A. vallecula.   D. epiglottic fossa.
  B. cricoid.   E. glottic opening.
  C. arytenoid fold.

_C_ 116. Which of the following is the only bone in the axial skeleton that does not articulate with another bone?
  A. the mandible   D. the thyroid
  B. the maxilla   E. the zygomatic bone
  C. the hyoid bone

_C_ 117. Which of the following correctly lists the order in which air passes through airway structures during inspiration?
  A. trachea, larynx, laryngopharynx, nasopharynx, nares
  B. nares, nasopharynx, trachea, laryngopharynx, larynx
  C. nares, nasopharynx, laryngopharynx, larynx, trachea
  D. laryngopharynx, nares, nasopharynx, larynx, trachea
  E. trachea, nares, laryngopharynx, larynx, nasopharynx

_D_ 118. The point at which the trachea divides into the two mainstem bronchi is called the:
  A. hilum.   D. carina.
  B. parenchyma.   E. pleura.
  C. vallecula.

_A_ 119. The mainstem bronchus that leaves the trachea at almost a straight angle is the right mainstem bronchus.
  A. True
  B. False

_E_ 120. The tissue covering each lung and the interior of the thorax is the:
  A. hilum.   D. carina.
  B. parenchyma.   E. pleura.
  C. vallecula.

_D_ 121. Which of the following is NOT one of the differences in respiration between pediatric patients and adults?
  A. The pediatric airway is smaller in all aspects.
  B. Pediatric ribs are softer and contribute less to respiration than those of adults.
  C. Children rely more on their diaphragms for breathing than adults do.
  D. The glottis is the narrowest point of the pediatric airway, while the cricoid cartilage is the narrowest point in adults.
  E. Children's teeth are softer and more prone to damage than those of adults.

_A_ 122. Internal respiration occurs in the:
  A. peripheral capillaries.   D. pulmonary capillaries.
  B. airway.   E. both C and D
  C. alveoli.

©2004 Pearson Education, Inc.
Intermediate Emergency Care: Principles & Practice

B 123. Which aspect of the respiratory cycle is passive?
- A. inspiration
- B. expiration
- C. neither A nor B
- D. both A and B
- E. both A and B, but only during stress

C 124. The oxygenated circulation that provides perfusion for the lung tissue itself flows through the:
- A. pulmonary arteries.
- B. pulmonary veins.
- C. bronchial arteries.
- D. bronchial veins.
- E. none of the above

A 125. The amount of nitrogen in the air is approximately:
- A. 79 percent.
- B. 4 percent.
- C. 0.4 percent.
- D. 0.04 percent.
- E. 0.10 percent.

E 126. The normal oxygen saturation of hemoglobin in blood as it leaves the lungs is about:
- A. 75 percent.
- B. 85 percent.
- C. 90 percent.
- D. 95 percent.
- E. 97 percent.

C 127. The majority of the carbon dioxide carried by the blood is:
- A. carried by the hemoglobin.
- B. dissolved in the plasma.
- C. transported as bicarbonate.
- D. found as free gas in the blood.
- E. carried as free radicals.

C 128. Which of the following will reduce the carbon dioxide levels in the blood?
- A. administration of bicarbonate
- B. administration of antacids
- C. hyperventilation
- D. high-flow oxygen
- E. hypoventilation

B 129. Which of the following would NOT increase the production of carbon dioxide?
- A. fever
- B. airway obstruction
- C. shivering
- D. metabolic acids
- E. exercise

A 130. The primary center controlling respiration is located in the:
- A. medulla.
- B. pons.
- C. spinal cord.
- D. cerebrum.
- E. cerebellum.

E 131. Which of the following is the secondary or backup stimulus that causes respiration to occur?
- A. an increase in pH of the blood
- B. a decrease in pH of the blood
- C. an increase in pH of the cerebrospinal fluid
- D. a decrease in pH of the cerebrospinal fluid
- E. reduced oxygen levels in the blood

C 132. The amount of air moved with one normal respiratory cycle is called:
- A. minute volume.
- B. alveolar air.
- C. tidal volume.
- D. dead air space.
- E. total lung capacity.

C 133. The volume of air contained in a normal inspiration is about:
- A. 150 mL.
- B. 350 mL.
- C. 500 mL.
- D. 6,000 mL.
- E. none of the above

_A_ 134. Which of the following abdominal organs is found in the left upper quadrant?
  A. spleen   D. sigmoid colon
  B. gallbladder   E. liver
  C. appendix

_C_ 135. Which of the following abdominal organs is found in the right lower quadrant?
  A. spleen   D. sigmoid colon
  B. gallbladder   E. liver
  C. appendix

_E_ 136. Which of the following abdominal organs is found in all of the abdominal quadrants?
  A. pancreas   D. sigmoid colon
  B. gallbladder   E. small bowel
  C. appendix

_E_ 137. Which of the following statements is TRUE regarding the digestive tract?
  A. It is a 25-foot-long hollow tube.   D. It moves food via peristalsis.
  B. It churns food.   E. all of the above
  C. It introduces digestive juices.

_B_ 138. In what order does digesting food pass through the digestive tract?
  A. duodenum, ileum, jejunum, colon   D. ileum, jejunum, colon, duodenum
  B. duodenum, jejunum, ileum, colon   E. colon, jejunum, ileum, duodenum
  C. jejunum, ileum, colon, duodenum

_A_ 139. The movement of digesting material through the digestive system occurs through a process called:
  A. peristalsis.   D. emulsification.
  B. chyme.   E. evisceration.
  C. peritonitis.

_E_ 140. The largest solid organ of the abdomen is the:
  A. spleen.   D. gallbladder.
  B. small bowel.   E. liver.
  C. pancreas.

_A_ 141. The delicate vascular organ that performs some immune functions is the:
  A. spleen.   D. gallbladder.
  B. small bowel.   E. liver.
  C. pancreas.

_B_ 142. The major functions of the urinary system include all of the following EXCEPT:
  A. maintenance of blood volume.
  B. control of development of white blood cells.
  C. regulation of arterial blood pressure.
  D. maintenance of the balance of electrolytes and blood pH.
  E. removal of many toxic wastes from the blood.

_A_ 143. BUN, or blood urea nitrogen, and creatinine are both measured in blood as part of assessment of kidney function.
  A. True
  B. False

_D_ 144. The enzyme that is produced by the kidney and is part of the physiologic response to low blood pressure is called:
  A. aldosterone.   D. renin.
  B. angiotensin.   E. progesterone.
  C. erythropoietin.

_B_ 145. The urethra in men is much shorter than it is in women, and this is one reason why there is a gender difference in the incidence of lower urinary tract infections.
  A. True
  B. False

©2004 Pearson Education, Inc.
Intermediate Emergency Care: Principles & Practice

_B_ 146. Which of the following structures is part of the external female genitalia?
  A. ovary
  B. perineum
  C. uterus
  D. vagina
  E. fallopian tube

_C_ 147. An elastic canal that connects the internal and external female genitalia is the:
  A. ureter.
  B. urethra.
  C. vagina.
  D. vulva.
  E. fallopian tube.

_E_ 148. The layer of the uterine wall where the fertilized egg implants is the:
  A. dermametrium.
  B. cyclometrium.
  C. myometrium.
  D. perimetrium.
  E. endometrium.

_A_ 149. Which of the following hormones is released by the ovaries?
  A. estrogen
  B. follicle-stimulating hormone
  C. gonadotropin
  D. luteinizing hormone
  E. thymosin

_B_ 150. The menstrual cycle generally lasts:
  A. 2 weeks.
  B. 28 days.
  C. 7 days.
  D. 9 months.
  E. 3 weeks.

_A_ 151. The onset of ovulation that establishes female sexual maturity is known as:
  A. menarche.
  B. menopause.
  C. menses.
  D. menstruation.
  E. menacme.

_C_ 152. The _____ phase of the menstrual cycle terminates with ovulation.
  A. ischemic
  B. menstrual
  C. proliferative
  D. secretory
  E. fallow

_D_ 153. Which process occurs during the proliferative phase of the menstrual cycle?
  A. drop in estrogen level
  B. rupture of small endometrial blood vessels
  C. shedding of the endometrium
  D. thickening of the endometrium
  E. the endometrium becomes pale

_C_ 154. The age range in which menopause generally occurs is:
  A. 35–40 years.
  B. 40–55 years.
  C. 45–55 years.
  D. 50–60 years.
  E. 60–65 years.

_C_ 155. Sperm cells are eliminated from a man's body after they move out of the testicles and pass through the following structures in first-to-last sequence:
  A. vas deferens, epididymis, urethra.
  B. ureter, epididymis, vas deferens, urethra.
  C. epididymis, vas deferens, urethra.
  D. epididymis, vas deferens, prostate gland, urethra.
  E. vas deferens, epididymis, prostate gland, urethra.

CHAPTER 3

Emergency Pharmacology

Part 1: Basic Pharmacology

Review of Chapter Objectives

Because Chapter 3 is lengthy, it has been divided into parts to aid your study. Read the assigned textbook pages, then progress through the objectives and self-evaluation materials as you would with other chapters. When you feel secure in your grasp of the content, proceed to the next part.

After reading this part of the chapter, you should be able to:

1. List the four main sources of drug products   p. 235

There are four main sources of drugs. They are plants, animals, minerals, and synthetic substances (laboratory).

2. Discuss the standardization of drugs and how they are classified.   p. 238

Drugs may contain the same active ingredient yet be far different in the way they are delivered to the body. To recognize this, an assay of the drug determines the amount and purity of the drug in the preparation. A bioassay determines the amount of drug that is available in a biological model and thereby establishes its bioequivalence, or relative therapeutic effectiveness compared with drugs with chemically equivalent compositions.

3. List the components of a drug profile.   p. 236

Names: The generic, trade, and sometimes the chemical names.
Classification: The broad group to which the drug belongs.
Mechanism of action: The way the drug causes it desired effects (its pharmacodynamics).
Indications: The conditions appropriate for the drug's administration.
Pharmacokinetics: How the drug is absorbed, distributed, and eliminated, including its onset and
    duration of action.
Side effects/adverse reactions: The drug's untoward or undesired effects.
Routes of administration: How the drug is given.
Contraindications: Conditions that make it inappropriate to administer a drug (including conditions in which administration is likely to cause a harmful outcome).
Dosage: The amount of drug that should be given.
How supplied: The typical concentrations and preparations of the drug.
Special considerations: How the drug may affect pregnant, pediatric, and geriatric patients.

©2004 Pearson Education, Inc.
Intermediate Emergency Care: Principles & Practice

4. Differentiate among the chemical, generic (nonproprietary), and trade (proprietary) names of a drug. pp. 234–235

The chemical name of a drug represents its chemical composition and molecular structure. An example is 7-chloro-1,3-dihydro-1-methyl-5-phenyl-2H-1,4-benzodiazepine-2-one.

The generic name of a drug is suggested by the original manufacturer and confirmed by the United States Adopted Name Council. An example, for which the chemical name is given above, is diazepam.

The brand, trade, or proprietary name of a drug is the name given the drug by a specific manufacturer. This name is a proper name and should be capitalized and may be followed by a trademark insignia. An example is Valium®, a brand name for diazepam.

5. Discuss the EMT-Intermediate's responsibilities and scope of management pertinent to the administration of medications, including special considerations for pregnant, pediatric, and geriatric patients. pp. 238–241

There are six basic "rights" of drug administration that indicate the EMT-I's essential responsibilities and practices. They are the right medication, the right dose, the right time, the right route, the right patient, and the right documentation.

The right medication. Ensure the medication is what is intended for the patient. Review your standing orders or, if an order is received from medical direction, repeat the order back to the physician so you are both clear on the medication, dose, route, and timing of the administration. Also examine the drug packaging to ensure it is the medication you wish to administer.

The right dose. Carefully calculate the dose (usually weight dependent) for the patient before you draw up the medication and again just before you administer it. Prehospital medications are usually packaged to accommodate a single administration. If the drug package you select has much more or less than you intend to use, recheck the packaging to ensure it is the right drug and right concentration and recheck your calculations to ensure the right dosage.

The right time. Usually prehospital medications are given rather rapidly and not on a schedule. Check the packaging and your protocols for administration rate and ensure you follow the sequencing, time intervals, and drip rates for emergency drugs.

The right route. While most emergency drugs are administered by the IV route, be aware of the alternate routes of drug administration, the drugs administered via those routes, and the circumstances requiring the use of those routes. With each medication administration, ensure you are using the right route.

The right patient. It is imperative to ensure that the patient is properly matched to medication. A patient/drug mismatch is an infrequent problem in prehospital care, but as EMS moves to the out-of-hospital environment, EMT-Is may be treating some patients on a routine basis. Always ensure that the medication order is for the patient you are attending.

The right documentation. Thoroughly document all aspects of patient care, including what drugs were administered in what dosage.

Pregnancy alters the mother's physiology and also adds a second party, the developing fetus, to the concerns regarding medication administration. The increased maternal heart rate, cardiac output, and blood volume can affect the onset and actions of many medications. Drugs may also alter fetal development and result in fetal injury, deformity, or death. During the third trimester, some drugs may pass through the placenta and affect the fetus directly.

Several anatomic and physiological differences between pediatric patients and adults result in differences in the ways drugs are absorbed and metabolized. Differences in gastric pH and emptying time and lower digestive enzyme levels in children change the way enteral medications are absorbed. A child's thinner skin causes topical agents to be absorbed more quickly. Lower plasma protein levels in children affect the availability of agents that usually bind to them. Higher water content in the neonate also affects drug absorption and distribution, as does the slower, then faster metabolism of the neonate and child, respectively. Organ maturity also affects drug metabolism and elimination. For children, drug administration is often guided by weight and in some cases guided by height (the Broselow tape).

With advancing age, the body's metabolism, gastric motility, decreased plasma proteins, reduced body fat and muscle mass, and depressed liver function all affect the absorption, metabolism, and elimination of drugs. Older patients are also likely to be on multiple medications for multiple diseases, thereby increasing the likelihood of adverse medication interactions.

6. List and describe general properties of drugs. pp. 247–249

- **Affinity** is the force of attraction between the drug and the receptor site.
- **Efficacy** is the drug's ability to cause its expected effect.
- An **agonist** is a drug that causes the expected effect when bound to the receptor site.
- An **antagonist** is a drug that does not cause the expected effect when bound to the receptor site.
- An **agonist-antagonist** is a drug that binds to a receptor site, causing some expected effects and blocking others.
- A **competitive antagonist** is a drug that causes some effects as it binds to a receptor site but blocks the binding of another drug.
- A **noncompetitive antagonist** is a drug that binds to and deforms a receptor site so other drugs cannot bind there.

7. List and describe liquid and solid, and gas drug forms. pp. 246–247

Drugs come in many different forms.

Liquid drug forms include the following:

- **Solutions** are drugs dissolved in a solvent, usually water- or oil-based.
- **Tinctures** are medications extracted using alcohol with some alcohol usually remaining.
- **Suspensions** are mixtures of a solvent and drug in which the solid portion will precipitate out.
- **Emulsions** are suspensions with an oily substance in the solvent that remains as globules even when mixed.
- **Spirits** are solutions of volatile drugs in alcohol.
- **Elixirs** are drugs mixed with alcohol and water, often with flavorings to improve taste.
- **Syrups** are solutions of sugar, water, and drugs.

Solid drug forms include the following:

- **Pills** are drugs that are shaped spherically for easily swallowing.
- **Powders** are drugs simply in a powder form.
- **Tablets** are powders compressed into a disk-like form
- **Suppositories** are drugs mixed with a wax-like base that melts at body temperature. They are usually inserted into the rectum or vagina.
- **Capsules** are gelatin containers filled with the drug powder or tiny pills. When the container dissolves, the drug is released into the gastrointestinal tract.

Gas drug forms include the following:

- **Oxygen** is the most common gas drug form.
- **Nitrous oxide** is used as an inhaled analgesic.

8. Differentiate between enteral and parenteral routes of drug administration. pp. 245–246

Enteral routes of administration are those that direct drugs into the gastrointestinal system and include oral (PO), orogastric or nasogastric tube (OG/ON), sublingual (SL), buccal, and rectal. Parenteral routes are routes of administration outside the gastrointestinal tract and include intravenous (IV), endotracheal (ET), intraosseous (IO), umbilical, intramuscular (IM), subcutaneous (SQ), inhalation/nebulization, topical, transdermal, nasal, instillation, and intradermal.

9. Describe mechanisms of drug action. pp. 247–249

How a drug interacts with the body to cause its effects is referred to as pharmacodynamics. Drugs induce their effects by binding to a receptor site, changing the physical properties of the body, chemically combining with other substances, or altering a normal metabolic pathway.

©2004 Pearson Education, Inc.
Intermediate Emergency Care: Principles & Practice

10. List and differentiate the phases of drug activity, including the pharmaceutical, pharmacokinetic, and pharmacodynamic phases. pp. 241–252

The pharmaceutical phase of drug activity addresses the drug's intrinsic characteristics such as how the drug dissolves or disintegrates once injected or ingested. Pharmacokinetics refers to the processes by which a drug is absorbed, distributed, biotransformed, and eliminated by the body. Pharmacodynamics is the mechanism (or mechanisms) by which a drug interacts with the body to accomplish its action.

11. Describe the processes called pharmacokinetics and pharmacodynamics, including theories of drug action, drug-response relationship, factors altering drug responses, predictable drug responses, iatrogenic drug responses, and unpredictable adverse drug responses. pp. 241–252

There are two important elements of pharmacology: how drugs are transported into or out of the body (pharmacokinetics) and how drugs interact with the body to cause their effects (pharmacodynamics).

Pharmacokinetics examines the absorption, distribution, biotransformation, and elimination of drugs.

For a drug to perform its action, it must first reach its site of action, a process referred to as **absorption.** While some drugs affect target tissue directly (like antacids in the stomach), most must first find their way to the bloodstream. Drugs administered directly into a venous or arterial vessel are quickly transported to the heart, mixed with the blood, and distributed throughout the body. A drug injected into the muscle tissue and, to a somewhat lesser degree, into the subcutaneous tissue, is transported quickly to the bloodstream because of the more than adequate circulation in these tissues. However, shock and hypothermia may slow the process, while fever and hyperthermia may speed it. Oral medications must survive the gastric acidity and be somewhat lipid soluble to be transported across the intestinal membrane. The differing acid content of the digestive tract also impacts the dissociation of the drug into ions that are more difficult to move into the circulation. And finally, the drug's concentration affects its uptake by the bloodstream and, ultimately, its distribution. The end result of the absorption process is the concentration of the drug in the bloodstream and its availability for activation of the target tissue, called its bioavailability.

Once a drug enters the bloodstream, it must be carried throughout the body and to its site of action. This term for this process is **distribution.** Many factors affect the release and uptake of a drug by the body's cells. Some drugs bind to the plasma proteins of the blood and are released over a prolonged period of time. An increase in the blood's pH may increase the rate of release of the drug, or competition from other drugs for binding sites may cause more of a drug to become available. Distribution of some drugs is dependent upon their ability to cross the blood-brain or placental barriers. Other drugs are easily deposited in fatty tissue, bones, and teeth.

Once in the body, drugs are broken down into metabolites in a process called **biotransformation.** This process makes the drug more or less active and can make the drug more water soluble and easier to eliminate. Some drugs are totally metabolized, some are partially metabolized, while still others are not metabolized at all. The liver is responsible for most biotransformation, while the lungs, kidneys, and GI tract do some limited biotransformation.

Elimination is the excretion of the drug in urine, expired air, or in feces. Renal excretion is the major mechanism for eliminating drugs from the body. Drugs are eliminated as the blood pressure pushes and filters blood through kidney structures. This effect is enhanced by special cells that "pump" (active transport) some metabolites into the tubules. Kidney reabsorption also plays a part in drug excretion. Protein-soluble molecules and electrolytes are easily absorbed, but the uptake may be affected by the blood's pH.

A drug's effects on the body are referred to as **pharmacodynamics.** Drugs may cause their effects by binding on a receptor site, by changing physical properties, by chemically combining with other substances, or by altering a normal metabolic pathway.

Most drugs effect their actions by binding to receptor sites, especially those of the autonomic nervous system. The drug either inhibits or stimulates the cells or tissue. The force of attraction of a drug is referred to as its **affinity.** Affinity becomes important when different drugs compete for a site. The drug's **efficacy** is its ability to cause the expected response. Binding to a receptor site causes a change within the cell and induces the drug's effect. However, some drugs may establish a chain-reaction effect whereby other drugs are released and cause the desired effect. The number of receptor sites may change as the drug becomes available and uses them, thereby reducing the drug's continuing effect. Chemicals that bind to the receptor and cause the expected response are termed **agonists. Antagonists** bind to the site and do not cause the expected response. Some drugs have both properties. Often drugs compete for receptor site in a process called **competitive antagonism,** while a situation in which a drug attaches to a receptor, effectively locking out other drugs, is termed **noncompetitive antagonism.** Permanent binding to a receptor site is **irreversible antagonism.**

Drugs may also act by modifying the physical properties of a part of the body. For example, the drug mannitol changes the blood's osmolarity and increases urine output.

Some drugs chemically combine with other substances to cause their desired effect. For example, antacids interact with the hydrochloric acid in the stomach to reduce the pH.

Other drugs act by altering normal biologic processes and the metabolic pathways. Such drugs are used to treat cancers and viral infections.

The **drug-response relationship** is the relationship between a drug's pharmaceutical, pharmacokinetic, and pharmacodynamic properties. It most commonly relates to the blood plasma level of the drug. Other important factors include the speed of onset, duration of action, minimum effective concentration, and biologic half-life. Another very important factor in the drug-response relationship is the **therapeutic index,** or the ratio between the drug's lethal and effective doses.

Factors altering drug response include the patient's age, body mass, sex, pathologic state, genetic factors, and psychological factors as well as environmental considerations and the time of administration. These factors may increase or decrease the drug's ability to generate its desired affect.

Responses to drug administration may include unintended responses, or **side effects.** These are care-provider induced (iatrogenic) and include allergic reactions, idiosyncratic (unique to an individual) reactions, tolerance, cross tolerance, tachyphylaxis, cumulative effects, dependency, drug interactions, drug antagonisms, summation, synergistic reactions (a result greater than the expected additive result of two drugs administered together), potentiation, and interference. Some of these effects may be predictable and desired and some may be unexpected.

12. **Discuss considerations for storing and securing drugs.**   **p. 247**

Temperature, humidity, ultraviolet radiation (sunlight), and time affect the potency of many drugs. It is important that they be stored under proper conditions and that they are rotated so they are utilized (or discarded) before their shelf life expires.

CASE STUDY REVIEW

This case study demonstrates the type of legal dilemma that many EMT-Is may encounter during their EMS responses.

The EMT-Is of EMS 117 are presented with a patient who is behaving bizarrely just before she becomes unconscious. They treat her, assuming that if she were conscious and alert she would recognize her need for treatment and consent to it (implied consent). Once she becomes conscious, she exercises her right to refuse treatment. The EMT-Is assess her and determine that she is able to make a rational decision and honor that decision. They recommend that she eat immediately to raise her glucose level and see her physician at the earliest opportunity. While all this seems reasonable, the EMT-Is are still exposed to legal responsibility for what happens to their patient after their care and release.

Some responsibility may fall upon the EMT-Is should their patient not obtain something to eat, suffer a later drop in blood-glucose level, and injure herself or others while driving. It is essential that the EMT-Is carefully explain to the patient that she was driving erratically and appeared intoxicated. They must identify that if she does not obtain something to eat, this behavior may occur again and cause her to do harm to herself or others. They should also explain that this incident indicates the need for a medical evaluation of her condition to assure that episodes like it do not occur again. She truly needs to see a physician immediately and her refusal of transport to the hospital is against their expert advice.

EMT-Is will further protect themselves by thoroughly documenting the incident. They must carefully identify what their assessment revealed and their reasons for administering dextrose. They must identify the results of their care (the patient becoming alert and oriented) and her subsequent refusal of further care. They must document that they encouraged her to go to the hospital with them and receive evaluation by a physician and that, when she refused, they had her speak with an on-line medical direction physician. They must document their advising her to obtain food immediately and to see her physician at the earliest opportunity. They will also document her agreement to go to the mini-mart and obtain food as well as her assurance that she has an appointment with her physician. Finally, they must have her sign a "release-from-liability" form and document by what criteria they determined she was rational and able to make that decision.

In a situation of this type, a good working relationship with the police might be helpful. The woman was clearly driving while impaired and is likely to receive a moving violation from the officer. Indicating to him the risk of a later fall in glucose level (if she does not eat) and a return to her erratic behavior might cause him to encourage the patient to ride with the EMT-Is to the hospital.

CONTENT SELF-EVALUATION

MULTIPLE CHOICE

_D_ 1. The study of drugs and their interactions with the body is:
   A. pharmaceutics.
   B. pharmacokinetics.
   C. pharmacodynamics.
   D. pharmacology.
   E. pharmacopedia.

_A_ 2. Which of the following types of drug names is 7 chloro-1,3-dihydro-1-methyl-5-phenyl-2H-1,4 benzodiazepine-2-one?
   A. chemical name
   B. generic name
   C. official name
   D. brand name
   E. common name

_B_ 3. Which of the following types of drug names is diazepam?
   A. chemical name
   B. generic name
   C. official name
   D. brand name
   E. common name

_A_ 4. Digitalis is an example of a drug derived from:
   A. a plant.
   B. an animal.
   C. a mineral.
   D. synthetic production.
   E. a lipid base.

_B_ 5. Bovine insulin is an example of a drug derived from:
   A. a plant.
   B. an animal.
   C. a mineral.
   D. synthetic production.
   E. a lipid base.

_B_ 6. The drug reference that presents manufacturer-provided drug information and some photos of drugs is the:
   A. _EMS Guide to Drugs._
   B. _Physician's Desk Reference._
   C. _AMA Drug Evaluations._
   D. _Monthly Prescribing Reference._
   E. all of the above

_C_ 7. The broad group to which a drug belongs is its:
   A. indication.
   B. pharmacokinetics.
   C. classification.
   D. mechanism of action.
   E. none of the above

_C_ 8. Conditions in which it is inappropriate to give a drug are referred to as its:
   A. mechanisms of action.
   B. indications.
   C. contraindications.
   D. side effects.
   E. special considerations.

_E_ 9. Which of the following drugs is classified as a Schedule II controlled substance?
   A. heroin
   B. morphine
   C. codeine
   D. diazepam
   E. B and C

_B_ 10. The assay of a drug in a preparation determines its:
   A. potency.
   B. amount and purity.
   C. effectiveness.
   D. availability in a biological model.
   E. effectiveness compared to other like drugs.

_E_ 11. The bioequivalence of a drug in a preparation refers to its:
   A. potency.
   B. amount and purity.
   C. effectiveness.
   D. availability in a biological model.
   E. effectiveness compared to other like drugs.

_E_ 12. Which of the following is NOT one of the six rights of medication administration?
   A. right dose
   B. right patient
   C. right documentation
   D. right time
   E. right mechanism

_A_ 13. Dosages of many emergency drugs are based upon patient weight, so unit dose packaging may not contain the right amount for every patient.
   A. True
   B. False

_B_ 14. Children are, for the most part, just small adults, so drug dosages just need to be reduced proportionally by weight.
   A. True
   B. False

_D_ 15. Which of the following is NOT true regarding the newborn patient?
   A. The neonate has less gastric acid than an adult.
   B. The neonate has diminished blood plasma levels.
   C. The neonate has immature renal and hepatic systems.
   D. The neonate has less body water than an adult.
   E. The neonate has lower enzyme levels than an adult.

_E_ 16. Drugs in which of the following FDA categories have demonstrated definite risks to the fetus?
   A. R
   B. A
   C. B
   D. C
   E. D

_D_ 17. Which of the following is NOT true regarding the geriatric patient?
   A. The geriatric patient has decreased gastrointestinal motility.
   B. The geriatric patient has decreased body fat.
   C. The geriatric patient has decreased muscle mass.
   D. The geriatric patient is more likely to be disease free.
   E. The geriatric patient has decreased liver function.

_A_ 18. Drugs do not confer any new properties on cells or tissues; they only modify or exploit existing functions.
   A. True
   B. False

©2004 Pearson Education, Inc.
Intermediate Emergency Care: Principles & Practice

C _____ 19. Which of the following is NOT one of the four basic processes of pharmacokinetics?
  A. absorption
  B. distribution
  C. receptor binding
  D. biotransformation
  E. elimination

B _____ 20. Which of the following represents an energy-consuming movement of ions against the concentration gradient?
  A. diffusion
  B. active transport
  C. osmosis
  D. filtration
  E. facilitated transport

D _____ 21. Which of the following represents movement of molecules across a membrane from an area of higher pressure to an area of lower pressure?
  A. diffusion
  B. active transport
  C. osmosis
  D. filtration
  E. facilitated transport

A _____ 22. The measure of the amount of a drug that is still active after it reaches the target organ is its:
  A. bioavailability.
  B. biotransformativity.
  C. metabolism.
  D. pro-drug effect.
  E. active distribution.

D _____ 23. Which of the following is NOT a significant medium for elimination of drugs from the body?
  A. urine
  B. respiratory air
  C. feces
  D. sweat
  E. all are significant

B _____ 24. Which of the following is NOT an enteral route of drug administration?
  A. oral
  B. umbilical
  C. buccal
  D. sublingual
  E. rectal

D _____ 25. Which of the following is the preferred route for medication administration in most emergencies?
  A. intramuscular
  B. inhalation
  C. endotracheal
  D. intravenous
  E. subcutaneous

A _____ 26. Drugs that are spherically shaped to be easy to swallow are:
  A. pills.
  B. suppositories.
  C. tablets.
  D. capsules.
  E. suspensions.

C _____ 27. Drugs that are powders compressed into disks are:
  A. pills.
  B. suppositories.
  C. tablets.
  D. capsules.
  E. suspensions.

C _____ 28. Preparations in which the solid does not dissolve in the solvent are:
  A. solutions.
  B. tinctures.
  C. suspensions.
  D. spirits.
  E. elixirs.

E _____ 29. Preparations made with alcohol and water solvent, often with flavorings, are:
  A. solutions.
  B. tinctures.
  C. suspensions.
  D. spirits.
  E. elixirs.

_C_ 30. Pharmacodynamics are best described as:
  A. interactions between drugs.
  B. the processes by which drugs are eliminated from the body.
  C. the effects of a drug on the body.
  D. the processes by which drugs bind to receptor sites.
  E. the process by which a drug is administered.

_C_ 31. The location where a drug combines with a protein, resulting in a biochemical effect, is a:
  A. second messenger.   D. agonist.
  B. antagonist.   E. protein block.
  C. receptor.

_B_ 32. A drug's ability to cause its expected response is referred to as its:
  A. affinity.   D. antagonism.
  B. efficacy.   E. equilibrium.
  C. agonism.

_D_ 33. A chemical that binds to a receptor site but does not cause the expected effect is a(n):
  A. partial-antagonist.   D. antagonist.
  B. competitive antagonist.   E. noncompetitive antagonist.
  C. agonist.

_B_ 34. A chemical that binds to a receptor site, causes the expected effect, and prevents other drugs from activating the receptor site is a(n):
  A. partial antagonist.   D. antagonist.
  B. competitive antagonist.   E. noncompetitive antagonist.
  C. agonist.

_C_ 35. The drug morphine sulfate is an example of a(n):
  A. agonist-antagonist.   D. antagonist.
  B. competitive antagonist.   E. noncompetitive antagonist.
  C. agonist.

_A_ 36. The drug nalbuphine (Nubain) is an example of a(n):
  A. agonist-antagonist.   D. antagonist.
  B. competitive antagonist.   E. noncompetitive antagonist.
  C. agonist.

_A_ 37. A drug reaction that is unique to an individual is referred to as:
  A. idiosyncrasy.   D. synergism.
  B. tachyphylaxis.   E. potentiation.
  C. antagonism.

_D_ 38. A drug reaction that is greater than expected from the administration of two drugs that have the same effect at the same time is referred to as:
  A. idiosyncrasy.   D. synergism.
  B. tachyphylaxis.   E. potentiation.
  C. antagonism.

_E_ 39. The time span between when a drug drops below its minimum effective concentration and its complete elimination from the body is its:
  A. onset of action.   D. biologic half-life.
  B. duration of action.   E. termination of action.
  C. therapeutic index.

_C_ 40. The ratio between a drug's lethal dose and its effective dose is its:
  A. onset of action.   D. biologic half-life.
  B. duration of action.   E. termination of action.
  C. therapeutic index.

CHAPTER 3

Emergency Pharmacology

Part 2: Nervous System Components

Review of Chapter Objectives

After reading this part of the chapter, you should be able to:

1. Review the specific anatomy and physiology pertinent to pharmacology. pp. 252–258

Drugs affect many systems of the body including the central nervous system, the autonomic nervous system, the cardiovascular system, the respiratory system, the gastrointestinal system, and the endocrine system. Drugs are also used to treat infectious disease and inflammation.

Central Nervous System Pharmacology
The central nervous system consists of the brain and spinal column and all neurons that both originate and terminate within these structures. Since this system is responsible for conscious thought and affects many bodily functions, it is the target for many drugs used in medical care. These agents include analgesics, anesthetics, antianxiety and sedative-hypnotic drugs, antiseizure and antiepileptic drugs, CNS stimulants, and psychotherapeutic drugs.

Autonomic Nervous System Pharmacology
The autonomic nervous system is located within the peripheral nervous system and consists of the sympathetic (fight-or-flight) and parasympathetic (feed-and-breed) systems. These systems are antagonistic and provide control over body functions. The autonomic nervous system controls virtually every organ and body structure not under conscious control and is responsible for maintaining the internal human environment. The nerves of the two systems do not actually touch other nerves or target organs. Messages are carried through the small space between them (synapse) via chemical messengers (neurotransmitters). Acetylcholine is the neurotransmitter at the target organs of the parasympathetic nervous system, while norepinephrine is the neurotransmitter at the target organs for the sympathetic nervous system.

Stimulation of the parasympathetic nervous system causes pupillary constriction, digestive gland secretion, decreased cardiac rate and strength of contraction, bronchoconstriction, and increased digestive activity. Cholinergic (effecting the acetylcholine receptors) drugs stimulate the parasympathetic nervous system and produce salivation, lacrimation, urination, defecation, gastric motility, and emesis (signs suggested by the acronym SLUDGE). They cause their actions directly by acting on the receptor sites (bethanechol and pilocarpine) or indirectly by inhibiting the degradation of acetylcholine (neostigmine and physostigmine). Anticholenergic (parasympatholytic) drugs oppose the actions of acetylcholine and the parasympathetic nervous system. Atropine is the prototype anticholinergic drug, while scopolamine (transdermal) is used to treat motion sickness, and ipratropium bromide (Atrovent) is inhaled to treat bronchoconstriction caused by asthma. Ganglionic blocking agents compete for the acetylcholine receptors at the ganglia and can effectively turn off the parasympathetic nervous system. Neuromuscular blocking agents produce a state of paralysis without inducing unconsciousness. Ganglionic stimulating agents (nicotine) stimulate the ganglia of both the parasympathetic and sympathetic nervous systems yet have no therapeutic purpose.

Stimulation of the sympathetic nervous system causes an increased heart rate and strength of contraction, bronchodilation, increased blood flow to the muscles, decreased blood flow to the skin and abdominal organs, decreased digestive activity, release of glucose stores from the liver, increased energy production, decreased digestive activity, and the release of epinephrine and norepinephrine. Sympathetic receptors include four adrenergic receptors (alpha 1, alpha 2, beta 1, and beta 2) and dopaminergic receptors. Alpha 1 stimulation causes peripheral vasoconstriction, mild bronchoconstriction, and increased metabolism. Alpha 2 stimulation prevents the over-release of norepinephrine at the synapse. Beta 1 stimulation exclusively affects the heart and causes increased heart rate, cardiac contractile force, automaticity, and conduction. Beta 2 stimulation causes bronchodilation and selective vasodilation. Dopaminergic stimulation causes increased circulation to the kidneys, heart, and brain. Sympathomimetic (adrenergic) drugs stimulate the effects of the sympathetic nervous system, while sympatholytic drugs block the actions of the sympathetic nervous system. Alpha 1 drugs increase peripheral vascular resistance, preload, and blood pressure. Alpha 1 agonists are used to control blood pressure or to control injury due to the infiltration of an alpha 1 drug. Beta 1 drugs stimulate the heart and are primarily used in cardiac arrest or cardiogenic shock. Beta 1 antagonists are used to control blood pressure, suppress tachycardia, and reduce cardiac workload in angina. Beta 2 agonists are used to treat asthma.

CONTENT SELF-EVALUATION

MULTIPLE CHOICE

E   1. Which of the following is NOT a division of the nervous system?
   A. central nervous system
   B. peripheral nervous system
   C. autonomic nervous system
   D. sympathetic nervous system
   E. antagonistic nervous system

A   2. Which nervous system controls motor functions?
   A. somatic
   B. autonomic
   C. sympathetic
   D. parasympathetic
   E. antagonistic

D   3. Which nervous system is responsible for the "feed-or-breed" response?
   A. somatic
   B. autonomic
   C. sympathetic
   D. parasympathetic
   E. antagonistic

B   4. Which nervous system works in opposition to the parasympathetic nervous system?
   A. central
   B. sympathetic
   C. autonomic
   D. somatic
   E. antagonistic

B   5. The agents that transport impulses through the synapse between neurons and between nerve cells and the target organs are called:
   A. neuroeffectors.
   B. neurotransmitters.
   C. intrasynaptic agents.
   D. neuroleptic ions.
   E. transport cells.

A   6. The cholinergic neurotransmitter is:
   A. acetylcholine.
   B. epinephrine.
   C. norepinephrine.
   D. muscarinic antagonist.
   E. muscarinic agonist.

A   7. Which neurotransmitter serves both the sympathetic and parasympathetic nervous systems?
   A. acetylcholine
   B. epinephrine
   C. norepinephrine
   D. dopamine
   E. none of the above

©2004 Pearson Education, Inc.
Intermediate Emergency Care: Principles & Practice

_D_ 8. A drug that stimulates the parasympathetic nervous system is called a(n):
A. sympatholytic.
B. sympathomimetic.
C. parasympatholytic.
D. parasympathomimetic.
E. antiemetic.

_D_ 9. A cholinergic drug is also which of the following:
A. a sympatholytic.
B. a sympathomimetic.
C. a parasympatholytic.
D. a parasympathomimetic.
E. an antiemetic.

_C_ 10. The acronym that describes the effects of cholinergic stimulation is:
A. SARIN.
B. 2-PAM.
C. SLUDGE.
D. ALPHA.
E. BETA.

_B_ 11. The effects of cholinergic stimulation include all of the following except:
A. salivation.
B. bradycardia.
C. defecation.
D. urination.
E. emesis.

_D_ 12. The prototype anticholenergic drug is:
A. epinephrine.
B. norepinephrine.
C. acetylcholine.
D. atropine.
E. dopamine.

_B_ 13. Neuromuscular blockade produces paralysis and amnesia to the event.
A. True
B. False

_A_ 14. Alpha 1 antagonist drugs are used almost exclusively to control hypertension.
A. True
B. False

_E_ 15. What effect does alpha stimulation have on the heart?
A. increases heart rate
B. increases automaticity
C. increases contractile strength
D. increases oxygen consumption
E. none of the above

_B_ 16. Which type of drug decreases cardiac contractility and heart rate?
A. beta 2 agonists
B. beta 1 antagonists
C. beta 1 agonists
D. alpha 1 antagonists
E. alpha 1 agonists

_D_ 17. The prototype beta blocker is:
A. isoproterenol.
B. dopamine.
C. atropine.
D. propranolol.
E. none of the above.

_D_ 18. Which of the following is NOT a naturally occurring catecholamine?
A. dopamine
B. epinephrine
C. norepinephrine
D. isoproterenol
E. A and C

_A_ 19. Which type of drug causes bronchodilation?
A. beta 2 agonists
B. beta 1 antagonists
C. beta 1 agonists
D. alpha 1 antagonists
E. alpha 1 agonists

_A_ 20. Beta blockers block both $beta_1$ and $beta_2$ receptors.
A. True
B. False

CHAPTER 3

Emergency Pharmacology

Part 3: EMT-Intermediate Medications

Review of Chapter Objectives

After reading this part of the chapter, you should be able to:

1. **List and describe the drugs that an EMT-Intermediate may administer in a pharmacological management plan according to local protocol.**   **pp. 259-269**

   At the back of this workbook you will find a series of pages with drug cards. Each card contains the name/class, description, indications, contraindications, precautions, routes of administration, and dosages for a drug commonly used in prehospital emergency care. Detach the cards and begin to use them as flash cards. This will help you learn essential information about the drugs you will use during your career as an EMT-I.

SPECIAL PROJECT

Crossword Puzzle

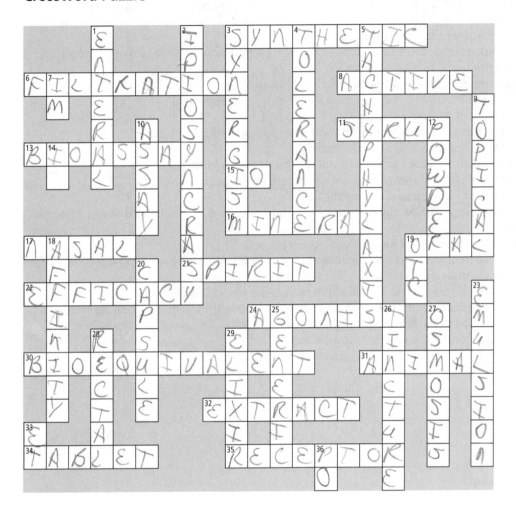

Across

3. Type of drug created in the laboratory
6. Movement of molecules across a membrane down a pressure gradient
8. _____ transport: mechanism to move a substance that requires energy
11. A sugar, water, and drug solution
13. Test that determines a drug's bioequivalency
15. Drug administration to the medullary spaces of bones (abbr.)
16. Generic term for the inorganic source of a drug
17. Route of drug administration via the nose
19. Route of drug administration via the mouth
21. Solution of a volatile drug in alcohol
22. A drug's ability to cause the expected response
24. An agent that binds to a receptor site to cause its intended response
30. Chemically equal to and having the same therapeutic effect as another drug
31. Generic term for the source of drugs extracted from living creatures
32. Drug drawn from a compound by withdrawing a carrier
34. A powder compressed into a disk-like form
35. A protein molecule on the cell wall to which a drug attaches, resulting in a biochemical effect

Down

1. Route of medication delivery via the gastrointestinal tract
2. Drug effect that is unique to an individual
3. Two drugs together producing a response greater than the expected sum of responses
4. Decreased response to the same amount of drug after repeated doses
5. Rapidly occurring tolerance to a drug
7. Route of drug administration that is slower than intravenous injection because the drug passes into the capillaries (abbr.)
9. Route of drug administration via the surface of the skin
10. Test to determine the amount and purity of a chemical in a preparation
12. Fine granular form of a drug
14. Preferred route of drug administration in most emergencies (abbr.)
18. Force of attraction between a drug and a receptor
19. Type of drugs available to the public without a prescription (abbr.)
20. Gelatin container filled with powder or small spheres of drug
23. Suspension of an oily substance in a solvent
25. Name for a drug, suggested by the manufacturer and confirmed by the United States Adopted Name Council
26. Form of a drug prepared by an alcohol extraction process
27. Movement of a solvent through a semipermeable membrane from an area of lower to one of higher solute concentration
28. Route of drug administration via the terminal end of the enteral route
29. Drug that is a combination of alcohol and water solvent, commonly mixed with flavorings
33. Oral route of drug administration (abbr.)
36. Endotracheal route of drug administration (abbr.)

©2004 Pearson Education, Inc.
Intermediate Emergency Care: Principles & Practice

CHAPTER 4

✳

Venous Access and Medication Administration

Part 1: Principles and Routes of Medication Administration

Review of Chapter Objectives

Because Chapter 4 is lengthy, it has been divided into parts to aid your study. Read the assigned textbook pages, then progress through the objectives and self-evaluation materials as you would with other chapters. When you feel secure in your grasp of the content, proceed to the next part.

After reading this part of the chapter, you should be able to:

1. **Review the specific anatomy and physiology pertinent to medication administration.**
   pp. 274–303

   Chapter 2 reviewed human anatomy as it pertains to the absorption, distribution, metabolization, and elimination of the drugs we use to treat disease and trauma. This chapter identifies the anatomy and physiology related to medication administration.

   The percutaneous routes of drug administration include transdermal and mucous membrane administration. Transdermal administration permits drug absorption through the skin via topical application in which the medication is slowly and steadily absorbed. Mucous membrane administration methods include sublingual, buccal, ocular, nasal, and aural administration, in which a drug is given under the tongue, between the cheek and gum, in the eye, into the nose, or into the ear respectively. Sublingual and buccal routes result in systemic absorption, while the remaining routes result in more local effects.

   Pulmonary administration introduces a drug by nebulizer or metered dose inhaler or through an endotracheal tube. All three methods direct the drug to the lung tissue for action; however, endotracheal administration is an emergency route for systemic administration.

   Enteral administration delivers a drug to the gastrointestinal tract, where it is absorbed. This is a relatively safe and simple route for drug administration and is the most common route for over-the-counter and prescription drug administration. The disadvantage of this route is that many factors can affect absorption including stress, diet, and metabolic rate. Liver function metabolizes some drugs, and a dysfunctional liver may alter the medication's metabolization or distribution. The enteral methods of administration include oral, gastric tube, and rectal administration. (Rectal administration is not subject to hepatic [liver] alteration.)

With parenteral administration, a drug is injected into the dermis (intradermal), the subcutaneous layer (subcutaneous), muscle (intramuscular), or veins (intravenous). The intradermal route provides little or no systemic absorption and is used for diagnostic testing and for the administration of local anesthetic. Subcutaneous injection promotes slow, sustained systemic absorption of a drug, while intramuscular injection permits systemic drug absorption at a moderate rate. Because intravenous drug administration injects the drug directly into the bloodstream, where it is directed to the heart, mixed with the returning venous blood, and then distributed systemically, it is the fastest parenteral administration route.

Anatomically, subcutaneous injections may be made into the skin regions over the deltoid muscle, the thighs, and, in some cases, the upper abdomen. Intramuscular injections may be given into the deltoid muscle, 2 inches below the acromial process; into the gluteal muscle, in the upper outer quadrant of the buttocks; into the anterolateral aspect of the thigh muscle (vastus lateralis); and into the central and lateral segment of the mid-thigh (rectus femoris).

2. Discuss legal aspects affecting medication administration, including the "six rights" of drug administration. pp. 274–276

The administration of the wrong medication or withholding the right medication or providing it in the wrong dose or by the wrong route can have catastrophic consequences. Hence, medication administration is an area of EMT-I practice where the EMT-I is exposed to legal liability. You must ensure that you receive informed and expressed consent from the patient (when possible), provide medications in strict compliance with system protocols and the direction of on-line medical direction, and follow proper administration techniques. Once a medication is administered, it is essential that you document the indication for the drug, any online authorization for the administration, the name of the person who delivered the drug, the drug name, dose, route and rate of delivery, and the resulting patient response, whether positive or negative. These actions will go a long way to limiting your liability in drug administration.

There are basically six rights of drug administration. They are the right patient, the right drug, the right dose, the right time, the right route, and the right documentation.

The right patient. Ensure that the patient is the right person and properly matched to the medication. This is an infrequent problem in prehospital care, but as EMS moves to the out-of-hospital environment, we may be treating some patients on a routine basis. Ensure the medication order is for the patient you are attending.

The right drug. Ensure the drug is what is intended for the patient. Review your standing orders or, if the order is received from medical direction, repeat ("echo") the order back to the physician so you are both clear on the drug, dose, route, and timing of the order. Also examine the drug packaging to ensure that it contains the medication you wish to administer and that the medication is still sterile, has not expired, and is not contaminated or discolored.

The right dose. Carefully calculate the exact dose (usually weight dependent) for the patient before you draw up the medication and again just before you administer it. If the drug package you select has significantly more or less of the drug than you intend to use, recheck the packaging to ensure it is the right drug and right concentration, and recheck your calculations to ensure the right dosage. Never overdose or underdose your patient.

The right time. Usually prehospital medications are given rather rapidly and not on a schedule. Check the packaging and your protocols for administration rates and ensure that you follow the sequencing, time intervals between, and drip rates for emergency drugs.

The right route. Specific drugs require specific routes of administration. While most emergency drugs are administered by the IV route, be aware of alternate drug administration routes, the drugs that can be administered by those routes, and the circumstances requiring the use of those routes. With each medication administration, ensure you are using the right route.

The right documentation. Documentation of drug administration is of paramount importance. You must carefully record the patient's condition (the circumstances that require the drug's administration), the drug name, dose, and route of administration, and who administered the

©2004 Pearson Education, Inc.
Intermediate Emergency Care: Principles & Practice

drug and at what time. It is also essential that you record the patient's response to the drug, whether good or bad.

3. **Discuss medical asepsis and the differences between clean and sterile techniques, and uses of antiseptics and disinfectants.**   pp. 275–276

Medical asepsis describes a medical environment free of pathogens. The most aseptic environment is a sterile one, one free of all living organisms. However, in prehospital care we frequently cannot attain such a state. We utilize equipment and supplies that are sterile when packaged and then use medically clean techniques to reduce the risk of spreading infection. These techniques include the use of disinfectants to kill microorganisms on equipment and in the ambulance and of antiseptics to reduce the bacterial load on the patient's skin when we utilize procedures like venipuncture.

Antiseptics are agents that are designed for topical use to destroy or inhibit pathogenic microorganisms already on living tissue. They are used to cleanse the skin before parenteral drug administration to prevent infection secondary to the needle stick.

Disinfectants are powerful agents that are toxic to living tissue. They are not designed for topical administration but for the direct cleaning of durable patient care equipment.

4. **Describe how body substance isolation (BSI) precautions relate to medication administration.**   p. 275

Any time there is the possibility of contact with body substances or patient wounds, you must use body substance isolation measures. Gloves, at a minimum, provide barrier protection to the care giver from possibly infectious material at the scene and to the patient from the care giver. Goggles and a mask also provide protection, as does hand washing after contact with a patient or possibly infected material.

5. **Describe the indications, equipment, techniques, precautions, and general principles of administering medications by inhalation routes.**   pp. 280–283

Pulmonary medications are administered via nebulizer, metered dose inhaler, and endotracheal tube. Drugs indicated for inhalation include those that cause bronchodilation, mucolytics, antibiotics, and topical steroids for respiratory emergencies, congestion, infection, and inflammation respectively.

A nebulizer aerosolizes a small volume of liquid (or dissolved) medication using oxygen, which is then inhaled into the lungs and absorbed quickly. The device is assembled (mouth piece, medication reservoir, oxygen port, relief valve, and oxygen tubing and source), and 3 to 5 ml of solution (or a medication dissolved in 3 to 5 ml of sterile water) is placed in the medication reservoir. Oxygen is set to run at 5 to 8 liters per minute (without a humidifier), and the mouthpiece is placed in the patient's mouth. The patient should hold the nebulizer and inhale slowly and deeply with each breath, then hold the breath for 1 to 2 seconds before exhaling. The patient should continue doing this until the medication is gone (about 3 to 5 minutes). For nebulized medications to be effective, the patient must have an adequate tidal volume and respiratory rate, although nebulizers can be connected to an endotracheal tube during positive pressure ventilation.

Metered dose inhalers are frequently used in patients with COPD and asthma to deliver agents to induce bronchodilation. The device consists of a pressurized medication canister, plastic shell and mouthpiece, and possibly a spacer. The patient self-administers the drug by assembling the inhaler, shaking it for 2 to 5 seconds, inverting it, placing the mouthpiece in the mouth, and sealing the lips against the mouthpiece. Then, during the beginning of a deep inhalation, the patient presses the canister downward to release a dose of medication. A second dose may be necessary. Nebulizers are preferable to metered dose inhalers in acute respiratory emergencies because they administer the drug over more time and are less dependent on a single deep inspiration.

Endotracheal administration of a drug involves expressing the drug down the endotracheal tube (in a volume of 10 ml and from 2 to 2.5 times the normal intravenous dose). Narcan, atropine, lidocaine, and epinephrine can be administered this way in an emergency when IV access is not otherwise available. Once the drug is injected down the endotracheal tube, the ventilator provides several deep ventilations to deliver the drug to the pulmonary tissue.

6. Differentiate among the different dosage forms of oral medications, and describe the equipment and general principles of their administration. pp. 284–288

Oral medications are introduced as capsules, tablets, pills, time release capsules, elixirs, emulsions, lozenges, suspensions, or syrups introduced into the oral cavity and swallowed with 4 to 8 ounces of water. This is the most common method of over-the-counter and prescription drug administration because of its ease of administration.

Administering oral medication is easy and the equipment used depends on the patient's status. A soufflé cup is a cup in which the solid med is placed too make it easy for the patient to self-administer. A medicine cup has volumetric measurements on the side for taking liquid doses. A medicine dropper is used for children or patients who do not tolerate other devices. A teaspoon is commonly used provided it is a measured teaspoon. An oral syringe, without a needle, can be used for liquid medications, and finally a plastic nipple may be used for infants.

General principles to consider when administering an oral medication include: taking BSI precautions, note if the med should be taken with food or on an empty stomach, have the patient sit upright when not contraindicated by their medical condition, after a liquid med give the patient 4–6 ounces of water, assure the patient has actually swallowed the medication and not hidden it in his mouth.

7. Describe the medications, equipment, techniques, precautions, and general principles of rectal medication administration. pp. 288–289

Rectal administration involves topical administration of a medication to the rectal mucosa and provides rapid predictable absorption. Use a syringe and 14-gauge needleless catheter (or small endotracheal tube) to introduce the medication into the rectum, then hold the buttocks closed to promote retention and absorption. A suppository is a soft, pliable form of drug that melts at body temperature and is inserted into the rectum for absorption. An enema is a liquid bolus of medication introduced through the rectum.

In the emergency setting due to the extreme vascularity of the rectum and its rapid drug absorption, if an IV line cannot be established your local protocols may allow administration of certain medications such as diazepam (Valium) for protracted seizures or aspirin for cardiac or neurological emergencies. This route may be more commonly used in the pediatric patient as oral meds are more difficult to administer in a child.

To administer a rectal medication in the emergent setting follow these steps:
- Confirm the indication for administration and dose and draw the correct quantity of med in a syringe.
- Place the hub of a 14-gauge Teflon catheter (removed from the angiocath) on the end of a needleless syringe.
- Insert the Teflon catheter into the patient's rectum and inject the medication in the lower part of the rectum. Administration higher in the rectum may result in the medication being absorbed by the veins that deliver the drug to the portal circulation.
- Withdraw the catheter and hold the patient's buttocks together to permit retention and absorption.

In the nonemergent setting suppositories or enemas are common methods for rectal administration of medication. If your responsibilities include nonemergent settings, you should be aware of the specific techniques for insertion of these devices and local protocols in your area. A suppository is a medication that is packaged in a soft pliable form that is refrigerated until used. When inserted they breakdown due to the warmth of the body temperature. An enema is typically a liquid bolus of medication that is injected into the rectum.

8. Describe the equipment, techniques, complications, and general principles for the preparation and administration of parenteral medication. pp. 289–303

Parenteral administration includes the routes utilizing needles to administer drugs into the tissues or vascular system—intradermal, subcutaneous, intramuscular, intravenous, and intraosseous

©2004 Pearson Education, Inc.
Intermediate Emergency Care: Principles & Practice

routes. Begin the parenteral administration process by cleansing the patient's skin at the injection site with an antiseptic such as alcohol or a betadine solution. The medication for injection is in solution and drawn up in a syringe, then injected with a needle (bevel up). For subcutaneous and intramuscular injection, consider injecting a 0.1-ml air bubble after the medication to limit leakage, and then massage the region to enhance absorption. Most emergency medications are injected via the intravenous route because of its rapid distribution throughout the body.

Intradermal drug administration calls for insertion of a 25- to 27-gauge needle at a 10- to 15-degree angle just into a segment of skin that is pulled taut. Slow injection of up to 1 ml of solution will create a small wheal of medication. Then remove the needle. Intradermal injection results in a very slow absorption rate greatly affected by local perfusion rates and is used for diagnostic testing and the administration of local anesthetics.

For subcutaneous administration, place a 24- to 26-gauge needle into a 1-inch "pinch" of the patient's skin at a 45-degree angle and inject no more than 1 ml of medication. The skin must be free of scarring, superficial nerves, blood vessels and tendons, tattoos, and bruising. Pulling the plunger back ensures that the needle is not in a blood vessel (aspiration of blood indicates a blood vessel entry). Subcutaneous injection may be given at many locations around the body, including the tissue under the tongue.

For intramuscular injections, use a 21- to 23-gauge needle inserted at a 90-degree angle into the deltoid (up to 2 ml), dorsal gluteal (up to 5 ml), vastus lateralis (up to 5 ml), or rectus femoris (up to 5 ml) muscle. Again, pulling back on the plunger ensures that the needle is not in a blood vessel. Intramuscular injection provides a predictable systemic absorption and is used for several prehospital drugs including glucagon and morphine. Careful placement of parenteral needles is important because of potential damage to nerves and arteries. Needles for intradermal, subcutaneous, and intramuscular injection are 3/8 to 1 inch in length.

9. **Describe disposal of contaminated items and sharps.**   p. 279

Sharps and contaminated materials pose a risk for the spread of infection. Do not recap needles unless absolutely necessary and, in such instance, do so using only one hand. Used needles represent a real risk for introducing pathogens from the patient's blood into someone stuck with the needle. Dispose of all needles in a puncture-proof biohazard container. Ensure all medical waste is placed in a biohazardous waste bag and is not left at the scene. Follow your service's biohazard exposure plan should you receive a needle stick.

10. **Synthesize a pharmacologic management plan including medication administration.**   pp. 273–275

As you care for patients with serious medical and trauma emergencies, you will often need to administer medications to them via the sublingual, oral, pulmonary, subcutaneous, intramuscular, intravenous, and intraosseous routes. The procedures described in this chapter must become an integral part of your patient management skills.

11. **Integrate pathophysiological principles of medication administration with patient management.**   pp. 273–275

Drug administration is a fundamental skill used in the treatment of the sick and injured. For medications to be effective, they must be safely delivered to the body by the appropriate route. Many different routes for drug delivery are available to the EMT-I; however, specific drugs require specific routes for administration. It is the responsibility of the EMT-I to know the best medication to give by the best route in the appropriate dose at the appropriate time to manage his patient's condition according to the treatment protocols and local medical direction. You have learned in this chapter, for example, that certain medications do not work well when administered orally to a patient in shock or by IM to a patient with poor distal perfusion. By integrating the pathophysiologic principles of medication administration with and understanding of your assessment of the patient's medical condition you will be able to better manage the patient's needs.

CASE STUDY REVIEW

Susan and Todd are presented with a typical emergency patient in this scenario. While Susan anticipated asthma from the patient's wheezing, her positioning, and her general appearance (all determined during the first impression of the patient), she is meticulous in her complete patient evaluation and determination of baseline vital signs, pulse oximetry, and patient (SAMPLE) history. This information is essential to identify the pathology affecting the patient and to identify and document the indications, and rule out possible contraindications, for medication administration.

Susan and Todd identify that the patient attempted to use a metered dose inhaler for relief from the asthma attack. Because of their knowledge of various medication administration techniques and their respective advantages and disadvantages, they know that in severe attacks of respiratory distress, the ventilatory exchange is poor and limits the effectiveness of the inhaler. They employ albuterol neb-ulization because the prolonged and humidified inhalation may be more effective in delivering the drug to the deeper respiratory tissue. They also recognize the seriousness of the attack and administer epinephrine subcutaneously to assure rapid delivery of a bronchodilator.

For each of these drug routes, Susan must be familiar with the specific equipment used, the location for injections, and the technique of drug injection and must recognize what common complications may be associated with a particular route of administration. Susan must also be able to calculate the proper dose of the drug and the volume of drug on hand that contains that dose.

During each medication administration, Susan must follow the proper protocol, identify the six rights of drug administration, and employ the appropriate technique to draw up and deliver the medication. She must also observe body substance isolation measures and aseptic and medically clean techniques, dispose of sharps, drug containers, and other biohazards properly, and document the indications, administration, and effects of each drug she used. While this is a complicated process, it will become second nature to you once you begin your career as a EMT-I.

CONTENT SELF-EVALUATION

MULTIPLE CHOICE

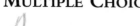

1. Medication administration is an important part of the medical care provided by EMT-Is.
   A. True
   B. False

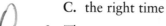

2. Which of the following is NOT one of the six rights of drug administration?
   A. the right dosage
   B. the right indication
   C. the right time
   D. the right documentation
   E. the right patient

3. The process you use to ensure you hear and correctly understand the medical direction physician's order to administer a medication is:
   A. protocol compliance.
   B. order confirmation with your partner.
   C. redundant physician orders.
   D. echoing the order back to the physician.
   E. asking the physician to repeat the order.

4. Which of the following must you know about the drugs you are authorized to administer?
   A. their usual dosages
   B. their contraindications
   C. their common side effects
   D. their routes of administration
   E. all of the above

A 5. When you administer drugs, which of the following body substance isolation measures should you always employ?
   - A. gloves
   - B. a mask
   - C. goggles
   - D. a gown
   - E. A and D

A 6. The condition in which a medical environment is free of all pathogens is described as:
   - A. asepsis.
   - B. uncontaminated.
   - C. medically clean.
   - D. disinfection.
   - E. none of the above

C 7. The environment that EMT-Is should strive to maintain while delivering prehospital emergency care is:
   - A. aseptic.
   - B. sterile.
   - C. medically clean.
   - D. disinfected.
   - E. none of the above

D 8. To cleanse the site of a parenteral injection, you would use a(n):
   - A. aseptic.
   - B. disinfectant.
   - C. detergent.
   - D. antiseptic.
   - E. dilutant.

A 9. When possible, you should recap needles:
   - A. as a last resort.
   - B. in a moving ambulance only.
   - C. except in a moving ambulance.
   - D. only when they have not been used on a patient.
   - E. when directed by a physician.

C 10. Documentation regarding the administration of a drug should include all of the following EXCEPT the:
   - A. time of administration.
   - B. route of administration.
   - C. class of drug administered.
   - D. positive patient responses.
   - E. negative patient responses.

E 11. Transdermal medications are provided in which of the following forms?
   - A. ointments
   - B. wet dressings
   - C. foams
   - D. lotions
   - E. all of the above

D 12. Which of the following factors can decrease the absorption rate with transdermal medication administration?
   - A. thin skin
   - B. overdose
   - C. penetrating solvents
   - D. peripheral vascular disease
   - E. all of the above

C 13. Which of the following is a common emergency drug administered sublingually?
   - A. sodium bicarbonate
   - B. epinephrine
   - C. nitroglycerin
   - D. aspirin
   - E. magnesium

C 14. The route in which a drug is administered between the cheek and gum is:
   - A. transdermal.
   - B. sublingual.
   - C. buccal.
   - D. aural.
   - E. inhalation.

E 15. Ocular medications are given for which conditions?
   - A. eye pain
   - B. eye infection
   - C. increased intraocular pressure
   - D. lubricating the eyelid
   - E. all of the above

_D_ 16. Ocular medications are most commonly administered:
- **A.** over the pupil.
- **B.** over the iris.
- **C.** over the sclera.
- **D.** into the conjunctival sac.
- **E.** all of the above

_B_ 17. Nasal administration of medication is used frequently because of its rapid absorption rate and systemic effects.
- **A.** True
- **B.** False

_B_ 18. The small volume nebulizer often used in prehospital emergency medical service administers what volume of medication?
- **A.** 1 to 2 ml
- **B.** 3 to 5 ml
- **C.** 5 to 10 ml
- **D.** 10 to 15 ml
- **E.** 15 to 20 ml

_B_ 19. The small volume nebulizer's major advantage over the metered dose inhaler is that the patient does not need an adequate tidal volume for effective medication delivery.
- **A.** True
- **B.** False

_C_ 20. The metered dose inhaler is activated to release its medication:
- **A.** just before the patient seals his lips to the mouthpiece.
- **B.** as the patient exhales.
- **C.** as the patient inhales.
- **D.** during both inhalation and exhalation.
- **E.** between inhalation and exhalation.

_A_ 21. Nebulizers and metered dose inhalers are advantageous in respiratory emergencies because they deliver their medication to the exact site of action.
- **A.** True
- **B.** False

_E_ 22. Endotracheal medication administration calls for drugs to be diluted to what volume?
- **A.** 1 ml
- **B.** 2 ml
- **C.** 3 ml
- **D.** 5 ml
- **E.** 10 ml

_A_ 23. Which of the following drugs is NOT administered via the endotracheal route?
- **A.** meperidine
- **B.** naloxone
- **C.** atropine
- **D.** lidocaine
- **E.** epinephrine

_B_ 24. Enteral medications are absorbed through the:
- **A.** liver.
- **B.** gastrointestinal tract.
- **C.** mucous membranes.
- **D.** portal system.
- **E.** accessory organs.

_A_ 25. Liver function is an important factor in the effectiveness of enteral drug administration.
- **A.** True
- **B.** False

_B_ 26. When using a medicine cup to measure an oral dose of medication, you should use what aspect of fluid level to determine the fluid volume?
- **A.** the highest point of the meniscus
- **B.** the lowest point of the meniscus
- **C.** between the high and low point of the meniscus
- **D.** one calibration below the lowest level of the meniscus
- **E.** none of the above

©2004 Pearson Education, Inc.
Intermediate Emergency Care: Principles & Practice

_A_ 27. The normal teaspoon holds about what volume of fluid?
A. 2 ml   D. 10 ml
B. 3 ml   E. 12 ml
C. 5 ml

_B_ 28. The advantage of rectal administration over the other enteral drug routes is that:
A. the rectal route is easier to administer drugs through.
B. there is no hepatic alteration of the drug.
C. the rectal route can absorb more medication.
D. rectal irritation is rare.
E. all of the above

_D_ 29. To inject a drug rectally you may use:
A. a large catheter with needle removed.
B. a special enema container with a rectal tip.
C. a small endotracheal tube attached to a syringe.
D. all of the above
E. none of the above

_B_ 30. A syringe should be chosen for drug administration that is slightly smaller than the volume of drug to be administered.
A. True
B. False

_B_ 31. The smaller the gauge of a hypodermic needle, the smaller the diameter of its lumen.
A. True
B. False

_B_ 32. What is the total dose of a drug contained in an ampule with 5 ml of a drug in a 0.3 mg/ml concentration?
A. 0.3 mg   D. 15 mg
B. 1.5 mg   E. none of the above
C. 5 mg

_A_ 33. Which of the following drug containers may contain multiple doses of a drug?
A. vial   D. preloaded syringe
B. ampule   E. medicated solutions
C. Mix-o-Vial

_A_ 34. Prior to drawing medication from a vial, you must first inject an equal volume of air into the vial.
A. True
B. False

_E_ 35. Which of the following must be cleansed with an alcohol swab before the drug is withdrawn?
A. vial   D. preloaded syringe
B. ampule   E. A and C
C. Mix-o-Vial

_A_ 36. The drug route that calls for insertion of the needle at 10 to 15 degrees is:
A. intradermal.   D. intraosseous.
B. subcutaneous.   E. none of the above
C. intramuscular.

_C_ 37. Which of the following is most likely to be an acceptable site for subcutaneous injection?
A. forearms   D. buttocks
B. calves   E. all of the above
C. abdomen

©2004 Pearson Education, Inc.
Intermediate Emergency Care: Principles & Practice

CHAPTER 4   _Venous Access and Medication Administration_   **101**

_D_ 38. Through which of the following routes should you inject no more than 1 ml of a drug?
   A. intradermal
   B. subcutaneous
   C. intramuscular
   D. A and B
   E. all of the above

_B_ 39. For intradermal and subcutaneous injections, the needle is inserted with the bevel down.
   A. True
   B. False

_A_ 40. At which of the following intramuscular injection sites should you administer a maximum of 2 ml of a drug?
   A. deltoid
   B. gluteal
   C. vastus lateralis
   D. rectus femoris
   E. both B and C

_D_ 41. When you pull back on the syringe plunger during subcutaneous or intramuscular injection and blood appears, you should:
   A. inject the drug.
   B. inject the drug followed by a small bubble of air.
   C. insert the needle 1 cm further.
   D. attempt the injection at another site.
   E. consider the appearance of blood insignificant.

_C_ 42. The drug route that calls for use of a 21- to 23-gauge needle is:
   A. intradermal.
   B. subcutaneous.
   C. intramuscular.
   D. intraosseous.
   E. none of the above

_D_ 43. The drug route that calls for use of a needle 3/8 to 1 inch long is:
   A. intradermal.
   B. subcutaneous.
   C. intramuscular.
   D. all of the above
   E. none of the above

_D_ 44. The recommended angle of insertion for the needle when administering an intramuscular injection is:
   A. 10 degrees.
   B. 15 degrees.
   C. 45 degrees.
   D. 90 degrees.
   E. between 10 and 15 degrees.

_B_ 45. After injecting an intramuscular drug, massaging the site is contraindicated because it will slow absorption.
   A. True
   B. False

©2004 Pearson Education, Inc.
Intermediate Emergency Care: Principles & Practice

CHAPTER 4

✳

Venous Access and Medication Administration

Part 2: Intravenous Access, Blood Sampling, and Intraosseous Infusion

Review of Chapter Objectives

After reading this part of the chapter, you should be able to:

1. **Describe the indications, equipment, techniques, precautions, and general principles of peripheral venous or external jugular cannulation.** **pp. 303–330**

Peripheral venous access is the preferable route for medication administration in the emergency prehospital setting. Most emergency drugs are administered this way because it provides a direct route into the venous system, then to the heart, where the drug and blood are further mixed, and then to the body as distributed by the arterial system. Vascular access can be obtained using a steel needle with a beveled sharp edge. Most commonly, an over-the-needle catheter is advanced into the vein, with the needle then withdrawn, leaving the catheter to permit introduction of drugs or fluid or withdrawal of blood for diagnostic testing. The veins of the hands, arms, antecubital fossa, feet, and legs and the external jugular veins are common sites for intravenous cannulation.

The equipment used for intravenous therapy includes a venous constricting band to help engorge the veins; the needle for venipuncture; an antiseptic to cleanse the site; administration tubing to direct and control fluid administration from an IV bag or a syringe to draw up, then administer medication; tape or commercial devices to secure the intravenous catheter; and bacteriostatic ointment to protect the site from infection. An ideal location for venipuncture is free of injury and with relatively prominent veins. The care giver should take appropriate body substance isolation measures before beginning the procedure. Then the venous constricting band is secured just proximal to the selected site and a vein is chosen. The area is cleansed with an alcohol or betadine swab, using concentric circles moving outward from the selected site. An over-the-needle catheter is selected, with 14- to 18-gauge for blood, thick medications such as glucose, or fluid volume administration or a 20- to 22-gauge catheter for pediatric or geriatric patients or patients who do not need a larger catheter. The catheter is directed, bevel up, through the skin at an angle of 10 to 30 degrees until a "pop" is felt or blood appears in the flash chamber. Once in the vein, the catheter is advanced an additional 0.5 cm and then the catheter is threaded into the vein. The needle is withdrawn, the constricting band is released, and the administration set or saline or heparin lock is attached. A small amount of fluid is run to ensure that the catheter is patent. Watch for edema around the site, which is suggestive of infiltration. Intravenous cannulation and infusion may result in local pain, infiltration, pyrogenic reactions, allergic reactions, catheter shear and embolism, inadvertent arterial puncture, circulatory overload, thrombophlebitis, thrombus formation, air embolism, and necrosis.

Fluid is infused through a venipuncture site to hydrate the patient or to keep the drug route open and quickly available. Most prehospital infusions use isotonic (same osmotic pressure as the plasma) solutions such as normal saline, 5 percent dextrose in water, or lactated Ringer's solution. These solutions flow through the administration set, where their rate of administration is regulated by adjusting the drip rate in a chamber. Most commonly 10 (macro) or 60 (micro) drops traveling through a drip chamber equal 1 milliliter. The administration set contains one or more injection ports to accommodate the administration of drugs or additional fluid administration. A special type of administration set is the measured volume administration set, which contains a calibrated chamber that will permit the discrete administration of a volume of fluid.

The external jugular vein is an alternate venous access site located on the lateral anterior neck. It is a large, easily found vein that permits venous access when other veins are collapsed due to hypovolemia or other vascular problems. It is close to the central circulation, so it provides almost immediate absorption of any drugs administered through it. The jugular vein can be engorged by placing digital pressure along the vein just above the clavical. External jugular cannulation is painful and risks damage to the airway or arterial structures in the neck.

2. **Describe the indications, equipment, techniques, precautions, and general principles of intraosseous needle placement and infusion.**   pp. 333–339

Intraosseous needle placement is indicated for the critical pediatric patient under 5 when you cannot establish other IV access sites or for the adult patient when you also cannot perform peripheral venous access because of disease or extreme hypovolemia. A special needle is introduced through the compact bone of the tibia and into the medullary space. There fluids or drugs are readily available for absorption and distribution by the venous system.

In the child, the needle is placed at 90 degrees to the tibial plateau, just medial and about two finger widths below the tibial tuberosity (the anterior bump just below the patella). Don gloves and cleanse the site with an antiseptic swab. With a firm twisting motion, introduce the needle into the bone for a few centimeters until you feel a "pop" or reduced resistance. Remove the trocar, attach a syringe, and draw back on the syringe to aspirate bone marrow and blood. Rotate the plastic disk to engage the skin and secure the needle. Connect the IV fluid administration set and secure the needle with bulky dressings and tape. Adult or geriatric IO administration uses the flat tibial plate just two finger widths above the medial malleolus. IO infusion may result in bone fracture, infiltration, growth-plate damage, pulmonary embolism, and the problems associated with venous cannulation. This site is not very effective for extensive fluid resuscitation in the adult.

3. **Describe the purpose, equipment, techniques, complications, and general principles for obtaining a blood sample.**   pp. 330–333

Blood composition, the presence of toxins, and blood gas levels are important values to determine for learning what is wrong with a patient. Since emergency care may alter these figures, it is sometimes important to draw blood in the prehospital setting. Blood is withdrawn from a vein through either a needle or catheter and is either directly placed in special containers (blood tubes) or into a syringe for distribution into the blood tubes. A large vein must be used, because the withdrawal of blood may collapse smaller veins. A needled vacutainer is introduced into an engorged vein and blood tubes are introduced, one at a time. The vacuum withdraws blood from the vein and into the tubes, which are then manually agitated to mix the blood with an anticoagulant (all but the red top tube). If a vacutainer is not available, 20 ml of blood may be drawn up in a syringe and distributed among the containers. It is important to fill the containers in order of red, blue, green, purple, and gray (as available), because they contain various anticoagulants and another order may cross-contaminate the blood.

©2004 Pearson Education, Inc.
Intermediate Emergency Care: Principles & Practice

CONTENT SELF-EVALUATION

MULTIPLE CHOICE

_E_ 1. Which of the following is an indication for intravenous administration?
A. fluid replacement
B. blood replacement
C. drug administration
D. need of blood for analysis
E. all of the above

_B_ 2. Both central venous and peripheral venous cannulation are common in prehospital care.
A. True
B. False

_E_ 3. Which of the following is a likely site for intravenous cannulation?
A. the hands
B. the arms
C. the legs
D. the neck
E. all of the above

_D_ 4. Which of the following is NOT a central venous vessel?
A. the internal jugular
B. the subclavian
C. the femoral
D. the antecubital
E. all of the above are central venous vessels

_B_ 5. The solution that contains large proteins is a(n):
A. colliod.
B. crystalloid.
C. isotonic.
D. hypotonic.
E. hypertonic.

_C_ 6. The solution that contains an electrolyte concentration close to that of plasma is a(n):
A. colliod.
B. crystalloid.
C. isotonic.
D. hypotonic.
E. hypertonic.

_E_ 7. The solution that contains an electrolyte concentration greater than that of plasma is a(n):
A. colliod.
B. crystalloid.
C. isotonic.
D. hypotonic.
E. hypertonic.

_D_ 8. One example of a hypotonic solution is:
A. normal saline.
B. lactated Ringer's solution.
C. plasmanate.
D. 5 percent dextrose in water.
E. dextran.

_E_ 9. The most desirable replacement for blood lost during trauma is:
A. normal saline.
B. lactated Ringer's solution.
C. plasmanate.
D. 5 percent dextrose in water.
E. none of the above

_E_ 10. Which intravenous fluid bag would you discard?
A. one that is cloudy
B. one that is discolored
C. one that is leaking
D. one that is expired
E. all of the above

_B_ 11. For optimal fluid delivery, the drip chamber should be how full?
A. 1/4
B. 1/3
C. 1/2
D. 2/3
E. none of the above

_A_ 12. The administration set most appropriate for administration of intravenous solutions for fluid replacement is the:
  A. macrodrip administration set.
  B. microdrip administration set.
  C. measured volume administration set.
  D. blood tubing set.
  E. none of the above

_D_ 13. The most common microdrip setting equaling 1 ml is:
  A. 10 gtts.   D. 60 gtts.
  B. 20 gtts.   E. none of the above
  C. 45 gtts.

_C_ 14. The administration set most appropriate for administration of a very specific volume of intravenous solution or drug is the:
  A. macrodrip administration set.
  B. microdrip administration set.
  C. measured volume administration set.
  D. blood tubing set.
  E. none of the above

_A_ 15. The major difference between blood tubing and a standard intravenous administration set is that blood tubing has a filter to remove clots and particulate matter.
  A. True
  B. False

_A_ 16. Blood is not administered with fluids like lactated Ringer's solution because such solutions increase blood's potential for coagulation.
  A. True
  B. False

_A_ 17. Many patients are prone to develop hypothermia during fluid administration.
  A. True
  B. False

_E_ 18. The most common intravenous cannula used in the prehospital setting is the:
  A. over-the-needle.   D. angiocatheter.
  B. through-the-needle.   E. A and D
  C. hollow needle.

_B_ 19. A needle gauge of 18 is smaller than a needle gauge of 22.
  A. True
  B. False

_B_ 20. A venous constricting band should be left in place no longer than:
  A. 1 minute.   D. 5 minutes.
  B. 2 minutes.   E. 10 minutes.
  C. 3 minutes.

_D_ 21. Leaving the constricting band on for too long is likely to cause:
  A. collapse of the vein.
  B. damage to the distal blood vessels.
  C. damage to the vessels under the band.
  D. changes in the distal venous blood.
  E. all of the above

_B_ 22. When cleansing the site for intravenous cannulation, you should make one swipe over the intended site with a betadine or alcohol swab.
  A. True
  B. False

©2004 Pearson Education, Inc.
Intermediate Emergency Care: Principles & Practice

_B_ 23. The angle of insertion for intravenous cannulation is:
    A. 10 degrees.   D. 60 degrees.
    B. 10 to 30 degrees.   E. 60 to 90 degrees.
    C. 45 degrees.

_B_ 24. After you feel the "pop" associated with intravenous cannulation, you should:
    A. advance the catheter.
    B. advance the needle 0.5 centimeter, then advance the catheter.
    C. advance the needle 1 centimeter, then advance the catheter.
    D. advance the needle 2 centimeters, then advance the catheter.
    E. withdraw the needle, then advance the catheter.

_A_ 25. You should consider using the external jugular vein as an IV access site only after you have exhausted other means of peripheral access or when the patient needs immediate fluid administration.
    A. True
    B. False

_C_ 26. During external jugular vein cannulation, the patient's head should be:
    A. moved to the sniffing position.   D. hyperextended.
    B. turned toward the side of access.   E. hyperflexed.
    C. turned away from the side of access.

_C_ 27. To fill the jugular access site and make the vessel easier to both locate and cannulate, you should:
    A. apply a venous constricting band, tightly.
    B. apply a venous constricting band, loosely.
    C. occlude the vein gently with a finger.
    D. perform the procedure without occluding the vein.
    E. have the patient take a deep breath and hold it.

_E_ 28. When establishing an IV with blood tubing, you must be careful to:
    A. fill the drip chamber 1/3 full.
    B. completely cover the blood filter with blood.
    C. fill the set with normal saline first.
    D. fill the drip chamber 3/4 full.
    E. both A and B above

_E_ 29. Which of the following is a factor that may affect intravenous flow rates?
    A. failure to remove a venous constricting band
    B. edema at the access site
    C. the cannula tip up against a vein valve
    D. a clogged catheter
    E. all of the above

_D_ 30. The complication of peripheral venous access in which a plastic embolus can form is:
    A. pyrogenic reaction.   D. catheter shear.
    B. pain.   E. all of the above
    C. thrombophlebitis.

_D_ 31. The most common cause of catheter shear is:
    A. cannulating thick veins.
    B. cannulating underneath the constricting band.
    C. withdrawing the needle from within the catheter.
    D. withdrawing the catheter from the needle.
    E. faulty catheter construction.

_B_ 32. If a blood clot appears to stop or slow intravenous fluid flow, forcefully inject a small amount of heparin into the catheter and continue the infusion.
    A. True
    B. False

_D_ 33. You should change a large (500- to 1,000-ml) infusion bag when the volume remaining in the bag is:
A. 10 ml.   D. 50 ml.
B. 20 ml.   E. 100 ml.
C. 30 ml.

_C_ 34. If air becomes entrained in the administration set when you are changing an IV bag or bottle, you should:
A. continue the infusion, because the volume of air is negligible.
B. discard the set and use a new one.
C. use a syringe placed between the bubbles and patient to withdraw the air.
D. reverse the fluid flow until the bubbles enter the fluid bag or drip chamber.
E. squeeze the tubing to push them into the drip chamber or bag.

_A_ 35. Never administer an intravenous drug infusion as the primary IV line.
A. True
B. False

_B_ 36. Which of the following is NOT true regarding infusion pumps?
A. They deliver fluids under pressure.
B. They are large and difficult to carry.
C. Most pumps contain alarms for occlusion.
D. Most pumps contain alarms for fluid source depletion.
E. They deliver fluids at precise rates.

_A_ 37. The reason venous blood sampling is important in the prehospital setting is that our interventions may alter the blood's composition or erase important information about it.
A. True
B. False

_B_ 38. The color of the blood tube container that must be drawn first is:
A. blue.   D. purple.
B. red.   E. gray.
C. green.

_B_ 39. Drawing blood and injecting it into the blood tubes in the wrong order may result in:
A. leaving the wrong volume of blood in a tube.
B. cross-contamination of the blood with anticoagulants.
C. depletion of the vacuum in the tubes at too early a stage.
D. coagulation in the last tubes to be filled.
E. all but C

_A_ 40. Do not use a blood tube after its expiration date because the anticoagulant and vacuum may have become ineffective.
A. True
B. False

_C_ 41. The device that accepts the blood tube to permit its filling is:
A. the leur lock.   D. the leur-sampling needle.
B. the Huber needle.   E. either A or C
C. the vacutainer.

_B_ 42. You should fill the blood tube to between a third and a half of its volume because the anticoagulant is measured for this amount of blood.
A. True
B. False

©2004 Pearson Education, Inc.
Intermediate Emergency Care: Principles & Practice

_C_ 43. When using a syringe to fill your blood tubes, you should draw a volume of blood of about:
- A. 5 ml.
- B. 10 ml.
- C. 20 ml.
- D. 35 ml.
- E. 50 ml.

_C_ 44. The complication from drawing blood in which red blood cells are destroyed is:
- A. hematocrit.
- B. hemoconcentration.
- C. hemolysis.
- D. hemotypsis.
- E. hematuria.

_A_ 45. Hemoconcentration occurs during drawing blood:
- A. when the constricting band is left in place too long.
- B. when blood is drawn back through a needle that is too small.
- C. with premature mixing of the anticoagulant.
- D. with too vigorous a mixing of the blood and anticoagulant.
- E. with too forceful an aspiration of blood into the syringe.

_A_ 46. When an IV catheter is withdrawn, place pressure on the venipuncture site with a sterile gauze pad for about 5 minutes.
- A. True
- B. False

_C_ 47. The intraosseous site of infusion is most commonly used for which category of patient?
- A. geriatric patients
- B. cardiac patients
- C. children under 5 years of age
- D. patients with non-skeletal injuries
- E. all of the above

_A_ 48. The proper site for intraosseous needle placement in the child is one to two finger widths:
- A. below and medial to the tibial tuberosity.
- B. below and lateral to the tibial tuberosity.
- C. above the medial malleolus.
- D. above the lateral malleolus.
- E. above and lateral to the tibial crest.

_D_ 49. Confirmation that you are in the medullary space is achieved by:
- A. feeling the bone "pop."
- B. pushing the needle 2 to 4 mm.
- C. aspirating bone marrow and blood.
- D. feeling resistance to the twisting of insertion.
- E. none of the above

_D_ 50. Complications of intraosseous cannulation include all of the following EXCEPT:
- A. pulmonary embolism.
- B. fracture.
- C. growth plate damage.
- D. aspiration of bone marrow.
- E. complete insertion.

SPECIAL PROJECT

Medication Administration—Personal Benchmarking

To administer medications to the patient experiencing a trauma or medical emergency, you must be familiar with the subcutaneous, intramuscular, and intravenous administration sites located around the body. By locating these various sites on your own body, you can become accustomed to the texture and feel of the various sites used for administration of medications and fluids. This personal benchmarking can help you identify these locations as you begin to treat patients.

Subcutaneous Injection Sites

Medications such as epinephrine are injected subcutaneously because of the slow, steady, and dependable absorption associated with that method. The hypodermic needle is inserted into a "pinch" of skin located on the proximal arm, lateral thigh, and, in some cases, the abdomen (as shown in the illustration on page 401 of the textbook). Examine each of these areas on yourself or a friend and locate possible administration sites where you can easily pinch the skin and feel it separate from the muscular tissue below. Inspect the tissue to assure it is free of superficial blood vessels, nerves, and tendons, and avoid areas of bruising, scar tissue, or tattoos.

Intramuscular Injection Sites

Medications such as glucagon and morphine are administered into the muscular tissue because it has both the ability to accept a relatively large (2 to more than 5 ml) amount of the drug and a moderate and predictable absorption rate. A hypodermic needle is inserted directly (at an angle of 90 degrees to the skin surface) through the skin and subcutaneous tissue and into the muscle mass directly beneath. Muscle masses for IM medication administration are chosen carefully to reduce the risk of injecting the drug into a blood vessel or nerve. Common IM sites include the deltoid muscle, the dorsal gluteal muscle, the vastus lateralis muscle and the rectus femoris muscle. These muscle locations are diagrammed on page 404 of your textbook. Palpate each muscle on yourself and a friend to identify the proper locations for IM needle insertions and medication administration. You should be able to feel the firm muscle mass as pictured on page 404 and locate the safe regions to inject medications. Avoid areas of scar tissue and bruises and try to select ones that are free of superficial blood vessels.

Intravenous Injection Sites

Most medications during prehospital care are administered through the intravenous route. This route allows rapid introduction of a drug into the bloodstream, where it is mixed with blood and then distributed throughout the body. The most common venipuncture sites include the veins of the back of the hand, the arm, the antecubital fossa, and the legs and the external jugular vein (see page 408 of the textbook). It is preferable to initiate an IV cannulation with the smallest vein needed at the most distal site, because infiltration or blood vessel injury limits the usefulness of the vein distal to the injury. Obtain a venous constricting band and place it just proximal to the area you will examine for veins. Wait a few seconds until the veins engorge with blood and become more prominent. Then look at the skin below the band for a prominent bump along the course of the vein and a possible bluish discoloration due to the accumulation of blood. Palpate the vessel and appreciate the spongy feel of the blood-filled tube. As you collapse the vessel with your finger pressure, you should feel it compress easily and form a hollow depression beneath your finger. Close your eyes and palpate a region, trying to locate veins by touch. In many patients you will not see the prominence of veins and may only have the characteristic feel of the skin's surface to go by. Palpate the antecubital fossa to locate the antecubital vein. Note that it is rather central in the fold of the elbow and has the spongy feel. This vessel may be the only one you can locate on the patient with severe hypovolemia.

Stand in front of a mirror and look for the external jugular vein. Turn your head to the side and place digital pressure on the jugular vein just above the clavicle. The vein should initially be collapsed and difficult to see in a standing patient, but occluding the vein should cause it to rapidly engorge and become prominent. Notice the course the vein takes as it travels down from the angle of the jaw to the clavicle.

Intraosseous Injection Sites

When other injection sites are unavailable in pediatric, geriatric, and adult patients, an alternative site is the tibia (intraosseous). This site has the advantages of permitting the injection of any intravenous drug or fluid and of being easily located when the patient is otherwise in vascular collapse and the veins are very difficult to find. It is only used when another intravenous site cannot be established. Two sites are used, the proximal site for the pediatric patient and the distal site for the adult or geriatric patient (see page 443 of the textbook). Locate the proximal site by identifying the prominent bump at the top of the tibia (the tibial tuberosity) and then locating the flat surface one to two finger widths below and medial to it. Locate the distal site by locating the medial malleolus (the medial prominence of the ankle) and then the flat surface one to two finger widths above and anterior to it (medial to the anterior tibial crest).

CHAPTER 4

✳

Venous Access and Medication Administration

Part 3: Medical Mathematics

Review of Chapter Objectives

After reading this part of the chapter, you should be able to:

1. **Review mathematical principles, equivalents, and conversions.**　　**pp. 339–342**

   The metric system's three fundamental units are grams, meters, and liters. If you know the prefixes and their numeric equivalents, you can easily convert measurements to smaller or larger units. To convert to a smaller unit multiply the original measurement by the numerical equivalent of the smaller measurement's prefix. To convert a measurement to a larger unit, divide the original measurement by the numerical equivalent of the smaller measurement's prefix.

   The metric system has replaced the traditional apothecary and household systems of measure although there are still some occasional holdovers that you may run into. The International thermometric scale measures temperature in degrees Celsius. The centigrade is slightly different from Celsius, yet based on a similar system of 100 equal parts. The more popular Fahrenheit measurement is still used but not the basis for medicine. Thus the EMT-I should learn to convert from Fahrenheit to Celsius and back again.

2. **Calculate oral and parenteral drug dosages for all emergency medications administered to adults, infants, and children.**　　**pp. 343–345**

   To calculate basic drug dosage, either oral or parenteral, you need to know the desired dose, the dose on hand, and the volume on hand. The desired dose is the specific quantity of medication needed. Dosages may be standard or calculated according to body weight or age. Concentration refers to weight per volume. A liquid medication's concentration is the drug's weight per volume of liquid in which it is dissolved. From the concentration, you can determine the dosage on hand and the volume on hand. Because you cannot see the desired dose dissolved in liquid, you must convert its weight to volume using the formula:

   $$\text{Volume to be administered} = \frac{\text{Volume on hand (desired dose)}}{\text{Dosage on hand}}$$

   Remember to express all weight and volume measurements with the same metric prefix.

©2004 Pearson Education, Inc.
Intermediate Emergency Care: Principles & Practice

3. Calculate intravenous infusion rates for adults, infants, and children. pp. 345–346

To deliver fluid or medication through an IV infusion, you must calculate the correct infusion rate in drops per minute. To calculate the correct IV infusion rate you must first know the administration tubing's drip chamber factor, as well as the volume on hand, desired dose, and dosage on hand. The correct formula to use is as follows:

$$\text{Drops/minute} = \frac{\text{Volume on hand} \times \text{drop} \times \text{drip factor} \times \text{desired dose}}{\text{Dosage on hand}}$$

Fluids being administered, either with or without medication, require a specific period of time to infuse. To calculate the time to infuse the following formula is used:

$$\text{Drops/minute} = \frac{\text{Volume to be administered (drip factor)}}{\text{Time in minutes}}$$

Remember that the dosages in infants and children are weight dependent and your calculation of their weight should be accurate.

SPECIAL PROJECT

PHARMACOLOGY (DRIP AND DRUG) MATH

Guide to Easier Drug Calculations

While there might be more rapid systems to calculate drip rates and concentrations, the following step-wise approach is designed to help you understand the math so you are able to solve almost any problem. While math is an essential skill for the EMT-I, most drip calculations are simple, standard, and easy to perform once you become familiar with the drugs and drip rates used in your system.

STEP I: Identify all known elements.

Elements for most drug dose calculations:

C = Concentration (g, mg, or µg per ml)
Dd = Desired dose
Va = Volume to be administered
Dh = Weight (Dose on hand) (g, mg, or µg)
Vh = Volume on hand (convert to ml)

Elements for most drip calculations:

R = Rate (either in gtts/min, gtts/min, or ml/min)
V = Volume (convert to ml)
T = Time (convert to minutes)
D = Drip conversion (gtts per ml)

STEP II: Select the proper formula.

The element that you don't know (and need to find) should be equal to the remainder of the formula.

Concentration = Dose on hand/Volume on hand   C = Dh/Vh
Dose on hand = Volume on hand × Concentration   Dh = Vh × C
Volume on hand = Dose on hand/Concentration   Vh = Dh/C

©2004 Pearson Education, Inc.
Intermediate Emergency Care: Principles & Practice

$$\text{Volume to be administered} = \frac{\text{Volume on hand} \times \text{Desired dose}}{\text{Dosage on hand}} \qquad Va = \frac{Vh \times Dd}{Dh}$$

$$\text{Dose on hand} = \frac{\text{Volume on hand} \times \text{Desired dose}}{\text{Volume to be administered}} \qquad Dh = \frac{Vh \times Dd}{Va}$$

$$\text{Desired dose} = \frac{\text{Volume to be administered} \times \text{Dosage on hand}}{\text{Volume on hand}} \qquad Dd = \frac{Va \times Dh}{Vh}$$

$$\text{Volume on hand} = \frac{\text{Volume to be administered} \times \text{Dosage on hand}}{\text{Desired dose}} \qquad Vh = \frac{Va \times Dh}{Dd}$$

Rate = Volume/Time (R = V/T)

Volume = Rate $\times$ Time (V = R $\times$ T)

Time = Volume/Rate (T = V/R)

STEP III: Convert all variables into common terms.

Use the drip conversion figure or other conversion formula to convert all values to metric and standard values.

Rate—into milliliters or milligrams/minute

Volume—into milliliters

Concentration—into milligrams/milliliter

Time—into minutes

Weight—into milligrams

STEP IV: Plug in the known values.

Complete the formula, inserting the values identified in Step I.

STEP V: Cancel out labels.

Cross multiply labels to cancel them out. The result should leave you with the label in terms of the unknown value.

$$\text{Volume} = \frac{\text{Rate} \times \text{Time}}{\text{min}} = \frac{X \text{ ml} \times Y \text{ } \cancel{\text{min}}}{\cancel{\text{min}}} = X \text{ ml} \times Y = X \times Y \text{ ml}$$

STEP VI: Do the mathematical operations.

Multiply, divide, add, or subtract as necessary.

$$3 \times 7 = 21 \qquad 3/7 = 0.43 \qquad 7 + 3 = 10 \qquad 7 - 3 = 4$$

STEP VII: Apply any needed conversions.

Use the mathematical conversions needed, such as the drip conversion, to determine the final answer. Ensure that your answer is provided in the form and label the question asks for.

$$\frac{X \text{ ml/min}}{\text{min}} \text{ using a } \frac{Y \text{ gtts/ml}}{\text{ml}} = X \text{ ml} \times \text{gtts} = \frac{X \times Y \text{ gtts}}{\text{min}} = X \times Y \text{ gtts/min}$$

There are two particular types of math used in prehospital care. One deals with continuous intravenous infusions (drip math) and the other deals with parenteral bolus or enteral administration (drug math). Included within this workbook are exercises for drip and drug math.

©2004 Pearson Education, Inc.
Intermediate Emergency Care: Principles & Practice

DRIP MATH WORKSHEET 1

Formulas

Rate = Volume/Time   ml/min = gtts per min/gtts per ml
Volume = Rate × Time   gtts/min = ml per min × gtts per ml
Time = Volume/Rate   ml = gtts/gtts per ml

Please complete the following drip math problems.

1. You are running a D_5W drip (60 gtts/ml) into a patient at 15 gtts/min. During a 25-minute trip to the hospital, how much fluid would you infuse?

    R - 15
    V =
    T - 25
    D - 60

    R×T $15 \times 25 = \frac{375}{60}$

2. Medical direction requests that you infuse 250 ml of a solution during a 1 hour transport. What rate do you need to set:

    A. for a 60 gtts/ml infusion set?

    R -
    V - 250
    T - 60
    D - 60

    $\frac{250}{60} = 4.17 \times 60$

    B. for a 10 gtts/ml infusion set?

    R -
    V - 250
    T - 60
    D - 10

    $\frac{250}{60} = 4.17 \times 10 = 41.70$

3. If a 50 ml bag of normal saline is hung and running through a 45 gtts/ml administration set at 32 drops per minute, how long will the fluid last?

    R - 32
    V - 50
    T -
    D - 45

    $32 = \frac{50 \times 45 ml}{time}$

4. If you are running a macro drip (10 gtts/ml) at 4 drops per second, how much fluid could you infuse in 45 minutes?

    R - 240
    V -
    T - 45
    D - 10

    $240 \times 45 = 10,800$
    $10,800 =$

5. Medical direction orders you to infuse 1.5 ml of a solution every minute. What drip rate would you set:

    A. with a 60 gtts/ml set?

    B. with a 45 gtts/ml set?

    C. with a 10 gtts/ml set?

DRUG MATH WORKSHEET 1

Formulas

Concentration = Dose on hand/Volume on hand $\qquad$ C = Dh/Vh

Dose on hand = Volume on hand × Concentration $\qquad$ Dh = Vh × C

Volume on hand = Dose on hand/Concentration $\qquad$ Vh = Dh/C

$$\text{Volume to be administered} = \frac{\text{Volume on hand} \times \text{Desired dose}}{\text{Dose on hand}} \qquad Va = \frac{Vh \times Dd}{Dh}$$

$$\text{Dose on hand} = \frac{\text{Volume on hand} \times \text{Desired dose}}{\text{Volume to be administered}} \qquad Dh = \frac{Vh \times Dd}{Va}$$

$$\text{Desired dose} = \frac{\text{Volume to be administered} \times \text{Dose on hand}}{\text{Volume on hand}} \qquad Dd = \frac{Va \times Dh}{Vh}$$

$$\text{Volume on hand} = \frac{\text{Volume to be administered} \times \text{Dose on hand}}{\text{Desired dose}} \qquad Vh = \frac{Va \times Dh}{Dd}$$

1 kg = 2.2 lb $\qquad$ 1 g = 1,000 mg $\qquad$ 1 mg = 1,000 μg

Please complete the following drug math problems.

1. What volume of atropine, provided as 1 mg in 5 ml, would you administer to provide 0.5 mg of drug to the patient?

2. The medical direction physician asks you to administer 40 mg of furosemide to a patient. It comes in an ampule with 80 mg in 4 ml. What volume will you administer?

3. What volume of epinephrine would you administer to provide a patient with 1 mg of the drug:

   A. if provided as a 1:1,000 solution? (1 g/1,000 ml)

   B. if provided as a 1:10,000 solution? (1 g/10,000 ml)

4. Protocol calls for the administration of 0.2 mg/kg of adenosine for a pediatric patient. Your patient weighs 6 kilograms, and the drug is supplied in a vial with 6 mg in 2 ml. What volume would you administer to your patient?

CHAPTER 5

✳

Airway Management and Ventilation

Review of Chapter Objectives

After reading this chapter, you should be able to:

1. **Review the anatomy and physiology of the respiratory system, specifically the upper and lower airway.** **(see Chapter 2, pp. 200–213)**

2. **Define the terms hypoxia, hypoxemia, pulsus paradoxus, gag reflex, and gastric distention.** **pp. 352, 354, 355, 367, 370**

   These terms are defined as followed:
   - **Hypoxia** is a decrease in cellular oxygen levels characterized by cyanosis.
   - **Hypoxemia** is an abnormally low arterial blood oxygen level.
   - **Pulsus paradoxus** is an abnormal drop in the BP more than 10 mm Hg occurring only during inspiration.
   - **Gag reflex** is the involuntary reflex to swallow and protect the glottic opening with the epiglottis when the back of the throat is stimulated. This reflex is lost in some patients with an altered mental state.
   - **Gastric distention** is the swelling of the stomach due to excessive fluid, food, or gas which can often lead to regurgitation and or vomiting. It can also put pressure underneath the diaphragm reducing the respiratory excursion during resuscitation. To limit or prevent gastric distention ventilate the patient with slow breaths that do not contain excessive volume and properly open the airway.

3. **Explain the primary objective of airway maintenance.** **p. 350**

   The primary objective of airway maintenance is to keep the airway open and clear (patent) so that oxygen can be carried to and carbon dioxide carried away from the alveoli and the capillary beds of the pulmonary tissue.

4. **Identify commonly neglected prehospital skills related to the airway.** **pp. 358–360**

   The manual maintenance of the airway, using the head-tilt/chin-lift or jaw-thrust maneuver, is one of the most important but often neglected prehospital airway skills. Proper use of these techniques helps ensure an adequate airway early in the care process.

5. **List factors that decrease oxygen concentrations in the blood and increase or decrease carbon dioxide production in the body.** **p. 352**

   Respiratory emergencies pose an immediate life threat to the patient. Respiratory difficulty may be due to airway obstruction, injury to the upper or lower airway structures, inadequate ventilation caused by worsening of an underlying lung disease and fatigue, or central nervous system problems that threaten the airway or respiratory effort.

6. Describe how to measure oxygen and carbon dioxide in the blood. pp. 357–360

Pulse oximetry is a non-invasive monitoring of the arterial oxygenation of the skin. It accurately reflects the oxygen delivery to the end organs, giving an ongoing evaluation of circulation and respiration. In prehospital care, the oximeter is quick and easy to use and provides an accurate and constant evaluation of the cardiorespiratory system.

Capnography is the measurement of exhaled carbon dioxide concentrations. Devices such as the end-tidal carbon dioxide detectors are commonly used to assess the proper placement of endotracheal tubes. Higher concentrations of carbon dioxide change the color of a sensitive paper or the digital readout of an electronic device.

7. List causes of upper airway obstruction and respiratory disease, and describe the modified forms of respiration. pp. 350–352, 354

Upper airway obstruction can be caused by interference with air movement through the upper airway. The tongue, foreign bodies, vomitus, blood, or teeth can all obstruct the upper airway. Patients with obstruction, yet adequate air exchange, can cough effectively; those with poor air exchange cannot. They often emit a high-pitched noise while inhaling (stridor), and their skin may be cyanotic. They also have increased breathing difficulty as well as choking, gagging, dyspnea, or dysphonia (difficulty speaking).

When assessing the patient with breathing difficulty observe for the following modified forms of respiration:
- **Coughing** is a forceful exhalation of a large volume of air from the lungs.
- **Sneezing** is a sudden forceful exhalation from the nose.
- **Hiccoughing** is a sudden inspiration caused by spasmodic contraction of the diaphragm with spastic closure of the glottis.
- **Sighing** is a slow, deep, involuntary inspiration followed by a prolonged expiration which hyperinflates the lungs to reexpands the atelectatic alveoli.
- **Grunting** is a forceful expiration that occurs against a partially closed epiglottis indicating respiratory distress.

8. Identify types of oxygen cylinders and pressure regulators (including a high-pressure regulator and a therapy regulator), and explain safety considerations of oxygen storage and delivery. p. 360

Oxygen is supplied in aluminum or steel compressed gas tanks in 400 liter (D), 660 liter (E), or 3,450 liter (M) volumes. Regulators are either high-pressure, which are used to transfer oxygen at high pressures from tank to tank, or therapy regulators, which are used for delivering oxygen to patients. The default pressure for therapy regulators is 50 psi.

Always handle oxygen cylinders carefully. Make sure they are properly secured so they do not drop and break the regulator. Oxygen cylinders are pressurized and can cause considerable damage. They should be hand tightened and not stored near any flammable substances. Make sure your cylinders have been hydrostat tested and are not allowed to completely empty. Check with your EMS agency on their SOP on refilling tanks.

9. Describe supplemental oxygen delivery devices, including their indications, contraindications, advantages, disadvantages, complications, liter flow range and concentrations of delivered oxygen. pp. 360–361

Supplemental oxygen devices include: nasal cannula, Venturi mask, simple face mask, partial rebreather mask, nonrebreather mask, and a small volume nebulizer. Specifics about these devices follow below:
- A nasal cannula provides up to 40% at flow rates up to 6 L/min. It should not be set at any higher flow as it may cause damage to the nasal mucous membranes. This device is well tolerated for long periods of time.
- A Venturi mask is a high-flow face mask designed to deliver precise oxygen concentrations regardless of the patient's rate and depth of breathing. Since the device is very accurate (24%, 28%, 35%, or 40%), it works well with COPD patients.

©2004 Pearson Education, Inc.
Intermediate Emergency Care: Principles & Practice

- A simple face mask is indicated in patients requiring moderate to high concentrations of oxygen in the 40% to 60% range when set at 6 to 10 L/min.
- A partial rebreather mask is indicated for the patients requiring moderate to high oxygen concentrations when satisfactory clinical results are not obtained with the simple face mask. The maximal flow rate is 10 L/min.
- A nonrebreather mask has one-way side ports and an attached reservoir bag so exhaled air exits the mask and inhaled air comes directly from the reservoir of 80–95% oxygen when the flow is set at 15 L/min.
- A small volume nebulizer is designed to deliver 3–5 cc of fluid medication that is delivered in aerosol form to the patient by the pressurized oxygen gas flowing through the fluid. This is often used as a bronchodilator treatment for an asthmatic patient.

10. Describe the use, advantages, and disadvantages of an oxygen humidifier.   **p. 361**

An oxygen humidifier is a device that has a sterile water reservoir though which the oxygen gas is bubbled up. This mist is especially helpful to the patient with croup, epiglottitis, or bronchiolitis as well as those patients receiving long-term oxygen therapy.

11. Explain the risk of infection to EMS providers associated with ventilation.   **pp. 366–368, 379, 396**

The EMT-I should always use BSI when ventilating or suctioning a patient. Oral secretions may contain infectious pathogens that can transmit communicable diseases such as hepatitis. If a patient has a productive cough he may transmit TB. Always follow your agency's exposure control plan and use your personal protective equipment when using airway adjuncts and ventilating a patient.

12. Describe the indications, contraindications, advantages, disadvantages, complications, and techniques for ventilating a patient: mouth-to-mouth; mouth-to-nose; mouth-to-mask; one-, two-, and three-person bag-valve mask; flow-restricted, oxygen-powered ventilation device; and automatic transport ventilator (ATV).   **pp. 361–365**

The EMT-I is taught to ventilate a patient several ways. It is helpful to know the advantages and disadvantages of each technique listed below:

- Mouth-to-mouth and mouth-to-nose ventilation are the most basic methods of rescue ventilation indicated when no other devices are available. They require no special equipment and both allow an adequate seal to provide effective ventilation with expired air that has approximately 17% oxygen. The major drawback is the potential for exposing the rescuer to communicable diseases through contact with blood and other body fluids.
- Mouth-to-mask ventilation is easy to employ, and many of the disposable masks are small enough that they can be carried in a pocket or a purse. Its advantage is that it can be used with a two-handed seal and adequate ventilation volume can be given to the patient. Many of the units have the ability to provide supplemental oxygen at a flow rate of 10 L/min, which will deliver approximately 50% to the patient. The rescuer should always be careful not to over inflate and potentially cause gastric distention to the patient.
- Bag-valve-mask devices have improved over the years. The most recent models have built-in colormetric capnometers on them. It is important to select the appropriate size BVM for the patient (neonatal, child, or adult) and to assure that there is no pediatric pop-off valve engaged in the BVM. Each BVM should be assembled with the appropriate oxygen reservoir system because without any oxygen attached the BVM will only deliver room air (21% oxygen). If the oxygen tubing is attached without the benefit of the complete reservoir system, it will only deliver approximately 60% to 70% oxygen. Since ventilated patients or those requiring ventilation assistance with a BVM need to have the highest concentration of oxygen available, the complete BVM reservoir system should be used. Doing so usually produces approximately 90% to 95% oxygen concentration at a liter flow of 15 L/min. The EMT-I doing the ventilations must carefully observe the chest for rise and fall with each inflation. If there is any leak

of gas around the mask, either felt or heard, the airway must be repositioned and the mask resealed because even small leaks will produce large volume deficits.

Using the BVM by yourself is difficult because your hands will tire unless the patient has an ET tube inserted. In that case it is not necessary to seal the mask. Studies have shown that the best way to use a BVM is with a minimum of two rescuers; one rescuer would seal the mask with two hands, and the other rescuer would squeeze the bag of the BVM while administering slow breaths. If there is trauma involved, a jaw-thrust maneuver is needed and a third rescuer will be needed to assist in stabilizing the head and neck. Be very careful not to squeeze too fast and produce high pressure "bursts" of air as this tends to produce high airway pressures and increase the chances of gastric distention. Remember to open the airway fully and ventilate slowly just like a patient actually breathes.

- Flow-restricted, oxygen-powered ventilation devices are sometimes called demand valves or manually triggered oxygen-powered ventilation devices. Such a device will deliver 100% oxygen to a patient at its highest flow rates (40 liters per minute maximum). The device can be attached to a mask or an ET tube and utilizes high pressure tubing that works off an oxygen regulator's high pressure port. It is important that the operator closely watch the chest rise and fall when ventilating the patient as it is very easy to over inflate and cause barotrauma, gastric distention, or regurgitation. This device is not recommended for use in patients under the age of 16 and should be used with care in patients who are intubated.

- Automatic transport ventilators are now available for use in prehospital care. They are designed to maintain a minute volume better than a BVM and often have an adjustable tidal volume and ventilatory rate. These devices can be particularly helpful for patients being transported between critical care units who need to be ventilated at a specific rate and volume. During a cardiac arrest situation, the ATV does allow chest compressions to be interposed between mechanical breaths.

13. Compare the ventilation techniques used for an adult patient to those used for pediatric patients. pp. 363–364

The differences in the pediatric patient's anatomy require some variation in ventilation technique. The child's flat nasal bridge makes mask seal more difficult. Simply pressing against the mask may obstruct the airway which is more compressible than an adult's. For BVM ventilation the bag size depends on the child's age. Consider using a length-based resuscitation tape (Broselow tape) to help determine the appropriate devices to use for resuscitating a child.

The mask seal is best achieved with a two-rescuer BVM technique using the jaw-thrust to maintain an open airway. Place the mask over the child's mouth and nose and avoid compressing the eyes. Using one hand, place your thumb on the mask at the apex and your index finger on the mask at the chin (C-grip). Apply gentle pressure downward on the mask to establish an adequate seal. Maintain the airway by lifting the bony prominence of the chin with the remaining fingers forming an E under the jaw. Avoid placing pressure on the soft area under the chin.

14. Define, identify, and describe a tracheostomy, a laryngectomy, a stoma, a tracheostomy tube, and how to ventilate and manage the airway of a patient with a stoma. pp. 397–398

Often patients who have had a laryngectomy or tracheostomy breathe through a stoma. These patients frequently have tracheostomy tubes, which consist of an inner and outer cannula, in place to keep the soft tissue stoma open. If a patient with a stoma needs ventilation, the bystander may use the mouth-to-stoma technique, while rescue personnel will generally use the BVM device. If you use the mouth-to-stoma technique, it is preferable to use a pocket mask to cover the stoma for protection from communicable disease. For either technique, locate the stoma site and expose it. Obtain a tight seal around the stoma site, and check for adequate ventilation. A pediatric mask usually works best. Be sure to seal the mouth and nose if you note air leaking from these sites which would indicate the patient was a partial laryngectomy since in a complete laryngectomy the trachea actually ends at the stoma.

15. **Describe a complete airway obstruction and related maneuvers.** pp. 350–352

Airway obstruction may be either partial or complete. When you cannot feel or hear airflow from the nose and mouth, or when the patient cannot speak (aphonia), breathe, or cough, his airway is completely obstructed. He will quickly become unconscious and die if you do not relieve the obstruction. The basic foreign body airway maneuvers should be followed according to the current standards of the American Heart Association. The procedure will involve a series of abdominal thrusts or chest thrusts depending on the age of the patient and if the patient is pregnant or obese.

16. **Define and explain the implications of partial airway obstruction with good and poor air exchange.** pp. 350–351

Obstruction of the airway by a foreign object or swelling may range from minor to complete. If the airway obstruction permits speech and coughing and you do not notice skin color changes, respiration is probably adequate and intervention may not be needed. However, if the patient has serious dyspnea, cannot speak or cough, is choking or gagging, and you notice skin color changes, intervention is necessary. Continued inadequate respiration will lead to increasing hypoxia.

   Causes of upper airway obstruction include:

- **Tongue**
  The most common cause of airway obstruction is the tongue. In the unconscious person or the supine patient, the lack of muscle tone allows the tongue to rest against the posterior pharynx and thereby obstruct the airway.
- **Foreign body aspiration**
  Large, poorly chewed lumps of food and objects aspirated by children commonly account for airway obstruction. The victim will often grasp his or her throat, a universal distress signal.
- **Laryngeal spasm**
  The glottis is the smallest part of the airway and may be responsible for obstruction secondary to spasm. Spasm may be caused by stimulation by a foreign object as during endotracheal intubation.
- **Laryngeal edema**
  As the glottis is the narrowest part of the adult airway, swelling will rapidly reduce the airway lumen size and restrict breathing. Restriction and obstruction may be caused by anaphylaxis, epiglottitis, or the inhalation of toxic substances, superheated steam, or smoke.
- **Trauma**
  Physical injury to the structures of the upper airway may result in loose objects such as the teeth, tissue, or clotted blood obstructing the airway. Further, blunt or penetrating trauma may result in collapse of the airway due to fracture or displacement of the larynx or trachea. Soft-tissue swelling may also restrict the lumen of the airway.

17. **Describe laryngoscopy for the removal of a foreign body airway obstruction.** p. 386

When the basic foreign body airway maneuvers are unsuccessful, the EMT- Intermediate should attempt direct laryngoscopy with a laryngoscope to visualize the epiglottis. It may be possible to see the obstruction, such as a bolus of meat, and then go in with a device, such as the Magill forceps to remove the piece of meat. This procedure should be done quickly in order to prevent the patient from going into cardiac arrest.

18. **Identify the different types of suction equipment, including catheters.** pp. 365–366

Many different suctioning devices are available. They may be handheld, oxygen-powered, battery-powered, or mounted (nonportable). The most commonly used suction catheters are either hard/rigid catheters (Yankauer or tonsil tip) or soft catheters (whistle tip).

19. **Explain the purpose, indications, techniques, and special considerations for suctioning the upper airway.** pp. 365–367

Suctioning is the use of pressures that are less than atmospheric to draw fluids and semi-fluids out of the airway. It should be used any time it can effectively remove material from the airway. Continuous suctioning should be avoided because it draws against the patient's ventilation

©2004 Pearson Education, Inc.
Intermediate Emergency Care: Principles & Practice

attempts and generally interrupts artificial ventilation of the apneic patient. Suctioning can be provided by an electric or a mechanical device.

20. Describe the technique of tracheobronchial suctioning in the intubated patient. pp. 366–367

You may have to suction some patients through an endotracheal tube or a tracheostomy tube to remove secretions or mucous plugs that can cause respiratory distress. You will need to use a sterile catheter and use a sterile technique to avoid contaminating the pulmonary system. Use only soft-tip catheters to avoid damaging structures, and be certain to prelubricate it. Once you have preoxygenated the patient with 100% oxygen, lubricate the catheter tip with a water-soluble gel and gently insert it until you feel resistance. Then apply suction for 10–15 seconds while extracting the catheter. Ventilation and oxygenation are essential immediately following this procedure.

21. Describe the indications, contraindications, advantages, disadvantages, complications, equipment, and technique for inserting a nasogastric tube and an orogastric tube. p. 367

Nasogastric tube insertion is recommended for the conscious patient, because it permits him or her to talk more easily. It is contraindicated if there is danger of skull fracture as the tube's placement could cause further injury. Both oral and nasal techniques may be used for gastric decompression when patient ventilation is restricted or there is danger of aspiration. The tube is measured for depth of insertion by measuring from the epigastrium to the angle of the jaw and then to the nares. Use a topical anesthetic spray, and then lubricate the distal tip and insert the tube through the nares and along the nasal floor or through the mouth along the midline. Advance the tube, encourage patient swallowing if possible, and then introduce 30 to 50 mL of air while listening over the epigastrium. The absence of gastric sounds and the inability to speak suggests tracheal placement and the need to re-attempt insertion.

22. Describe manual airway maneuvers. pp. 368–370

- Head-tilt/chin-lift maneuver
  To execute the head-tilt/chin-lift airway maneuver, the rescuer places one hand on the patient's forehead, gently tilting the head back, while the other engages the mandible, displacing it anteriorly.
- Jaw-thrust maneuver
  During the jaw-thrust (or the triple-airway) maneuver, the rescuer places his fingers on the patient's lateral mandible, displacing it anteriorly while the thumbs displace it inferiorly. The maneuver may rotate the head and extend the neck. If spinal injury is suspected, the head should not be tilted backward (use the modified jaw-thrust).
- Modified jaw-thrust maneuver
  The modified jaw-thrust (for the trauma patient) requires that the jaw-thrust maneuver be modified by manually securing the head in a neutral position while the mandible is displaced forward.

23. Describe the indications, contraindications, advantages, disadvantages, complications, and techniques for inserting the oropharyngeal and nasopharyngeal airways. pp. 370–374

The oropharyngeal airway (OPA) is easily placed in the mouth of a patient who does not have a gag reflex to help hold the tongue away from the back of the throat. When properly positioned, this device has several advantages:

- It is easy to place using proper technique.
- Air can pass around and through the device.
- It helps prevent obstruction by the teeth and lips.
- It helps manage unconscious patients who are breathing spontaneously or need mechanical ventilation.
- It makes suction of the pharynx easier, as a large suction catheter can pass on either side of the device.

- It serves as an effective bite block in case of seizures or to protect the endotracheal tube.

The disadvantages to the OPA are as follow:
- It does not isolate the trachea or prevent aspiration.
- It cannot be inserted when the teeth are clenched. It may obstruct the airway if not inserted properly.
- It is easily dislodged.
- Return of the gag reflex may produce vomiting.

To insert the OPA, simply select the proper size that extends from the center of the mouth to the angle of the jaw or the corner of the mouth to the earlobe. Then, provided the patient has no neck trauma, hyperextend the neck and open the mouth to assure there are no visible obstructions present. Next assure the patient has effective ventilation volume. If indicated, ventilate with 100% oxygen. Grasp the patient's jaw and lift anteriorly. With your other hand, hold the airway at its proximal end and insert it into the patient's mouth. Make sure the curve is reversed, with the tip pointing toward the roof of the mouth. Once the tip reaches the level of the soft palate, gently rotate the airway 180 degrees until it comes to rest over the tongue. Verify appropriate position of the airway. Clear breath sounds and chest rise indicate correct placement. Hyperventilate the patient with 100 % oxygen, if needed.

The nasopharyngeal airway (NPA) is an uncuffed tube made of soft rubber or plastic. The NPA follows the natural curvature of the nasopharynx and may be used in patients with altered mental states who still have a gag reflex. The NPA's advantages are:
- It can be rapidly inserted and safely placed blindly.
- It bypasses the tongue, providing a patent airway.
- You may use it in the presence of a gag reflex.
- You may use it when the patient has suffered injury to his oral cavity (anything from trauma to the mandible to significant soft tissue damage to the tongue or pharynx).
- You may suction through it.
- You may use it when the patient's teeth are clenched.

The disadvantages of the NPA are as follows:
- It is smaller than the OPA.
- It does not isolate the trachea.
- It is difficult to suction through it.
- It may cause severe nosebleeds if inserted too forcefully.
- It may cause pressure necrosis of the nasal mucosa.
- It may kink and clog, obstructing the airway.
- Inserting it is difficult if nasal damage (old or new) is present.
- You may not use it if the patient has or is suspected to have a basilar skull fracture.

To insert the NPA, select the proper size NPA which is slightly smaller than the patient's nostril. If the patient has no history of trauma, then hyperextend his head and neck. Assure or maintain effective ventilation. If needed, hyperventilate the patient with 100% oxygen. Lubricate the exterior of the tube with a water-soluble gel to prevent trauma during insertion. If possible, use a lidocaine gel in the alert or responsive patient; its anesthetic effect on the mucosa will make insertion more comfortable. Push gently up on the tip of the nose and pass the tube into the right nostril. If the septum is deviated and you cannot easily insert the tube into the right nostril, use the left nostril. With the bevel oriented toward the septum, insert the tube gently along the nasal floor, parallel to the mouth. Verify appropriate position of the airway. Clear breath sounds and chest rise indicate correct placement. Also, feel at the airway's proximal end for airflow on expiration. Hyperventilate the patient with 100% oxygen, if needed.

24. Describe Sellick's maneuver and the use of cricoid pressure during intubation.   pp. 369–370

To help prevent regurgitation and reduce gastric distention, Sellick's maneuver applies gentle pressure posteriorly on the anterior cricoid cartilage. Since the esophagus lies just behind the cricoid cartilage, this maneuver will effectively close the esophagus to pressures as high as 100 cm/H2O. It also facilitates intubation by moving the larynx posterior, bringing it into view.

25. Differentiate endotracheal intubation from other methods of advanced airway management. p. 374

Endotracheal intubation is considered the gold standard of airway management. It is the preferred method of airway management as it is the only procedure that effectively isolates the trachea. In some EMS systems endotracheal intubation is not available. These systems use other airway devices such as the Esophageal Tracheal CombiTube (ETC), Pharyngeo-tracheal Lumen (PtL) airway, or Laryngeal Mask Airway (LMA).

26. Describe the indications, contraindications, advantages, disadvantages, and complications of endotracheal intubation. pp. 379–382

Indications for endotracheal intubation include respiratory or cardiac arrest; unresponsiveness without a gag reflex; inability to protect the airway, resulting in an increased risk of aspiration and obstruction due to foreign bodies, trauma, burns, or anaphylaxis. Endotracheal intubation also improves oxygenation and ventilation in patients with extreme lower airway difficulty. Some lower airway indications include severe respiratory distress due to diseases such as asthma, COPD, CHF, or pneumonia, as well as pneumonia, hemothorax, or hemopneumothorax with respiratory difficulty.

The advantages of endotracheal intubation are that it:
- Isolates the trachea and permits complete control of the airway.
- Impedes gastric distention by channeling air directly into the trachea.
- Eliminates the need to maintain a mask seal.
- Offers a direct route for suctioning of the respiratory passages.
- Permits administration of the medications lidocaine, epinephrine, atropine, and naloxone via the ET tube.

The disadvantages of endotracheal intubation include:
- Requires considerable training and experience.
- Requires specialized equipment.
- Requires direct visualization of the vocal cords.
- Bypasses the upper airway's function of warming, filtering, and humidifying the inhaled air.

Intubation presents a number of potential complications, such as a right main stem intubation or an esophageal intubation. Properly attending to detail and taking appropriate precautions will help you to avoid these problems. Always document proper tube placement and lung sounds with multiple methods before and after every patient movement and use an end tidal CO_2 monitor (capnometer).

27. Describe the visual landmarks for direct laryngoscopy. pp. 382–386

To insert an endotracheal tube, it is necessary to place the patient in the sniffing position and then insert the laryngoscope into the mouth to lift the tongue and mandible anteriorly so the vocal cords can be visualize. If a curved laryngoscope is used, the tip must be placed in the vallecula, which when lifted anteriorly, will help move the epiglottis away from the glottic opening. If a straight blade is used, the epiglottis is actually lifted along with the tongue and jaw as the structures are moved anteriorly to expose the glottic opening. Once the glottic opening is exposed, the vocal cords can be seen and the ET tube is passed about 1–2 cm past the cuff on the tube. If you cannot visualize the vocal cords, the procedure may not be successful.

28. Describe the methods of assessing, confirming, and securing correct placement of an endotracheal tube (ETT). pp. 385–386

The most reliable method of confirming proper ETT placement is direct visualization of its passage through the vocal cords. Following ETT placement, watch to be sure that the patient's chest rises with ventilations. If the ETT is misplaced in the esophagus, the chest will not rise. You should auscultate for breath sounds. Their equal presence over both sides (apices and bases) of the chest and their absence over the epigastrium help to confirm proper ETT placement. It is important to assure proper ETT placement. Allegations of improperly placed endotracheal tubes

are a major reason for EMT-I malpractice suits. Because of this, it is important to verify and document proper ETT placement. In fact, it is ideal to verify and document at least three different indicators of proper placement. These may include:
- Visualization of the tube passing between the cords.
- Presence of bilateral breath sounds.
- Absence of breath sounds.
- Positive end-tidal CO_2 change on capnometer.
- Verification of endotracheal placement by an esophageal detector device.
- Presence of condensation inside the ETT.
- Absence of vomitus inside the ETT.
- Absence of phonation, or vocal sounds, once the tube is placed.

Traditionally ETT have been secured by adhesive tape. It is strongly advised that a commercially available and sterile tube restraint be used to tie the tube in place and keep the ETT from moving from its original

29. Describe the indications, contraindications, advantages, disadvantages, complications, equipment, and technique for extubation.   **pp. 390–391**

Infrequently, an intubated patient will awaken and be intolerant of the ETT. If the patient is clearly able to protect his airway and can accomplish adequate spontaneous respirations and is not under the influence of any sedating agents, and if reassessment indicates the problem that led to ETT is resolved, extubation may be indicated. However, you must consider the high risk of laryngospasm, involuntary closure of the glottis upon extubation, especially in the awake patient. Laryngospasm may prohibit successful reintubation attempts.

To perform field extubation:
- Continue BSI. Ensure patient's oxygenation. A method for accomplishing this in the field is to be certain that the patient's mental status, skin color, and pulse oximetry are optimal on room air with the ETT in place.
- Prepare intubation equipment and suction.
- Confirm patient responsiveness.
- Suction the patient's oropharynx.
- Deflate the ETT cuff.
- Remove the ETT upon cough or expiration.
- Provide supplemental oxygen as indicated.
- Reassess the adequacy of the patient's ventilation and oxygenation.

30. Describe methods of endotracheal intubation in the pediatric patient.   **pp. 386–390**

While the indications, procedures, and precautions for airway management in children are fundamentally the same as in adult, you must take additional precautions and remember several significant differences. These concerns revolve around variances in anatomy.

A straight laryngoscope blade is preferred for most pediatric patients, although straight or curved may be useful for adolescents. A guide for sizing ET tubes is to use the formula ETT size:

(mm) = (Age in years + 16)/4

Also remember that infants and small children have greater vagal tone than adults. Therefore, laryngoscopy and passage of an endotracheal tube are more likely to precipitate a vagal response, dramatically slowing the child's heart rate and decreasing cardiac output and BP. The indications for endotracheal intubation in a pediatric patient are the same as those for adults.

31. Describe the indications, contraindications, advantages, disadvantages, complications, equipment, and techniques for using a dual lumen airway.   **pp. 391–395**

The Esophageal Tracheal CombiTube (ETC) is a dual-lumen airway with a ventilation port for each lumen. The longer, blue port is the distal port; the shorter, clear port is the proximal port, which terminates in the hypopharynx. The ECT has two inflatable cuffs: a 15 ml cuff just proximal to the distal port and a 100 ml cuff just distal to the proximal port. It is inserted blindly through the mouth into the posterior oropharynx and then gently advanced. Upon insertion, one port enters the trachea and the other enters the esophagus. To determine which port has entered the trachea and is to be ventilated, first ventilate the longer external port, since esophageal insertion is highly likely. Now auscultate the chest. If you hear breath sounds over the chest and none over the stomach, continue ventilating through the longer external port. If you hear ventilation sounds over the stomach without breath sounds over the chest, stop ventilating through the longer port and attach the bag-valve device to the shorter port. The distal cuff isolates the distal port, and the larger proximal cuff isolates the proximal port, encouraging air that is insufflated into the hypopharynx to enter the trachea.

Advantages of the ETC include:
- It provides alternative airway control when conventional intubation techniques are unsuccessful or unavailable.
- Insertion is rapid and easy.
- Insertion does not require visualization of the larynx or special equipment.
- The pharyngeal balloon anchors the airway behind the hard palate.
- The patient may be ventilated regardless of tube placement (esophageal or tracheal).
- It significantly diminishes gastric distention and regurgitation.
- It can be used on trauma patients, since the neck can remain in neutral position during insertion and use.
- If the tube is placed in the esophagus, gastric contents can be suctioned for decompression through the distal port.

Disadvantages of the ETC include:
- Suctioning tracheal secretions is impossible when the airway is in the esophagus.
- Placing an endotracheal tube is very difficult with the ETC in place.
- It cannot be used in conscious patients or in those with a gag reflex.
- The cuffs can cause esophageal, tracheal, and hypopharyngeal ischemia.
- It does not isolate and completely protect the trachea.
- It cannot be used in patients with esophageal disease or caustic ingestions.
- It cannot be used with pediatric patients.
- Placement of the CombiTube is not foolproof—errors can be made if assessment skills are not adequate.

32. Describe the special considerations in airway management and ventilation for patients with facial injuries. pp. 386–387

If a patient has facial injuries the airway management techniques must involve in-line manual stabilization of the head and neck and utilize the jaw thrust. To pass an ETT it will be necessary to limit the neck movement and utilize a second rescuer to stabilize the neck and apply a collar. Nasal airways will be contraindicated if the patient had a potential skull fracture. It is essential that the patient's airway be protected especially since the trauma patient will need to be immobilized to a long spine board in the supine position. Should the patient vomit at any time it would be the EMT-I's responsibility to assure the airway would remain patent at all times.

CASE STUDY REVIEW

This study focuses on the variety of techniques that EMT-Is might be called on to employ to ensure the management of a patient's airway and breathing in an emergency situation.

Crystal and Charlie attend a trauma patient with a mechanism of injury suggesting serious internal injuries. They are immediately obligated to employ spinal precautions, requiring that they position the patient's head and neck in the neutral position and maintain that positioning. As they move to the airway evaluation portion of the initial assessment, Crystal hears gurgling and attempts to clear the airway with positioning (displacing the jaw forward while maintaining the spinal immobilization) and suction. Airway maintenance is more difficult in this trauma patient because of the inability to extend his head and neck due to the potential for spine injury. The landmarks for endotracheal intubation are

©2004 Pearson Education, Inc.
Intermediate Emergency Care: Principles & Practice

also more difficult to visualize because the head cannot be brought to the sniffing position and because there is likely to be some blood in the airway. Crystal needs to be very careful to assure and confirm proper tube placement because unrecognized esophageal placement is deadly.

Charles employs Sellick's maneuver, placing posterior pressure on the cartilage ring (cricoid cartilage) at the base of the larynx. This pressure compresses the esophagus between the cricoid cartilage and the vertebral column, holding it closed and thereby preventing any passage of emesis upward and into the pharynx. This procedure will also displace the larynx, somewhat posteriorly, making it easier to visualize during an intubation attempt. Charles must maintain this pressure until the patient is intubated because relaxing it may release emesis into the pharynx.

Once the endotracheal tube is placed, both Charles and Crystal must carefully assure it is properly located. All signs demonstrate that the ventilations are effective, including bilateral and equal lung sounds with each breath, increasing oxygen saturation, and color change from the end-title CO_2 detector. Charles and Crystal will carefully secure the tube in place and note the depth of insertion by recording the number on the side of the endotracheal tube. A real danger in prehospital care is the unnoticed dislodging of an endotracheal tube during C-collar placement, immobilization to the long spine board, movement of the patient to the long spine board, or while loading or unloading the patient from the ambulance. Again, the consequence of unrecognized endotracheal tube displacement is patient death. Crystal and Charles will check the breath sounds, oximetry, and the end-tidal CO_2 detector after each move and frequently during their care and transport.

Crystal employs a glucose test to rule out hypoglycemia, which could account for the unconsciousness and because hypoglycemia is detrimental in the head injury patient.

CONTENT SELF-EVALUATION

MULTIPLE CHOICE

_A_   1. Which of the following is the most common cause of upper airway obstruction?
- A. the tongue
- B. foreign bodies
- C. trauma
- D. laryngeal swelling
- E. aspiration of blood or vomitus

_C_   2. All of the following conditions may cause reduced inspiratory volumes EXCEPT:
- A. pneumothorax.
- B. asthma.
- C. high inspired oxygen concentrations.
- D. respiratory muscle paralysis.
- E. emphysema.

_B_   3. The normal respiratory rate for an adult at rest is:
- A. 8 to 12.
- B. 12 to 20.
- C. 18 to 24.
- D. 24 to 32.
- E. 40 to 60.

_B_   4. Which of the following is a breathing pattern associated with flail chest?
- A. abdominal breathing
- B. paradoxical breathing
- C. diaphragmatic breathing
- D. intercostal retraction
- E. both A and C

_B_   5. It is unlikely that a patient will have significant hypoxia and not display cyanosis.
- A. True
- B. False

_E_   6. Which modified form of respiration is designed to expand alveoli that may have collapsed during periods of inactivity or rest?
- A. coughing
- B. sneezing
- C. hiccoughing
- D. grunting
- E. sighing

_D_ 7. The respiratory pattern that presents with deep and rapid respirations is:
   A. apneustic respirations.
   B. Cheyne-Stokes respirations.
   C. Biot's respirations.
   D. central neurogenic hyperventilation.
   E. agonal respirations.

_A_ 8. Stridor is most commonly associated with:
   A. laryngeal constriction or edema.
   B. the tongue blocking the airway.
   C. narrowing of the bronchioles.
   D. fluids within the airway.
   E. foreign bodies in the lower airway.

_C_ 9. The absence of CO_2 in exhaled air, as identified by a capnometer or end-expiratory CO_2 detector, suggests:
   A. ventilation is not deep enough.
   B. ventilations are not occurring fast enough.
   C. the endotracheal tube may be in the esophagus.
   D. the oxygen percentage of inspired air is insufficient.
   E. all of the above

_C_ 10. Which of the devices listed below delivers the highest concentration of oxygen to the patient?
   A. nasal cannula
   B. simple face mask
   C. nonrebreather mask
   D. Venturi mask
   E. A and D

_D_ 11. Which of the devices below delivers the most controlled concentration of oxygen to a patient?
   A. nasal cannula
   B. simple face mask
   C. nonrebreather mask
   D. Venturi mask
   E. B and C

_D_ 12. The bag-valve mask with an oxygen supply attached and oxygen flowing at 15 L per minute delivers what percentage of oxygen to the patient?
   A. 21 percent
   B. 40 to 60 percent
   C. 60 to 80 percent
   D. 90 to 95 percent
   E. 99.9 percent

_D_ 13. One rescuer bag-valve masking is difficult to perform effectively because:
   A. it is difficult to maintain proper airway positioning.
   B. it is difficult to maintain mask seal.
   C. it is difficult to squeeze the bag.
   D. all of the above
   E. none of the above

_A_ 14. Hazards of using the demand valve to ventilate a patient include all of the following EXCEPT:
   A. oxygen toxicity.
   B. gastric distention.
   C. pulmonary barotrauma.
   D. pneumothorax.
   E. subcutaneous emphysema.

_D_ 15. Which of the following is NOT an advantage of automatic ventilators?
   A. They free a rescuer when the patient is not breathing.
   B. They are convenient and easy to use.
   C. They are dependable.
   D. They can be used on children younger than age 5.
   E. They are lightweight and tolerant to temperature extremes.

©2004 Pearson Education, Inc.
Intermediate Emergency Care: Principles & Practice

_E_ 16. Which of the following is a part of suctioning the stoma patient?
A. pre-oxygenating with 100 percent oxygen
B. injecting 3 mL of saline
C. inserting the catheter until resistance is met
D. withdrawing the catheter while the patient exhales or coughs
E. all of the above

_B_ 17. Which of the following is <u>NOT</u> indicated when suctioning through the endotracheal tube?
A. Insert the catheter until you meet resistance.
B. Suction only during insertion.
C. Pre-oxygenate the patient.
D. Rotate the suction catheter while suctioning.
E. Suction no longer than 10 to 15 seconds.

_C_ 18. Nasogastric tube placement is indicated in a patient:
A. with facial fractures.
B. with a possible basilar skull fracture.
C. who is awake.
D. for whom a relatively large gastric tube is indicated.
E. all of the above

_B_ 19. In the head-tilt/chin-lift maneuver, the fingers under the chin should apply a firm pressure to ensure the jaw remains closed.
A. True
B. False

_C_ 20. The intent behind employing Sellick's maneuver is to:
A. displace the diaphragm.
B. increase venous return.
C. prevent regurgitation.
D. clear an airway obstruction.
E. increase blood flow to the brain.

_D_ 21. Which of the following is an advantage of the nasopharyngeal airway over the oropharyngeal airway?
A. It has a larger diameter.
B. It is easier to insert.
C. It is blocked less frequently by vomitus.
D. It does not stimulate the gag reflex as strongly.
E. It can be used with a BVM.

_B_ 22. Insertion of the nasopharyngeal airway directs the soft rubber tube:
A. directly up and into the nostril.
B. directly along the floor of the nasal cavity.
C. into the left nostril, most frequently.
D. laterally along the side of the nasal cavity.
E. directly into the vallecula space.

_A_ 23. The airway adjunct that acts primarily by displacing the tongue forward is the:
A. oropharyngeal airway.
B. LMA airway.
C. endotracheal tube.
D. nasopharyngeal airway.
E. esophageal gastric tube airway.

_A_ 24. The preferred technique of insertion for the oropharyngeal airway in pediatric patients calls for inserting the airway using a tongue blade without rotating the device.
A. True
B. False

C 25. The airway technique preferred for use with the patient who is unconscious is:
A. the oropharyngeal airway. D. nasotracheal intubation.
B. the nasopharyngeal airway. E. EGTA.
C. endotracheal intubation.

B 26. The light of the laryngoscope should be a bright yellow and flicker slightly when pressure is placed on the blade.
A. True
B. False

C 27. The tip of the curve of the Macintosh laryngoscope blade is designed to fit into the:
A. nasopharynx. D. arytenoid fossa.
B. glottic opening. E. epiglottis.
C. vallecula.

C 28. The laryngoscope blade considered to be best designed for intubation of the pediatric patient is:
A. the Macintosh blade. D. either B or C
B. the curved blade. E. none of the above
C. the straight blade.

B 29. The pilot balloon of the endotracheal tube should be very firm to ensure there is a good seal between the tube and the interior of the trachea.
A. True
B. False

A 30. The major purpose for using a malleable stylet during endotracheal intubation is to:
A. maintain a pre-set curve in the tube.
B. keep the tube's lumen open.
C. stiffen the tube so it can be pushed through the glottis.
D. prevent foreign matter from entering the tube.
E. all of the above

E 31. Which of the following is NOT an indication for endotracheal intubation?
A. respiratory arrest
B. cardiac arrest
C. inability to protect the airway
D. obstruction due to foreign object, swelling, or burns
E. severe epiglottitis

B 32. When using the laryngoscope to visualize the glottis, it is best to use the teeth as a fulcrum to increase your ability to lift the tissue.
A. True
B. False

B 33. To reduce the risk of hypoxia, limit attempts at intubation to no more than:
A. 15 seconds. D. 60 seconds.
B. 30 seconds. E. 80 seconds.
C. 45 seconds.

D 34. Which of the following is NOT an indication for esophageal intubation?
A. absence of chest rise with ventilation
B. gurgling sound over the epigastrium
C. a falling pulse oximetry reading
D. skin color turning pink
E. increasing resistance to ventilatory effort

©2004 Pearson Education, Inc.
Intermediate Emergency Care: Principles & Practice

_E_ 35. Upon placing the endotracheal tube, you hear very faint breath sounds and some gurgling over the epigastric region. You should next:
A. advance the tube slightly.
B. withdraw the tube slightly.
C. inflate the cuff and auscultate again.
D. ventilate more forcibly.
E. remove the tube and re-intubate.

_A_ 36. Upon placing the endotracheal tube in a patient, you determine that you can only auscultate breath sounds on the right side. You should next:
A. withdraw the tube a few centimeters.
B. withdraw the tube completely.
C. pass the tube a few centimeters further.
D. secure the tube and ventilate more aggressively.
E. check the mask seal.

_C_ 37. The purpose of the cuff on the end of the endotracheal tube is to:
A. help guide the tube to its proper location.
B. prevent dislodging of the tube after it is correctly placed.
C. seal the airway.
D. center the tube in the trachea.
E. widen the opening of the vocal cords.

_C_ 38. What volume of air is used to inflate the cuff of an endotracheal tube?
A. 2 to 4 mL
B. 4 to 6 mL
C. 5 to 10 mL
D. 10 to 15 mL
E. 15 to 25 mL

_E_ 39. Confirmation of proper endotracheal tube placement is achieved by:
A. visualizing the tube passing through the glottis.
B. hearing clear and bilaterally equal breath sounds.
C. noting the absence of gastric sounds with ventilation.
D. observing condensation on the endotracheal tube with exhalation.
E. any three of the above

_A_ 40. Which of the following is NOT a standard procedure when performing endotracheal intubation in bright daylight using the transillumination technique?
A. cutting the tube to 35 to 37 cm
B. conforming the stylet and tube to a "hockey-stick" configuration
C. placing the stylet in the ETT and locking the ETT in place at its proximal end
D. lifting the patient's tongue and jaw forward with your fingers
E. advancing the tube/stylet into the mouth and advancing it into the hypopharynx

_B_ 41. In the intubation of children under 8 years old, it is recommended that the EMT-I use:
A. a cuffed endotracheal tube and a straight laryngoscope blade.
B. an uncuffed endotracheal tube and a straight laryngoscope blade.
C. a cuffed endotracheal tube and a curved laryngoscope blade.
D. an uncuffed endotracheal tube and a curved laryngoscope blade.
E. an uncuffed endotracheal tube and digital technique.

_B_ 42. Because of the anterior location of the glottic opening, it is essential to use a stylet with the endotracheal tube during pediatric intubation.
A. True
B. False

_A_ 43. The primary danger associated with extubation is:
A. laryngospasm.
B. aspiration.
C. fasciculations.
D. tracheal damage.
E. vomiting.

©2004 Pearson Education, Inc.
Intermediate Emergency Care: Principles & Practice

CHAPTER 5 Airway Management and Ventilation 131

_A_ **44.** The major disadvantage to the use of the Esophageal Tracheal CombiTube is that:
  A. it may be difficult to seal.
  B. the tube must be in the trachea.
  C. it is associated with gastric distention and vomiting.
  D. it cannot be used in the trauma patient.
  E. it is somewhat time-consuming to insert.

_E_ **45.** Which of the following are features of the PtL airway?
  A. It can be inserted blindly.
  B. It can seal off the nasal and oral cavities.
  C. The patient can be ventilated regardless of whether the tube is in the trachea or esophagus.
  D. It can be inserted without moving the cervical spine.
  E. All of the above

©2004 Pearson Education, Inc.
Intermediate Emergency Care: Principles & Practice

Intermediate Emergency Care: Principles & Practice

Division 2
Patient Assessment

CHAPTER 6
*
History Taking

Review of Chapter Objectives

After reading this chapter, you should be able to:

1. Describe the factors that influence the EMT-Intermediate's ability to collect medical history. pp. 401–405, 413–416

For successful history taking, establish a rapport with the patient to gain his confidence and to set the stage for investigation of the chief complaint and medical history. Factors that will help in establishing rapport include:

- Well-groomed initial appearance
- Positive body language
- Good eye contact with the patient
- Professional demeanor
- Demonstration of interest in the patient

Your introduction should convey your interest in helping the patient and begin the two-way communication. It should convey your care and compassion for the patient and begin to build his trust in you.

Once you have introduced yourself and established your intent to help the patient, begin your questioning. Determine the formal chief complaint and investigate the current and past medical history. Pose questions in a way the patient understands, using terminology and the English language at the patient's level of comprehension.

Questioning frequently involves asking the patient personal, and possibly embarrassing, questions. At such times, ask these questions in a sensitive, nonthreatening way. "Ease into" the discussion of sensitive topics and use questions that are nonjudgmental. You may suggest to the patient that the issue of concern to him is common to many people in our society. Practice in questioning will help you develop the most effective approach. Be prepared to explain that the answers to questions are used for the patient's care and are not communicated beyond the necessary care providers.

2. Describe the structure, purpose, and techniques for obtaining a comprehensive patient history. pp. 401–416

The comprehensive health history establishes a relationship between you and the patient and draws out pertinent information about the patient's medical history. This information may explain the current problem or guide further care in either the prehospital or in-hospital settings. The comprehensive patient history is gained by investigative questioning of the patient about past and current medical problems, including the chief complaint, the present illness (OPQRST-ASPN), the past medical history, current health status, and a review of systems.

3. Discuss the importance of using open-ended and closed-ended questions. p. 403

Open-ended questions provide the patient with the opportunity to respond to your question with an unguided, spontaneous answer. An example is "What happened to cause you to call for an ambulance?" or "Describe what you had for lunch." Closed, or direct, questions guide the patient to an answer of yes or no or some other short response. The question does not allow for an explanation of the circumstance. Examples of closed or direct questions are "Do you have any chest pain?" and "Does it hurt to breathe?"

4. Describe the use of, and differentiate between facilitation, reflection, clarification, empathetic responses, confrontation, and interpretation. pp. 404–405

There are several feedback techniques to use during an interview, including:

Facilitation—encouraging the speaker to provide more information
Clarification—asking the speaker to help you understand confusing parts of his or her response
Empathetic responses—showing you understand the patient
Confrontation—focusing the speaker on a particular part of his or her response
Interpretation—relating your interpretation of the speaker's information

5. List the components of a history of an adult patient. p. 406

The comprehensive patient history includes the following:
- Preliminary data (age, race, sex, etc.)
- The chief complaint
- The present illness or problem (including investigation of onset, provocation, quality, region/ radiation, severity, time, as well as associated symptoms and pertinent negatives—OPQRST-ASPN)
- Past medical history (including the patient's general health, childhood and adult illnesses, psychiatric illness, serious accidents or injuries, and surgeries and hospitalizations)
- Current health status (including patient medications, allergies, use of tobacco, alcohol, and drugs, diet, recent screening tests and immunizations, exercise, leisure and sleep patterns, and environmental hazard/safety measures, family history, and psychosocial history)
- A review of systems (including, as appropriate, general physical information; skin; head, eyes, ears, nose, throat (HEENT); respiratory, cardiac; gastrointestinal; urinary; genital; peripheral vascular; musculoskeletal; neurologic; hematologic; endocrine; psychiatric)

6. List and describe the strategies to overcome situations that represent special challenges in obtaining a medical history. pp. 413–416

Silent patient. Be patient yourself. Speak reassuringly. Gently shake the patient. Consider a neurologic problem.
Overly talkative patient. Focus the patient on the important areas. Summarize what he or she says. Be patient.
Numerous symptoms. Be more clear in questioning; suspect an emotional problem.
Anxious patient. Encourage free conversation and reassure the patient.
Patient needing reassurance. Ask about his anxieties. Offer emotional support.
Anger and hostility. Accept the patient's responses without becoming defensive or angry.
Intoxicated patient. Be friendly and nonjudgmental. Listen to what the patient says, not how he says it. Make your safety and scene safety priorities.
Crying patient. Be patient. Accept the crying as a natural venting of emotions and be supportive.
Depression. Recognize the condition as a serious medical problem. Ask the patient whether he has had suicidal thoughts.
Sexually attractive or seductive patient. Maintain a professional relationship. Try to have a partner present.
Confusing behaviors or histories. Suspect mental illness, dementia, or delirium. Pay careful attention to the patient's mental status. Be reassuring.
Patient of limited intelligence. Try to evaluate the patient's mental abilities. Show genuine interest and establish a positive relationship. Elicit what information you can.
Language barriers. Seek out an interpreter. Be aware that important information is likely to be lost in translation.

Patient with hearing problems. Speak to the patient's best ear. If he reads lips, position yourself directly in front of him in good lighting, and speak slowly in a low-pitched voice. Consider writing your questions.

Patient who is blind or has limited vision. Identify yourself immediately and explain why you are there. Explain what you are doing before you do it.

Family and friends. If gaining pertinent information directly from the patient is difficult, talk to family members or friends on the scene.

CASE STUDY REVIEW

This case study draws attention to the value of the information gathered during the patient history and the process by which it is obtained.

The investigation of the chief complaint, associated symptoms, and the past medical history is extremely important both in determining what is wrong with your patient and then in guiding your provision of care. The circumstances of the emergency and the patient's presentation may confound you unless you employ a relatively standard, systematic approach to patient questioning, but one flexible enough to adapt to different circumstances. In a trauma emergency, you examine the mechanism of injury to determine what happened, while with a medical patient you must investigate the current and past medical history in depth.

EMT-I supervisor John Mason is presented with an "elderly man with abdominal pain." He begins his investigation of the history by introducing himself, identifying his role at the scene, and expressing his desire to help Mr. Sabau. He also asks for and uses Mr. Sabau's name to place the conversation on a more comfortable and personal level.

John first determines the patient's chief complaint, the problem that led him to call for the ambulance. (This may differ from the primary problem in some cases.) In this case, the chief complaint is, "My stomach hurts." John then quickly investigates the complaint by asking questions. The questions he asks are extensive and systematically examine the patient's symptoms. Note that these questions follow the acronym OPQRST-ASPN. John questions about Onset (What were you doing when it started? Did it come on suddenly?), Provocation/Palliation (Does anything make it better or worse?), Quality (Can you describe how it feels?), Radiation (Can you point to the area that hurts? Does the pain travel anywhere else?), Severity (How bad is it? On a scale of ten, with ten being the worst pain you have ever felt, how would you rate this pain?), Time (When did it start? Is it constant or does it come and go?), Associated Symptoms and Pertinent Negatives (Are you nauseous and have you vomited? Have you experienced a change in your bowel habits? Do you have any difficulty breathing?). As John asks these questions, he leans forward and repeats parts of the patient's answers to show his interest and involvement.

The approach that John uses assures an ordered and in-depth investigation of all elements of the patient's history. At the emergency scene, there is much going on and often a sense of urgency. However, taking the few moments to inquire systematically about the patient's presentation assures that you have the essential information to begin forming a differential field diagnosis.

Based on what he has discovered, John begins to form his differential field diagnosis. While the history of pain right after eating and upper right quadrant pain suggest gall bladder problems (cholecystitis), John suspects a broader list of potential problems. This keeps him from forming tunnel vision. As he moves to investigate the past medical history, he asks questions to support or rule out these other problems.

John questions Mr. Sabau about his past medical history and gains further information about pain after eating fatty foods, indigestion, and alcohol consumption. The patient's denials of bloody emesis and stools are pertinent negatives that help John rule out other possible diagnoses. This information also helps him confirm a final field diagnosis of gall bladder problems. With the facts that support his evaluation, John conveys the results of his patient questioning to Dr. Zehner at the emergency department. The laboratory findings support the field diagnosis, and Mr. Sabau is quickly moved to surgery.

CONTENT SELF-EVALUATION

MULTIPLE CHOICE

Pg. 400

A   1. In the majority of medical cases, the basis of the EMT-I's field diagnosis is the:
- A. chief complaint.
- B. index of suspicion.
- C. mechanism of injury.
- D. patient history.
- E. vital signs.

A   2. Always accept information from previous caregivers gratefully, but briefly reconfirm it with the patient.
- A. True
- B. False

A   3. Always use appropriate language during the interview to establish a closer, more trusting relationship.
- A. True
- B. False

B   4. It is best to form a prearranged list of specific questions to assure you cover all bases while interviewing your patient.
- A. True
- B. False

C   5. The process of encouraging the patient to provide details about his condition is called:
- A. empathy.
- B. confrontation.
- C. reflection.
- D. clarification.
- E. facilitation.

B   6. The reason (pain, discomfort, or dysfunction) that the patient or other person summons emergency medical services is termed the:
- A. primary problem.
- B. chief complaint.
- C. nature of the illness.
- D. mechanism of injury.
- E. none of the above

A   7. The underlying cause of the patient's pain, discomfort, or dysfunction is called the:
- A. primary problem.
- B. chief complaint.
- C. nature of the illness.
- D. mechanism of injury.
- E. none of the above

B   8. Any activity that alleviates a patient's symptoms would fit under which element of the OPQRST–ASPN mnemonic for the history of the current illness?
- A. O
- B. P
- C. Q
- D. R
- E. S

C   9. Which of the following is an important part of the past medical history?
- A. radiation of the pain
- B. last oral intake
- C. surgeries or hospitalizations
- D. quality of the pain
- E. all of the above

E   10. A medication not taken as prescribed may account for medical problems due to which of the following?
- A. over-medication
- B. under-medication
- C. allergic reaction
- D. untoward reaction
- E. all of the above

C   11. Allergies should be expected for all of the following EXCEPT:
- A. the "caine" family.
- B. tetanus toxoid.
- C. glucose.
- D. narcotics.
- E. both A and B

___D___ 12. A patient who has smoked 21 packs of cigarettes a week for 10 years has a pack history of:
- **A.** 21 pack/years.
- **B.** 70 pack/years.
- **C.** 7 pack/years.
- **D.** 30 pack/years.
- **E.** 10 pack/years.

___B___ 13. Which of the following is NOT a system examined during the review of systems?
- **A.** skin
- **B.** lymphatic system
- **C.** musculoskeletal system
- **D.** hematologic system
- **E.** endocrine system

___A___ 14. Which step below would you attempt with the patient who suddenly goes silent?
- **A.** Stay calm and observe for nonverbal clues.
- **B.** Arrange for air medical transport.
- **C.** Terminate the interview immediately.
- **D.** Attempt to walk the patient back and forth a few times.
- **E.** Rapidly provide oral glucose.

___A___ 15. Crying is a form of venting emotional stress; be patient and provide a patient who is crying with supportive remarks.
- **A.** True
- **B.** False

MATCHING

Classify each question or statement under the OPQRST category that best applies by writing the letter of the category in the space provided.

- **O.** Onset
- **P.** Provocation/palliation
- **Q.** Quality
- **R.** Region/radiation
- **S.** Severity
- **T.** Time

___S___ 16. How does this compare to the worst pain you have ever felt?

___P___ 17. Does rest lessen your pain?

___R___ 18. Point to where you feel pain.

___Q___ 19. Does this pain feel crushing in nature?

___P___ 20. Does deep breathing increase the pain?

___O___ 21. Did this pain begin suddenly or gradually?

___R___ 22. Where does this pain travel to?

___T___ 23. When did the first symptoms begin?

___Q___ 24. Describe how the pain feels.

___O___ 25. Were you walking or running when this pain first began?

CHAPTER 7

*

Techniques of Physical Examination

Review of Chapter Objectives

After reading this chapter, you should be able to:

1. **Define and describe the techniques of inspection, palpation, percussion, and auscultation.** pp. 420–424

   Inspection is the process of informed observation, viewing the patient for anatomical shape, coloration, and movement. It is the least invasive examination tool, yet may provide the most patient information.

   Palpation is the use of touch to gather information regarding size, shape, position, temperature, moisture, texture, movement, and response to pressure. The fingertips are most sensitive, while the palm best evaluates vibration and the back of the hand, temperature.

   Percussion is the production of a vibration in tissue to elicit sounds. These sounds—dull, resonant, hyperresonant, tympanic, and flat—identify the nature of the tissue underneath. The vibration is generated by striking the first knuckle of a finger placed against the area to be percussed with the fingertip of the other hand.

   Auscultation is listening for sounds within the body, most frequently with a stethoscope. The intensity, pitch, duration, quality, and timing of sounds in the patient's lungs, heart, blood vessels, and intestines are compared against normal sounds.

2. **Review the significance of and the procedures for taking vital signs.** pp. 424–427

   Pulse is the wave of pressure generated by the heart as it expels blood into the arterial system. It is measured by palpating a distal artery (or auscultated during blood pressure determination) and is evaluated for rate, rhythm, and quality (strength). The normal pulse is strong, regular, and has a rate of between 60 and 80 beats per minute.

   Respiration is the movement of air through the airway and into and out of the lungs. It is evaluated by observing and/or feeling chest excursion and listening to air movement. The rate, effort, and quality (depth and pattern) of respirations are determined. Normal respiration moves a tidal volume of 500 mL at a rate of 12 to 20 times per minute with symmetrical chest wall movement.

   Blood pressure is the force of blood against the arterial wall during the cardiac/pulse cycle. It is measured using a sphygmomanometer (blood pressure cuff) and stethoscope. The maximum or systolic blood pressure—the reading obtained when the ventricles contract, the lower or diastolic blood pressure—the reading obtained when the ventricles relax, and the difference between them, the pulse pressure, are evaluated. The systolic pressure is usually between 100 and 135, and the diastolic, between 60 and 80.

   Temperature is the body core temperature and is the product of heat-creating metabolism and body heat loss. It is measured by a glass or electronic thermometer placed in the axilla, mouth, or rectum. Normal body temperature is 98.6°F (37°C).

©2004 Pearson Education, Inc.
Intermediate Emergency Care: Principles & Practice

3. Describe the evaluation of mental status.

pp. 468–469

The evaluation of the mental status begins with your interview. The evaluation permits you to determine your patient's level of responsiveness, general appearance, behavior, and speech. You specifically look at his appearance and behavior, speech and language skills, mood, thought and perception, insight and judgment, and memory and attention.

4. Evaluate the importance of a general survey.

pp. 430–436

The general survey is the first part of the comprehensive exam. It is made up of your evaluation of the patient's appearance—including level of consciousness, expression, state of health, general characteristics (weight, height, etc.), posturing, dress, grooming, etc.—the vital signs, and additional assessments such as pulse oximetry, cardiac monitoring, and blood glucose determination. The survey helps you form a general impression of your patient's health.

5. Describe the examination of the following body regions, differentiate between normal and abnormal findings, and define the significance of abnormal findings:

Skin, hair, and nails

pp. 436–437

Observe the skin carefully for color, especially in the nail beds, lips, conjunctiva, and mucous membranes of the mouth. Pink skin reflects good oxygenation, while pale skin reflects poor blood flow from hypovolemia, hypothermia, compensatory shock, or anemia. A bluish-colored skin, cyanosis, suggests blood is low in oxygen. A yellow sclera or general discoloration, jaundice, is due to liver failure. Other skin observations may include petechiae, small round, flat purplish spots caused by capillary bleeding from a variety of etiologies, and ecchymosis, a larger, black-and-blue discoloration that is often the result of trauma or bleeding disorders. Moisture, temperature, texture, mobility, and turgor are also evaluated. Skin lesions are disruptions in normal tissue that may take on almost any shape, color, or arrangement.

Inspect and palpate the hair to determine color, quality, distribution, quantity, and texture and inspect and palpate the scalp for scaling, lesions, redness, lumps, or tenderness. Generalized hair loss may reflect chemotherapy; failure to develop normal hair patterns may be caused by a pituitary or hormonal problem; and unusual facial hair in women suggests a hormonal imbalance. Mild scalp flaking suggests dandruff; heavy scaling, psoriasis; and greasy scaling, seborrheic dermatitis. Lice eggs (nits) may be found firmly attached to the hair shafts. Normal hair texture is smooth and soft in Caucasians; in people of African descent, the texture is coarser. Dry, brittle, or fragile hair is abnormal.

Inspect the finger and toenails for color. Note any discolorations, lesions, ridging, grooves, depressions, or pitting. Depressions suggest systemic disease. Compress the nail and bed to determine its adherence and look for nail hygiene. Any bogginess suggests cardiorespiratory disease.

Head, scalp, and skull

pp. 437–439

Observe and palpate the skull and facial region for symmetry, smoothness, wounds, bleeding, size, and general contour. Examine the hair and scalp as described above. Check the eyes for bilateral periorbital and mastoid ecchymosis, "raccoon eyes" and "Battle's sign," respectively. They suggest basilar skull fracture and occur an hour or so after injury. Palpate the facial region for crepitation, false motion, or instability suggesting fracture. Evaluate the temporomandibular joint for pain, tenderness, swelling, and range of motion. Have the patient open and close his mouth and jut and retract his jaw. Any loss of normal function suggests injury.

Eyes, ears, nose, mouth, and pharynx

pp. 439–443

Examine for visual acuity, then evaluate for peripheral vision. While the patient faces you, have him look at your nose while you extend your arms, bend your elbows and wiggle the fingers. If he notices the fingers moving in all four directions (up, down, left, and right) for each eye, his peripheral vision is grossly normal. Inspect the eyes for symmetry, shape, inflammation, swelling, misalignment (disconjugate gaze), lesions, and contour. Examine the eyelids, open and closed, for swelling, discoloration, droop (ptosis), styes, and lash positioning. Observe the tearing or dryness of the eyes. Gently retract the lower eyelid while asking the patient to look through a range of motion. Examine the sclera for signs of irritation, cloudiness, yellow discoloration (jaundice), any nodules, swelling, discharge, or hemorrhage into the scleral tissue. With an oblique light source, inspect the cornea for opacities. Inspect the size, shape, symmetry, and reactivity of the pupils. Note the pupils' direct and consensual response to increased light intensity. A sluggish pupil suggests pressure on CN-III; bilateral sluggishness suggests global hypoxia or depressant drug action. Constricted pupils suggest opiate overdose, while dilated and fixed pupils reflect brain anoxia. Ask the patient to focus on your finger close at hand, then move the hand to his nose, then away. The eyes should converge, while the pupils should constrict slightly. Then have him follow your finger as you move it through an "H" pattern. The eyes should move smoothly together. Nystagmus is a jerky movement at the distal extremes of ocular movement. Gently touch the cornea with a strand of cotton. The patient should respond with a blink. Using an ophthalmoscope, look into the eye's anterior chamber for signs of blood (hyphema), cells, or pus (hypopyon), and check the cornea for lacerations, abrasions, cataracts, papilledema (from increased ICP), vascular occlusions, and retinal hemorrhage.

Examine the ears by looking for symmetry from in front of the patient, then examine each ear separately. Examine the external portion (auricle) for shape, size, landmarks, and position on the head. Examine the surrounding area for deformities, lesions, tenderness, and erythema. Pull the helix upward and outward, press on the tragus and on the mastoid process and note any discomfort or pain suggesting otitis or mastoiditis. Some pain may be associated with toothache, a cold, sore throat, or cervical spine injury. Inspect the ear canal for discharge (pus, mucus, blood, or cerebral spinal fluid [CSF]) and inflammation. Trauma can account for blood, mucus, and CSF in the ear canal. Check hearing acuity by covering one ear and whispering, then speaking into the other. Hearing loss may be accounted for by trauma, accumulation of debris (often cerumen), tympanic membrane rupture, drug use, and prolonged exposure to loud noise. Visualize the inner canal with the otoscope. With the largest speculum that will fit the canal, turn the patient's head away from you, pull the auricle slightly up and backward, and insert the otoscope. Inspect for wax (cerumen), discharge, redness, lesions, perforations, and foreign bodies. Then focus on the tympanic membrane. It should be a translucent pearly gray. Color changes suggest fluid behind the eardrum or infection. Also check for bulging, protractions, or perforations.

Visualize the patient's nose from the front and sides to determine any asymmetry, deviation, tenderness, flaring, or abnormal color. Tilt your patient's head back slightly and examine the nostrils. Insert the otoscope and check for deviation of the septum and perforations. Examine the nasal mucosa for color, and the color, consistency, and quantity of drainage. Rhinitis (a runny nose) suggests seasonal allergies; a thick yellow discharge, infection; and blood, epistaxis from trauma or a septal defect. Test each side of the nose for patency by occluding the other side during a breath. There is normally some difference in patency between the sides. Palpate the frontal sinuses for swelling and tenderness.

Begin assessment of the mouth by observing the lips for color and condition. They should be pink, smooth, symmetrical, and without lesions, swelling, lumps, cracks, or scaliness. Using a bright light and tongue blade, examine the oral mucosa for color, lesions, white patches, or fissures. The mucosa should be pinkish-red, smooth, and moist. The gums should be pink with clearly defined margins around the teeth. The teeth should be well formed and straight. If the gums are swollen, bleed easily, and are separated from the teeth, suspect periodontal disease. Ask the patient to stick his tongue out and note its velvety surface. Hold the tongue with a 2″ × 2″ gauze pad and inspect all sides and the bottom. All surfaces should be pink and smooth. Then examine the pharynx and have the patient say "aaaahhh" while you hold the tongue down with a tongue blade. Watch the movement of the uvula and the coloration and condition of the palatine tonsils and posterior pharynx. Look for any pus, swelling, ulcers, or drainage. Also notice any odors including alcohol, feces (bowel obstruction), acetone (diabetic ketoacidosis), gastric contents, coffee-grounds-like material (gastric hemorrhage), pink-tinged sputum (pulmonary edema), or the smell of bitter almonds (cyanide poisoning).

Neck   pp. 443–445
Inspect your patient's neck for symmetry and visible masses. Note any deformity, deviations, tugging, scars, gland enlargement, or visible lymph nodes. Examine for any open wounds and cover them with an occlusive dressing. Examine the jugular veins for distention while the patient is seated upright and at a 45° incline. Palpate the trachea to assure it is inline. Palpate the thyroid

while the patient swallows to assure it is small, smooth, and without nodules. Palpate each lymph node to determine size, shape, tenderness, consistency, and mobility. Tender, swollen, and mobile nodes suggest inflammation from infection, while hard and fixed ones suggest malignancy.

Thorax (anterior and posterior)   pp. 445–450

To assess the chest, you need a stethoscope with a bell and diaphragm. Expose the entire thorax with consideration for the patient's dignity and modesty, and inspect, palpate, percuss, and auscultate. Compare findings from one side of the chest to the other and from posterior to anterior. Look for general shape and symmetry as well as for the rate and pattern of breathing. Observe for retractions and the use of accessory muscles (suggestive of airway obstruction or restriction), and palpate for deformities, tenderness, crepitus (suggestive of rib fracture), and abnormal chest excursion (suggestive of flail chest or spinal injury). Feel for vibrations associated with air movement and speech. Percuss the chest for dullness (hemothorax, pleural effusion, or pneumonia), resonance, and hyperresonance (pneumothorax or tension pneumothorax). Finally, auscultate the lung lobes for normal breath sounds, crackles (pulmonary edema), wheezes (asthma), rhonchi, stridor (airway obstruction), and pleural friction rubs.

Arterial pulse including rate, rhythm, and amplitude   pp. 449–450

Locate a soft and pulsing carotid artery in the neck, just lateral to the cricoid cartilage to avoid pressure on the carotid sinus. Carefully press down until the pulse wave just lifts your finger off the artery. Determine the rate and carefully evaluate for regularity. Irregularity may be caused by dysrhythmia, while variation in strength may be due to such phenomena as pulsus paradoxus, increasing strength with exhalation and decreasing with inhalation. Also note any thrills (humming or vibration) and listen with the stethoscope for bruits (sounds of turbulent flow).

Jugular venous pressure and pulsations   pp. 449–450

Examine the anterior neck and locate the jugular veins. Position your patient with his head elevated 30° and turned away from you. Look for pulsation just above the suprasternal notch. Identify the highest point of pulsation and measure the distance from the sternal angle. The highest point of pulsation is usually between 1 and 2 cm from the sternal angle. (Distention when the patient is elevated at higher angles may reflect tension pneumothorax or pericardial tamponade, while flat veins at lower angles may suggest hypovolemia.)

Heart   pp. 449–451

The normal heart produces a "lub-dub" sound heard through the disk of the stethoscope with each cardiac contraction. The "lub" and "dub" may split when valves close out of sync, "la-lub-dub" reflects an S_1 split while "lub-da-dub" is an S_2 split. S_2 splitting is normal in children and young adults, though abnormal in older adults if expiratory or persistent splitting occurs. S_3 splitting produces a "lub-dub-dee" cadence like the word "Kentucky." It occurs commonly in children and young adults, but reflects blood filling a dilated ventricle and may suggest ventricular failure in the patient over 30. The S_4 heart sound is the "dee" sound of "dee-lub-dub" with a cadence similar to the word "Tennessee." It develops from vibrations as the atrium pushes blood into a ventricle that resists filling, suggestive of heart failure.

Abdomen   pp. 450–452

Question your patient regarding any pain, tenderness or unusual feeling, and recent bowel and bladder function. Carefully inspect the area for scars, dilated veins, stretch marks, rashes, lesions, and pigmentation changes. Discoloration around the umbilicus (Cullen's sign) or over the flanks (Grey-Turner's sign) suggest intra-abdominal hemorrhage. Assess the size and shape of the abdomen, determining whether it is scaphoid (concave), flat, round, or distended, and look for any bulges or hernias. Ascites result in bulges in the flanks and across the abdomen suggesting congestive heart or liver failure, while suprapubic bulges suggest a full bladder or pregnant uterus. Look also for any masses, palpations, or peristalsis. A slight vascular pulsing is normal, but excessive movement suggests an aneurysm. Auscultate and percuss as described earlier. Then depress each quadrant gently and release. Look for patient expression or muscle guarding suggestive of injury or peritonitis.

Male and female genitalia
pp. 452–454

Assure patient privacy, a warm environment, and patient modesty during the exam; also be sure the patient has emptied his or her bladder before beginning. Expose only those body areas that you must, and explain what you are going to do before you do it. Inspect the genitalia for development and maturity. Visually inspect the mons pubis, labia, and perineum of the female patient for swelling, lesions, or irritation suggestive of a sebaceous cyst or sexually transmitted disease. Check the hair bases for small red maculopapules suggestive of lice. Retract the labia and inspect the inner labia and urethral opening. Examine for a white curdy discharge (fungal infection) or yellow-green discharge (bacterial infection). For the male, inspect the penis and testicles, noting inflammation and lesions suggestive of sexually transmitted disease. Check for lice and examine the glans for degeneration, inflammation, or discharge. Yellow discharge is reflective of gonorrhea.

Peripheral vascular system
pp. 465–467

Examine the upper, then the lower extremities and compare them, one to another, for the following: size, symmetry, swelling, venous congestion, skin and nailbed color, temperature, skin texture, and turgor. Yellow brittle nails, swollen digit ends (clubbing), or poor nailbed color suggest chronic arterial insufficiency. Assess the distal circulation, noting the strength, rate, and regularity of the pulse and comparing pulses bilaterally. If you have difficulty palpating a pulse or can't find one, palpate a more proximal site. Feel the spongy compliance of the vessels, note their coloration, and examine for inflammation along the vein, indicative of deep vein thrombosis. Gently feel for edema and pitting edema in each distal extremity.

Extremities
pp. 454–462

Advancing age causes changes in the musculoskeletal system including shortening and increased curvature of the spine, a reduction in muscle mass and strength, and a reduction in the range of motion. Observe the patient's general posture, build, and muscular development as well as the movement of the extremities, gait, and position at rest. Then inspect all regions of the body for deformities, symmetry and symmetrical movement, joint structure, and swelling, nodules, or inflammation. Deformities are often related to misaligned articulating bones, dislocations, or subluxations. Impaired movement is usually related to arthritis; nodules related to rheumatic fever or rheumatoid arthritis; and redness related to gout, rheumatic fever, or arthritis. Compare dissimilar joints to determine what structures might be affected. Assess range of motion by moving the limb, ask the patient to move the limb, and then ask the patient to move the limb against resistance. Note any asymmetry and inequality between active and passive motion. Also examine for crepitation (a grating vibration or sound) that may suggest arthritis, an inflamed joint, or a fracture. Avoid manipulating a deformed or painful joint. Perform a physical exam on each joint, moving it through its normal range of motion and noting any deformities, limited or resistant movement, tenderness, and swelling.

Nervous system
pp. 467–472

To evaluate mental status and speech, examine your patient's appearance and behavior, speech and language, mood, thoughts and perceptions, and memory and attention. Observe the patient's appearance and behavior, level of consciousness, posture and motor behavior, appropriateness of dress, grooming and personal hygiene, and the patient's facial expression. Note any abnormal speech pattern and observe the patient's attitude toward you and others expressed both verbally and non-verbally. Note any excessive emotion or lack of emotion. Assess the patient's thoughts and perceptions. Are they realistic and socially acceptable? Question for any visions, voices, perceived odors, or feelings about things that are not there. Examine the patient's insights and judgments to determine if he knows what is happening. Assess the patient's memory and attention and determine his orientation to time, place, and person (sometimes considered as person and own person). Then test immediate, recent, and remote memory. Any deviation from a normal and expected response is to be noted and suggests illness or psychiatric problem.

Begin the examination of the motor system by observing the patient for symmetry, deformities, and involuntary movements. Tremors or fasiculations while the patient is at rest suggest Parkinson's disease, while their occurrence during motion suggests postural tremor. Determine muscle bulk, which is classified as normal, atrophy, hypertrophy, or pseudotrophy (bulk without strength as in muscular dystrophy). Unilateral hand atrophy suggests median or ulnar nerve paralysis. Check tone by moving a relaxed limb through a range of motion. Describe any flaccidity or rigidity and then examine muscle strength starting with grip strength and continuing through all limbs. Again note any asymmetry (the patient's dominant side should be slightly stronger). Observe the patient's gait and have him walk a straight line (heel to toe). Any ataxia suggests cerebellar disease, loss of position sense, or intoxication. Also have the patient walk on his toes, then heels, hop on each foot, and then do a shallow knee bend. Perform a Romberg test (have him stand with his feet together and eyes closed for 20 to 30 seconds). Any excessive sway (a positive Romberg test) suggests ataxia from loss of position sense, while inability to maintain balance with eyes open represents cerebellar ataxia. Ask the patient to hold his arms straight out in front with his palms up and eyes closed. Pronation suggests mild hemiparesis, drifting sideways or upward suggests loss of positional sense. Ask your patient to perform various rapid alternating movements and observe for smoothness, speed, and rhythm. The dominant side should perform best, and any slow, irregular or clumsy movements suggest cerebellar or extrapyramidal disease. Have your patient touch his thumb rapidly with the tip of the index finger, place his hand on his thigh and rapidly alternate from palm up to down, and assess for point-to-point testing (touch his nose, then your index finger several times rapidly, or, for the legs, have him touch heel to knee, then run it down the shin). Any jerking, difficulty in performing the task, or tremors suggest cerebellar disease. For position testing, have the patient perform the leg test with his eyes closed.

Evaluate the sensory system by testing sensations of pain, light touch, temperature, position, vibration, and discrimination. Compare responses bilaterally and from distal to proximal, then associate any deficit discovered with the dermatome it represents. Test superficial and deep tendon reflexes and note a dulled (cord or lower neuron damage) or hyperactive response (upper neuron disease).

6. Describe the assessment of respiration and the characteristics of breath sounds.   pp. 424–426

Have your patient breathe more deeply and slowly than normal with an open mouth. Using the stethoscope's disk, auscultate each side of the chest from the apex to the base every 5 cm, listening at each location for one full breath.

Normal breath sounds are the quiet sounds (almost low-pitched sighs) of air moving. Abnormal breath sounds are termed adventitious, and include the following. Any crackles (a light crackling, popping, non-musical sound) suggest fluid in the smaller airways. Late inspiratory crackles suggest heart failure or interstitial lung disease, while early crackles suggest heart failure or chronic bronchitis. Wheezes (more musical notes) denote obstruction of the smaller airways. The closer they appear to inspiration, the more serious the obstruction is. Stridor is a high-pitched, loud inspiratory wheeze reflective of laryngeal or tracheal obstruction. Grating or squeaking sounds describe pleural friction rubs and occur as the pleural layers become inflamed, then rub together. You may also listen for sound transmission while the patient speaks. Bronchophony occurs when you hear the words "ninety-nine" abnormally clearly through the stethoscope, a suggestion that blood, fluid, or a tumor has replaced normal tissue. Assess for whispered pectoriloquy by asking the patient to whisper "ninety-nine"; unusually clear sounds indicate an abnormal condition. Egophony occurs when you can hear the sound of long "e" as "a" when vocal resonance is abnormally increased.

7. Describe percussion of the chest and differentiate the percussion notes and their characteristics.   pp. 445–449

Percuss both the anterior and posterior chest surfaces, examining for resonant (normal), hyperresonant (air-filled pneumothorax or tension pneumothorax) or dull sounds. Percuss both sides symmetrically from the apex to the base at 5 centimeter intervals, avoiding the scapula. Determine the boundaries of any hyperresonance or dullness.

Percussion provides three basic sounds; dull, resonant, and hyperresonant. Dull reflects a density and is a medium-pitched thud. It is usually caused by a dense organ (like the liver) or fluid, like blood, underneath. Resonant sounds are generally associated with a less dense tissue, like the lungs, and are lower-pitched and longer lasting sounds. Hyperresonant sounds reflect air, or air under pressure, and are the lowest-pitched sounds and the ones that diminish in volume most slowly.

Patient Assessment

8. **Describe the general guidelines of recording examination information.** pp. 476–477

Use a standard format to organize the information. Use appropriate medical terminology and language. Present your findings legibly, accurately, and truthfully, remembering that your record will become a legal document. Include all data discovered in your assessment.

The standard organization for medical documentation is the S (Subjective), O (Objective), A (Assessment), and P (Plan) format (SOAP format):

Subjective information is what your patient or others tell you, including the chief complaint and the past and present medical history.
Objective information is that which you observe or determine during the scene size-up, initial assessment, focused history and physical exam, detailed assessment, and ongoing assessments.
Assessment summarizes the findings to suggest a field diagnosis.
Plan is the further diagnosis, treatment, and patient education you intend to offer.

9. **Discuss the examination considerations for an infant or child.** pp. 472–476

Children are not small adults, but patients with special physiological and psychological differences. In general, remain calm and confident, establish a rapport with the parents, and have them help with the exam. Provide positive feedback to both the child and parents.

The transition from newborn to adulthood is a continuum of development, both physically and emotionally. When assessing pediatric patients, keep the following differences from adults in mind:

The bones of the skull do not close until about 18 months and joints remain cartilaginous until 5 years.
The child's airway is narrow and will be more quickly and severely obstructed than the adult's.
Instead of listening for verbal complaints, note the child's eyes, expression, and the degree of activity it takes to distract him from the problem as an indication of its seriousness.
Rib fractures are rare due to the cartilaginous nature of the ribs, though the tissue underneath is more prone to injury.
The liver and spleen are proportionally large and are more subject to injury.
Children are more likely to experience bone injury rather than ligament and tendon injury.
Normal vital signs for children will change through the stages of their development.

CASE STUDY REVIEW

The case Ssudy demonstrates the value a good physical exam has in helping you determine the nature of a patient's medical problem when their symptoms are non-specific.

Here Tony is presented with an elderly patient who "just can't seem to stand up." Tony, through questioning, tries to rule out heart attack and respiratory problems and investigates Mr. Scalisi's past medical history. His current medications suggest a cardiac history, and Tony is very aware that many elderly patient experience heart attacks without overt signs and symptoms (the silent MI).

Since the transport is expected to take a relatively long time, Tony has the luxury of performing a detailed and extensive physical exam. His exam includes a thorough visual evaluation of each body region followed by gentle palpation and auscultation where warranted. All physical findings are unremarkable. He then performs a complete neurological exam, starting with a mental status evaluation. Nick is alert and oriented X3 with clear and well composed and articulated speech.

The motor function exam reveals slumping to the left with tremors only noted at the end of fine motor movement. As coordination is tested, Tony observes Nick's inability to perform several activities on the left side. Because Tony's findings involve the extrapyramidal tracks, they strongly suggest a same-sided (left sided) lesion. Tony's field diagnosis is impressive, especially since the signs of the problem are limited and only brought to note through a very thorough and complete physical exam.

A careful and detailed examination, such as that performed by Tony, will provide you with a great deal of information about your patient's condition. In many cases you may not be able to identify the exact problem affecting your patient but the information you gain may be invaluable to the emergency physician when you arrive at the ED. It can also be used to rule out many likely conditions that might otherwise be affecting your patient. With time and experience, you will find it easier to identify possible patient problems and an increasing reliability in your field diagnosis.

CONTENT SELF-EVALUATION

MULTIPLE CHOICE

_A_ 1. A normal pulse quality would be reported as:
   A. 0.   D. 3+.
   B. 1+.   E. 4+.
   C. 2+.

_A_ 2. Which of the following is NOT a sign of proximal arterial occlusion?
   A. thrills   D. poor color in the fingertips
   B. pulse deficit   E. slow capillary refill
   C. cold limb

_D_ 3. Pitting edema that depresses 1/2 to 1 inch is reported as:
   A. 0.   D. 3+.
   B. 1+.   E. 4+.
   C. 2+.

_E_ 4. The pitting of edema will usually disappear within how many seconds after the release of pressure?
   A. 2   D. 8
   B. 4   E. 10
   C. 6

_A_ 5. A patient who is drowsy but answers questions is considered to be:
   A. lethargic.   D. comatose.
   B. obtunded.   E. none of the above
   C. stuporous.

_E_ 6. Normal speech is:
   A. inflected.   D. varies in volume.
   B. clear and strong.   E. all of the above
   C. fluent and articulate.

_E_ 7. The term dysphonia refers to which of the following?
   A. defective speech caused by motor deficits
   B. voice changes due to vocal cord problems
   C. defective language due to neurologic problem
   D. voice changes due to aging
   E. none of the above

_E_ 8. The term aphasia refers to which of the following?
   A. defective speech caused by motor deficits
   B. voice changes due to vocal cord problems
   C. defective language due to a neurologic problem
   D. voice changes due to aging
   E. none of the above

_A_ 9. The twitching of small muscle fibers is:
   A. spasm.   D. fasciculations.
   B. tics.   E. atrophy.
   C. tremors.

_D_ 10. In cases of muscular dystrophy, the patient's muscles:
   A. increase in size.   D. decrease in strength.
   B. decrease in size.   E. both A and D
   C. increase in strength.

_B_ 11. During your testing of a patient's muscle strength, you notice one side to be slightly stronger than the other. This is a normal finding.
A. True
B. False

_____ 12. An area of skin innervated by a specific peripheral nerve root is a(n):
A. afferent region.
B. sensory topographic region.
C. myotome.
D. dermatome.
E. both A and C

_____ 13. The score on the muscle strength scale that describes a patient able to perform active movement against gravity is:
A. 5.
B. 4.
C. 3.
D. 2.
E. 1.

_____ 14. To assess the sensory system, you must test for:
A. pain.
B. light touch.
C. temperature.
D. dermatome.
E. A, B, and C

_E_ 15. In caring for the ill or injured child, it is important to be which of the following?
A. confident
B. direct
C. honest
D. calm
E. all of the above

_D_ 16. Which of the following is NOT recommended as part of the assessment and care for an ill or injured child?
A. Separate the patient from the parents if possible.
B. Give the patient a toy or object to play with.
C. Elicit a parent's help in obtaining a history.
D. Perform invasive procedures late in the assessment if possible.
E. Provide feedback and reassurance.

_C_ 17. The soft spots in the skull, called fontanelles, close at about what age?
A. 6 months
B. 12 months
C. 18 months
D. 24 months
E. 30 months

_E_ 18. Bulging along the sutures of the skull of a young child suggests which of the following?
A. dehydration
B. reduced venous pressure in the jugular veins
C. decreased arterial pressure
D. arterial blockage to the cerebrum
E. none of the above

_B_ 19. Because the tissue of the child's upper airway is so flexible, injuries, infections, or minor obstructions do not adversely affect it as seriously as they would an adult's.
A. True
B. False

_A_ 20. Which of the following statements regarding the chest of an infant or small child is FALSE?
A. Children have a less mobile mediastinum than adults.
B. The chest is rather elastic.
C. The chest is rather flexible.
D. Chest fractures are less likely.
E. The chest is comprised of more cartilage than the adult's.

©2004 Pearson Education, Inc.
Intermediate Emergency Care: Principles & Practice

_B_ 21. Because of the structure of the thoracic cage, the child is less likely to develop tension pneumothorax than the adult.
   A. True
   B. False

_B_ 22. The normal respiratory rate for an infant is:
   A. 30 to 50 breaths per minute.
   B. 30 to 60 breaths per minute.
   C. 24 to 40 breaths per minute.
   D. 22 to 34 breaths per minute.
   E. 18 to 30 breaths per minute.

_A_ 23. The normal systolic blood pressure for the newborn is:
   A. 60 to 90.
   B. 87 to 105.
   C. 95 to 105.
   D. 95 to 110.
   E. 112 to 128.

_D_ 24. Which of the following is NOT true regarding the abdomen of the child?
   A. The liver is proportionally larger than the adult's.
   B. The spleen is proportionally larger than the adult's.
   C. The abdominal muscles provide less protection than the adult's.
   D. The abdomen rarely bulges at the end of inspiration.
   E. Inguinal hernias are common in young children.

_E_ 25. Which of the following statements is true regarding the recording of examination findings?
   A. The patient care report is only as good as the accuracy, detail, and depth you provide.
   B. The patient chart is a legal document.
   C. The absence of an expected sign in a patient may be just as important as its presence.
   D. The universally accepted organization for recording patient information is SOAP.
   E. all of the above

_D_ 26. A likely location to notice retraction during forced inspiration is:
   A. the suprasternal notch.
   B. the intercostal spaces.
   C. the supraclavicular space.
   D. all of the above
   E. none of the above

_B_ 27. The type of motion associated with a free segment of the chest where the segment moves opposite to the rest of the chest during breathing is:
   A. symbiotic.
   B. paradoxical.
   C. antagonistic.
   D. retractive.
   E. traumatic.

_E_ 28. During the palpation of the chest, you should feel for which of the following?
   A. tenderness
   B. deformities
   C. depressions
   D. asymmetry
   E. all of the above

_B_ 29. During the check for chest excursion, the distance between your thumbs should increase by what amount during the patient's inspiration?
   A. 2 cm
   B. 3 to 5 cm
   C. 5 to 6 cm
   D. 10 to 12 cm
   E. the hands should not move

_____ 30. Tripodding and finger clubbing are signs of which of the following conditions?
   A. pneumonia
   B. pneumothorax
   C. pleural effusion
   D. chronic lung disease
   E. all of the above

_C_ 31. Which condition is most likely to cause an area of the lung that is dull to percussion?
  A. pneumothorax
  B. tension pneumothorax
  C. hemothorax
  D. pericardial tamponade
  E. friction rubs

_C_ 32. Light popping, nonmusical sounds heard in the chest during inspiration are known as:
  A. rhonchi.
  B. stridor.
  C. crackles.
  D. wheezes.
  E. none of the above

_B_ 33. Stridor is a high pitched inspiratory sound. It indicates a partial obstruction of the larynx or trachea.
  A. True
  B. False

_E_ 34. The "lub" of the heart sounds represents which event of the cardiac cycle?
  A. ejection of blood from the ventricles
  B. ventricular contraction
  C. ventricular filling
  D. closing of the aortic and pulmonic valves
  E. closing of the tricuspid and mitral valves

_D_ 35. An eccyhmotic discoloration over the umbilicus is:
  A. Grey-Turner's sign.
  B. borborygami.
  C. Hering-Breuer sign.
  D. Cullen's sign.
  E. none of the above

_E_ 36 Which abdominal quadrant should you palpate last?
  A. the left upper quadrant
  B. the right upper quadrant
  C. the left lower quadrant
  D. the right lower quadrant
  E. any quadrant with pain

_B_ 37. The sound or feeling caused by unlubricated bone ends rubbing together is:
  A. palpable fremitus.
  B. crepitation.
  C. bruit.
  D. friction rub.
  E. the pooh-pooh sign.

_B_ 38. Carpal tunnel syndrome involves which nerve?
  A. brachial
  B. median
  C. radial
  D. ulnar
  E. olecranon

_B_ 39. A lateral curvature of the spine is:
  A. lordosis.
  B. scoliosis.
  C. kyphosis.
  D. spina bifida.
  E. none of the above

_E_ 40. Tenderness at a vertebral process and in the surrounding musculature of the lumbar spine is most likely due to:
  A. vertebral process fracture.
  B. ligamentous injury.
  C. paravertebral muscular spasm.
  D. herniated intervertebral disk.
  E. none of the above

_A_ 41. Of the physical examination techniques used in prehospital care, which is the least invasive?
  A. inspection
  B. auscultation
  C. palpation
  D. percussion
  E. C and D

©2004 Pearson Education, Inc.
Intermediate Emergency Care: Principles & Practice

__B__ 42. "Crackles" would be found using which of the following assessment techniques?
   A. palpation
   B. auscultation
   C. inspection
   D. percussion
   E. none of the above

__A__ 43. "Guarding" would be discovered using which of the following assessment techniques?
   A. palpation
   B. auscultation
   C. inspection
   D. percussion
   E. none of the above

__C__ 44. Which of the following techniques should be performed first during the physical examination?
   A. palpation
   B. auscultation
   C. inspection
   D. percussion
   E. none of the above

__B__ 45. Which part of the hands and fingers is best suited to evaluate tissue consistency?
   A. tips of the fingers
   B. pads of the fingers
   C. palm of the hand
   D. back of the hands or fingers
   E. none of the above

__C__ 46. Which part of the hands and fingers is best suited to evaluate vibration?
   A. tips of the fingers
   B. pads of the fingers
   C. palm of the hand
   D. back of the hands or fingers
   E. none of the above

__A__ 47. Noticing areas of warmth during palpation might reflect an injury before significant edema and discoloration develop.
   A. True
   B. False

__A__ 48. The booming sound produced by percussing an air-filled region is:
   A. hyperresonance.
   B. dull.
   C. resonance.
   D. flat.
   E. none of the above

__C__ 49. The only region where you perform auscultation as other than the last step of assessment is the:
   A. anterior thorax.
   B. neck.
   C. abdomen.
   D. peripheral arteries.
   E. posterior thorax.

__B__ 50. A heart rate above 100 is known as a:
   A. bradycardia.
   B. tachycardia.
   C. hypercardia.
   D. tachypnea.
   E. bradypnea.

__C__ 51. One likely cause of bradycardia is:
   A. fever.
   B. pain.
   C. parasympathetic stimulation.
   D. fear.
   E. blood loss.

__A__ 52. Which of the following is NOT an aspect of pulse evaluation?
   A. volume
   B. rhythm
   C. quality
   D. rate
   E. none of the above

©2004 Pearson Education, Inc.
Intermediate Emergency Care: Principles & Practice

_____ 53. Normal exhalation is:
   A. an active process involving accessory muscles.
   B. an active process involving the diaphragm and intercostal muscles.
   C. active in its early stages and passive in later stages.
   D. passive in its early stages and active in later stages.
   E. a passive process.

_____ 54. For a patient with an airway obstruction, exhalation is likely to be:
   A. an active process involving accessory muscles.
   B. an active process involving only the diaphragm and intercostal muscles.
   C. active in its early stages and passive in later stages.
   D. passive in its early stages and active in later stages.
   E. a passive process.

_____ 55. The amount of air a patient moves into and out of his lungs in one breath is the:
   A. normal volume.   D. tidal volume.
   B. respiratory volume.   E. minute volume.
   C. residual volume.

_____ 56. The pressure of the blood within the blood vessels while the ventricles are relaxing is the:
   A. Korotkoff blood pressure.   D. asystolic blood pressure.
   B. systolic blood pressure.   E. atrial blood pressure.
   C. diastolic blood pressure.

_____ 57. The diastolic blood pressure represents a measure of:
   A. systemic vascular resistance.   D. the strength of ventricular contraction.
   B. the cardiac output.   E. relative blood volume.
   C. the viscosity of the blood.

_____ 58. Which of the following are likely to influence a patient's blood pressure?
   A. anxiety   D. eating
   B. position (lying, sitting, standing)   E. all of the above
   C. recent smoking

_____ 59. Generally, hypertension in a healthy adult is any blood pressure higher than:
   A. 120/80.   D. 180/100.
   B. 140/90.   E. 200/100.
   C. 160/90.

_____ 60. What is the pulse pressure in a patient with the following vital signs: pulse 82 and strong; respirations 14 and full: and blood pressure 144/96?
   A. 14   D. 96
   B. 40   E. 120
   C. 48

_____ 61. In the tilt test, what vital sign change is a positive sign of hypovolemia?
   A. blood pressure drops by 10 to 20 mmHg
   B. blood pressure rises by 10 to 20 mmHg
   C. pulse rate drops by 10 to 20 beats per minute
   D. pulse rate rises by 10 to 20 beats per minute
   E. either A or D

_____ 62. Hyperthermia can result from all of the following EXCEPT:
   A. high environmental temperatures. D. drugs.
   B. infections.   E. increases in metabolic activity.
   C. reduced metabolic activity.

_____ 63. What technique of stethoscope use best transmits low-pitched sound to the ear?
A. light pressure on the diaphragm
B. firm pressure on the diaphragm
C. moderate pressure on the bell
D. light pressure on the bell
E. strong pressure on the bell

_____ 64. The bell of a stethoscope is best for listening to the sounds of:
A. blood vessel bruits.
B. the blood pressure.
C. the heart.
D. the lung.
E. none of the above

_____ 65. Which of the following is NOT a characteristic of a good stethoscope?
A. thick, heavy tubing
B. long tubing (70 to 100 cm)
C. snug-fitting earpieces
D. a bell with a rubber-ring edge
E. all of the above

_____ 66. Generally, each narrow line on a sphygmomanometer represents what pressure difference?
A. 1 mmHg
B. 2 mmHg
C. 4 mmHg
D. 5 mmHg
E. 10 mmHg

_____ 67. If a patient has a regular and strong pulse, you should determine the pulse rate by assessing the number of beats in:
A. two minutes and dividing by 2.
B. three minutes.
C. 30 seconds and multiplying by 2.
D. 15 seconds and multiplying by 4.
E. 10 seconds and multiplying by 5.

_____ 68. Use of which of the following pulse points is recommended with a small child?
A. radial
B. brachial
C. carotid
D. popliteal
E. dorsalis pedis

_____ 69. It is important to attempt to evaluate your patient's respiratory rate and volume without his being aware of it.
A. True
B. False

_____ 70. The proper position of the patient's arm when taking the blood pressure is:
A. arm slightly flexed.
B. palm up.
C. fingers relaxed.
D. clothing removed from the upper arm.
E. all of the above

_____ 71. The sphygmomanometer should be inflated to what level beyond the point at which the patient's radial pulse disappears?
A. 10 mmHg
B. 20 mmHg
C. 30 mmHg
D. 40 mmHg
E. between B and C

_____ 72. The first blood pressure reading is the systolic blood pressure.
A. True
B. False

_____ 73. When using the oral glass thermometer, it should be left in the mouth for what period of time?
A. 30 to 45 seconds
B. 30 to 60 seconds
C. 1 to 2 minutes
D. 2 minutes
E. 3 to 4 minutes

_D_ 74. The normal patient oxygen saturation without supplemental oxygen at sea level should be:
- A. between 90 to 95 percent.
- B. below 95 percent.
- C. 100 percent.
- D. 96 to 100 percent.
- E. below 90 percent.

_B_ 75. A patient suffering from carbon monoxide poisoning will likely have a pulse oximetry reading that is:
- A. accurate.
- B. falsely high.
- C. falsely low.
- D. erratic and inaccurate.
- E. unreadable.

_D_ 76. The ECG of a cardiac monitor can tell you all of the following EXCEPT:
- A. the heart rate.
- B. the sequence of cardiac events.
- C. the timing of cardiac events.
- D. the pumping ability of the heart.
- E. both A and C

_E_ 77. Evaluation of the skin involves evaluating its:
- A. moisture.
- B. temperature.
- C. turgor.
- D. color.
- E. all of the above

_A_ 78. Pale skin is least likely to be caused by which of the following?
- A. increased deoxyhemoglobin
- B. a cold environment
- C. shock compensation
- D. anemia
- E. hypovolemic shock

_B_ 79. Which of the following skin discolorations represents a yellow hue?
- A. cyanosis
- B. jaundice
- C. eccyhmosis
- D. erythema
- E. pallor

_D_ 80. Thick skin often occurs with eczema and which of the following?
- A. dandruff
- B. nits
- C. seborrheic dermatitis
- D. psoriasis
- E. none of the above

_A_ 81. The blueish discoloration around the orbits of the eyes, suggestive of a basilar skull fracture, is called:
- A. "racoon eyes."
- B. "Battle's sign."
- C. periorbital ecchymosis.
- D. retroauricular ecchymosis.
- E. either A or C

_E_ 82. The characteristic of the unaffected eye responding to stimuli in the affected eye is:
- A. consenual response.
- B. direct response.
- C. simultaneous response.
- D. ipsilateral response.
- E. none of the above

_B_ 83. About 20 percent of the population have a noticeable difference in the size of the pupils, a condition called:
- A. hyphema.
- B. anisocoria.
- C. glaucoma.
- D. hypopyon.
- E. none of the above

_E_ 84. Otorrhea is a discharge from the ear that may contain:
- A. pus.
- B. mucus.
- C. blood.
- D. cerebrospinal fluid.
- E. all of the above

_A_ 85. The term for a common nosebleed is:
- A. epistaxis.
- B. otorrhea.
- C. rhinorrhea.
- D. rhinitis.
- E. none of the above

©2004 Pearson Education, Inc.
Intermediate Emergency Care: Principles & Practice

SPECIAL PROJECTS

Vital Signs

For each of the following vital signs, list the normal range of values and any other important considerations in their evaluation.

Pulse:

_____
_____
_____

Respirations:

_____
_____
_____
_____
_____
_____
_____

Blood pressure:

_____
_____
_____
_____
_____
_____
_____
_____

Temperature:

_____
_____
_____
_____
_____
_____
_____
_____

Physical Assessment—Personal Benchmarking

To perform the physical assessment of a patient, you will need to use the skills of inspection, palpation, auscultation, and percussion. You must not only master each of these skills but also learn to recognize normal and abnormal patient presentations. Often the distinction between normal and abnormal is very small and difficult to recognize without extensive experience. It is also difficult to maintain the ability to differentiate between normal and abnormal signs unless you practice the skill regularly. To help in skills maintenance, use yourself as a physiologic model upon which to practice assessment techniques and as a benchmark against which you can measure your patients' responses.

Pulse location and evaluation: Review page 424 of the text.

Palpate each of the following arteries for the location, rate, and strength of pulsation.

Radial—wrist, thumb side
Ulnar—wrist, little finger side
Brachial—medial aspect, just above the elbow
Carotid—just lateral of the trachea (palpate both)
Femoral—half the distance between the anterior iliac crest (the bone the belt sits on) and the
    symphysis pubis (just below the inguinal ligament)
Popliteal—just behind and below the knee
Posterior tibial—below the medial malleolus (ankle bone)
Dorsalis pedis—on top of the foot

Locate each of these pulses on yourself, but realize that you are healthy and perfusing well. It is more difficult to find and evaluate these distal pulses on patients, especially the pulses on the lower extremities and those of patients with serious medical or trauma-induced problems. Remember to place the pads of your fingers lightly over the artery and increase the pressure until you feel the strongest impulse. Rate each pulse from 0 to 3+ (with 0 = absent, 1+ = weak or thready, 2+ = normal, 3+ = bounding). Practice finding and rating the pulses quickly. These skills will be invaluable when you go to assess your patients.

You might try counting a pulse in your arm or forearm while driving or riding in a car. The vibration of travel makes the task much harder and simulates pulse evaluation in a moving ambulance. It might also be helpful to assess the pulses of friends and fellow emergency care workers to gain invaluable practice.

Auscultation: You need a stethoscope for this exercise.

Take the diaphragm of the stethoscope and apply it to the skin of your chest or abdomen. If you do not warm it first, you will be quite surprised at how cold it feels. Remember this as you are auscultating your patients' chests and abdomens.

Practice using the disk and diaphragm to assure you know which setting sends bell sounds to your ears and which sends diaphragm sounds. Listen to the different sounds found at various locations around the chest and abdomen. Increase the pressure on the bell from gentle for low sounds to strong pressure for high-pitched sounds. You might also practice listening with the television on at various volume levels. This simulates background noise at the emergency scene and demonstrates how difficult it can be to assess breath, heart, and bowel sounds in the field.

©2004 Pearson Education, Inc.
Intermediate Emergency Care: Principles & Practice

Lung sounds: Review page 423.

Listen to lung sounds in each of the five lung lobes. Remember that your patient's position will be reversed, his left lobes will be to your right. Take slow, deep breaths with your mouth open and listen for the faint noise of air moving through the small airways (normal or vesicular breath sounds). If you have a chance to auscultate your chest when you are experiencing the congestion of a cold, you may hear crackles or wheezes.

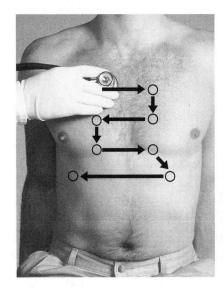

Then, auscultate the trachea at the suprasternal notch. Listen to the sounds, then move the diaphragm downward and laterally toward the lung fields. You will notice the quality of the sounds change as you move through the bronchial and bronchovesicular areas. Speak as you auscultate and notice how the speech sounds. It should be muffled, though you will hear it more clearly than when performing it on a patient because some sound is transmitted through the bones of the face and skull in addition to the stethoscope.

Heart sounds: Review pages 449–450.

Review the accompanying illustration to identify the proper locations for auscultating the heart sounds. With each sound, increase the pressure on the bell from very light to heavy and appreciate the changing quality of the sounds. You might also palpate the carotid artery and then the radial pulse while auscultating to note the synchronization and delay between the sounds and pulse. Listen for the S_1 and S_2 sounds (the "lub-dub") of the normal heart.

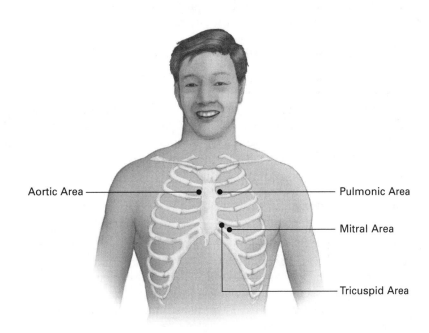

©2004 Pearson Education, Inc.
Intermediate Emergency Care: Principles & Practice

CHAPTER 8

Patient Assessment in the Field

Review of Chapter Objectives

After reading this chapter, you should be able to:

1. **Recognize hazards/potential hazards associated with the medical and trauma scene.**　　　　pp. 481–488

   During the scene size-up, you must examine the scene before you arrive at the patient's side. It is a time to evaluate and prepare for hazards including blood, fluids, airborne pathogens, and other conditions that may threaten your life or health. These conditions include the hazards of fire, structural collapse, traffic, unstable surfaces, electricity, broken glass, or jagged metal. Hazardous materials can involve chemical spills, radiation, and toxic environments. Finally, scene hazards can also include violent, disturbed, or unruly bystanders or patients. These hazards are not limited to the trauma scene but may be found at many medical scenes as well.

2. **Identify unsafe scenes and describe methods for making them safe.**　　　　pp. 481–488

   Your responsibility at the emergency scene is to recognize hazards including fire, structural collapse, traffic, unstable surfaces, electricity, broken glass, jagged metal, and hazardous materials and then act appropriately to protect yourself, other rescuers, and your patient. Unless you are specially trained and equipped to handle a specific hazard, do not enter the scene. In most cases, you will rely on the fire department, rescue service, police department, power company, hazmat team, or other specially trained personnel to secure the scene before you enter. If there is ever a question of whether a scene is safe or unsafe, do not enter the scene.

3. **Discuss common mechanisms of injury/nature of illness.**　　　　pp. 489–491

   Trauma is induced by a mechanism of injury through which forces enter the body and do physical harm. Common mechanisms include blunt trauma—for example, vehicle crashes (auto, recreational, watercraft, and bicycle), pedestrian vs. vehicle impacts, falls—and penetrating trauma—for example, gunshot and knife wounds. Medical problems have a related cause called the nature of the illness. The scene can provide evidence as to the nature of the illness. Examples include the presence of nebulizers, which suggest asthma, drug paraphernalia, which suggest overdose, and medications, which suggest preexisting cardiac or other problems.

4. **Discuss the reason for identifying the total number of patients at the scene.**　　　　pp. 488–489

   Determining the number of patients at a scene is important to assure that the needed resources are summoned to the scene and that every patient is cared for. At each and every scene, you should ask yourself, "Could there be others who are injured or ill?" While at the trauma scene it is common to find a patient wandering among the bystanders, the medical scene can have "hidden patients" too. The wife of a cardiac arrest patient, for example, may herself become a patient because of the emotional stress of the incident. Knowing the number of patients can help you gauge whether on-scene resources are adequate or whether you need to request that additional

©2004 Pearson Education, Inc.
Intermediate Emergency Care: Principles & Practice

units and manpower be dispatched to the scene. The earlier this request is made, the quicker those resources will arrive.

5. Organize the management of a scene following size-up.   **pp. 481–488**

The management of the scene following the scene size-up includes requesting both the appropriate units and personnel to manage scene hazards and the appropriate number and care levels of ambulances and personnel to treat the patients. You must also take the necessary steps to assure overall scene safety and to protect yourself, the patient, other scene personnel, and bystanders. The scene size-up also prepares you to manage the care of the patient by helping you recognize the mechanism of injury and anticipate injuries (index of suspicion) or by recognizing the nature of the illness.

6. Explain the reasons for identifying the need for additional help or assistance during the scene size-up.   **pp. 481, 484–488**

Multiple patients at the emergency scene can rapidly overwhelm your ability to provide effective care. If you wait until you are at a patient's side before calling for additional help, you may be distracted from making the call and delay an effective response. In cases where the number of patients far outstrips your ability to provide care, you may need to initiate a mass casualty response.

7. Summarize the reasons for forming a general impression of the patient.   **pp. 491–493**

The initial general impression of your patient takes into account the patient's age, gender, race, and other factors that will help you determine the seriousness of the problem and establish your priorities for patient care and transport. As you learn more about the patient through the initial assessment and the focused history and physical assessment, you will refine and improve on the accuracy and depth of the general impression. As you develop your general impression of the patient early in the assessment process, you can also begin to establish a rapport with him or her, explaining why you are there, what will be happening to him or her, and giving the patient the opportunity to refuse care.

8. Discuss methods of assessing mental status/levels of consciousness in the adult, infant, and child patient.   **pp. 493–494**

Initially determine the patient's mental status by categorizing him according to the AVPU system. Using this method, the patient is classified either **A**lert, responsive to **V**erbal stimuli, responsive to **P**ainful stimuli, or **U**nresponsive. You can further refine the evaluation by questioning the patient to determine orientation to place, time, and person and by differentiating his or her response to pain into purposeful and purposeless movement and decerebrate and decorticate posturing. An alert response for the infant or child is difficult to assess because of that patient's limited speech capabilities. Evaluate pediatric patients for activity and curiosity, being aware that the quiet child is often a seriously ill or injured one.

9. Discuss methods of assessing and securing a patient's airway.   **pp. 494–496**

The patient who is speaking clearly (or the child or infant who is crying loudly) has a patent airway. For other patients, position your head at the patient's mouth and look, listen, and feel for air moving through the airway. If you detect no movement, open the airway by using either the jaw thrust (in patients with trauma and suspected spine injury) or the head-tilt/chin-lift. Suction any fluids from the airway and remove obstructions using the Heimlich maneuver or laryngoscopy with Magill forceps. Secure the airway, as needed, with an oral or nasal airway, endotracheal intubation, or creation of a needle or surgical airway. When you have a pediatric patient, be sure to position the head and neck properly (using slight extension and padding under the shoulders), taking account of the differences in the pediatric anatomy. Also, reduce the size of the airways, laryngoscope blades, and endotracheal tubes you use with these patients.

10. **State reasons for taking spinal precautions for the trauma patient.** pp. 492–493

The spinal cord is the major communication distribution and collection conduit for the central nervous system. It is protected by the spinal column, the bony and flexible structure that runs from the base of the skull to just below the pelvis. If the column is injured, it may become unstable and permit injury to the spinal cord. Because injuries to the cord have such serious consequences, you should immobilize the spine early in your assessment and care to protect this essential communication pathway. Its immobilization will not harm the patient, while uncontrolled movement can cause permanent spinal cord injury.

11. **Describe methods for assessing respiration.** pp. 496–497

If your patient is speaking clearly (or if an infant or child patient is crying loudly) presume the airway is clear. Otherwise, listen for the sounds of airway restriction or obstruction, such as gurgling, stridor, or wheezes. If airway sounds are absent, place your ear at the patient's mouth while you listen, watch, and feel for air movement through it. If there is any doubt about airway patency, position the head with the jaw thrust or head-tilt/chin-lift. With a child, do not hyperextend the neck as this may block the airway. You may have to place padding behind the shoulders of a small child or infant to maintain proper head positioning.

12. **Describe methods for assessing circulation, including assessing for external bleeding.** p. 497

The initial assessment provides you with a general impression of the patient, a determination of the patient's mental status, and an evaluation of the airway, breathing, and circulation. This information indicates the status of the patient's respiration/oxygenation and circulation. It also indicates the patient's level of consciousness and the perfusion of the body's most important end-organ, the brain.

The patient with the potential for external hemorrhage must be assessed to determine both the nature and the extent of the blood loss. Any significant external hemorrhage must be halted and the amount of loss approximated to help prevent hypovolemia and to determine what effects the loss will have on the patient's body.

13. **Describe normal and abnormal findings when assessing skin color, temperature, and condition.** p. 497

Normal skin is warm, moist, and pink in color (in light-skinned people), reflecting good perfusion. The body's compensation for shock results in vasoconstriction, which produces mottled, cyanotic, pale or ashen skin color, and skin that is cool to the touch. Capillary refill times may exceed 3 seconds, though this may be due to a number of preexisting conditions in adults.

14. **Explain the reason and process for prioritizing a patient for care and transport.** pp. 500–501

At the conclusion of the initial assessment, you must determine your patient's priority, which will indicate how to proceed with assessment, care, and transport. With a seriously ill or injured patient, perform a rapid head-to-toe assessment. With a stable medical or trauma patient, perform a focused history and physical exam. You will also need to determine the priority for transport—either immediate transport with care rendered en route or with most care provided at the scene followed by transport.

15. **Describe orthostatic vital signs and evaluate their usefulness in assessing a patient in shock.** p. 516

The test for orthostatic vital signs, also called the tilt test, evaluates vital signs (blood pressure and pulse rate) before and after moving the patient from the supine to the seated, then to the full standing position. If after 30 to 60 seconds either the blood pressure drops by more than 10 mmHg or the pulse rate rises by more than 10, consider the test positive and suspect hypovolemia. (Note that the change in pulse rate is the more sensitive indicator.) Do not use this test when other indicators of shock are present as it places stress on the cardiovascular system.

©2004 Pearson Education, Inc.
Intermediate Emergency Care: Principles & Practice

16. Describe physical examination of the medical patient. pp. 511–517

The medical patient physical exam evaluates the head, ears, eyes, nose, and throat (HEENT), chest, abdomen, pelvis, extremities, posterior surface, and vital signs discretely, looking for illness or disease signs. The exam may be modified to meet the specific patient complaints of chest pain, respiratory distress, altered mental status, and acute abdomen. The medical patient exam may also include the results of pulse oximetry as well as cardiac and glucose level monitoring.

17. Differentiate between the assessment for a patient who has an unresponsive, altered mental status, and an assessment of other medical patients. pp. 511–517

Responsive and unresponsive medical patients are examined in much different fashions. The **responsive patient** can provide information regarding his or her chief complaint, history of the present illness, past medical history, and current health status. This information, along with a physical exam focused on the areas of expected signs, provides the information necessary to make a field diagnosis.

The **unresponsive patient** cannot provide this information, and the care giver must garner it from family and bystanders and through a more intensive and comprehensive physical examination.

The **patient with an altered mental status** is assessed like the unresponsive patient, though some information may be obtained from the patient. The information may not be reliable, hence the need for a more comprehensive physical exam.

18. Discuss the reasons for reconsidering the mechanism of injury. pp. 503–505

After the initial and rapid trauma assessments or focused history and physical exam, you have gathered enough information about your patient to determine if the mechanism of injury (and your resulting index of suspicion for associated injuries) agree with your assessment findings. If they do, maintain your priority for care and transport. If they do not agree, reevaluate your index of suspicion and the physical findings and possibly adjust your patient's priority. If you do alter your patient's priority, always err on the side of precaution.

19. Explain why patients should receive a rapid trauma assessment. p. 503

Every patient with a significant mechanism of injury, an altered level of consciousness, or multiple body-system traumas should receive the rapid trauma assessment. These patients are likely to have serious internal injuries and/or hemorrhage. However, the signs and symptoms of serious injury and shock are often hidden by other, more gruesome or painful injuries or by the body's compensatory mechanisms. Without maintaining a high index of suspicion for serious injury and evaluating the patient via the rapid trauma assessment, you are likely to overlook the patient with serious and life-threatening injury.

20. Describe physical examination of the trauma patient. pp. 503–510

The physical assessment of the trauma patient begins during the initial assessment with the check of the ABCs and then branches to either the rapid trauma assessment or focused history and physical exam. The patient with a serious mechanism of injury, altered mental status, or multi-system trauma receives a rapid trauma assessment, a fast, systematic physical exam evaluating body regions where serious or life-threatening problems are likely to occur. This assessment is a rapid evaluation of the critical structures and regions of the head (HEENT), neck, chest, abdomen, pelvis, extremities, posterior body, and vital signs. The patient with isolated trauma has an assessment directed at the areas of expected injury or patient complaint.

21. Describe the elements of the rapid trauma assessment and discuss their evaluation. pp. 503–510

Each region of the body is inspected, palpated, and, as appropriate, auscultated and percussed to identify the signs of injury (DCAP-BTLS and crepitation). For each region, the specific assessment considerations include the following:

©2004 Pearson Education, Inc.
Intermediate Emergency Care: Principles & Practice

Evaluate the **head** for any signs of serious bleeding and deformity from skull fracture. Also check for discharge from the ears and nose, for the stability of the facial bones, and for the patency of the airway.

Evaluate the **neck** for lacerations involving the major blood vessels and serious hemorrhage and possible air embolism. Examine the jugular veins for abnormal distention and palpate the position and any unusual motion of the trachea. Also examine for subcutaneous emphysema and then any evidence of spinal trauma.

Evaluate the **chest** for signs of respiratory distress, including use of accessory muscles and retractions, and any signs of open wounds. Also observe the motion of the chest. Chest excursion should be bilaterally equal and symmetrical. Palpate for signs of clavicular or costal fracture and subcutaneous emphysema. Erythema may be present, but the frank ecchymotic discoloration of a contusion takes time to develop. Auscultate the lungs at the mid-axillary line for bilaterally equal breath sounds.

Evaluate the **abdomen** for exaggerated abdominal wall motion, and inspect and palpate for signs of injury, noting rigidity, guarding, tenderness, and rebound tenderness.

Evaluate the **pelvis** for signs of injury and apply pressure directed posteriorly and medially to the iliac crests and pressure directed posteriorly to the symphysis pubis to check for pelvic instability.

Evaluate the **extremities** for signs of injury, distal circulation, and innervation.

Evaluate the **posterior body** for signs of injury, and be especially watchful for potential signs of spinal injury.

Evaluate **vital signs,** first to establish a baseline, and then to obtain other readings to compare to that baseline. Evaluate direct pupil response to light during the rapid trauma assessment, but evaluate the other pupillary responses during more specific and directed evaluation.

Gather a patient **history** while you perform the rapid trauma assessment. This should include the elements of the SAMPLE assessment (Signs/Symptoms, Allergies, Medications, Past medical history, Last oral intake, and Events preceding the incident).

22. Identify cases when the rapid assessment is altered or suspended to provide patient care. pp. 503–505

The rapid trauma assessment is interrupted to provide patient care whenever you identify any life-threatening condition that can be quickly addressed. Just as you would suction the airway when you find it full of fluids during the initial assessment, you might provide pleural decompression during the rapid trauma assessment when you notice a developing tension pneumothorax. You might also administer oxygen to a patient who begins to display dyspnea and accessory muscle use during your chest examination. Other examples might include employing the PASG for the patient with the early signs of shock compensation and an unstable pelvic fracture found during the pelvic assessment or immediate provision of spinal immobilization upon noticing a neurologic deficit during the extremity exam.

23. Discuss the reason for performing a focused history and physical exam. pp. 501, 511, 517

The focused history and physical exam is the third step (following the scene size-up and initial assessment) of the patient assessment process. It is an assessment directed at the areas where the signs of serious injury or illness are expected. It also draws upon a quick history to identify information supporting a specific diagnosis and elements critical to the continued care of the patient. The focused history and physical exam takes you quickly toward determining the nature of the illness or the existence of serious and specific injuries. It is performed in different ways for trauma patients with significant injuries or mechanisms of injury, trauma patients with isolated injuries, responsive medical patients, and unresponsive medical patients.

24. Describe when and why a detailed physical examination is necessary and identify its components. pp. 519–525

The detailed assessment is a combination of a detailed history and a comprehensive physical exam either to identify or to learn more about the effects of an illness or injury on the body. It, in its entirety, is employed only when all other assessment and care procedures have been performed,

©2004 Pearson Education, Inc.
Intermediate Emergency Care: Principles & Practice

most likely during transport to the hospital and then only for patients with serious trauma or disease. Since the seriously ill or injured patients require constant care, this assessment is rarely performed in the prehospital setting. However, portions of the detailed physical exam are frequently employed to examine specific body regions, looking for expected signs of illness or injury.

The detailed physical exam involves a comprehensive evaluation of each body region using the skills of inspection, palpation, auscultation, and percussion. It begins at the head and progresses downward to the extremities and includes the following:

Head. Inspect and palpate for any skull or facial asymmetry, deformity, instability, tenderness, unusual warmth, or crepitation. Look for the development of Battle's sign and periorbital ecchymosis.

Eyes. Carefully inspect the eye for shape, size, coloration, and foreign bodies as well as pupillary equality, light reactivity, consensual movement, and visual acuity.

Ears. Examine the external ear for signs of injury and the ear canal for hemorrhage or discharge.

Nose and sinuses. Palpate the external aspect of the nose and examine the nares for signs of injury, hemorrhage, discharge, and flaring. The nasal mucosa is rich in vasculature and may bleed heavily.

Mouth and pharynx. Examine the oral cavity for signs of injury and the potential for airway compromise. Notice any fluids or odors and examine tongue movement for signs of cranial nerve injury.

Neck. Briefly inspect the neck for signs of injury with special attention to open wounds and possible severe hemorrhage and air embolism. Palpate the trachea to identify any unusual movement and examine for jugular vein distention.

Chest and lungs. Observe the patient's breathing for symmetrical chest movement and respiratory pattern. Note any accessory muscle use, and auscultate and percuss for unusual findings. Look for signs of injury, and palpate for crepitation and tenderness.

Cardiovascular system. Look to the skin for pallor, and palpate a pulse for rate, rhythm, and strength. Auscultate for heart sounds, and locate the point of maximal impulse.

Abdomen. Inspect and palpate for signs of injury and rebound tenderness, rigidity, and guarding.

Pelvis. Observe the area, then place medial and posterior pressure on the iliac crests and posterior pressure on the symphysis pubis.

Genitalia. As needed, examine these organs for hemorrhage and, in the male, priapism.

Anus and rectum. If hemorrhage is present, inspect the anus and rectum and apply direct pressure to halt bleeding.

Peripheral vascular system. Inspect all four extremities, observing and palpating for signs of injury and skin color, moisture, temperature, and capillary refill to assure distal circulation.

Musculoskeletal system. Palpate the musculature of the extremities, feeling for differences in muscle tone and the flexibility and the active and passive range of motion in joints.

Nervous system. Evaluate the nervous system by examining the following:
- **Mental status and speech.** Assess the patient's level of consciousness and orientation and compare these findings to earlier ones. Note speech patterns and the patient's appropriateness of dress and actions.
- **Cranial nerves.** Test the discrete cranial nerves that have not already been tested.
- **Motor system.** Inspect the patient's general body structure, positioning, muscular development, and coordination.
- **Sensory system.** Test for ability to sense pain, touch, position, temperature, and vibration over the extremities, and as necessary, the dermatomes.
- **Reflexes.** Test deep tendon reflexes with a reflex hammer, noting heightened or diminished responses. Test superficial abdominal reflexes and plantar response.

Vital signs. Repeat the evaluation of the vital signs including blood pressure, pulse, respiration, temperature, and pupillary response.

25. Explain what additional care is provided while performing the detailed physical exam.
pp. 519–525

Since the complete detailed physical exam is an elective assessment, any time a significant sign of injury or the patient's condition suggests a care step, perform that step. The same principle applies

Patient Assessment

when a portion of the comprehensive physical exam is performed on a discrete body region after the focused history and physical exam.

26. Distinguish between the detailed physical exam that is performed on a trauma patient and that of the medical patient. pp. 519–525

The detailed physical exam for the trauma patient focuses evaluation on the areas where signs of injury are expected based upon the mechanism of injury analysis or the patient's complaints (for example, examination for signs of anterior chest injury when an auto steering wheel is deformed). The detailed physical exam for the medical patient is directed to the areas of patient complaint as well as those areas where the signs of an expected illness might be found (for example, an examination for pitting edema in the dependent areas with the congestive heart failure patient). The history component of the assessment also differs with trauma and medical patients. With the trauma patient, you may gather an abbreviated (SAMPLE) history, while with the medical patient, you may perform a more in-depth history evaluation as described in Chapter 6, "History Taking."

27. Differentiate between patients requiring a detailed physical exam and those who do not. p. 519

The patients who receive a complete detailed physical exam are patients with serious medical or trauma injuries. They receive the detailed physical exam during transport to the hospital after other important care measures have been employed. They represent a very small percentage of patients that you will treat because seriously ill or injured patients often require almost continuous care. *Portions* of the detailed exam will, however, be performed on many patients, and these portions will be directed at a body region where signs of injury or illness are expected. Patients receiving portions of the detailed exam include those with isolated injuries and those patients with stable medical problems. Seriously ill or injured patients may receive a detailed exam aimed at discovering significant signs of the pathology generally associated with cardiac, respiratory, vascular, abdominal, musculoskeletal, or nervous system problems.

28. Describe the components of the ongoing assessment, and discuss the rationale for repeating the initial assessment. pp. 525–528

The components of the ongoing assessment include reassessment of the pertinent elements of the initial assessment, focused history and physical exam or rapid trauma assessment, and vital signs and include:

Mental status. Quickly reevaluate the patient's mental status to determine AVPU status or level of orientation.

Airway patency/breathing rate and quality. Perform a quick check of airway patency and breathing rate, volume, and quality to assure respiration is adequate.

Pulse rate and quality. Quickly reevaluate the pulse rate, strength, and regularity to assure they remain within normal limits.

Skin condition. Quickly check the skin for moisture, temperature, and capillary refill to monitor distal perfusion.

Vital signs. Reassess blood pressure and temperature (along with pulse and respiration) and compare to baseline findings to determine whether the patient's condition is improving, deteriorating, or remaining the same.

Focused assessment. Quickly reevaluate the signs of injury/illness to identify any changes. This may include reevaluating pertinent negatives to rule out an evolving problem.

Effects of interventions. Repeat the ongoing assessment soon after any major intervention to determine the intervention's impact on the patient's condition.

Transport priorities. Based upon the findings of the ongoing assessment, either confirm or modify the patient's priority for care and transport.

The initial assessment, with its examination of mental status and evaluation of the airway, breathing, and circulation, contains crucial elements of continuing patient assessment. These components of the initial assessment can quickly tell you when the patient is suffering from a life-

©2004 Pearson Education, Inc.
Intermediate Emergency Care: Principles & Practice

threatening or serious problem and can help you monitor the patient's need for care. For this reason, these components are an integral part of any ongoing assessment.

29. Describe trending of assessment components.   pp. 525–528

Trending of the elements of the ongoing assessment—comparing of sequential findings—will suggest whether your patient's condition is improving, deteriorating, or remaining the same. This information prompts you to modify your priorities for patient care and transport, and may ultimately cause you to modify your field diagnosis.

30. Discuss medical identification devices/systems.   p. 509

Examine the patient's wrists, ankles, and neck for medical alert jewelry reflecting preexisting medical conditions such as diabetes, epilepsy, allergies, use of medications, and the like. Also check the wallet or purse for such information. This information may help you and the emergency department in prescribing care for the patient.

CASE STUDY REVIEW

This case study gives you the opportunity quickly to identify and review the elements of the patient assessment process. The process involves the scene size-up, initial assessment, focused history and physical exam, detailed exam, and ongoing assessments.

Even before Chris arrives at the scene, she uses the time available to her to review the elements of the scene size-up and her expected assessment and care. She identifies the likely mechanism of injury as a fall from a great height with an impact on an unforgiving surface. She suspects very serious injuries and the need for rapid assessment and care. Given the expected mechanism of injury, Chris may alert the trauma center to let them know of the incident and, if she is more than 15 minutes away from the center, might also put the helicopter service on standby.

As Chris arrives, she sizes up the scene and quickly determines that the dispatch information was correct. She dons her gloves to protect against the dangers of body substance contamination and requests additional help from the fire department. She also recognizes that this is not likely to be a hazardous scene but that she may have to contend with curious onlookers and those who are made emotionally distraught by the sight of blood and gore. Finally, Chris considers the mechanism of injury to help her anticipate injuries. Given the circumstances, Chris expects numerous broken bones, internal injuries, and head and spine trauma in this patient.

As Chris moves to the patient's side, she begins the initial assessment. She already has a general impression of the patient's condition, and it is not good. She builds upon this impression as the assessment continues. She immediately directs Nick to hold cervical spine stabilization as one of the first steps in the initial assessment. He continues manual stabilization until the patient is fully immobilized by mechanical means later on. Chris determines the patient is completely unresponsive and then moves to assess the ABCs. The airway is cleared, respirations are supported, and Chris begins treating the patient for shock. These actions are essential to sustain life, and Chris does not delay her initial assessment to care for any non-life-threatening injuries.

With the airway, breathing, and circulation stabilized, Chris moves to the rapid trauma assessment, a form of the focused history and physical exam. Here she concentrates her patient evaluation on possible critical injuries. She examines the head, neck, chest, abdomen, pelvis, and extremities and notes the depressed skull fracture, the rigid abdomen, and the pelvic and femur fractures. She also notes pertinent negatives (expected but not substantiated findings) like the absent signs of pneumothorax. Since this is a critical trauma patient, transport and life-sustaining interventions are the highest priorities, and Chris does not perform a detailed physical exam. Doing so would extend the time at the scene and probably not suggest any care steps that Chris and Nick are not already planning. The care team determines that their patient is critical and needs the services of a trauma center. They make arrangements to expedite transport.

Once the patient is on the way to the trauma center and all critical interventions have been performed, Chris provides an ongoing assessment. She quickly reevaluates the level of responsiveness,

ABCs, vital signs, and the patient's signs and symptoms. She documents the results to track the patient's progress during her care—Is the patient improving, deteriorating, or remaining the same? Since the patient is critical, Chris performs the ongoing assessment every 5 minutes. (She would perform it every 15 minutes or so for a nonserious patient.) She also employs the ongoing assessment whenever her team performs an invasive procedure or anytime they notice a change in a patient sign or symptom.

CONTENT SELF-EVALUATION

MULTIPLE CHOICE

1. As an EMT-I, you will certainly never perform a comprehensive history and physical exam in the acute setting.
   A. True
   B. False

2. Which component of the patient assessment process will be performed during patient transport?
   A. scene survey
   B. initial assessment
   C. focused history and physical exam
   D. detailed physical exam
   E. ongoing assessment

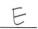

3. After the scene size-up and if necessary, you should inform the dispatcher of:
   A. the nature of the medical or trauma emergency.
   B. what resources you need.
   C. the phone number at which you can be reached.
   D. what actions you and your crew are taking.
   E. all of the above except C

4. Which of the following is NOT a component of the scene size-up?
   A. body substance isolation
   B. general impression of the patient
   C. location of all patients
   D. mechanism of injury/nature of the illness analysis
   E. scene safety

5. Which of the following body substance isolation devices will you employ with every patient you treat?
   A. latex or vinyl gloves   D. gown
   B. protective eyewear   E. both B and C
   C. face mask

6. Whenever you plan to intubate a patient, you should wear:
   A. latex or vinyl gloves and a gown.
   B. protective eyewear, a gown, and a face mask.
   C. latex or vinyl gloves, protective eyewear, and a face mask.
   D. protective eyewear and a gown.
   E. latex or vinyl gloves.

7. The HEPA respirator is designed to filter out which of the following pathogens that may be encountered when providing prehospital emergency care?
   A. tuberculosis   D. the flu
   B. small pox   E. tetanus toxoid
   C. anthrax

©2004 Pearson Education, Inc.
Intermediate Emergency Care: Principles & Practice

_E_   8. The intent of the safety analysis portion of the scene survey is to assure the safety of:
   A. the patient.
   B. bystanders.
   C. fellow responders.
   D. yourself.
   E. all of the above

_E_   9. To properly handle a scene safety issue, you must be:
   A. properly trained.
   B. properly equipped.
   C. properly clothed.
   D. prepared to attempt rescue procedures in which you have not been trained.
   E. A, B, and C above

_C_ 10. Potential hazards to rule out before entering the scene include all of the following EXCEPT:
   A. fire.
   B. electrocution.
   C. contamination with blood.
   D. structural collapse.
   E. broken glass and jagged metal.

_A_ 11. When called to a shooting or domestic disturbance, until the police arrive and secure the scene you should remain:
   A. outside the neighborhood.
   B. outside the residence.
   C. just down the street.
   D. at the door but don't enter.
   E. either B or C

_D_ 12. At which of the following incidents would you NOT expect to discover more than one patient in your scene size-up?
   A. a two-car accident
   B. a carbon monoxide poisoning in a home
   C. a car crash in which a child seat and diaper bag are visible
   D. a fall out of a tree
   E. a hazardous materials spill in a high-school chemistry lab

_B_ 13. You should delay the call for additional ambulances until you begin your initial assessment because you will not have enough information to determine the needs of the scene until then.
   A. True
   B. False

_A_ 14. The two important functions that must begin immediately in the mass-casualty situation are:
   A. triage and incident command.
   B. rescue and triage.
   C. fire fighting and rescue.
   D. incident command and extrication.
   E. incident command and scene isolation.

_B_ 15. The responsibilities of incident command at a disaster scene include all of the following EXCEPT:
   A. performing a scene size-up.
   B. triaging initial patients for care.
   C. determining the need for additional resources.
   D. radioing for additional equipment and personnel.
   E. directing in-coming crews.

_D_ 16. The responsibilities of the triage person at the disaster scene include all of the following EXCEPT:
   A. determining a patient's priority for immediate transport.
   B. determining a patient's priority for delayed transport.
   C. performing simple, but life-saving procedures.
   D. providing intensive care on salvageable patients.
   E. all of the above

_E_ 17. The mechanism of injury analysis examines:
  A. body locations affected.   D. nature of the crash forces.
  B. strength of the crash forces.   E. all of the above
  C. direction of the crash forces.

_C_ 18. The index of suspicion is best defined as:
  A. patient priority for care based on the MOI.
  B. anticipation of the nature of forces involved in an accident.
  C. anticipation of injuries based upon the MOI.
  D. anticipation of degree of injury based on the patient's appearance.
  E. none of the above

_E_ 19. The nature of the illness is determined from information you receive from:
  A. the patient.   D. scene clues.
  B. the patient's family.   E. all of the above
  C. bystanders.

_C_ 20. The initial assessment includes all of the following EXCEPT:
  A. forming a general impression of the patient.
  B. stabilizing the cervical spine as needed.
  C. immobilizing of fractures.
  D. assessing the airway.
  E. assessing the circulation.

_A_ 21. The general patient impression is based upon all of the following EXCEPT:
  A. blood pressure.   D. the environment.
  B. mechanism of injury.   E. your instincts.
  C. chief complaint.

_E_ 22. Which of the following is NOT a purpose served by your initial introduction to the patient?
  A. identifying yourself
  B. identifying your reason for being there
  C. establishing your level of training
  D. giving the patient an opportunity to refuse care
  E. obtaining informed consent

_C_ 23. During the initial assessment, the cervical spine should be stabilized:
  A. after the airway is established.
  B. just before you attempt artificial ventilation.
  C. immediately, if suggested by the MOI.
  D. after the circulation check.
  E. as the last step of the initial assessment.

_A_ 24. Which of the following conditions does NOT normally cause an altered mental status?
  A. eupnea   D. poisoning
  B. drug overdose   E. sepsis
  C. head injury

_C_ 25. A patient who only moves his arm when firmly pinched between the thumb and first finger and shows no other responses will be classified as which of the following under the AVPU system?
  A. A   D. U
  B. V   E. cannot be determined with the
  C. P   information at hand

_A_ 26. A patient who is disoriented and confused would be classified as which of the following under the AVPU system?
  A. A   D. U
  B. V   E. cannot be determined with the
  C. P   information at hand

©2004 Pearson Education, Inc.
Intermediate Emergency Care: Principles & Practice

_B_ **27.** Stridor can usually be caused by all of the following EXCEPT:

    A. infection.   **D.** severe swelling.

    B. gastric distress.   **E.** allergic reaction.

    C. foreign body.

_D_ **28.** For stridor that is caused by respiratory burns, the care procedure most likely to maintain the airway is:

    A. suctioning.

    B. blow-by oxygen and a quiet ride to the hospital.

    C. a surgical airway.

    D. early endotracheal intubation.

    E. vasoconstrictor medications.

_A_ **29.** A patient with abnormally deep respirations is said to be:

    A. hyperpneic.   **D.** bradypneic.

    B. tachypneic.   **E.** hypopneic.

    C. eupneic.

_C_ **30.** The presence of a radial pulse suggests that the systolic blood pressure is at least:

    A. 60 mmHg.   **D.** 100 mmHg.

    B. 70 mmHg.   **E.** 120 mmHg.

    C. 80 mmHg.

_C_ **31.** The focused history and physical exam is conducted differently for the four different categories of patients. Which of the following is NOT one of those categories?

pg 50i

    A. responsive medical patient

    B. unresponsive medical patient

    C. pediatric patient with altered consciousness

    D. trauma patient with an isolated injury

    E. trauma patient with a significant mechanism of injury

_D_ **32.** Which of the following is NOT a mechanism of injury that calls for rapid transport to the trauma center?

    A. ejection from a vehicle

    B. vehicle rollover

    C. severe vehicle deformity in a high-speed crash

    D. fall from less than 20 feet

    E. bicycle collision with loss of consciousness

_B_ **33.** The decision to provide rapid transport of a patient to the trauma center is predicated upon either the mechanism of injury or the:

    A. blood pressure reading.   **D.** ongoing assessments.

    B. physical signs of trauma.   **E.** none of the above

    C. pulse oximetry reading.

_A_ **34.** If you arrive at your patient's side only moments after the accident, he or she may not have lost enough blood to demonstrate the signs of shock.

    A. True

    B. False

_E_ **35.** Which of the following body regions is examined during the rapid trauma assessment?

    A. head   **D.** thorax

    B. neck   **E.** all of the above

    C. pelvis

_A_ **36.** The "B" of DCAP-BTLS stands for:

    A. burns.   **D.** bilateral injury.

    B. bumps.   **E.** bruises.

    C. blemishes.

D___ 37. Which of the following is NOT represented within the DCAP-BTLS mnemonic?
   A. contusions
   B. abrasions
   C. burns
   D. crepitation
   E. swelling

A___ 38. Scalp wounds tend to bleed heavily because:
   A. there is a lack of a protective vasospasm mechanism.
   B. the hair helps continue the blood loss.
   C. the close proximity of the skull permits blood to flow quickly outward.
   D. direct pressure is difficult to apply.
   E. both A and C

B___ 39. Subcutaneous emphysema is best described as:
   A. a grating sensation.
   B. air trapped under the skin.
   C. air leaking from the respiratory system.
   D. retraction of the tissues between the ribs.
   E. fluid accumulation just beneath the skin.

C___ 40. Suprasternal and intercostal retractions are caused by:
   A. tension pneumothorax.
   B. subcutaneous emphysema.
   C. airway obstruction or restriction.
   D. flail chest.
   E. either B or D

B___ 41. To assure adequate air exchange for the patient with a flail chest, you should:
   A. perform a needle decompression.
   B. assist ventilations with a BVM and oxygen.
   C. apply oxygen only.
   D. perform an endotracheal intubation.
   E. cover the wound with an occlusive dressing.

D___ 42. When assessing the pelvis for possible fracture, you should apply:
   A. anterior pressure on the iliac crests.
   B. lateral pressure on the symphysis pubis.
   C. firm pressure on the lower abdomen.
   D. medial and posterior pressure on the iliac crests.
   E. pressure to move the hips to the flexed position.

B___ 43. Your finding that a patient is able to move a limb, but the limb is cool, pale, and without a pulse is consistent with:
   A. neurologic compromise.
   B. vascular compromise.
   C. both a vascular and neurologic compromise.
   D. spinal injury.
   E. peripheral nerve root injury.

D___ 44. The "A" of the SAMPLE history stands for:
   A. alcohol consumption.
   B. adverse reactions.
   C. attitude.
   D. allergies.
   E. none of the above

C___ 45. With a patient who has a crushing injury to his index finger received when it was caught in a closing door, which form of patient assessment would be most reasonable?
   A. the rapid trauma assessment and a quick history
   B. the rapid trauma assessment and a detailed history
   C. a quick history and a physical exam focused on the injury
   D. a detailed patient history and a physical exam focused on the injury
   E. a detailed physical exam

©2004 Pearson Education, Inc.
Intermediate Emergency Care: Principles & Practice

_E_ **46.** While gathering the history of a chest pain patient, you will likely:
  A. attach a cardiac monitor.
  B. administer oxygen.
  C. take vital signs.
  D. start an IV, if appropriate.
  E. all of the above

_D_ **47.** The pain or discomfort that caused the patient to call you to his or her side is called the:
  A. presenting problem.
  B. differential diagnosis.
  C. field diagnosis.
  D. chief complaint.
  E. present illness.

_B_ **48.** A patient statement that "deep breathing makes my chest hurt" represents which element of the OPQRST-ASPN mnemonic for investigation of the chief complaint?
  A. O
  B. P
  C. R
  D. S
  E. PN

_C_ **49.** The jugular veins in a patient with normal cardiovascular function remain full or distended up to which of the following degrees of patient tilt?
  A. 15 degrees
  B. 30 degrees
  C. 45 degrees
  D. 60 degrees
  E. 90 degrees

_A_ **50.** If you hear bilateral rales on inspiration when auscultating a patient's chest, you should suspect:
  A. congestive heart failure.
  B. bronchospasm.
  C. asthma.
  D. chronic obstructive pulmonary disease.
  E. all of the above

_D_ **51.** In a patient who displays hyperresonance to percussion, you should suspect:
  A. pleural effusion.
  B. pulmonary edema.
  C. pneumonia.
  D. emphysema.
  E. none of the above

_B_ **52.** Examine a patient for unusual pulsation of the descending aorta:
  A. just right of the umbilicus.
  B. just left of the umbilicus.
  C. along a line from the umbilicus to the middle symphysis pubis.
  D. just beneath the zyphoid process.
  E. anywhere in the abdomen.

_E_ **53.** Accumulation of fluid within the abdominal cavity is common in patients with:
  A. hypovolemia.
  B. aortic aneurysm.
  C. emphysema.
  D. gastric ulcer disease.
  E. cirrhosis of the liver.

_B_ **54.** A patient in whom unequal pupils are a normal condition displays:
  A. Cullen's sign.
  B. anisocoria.
  C. consensual response.
  D. accommodation.
  E. Bell's palsy.

_E_ **55.** Vital signs provide the assessing EMT-I with:
  A. a window into what is happening with the patient.
  B. an objective capsule of the patient's clinical status.
  C. possible indications of severe illness.
  D. possible indications of the need to intervene.
  E. all of the above

_A_ 56. A pulse oximetry reading of 88 percent would indicate the need for:
   A. aggressive airway and ventilatory care.
   B. only the administration of blow-by oxygen.
   C. only some repositioning of the patient's head.
   D. no care at this point.
   E. careful monitoring of the patient for further deterioration.

_E_ 57. The type of patient most likely to receive the most comprehensive assessment is:
   A. the severe trauma patient.   D. the unresponsive medical patient.
   B. the minor trauma patient.   E. both A and D
   C. the responsive medical patient.

_A_ 58. EMT-Is employ the complete detailed physical assessment at the scene:
   A. rarely.
   B. occasionally.
   C. frequently.
   D. rarely in trauma patients, frequently in medical patients.
   E. frequently in trauma patients, rarely in medical patients.

_A_ 59. Reflexes not likely to be tested during the detailed physical exam are the:
   A. clavicular.   D. Achilles.
   B. biceps.   E. abdominal plantar.
   C. triceps.

_E_ 60. Serial ongoing assessments will facilitate:
   A. reassessment of the patient.
   B. revision of the field diagnosis.
   C. changes in the management plan.
   D. documentation of the effects of interventions.
   E. all of the above

LISTING

List the components of patient assessment in the order they would be performed in the field.

61. BSI / SCENE SIZE-UP
62. INITIAL ASSESSMENT
63. FOCUSED HISTORY + PHYSICAL EXAM
64. DETAILED PHYSICAL EXAM
65. ONGOING ASSESSMENT

©2004 Pearson Education, Inc.
Intermediate Emergency Care: Principles & Practice

CHAPTER 9

✳

Clinical Decision Making

Review of Chapter Objectives

After reading this chapter, you should be able to:

1. **Compare the factors influencing medical care on scene to other medical settings.** pp. 531–532

   Most health-care providers function in very controlled and supportive environments. The EMT-I carries out the skills of other health-care providers, but he often does so in hostile and adverse conditions. EMT-Is perform assessments, form field diagnoses, and devise and employ patient management plans at the scenes of emergencies in spite of poor weather, limited ambient light, limited diagnostic equipment, and few support personnel. The EMT-I also must perform these skills under extreme constraints of time and often without on-scene consultation and supervision.

2. **Differentiate among critical life-threatening, potentially life-threatening, and non-life-threatening patient presentations.** p. 532

   Critical life-threatening presentations include major multisystem trauma, devastating single system trauma, end-stage disease presentations, and acute presentations of chronic disease. These patients may present with airway, breathing, neurological, or circulatory (shock) problems and demand aggressive resuscitation.

   Potential life-threatening presentations include serious multisystem trauma and multiple disease etiologies. Patient presentation generally includes moderate to serious distress. The care required is sometimes invasive but generally supportive.

   Non-life-threatening presentations are isolated and uncomplicated minor injuries or illness. The patient is stable without serious signs or symptoms or the need for aggressive intervention.

3. **Evaluate the benefits and shortfalls of protocols, standing orders, and patient care algorithms.** pp. 532–534

   Protocols are written guidelines identifying the specific management of various medical and trauma patient problems. They may also be developed for special situations such as physician-on-the-scene, radio failure, and termination of resuscitation. They provide a standard care approach for patients with "classical" presentations. They do not apply to all patients or to patients who present with multiple problems and should not be adhered to so rigidly as to limit performance in unusual circumstances.

   Standing orders are protocols that an EMT-I can perform before direct on-line communication with a medical direction physician. They speed emergency care but may not address the atypical patient.

   Patient care algorithms are flowcharts with lines, arrows, and boxes that outline appropriate care measures based on patient presentation or response to care. They are generally useful guides and encourage uniform patient care, but again, they do not adequately address the atypical patient.

4. **Define the components, stages, and sequences of the critical-thinking process for EMT-Intermediates, and apply the fundamental elements.**   pp. 534–540

Components of critical thinking include the following:

Knowledge and Abilities
Knowledge and abilities comprise the first component of critical thinking. Your knowledge of prehospital emergency care is the basis for your decisions in the field. This knowledge comes from your classroom, clinical, and field experience. It is used to sort out your patient's presentation to determine the likely cause of the problem and to select the appropriate care skills. Your abilities are the technical skills you employ to assess or care for a patient.

Useful Thinking Styles
- **Reflective vs. Impulsive Situation Analysis.** Reflective analysis refers to taking time to deliberately and analytically contemplate possible patient care, as might occur with unknown medical illness. Impulsive analysis refers to the immediate response that the paramedic must provide in a life-threatening situation, as might be required with decompensating shock or cardiac arrest.
- **Divergent vs. Convergent Data Processing.** Divergent data processing considers all aspects of a situation before arriving at a solution and is most useful with complex situations. Convergent data processing focuses narrowly on the most important aspects of a situation and is best suited for uncomplicated situations that require little reflection.
- **Anticipatory vs. Reactive Decision Making.** With anticipatory decision making, you respond to what you think may happen to your patient. With reactive decision making, you provide a care modality once the patient presents with a symptom.

Thinking under Pressure
Thinking under pressure is a difficult but frequent challenge of prehospital emergency medicine. The "fight or flight" response may diminish your ability to think critically to such an extent that you are only able to respond at the pseudo-instinctive level, with preplanned and practiced responses (like the mental checklist) that are performed almost without thought. One example of a mental checklist includes the following steps:

Scan the situation by standing back and looking for subtle clues to the patient's complaint or problem.

Stop and think of both the possible benefits and side effects of each of your care interventions.

Decide and act by executing your chosen care plan with confidence and authority.

Maintain control of the scene, patient care, and your own emotions, even under the stress of a chaotic scene.

Reevaluate your patient's signs and symptoms and your associated care plan and make changes as the situation changes.

5. **Describe the effects of the "fight or flight" response and its positive and negative effects on a EMT-Intermediate's decision making.**   pp. 537–538

The "fight or flight" response is the intense activation of the sympathetic branch of the autonomic nervous system. Secretion of the system's major hormone, epinephrine, causes an increase in heart rate and cardiac output. It raises respiratory rate and volume, directs blood to the skeletal muscles, dilates the pupils (for distant vision), and increases hearing perception. However, the increased epinephrine may diminish critical thinking ability and concentration, impairing your ability to perform well in an emergency unless you raise your assessment and care skills to a pseudo-instinctive level, at which point acting under the pressure of an emergency becomes second nature.

6. **Develop strategies for effective thinking under pressure.**   pp. 537–538

Form a concept. Gather enough information from your first view of the patient and scene size-up to form a general impression of the patient's condition and the likely cause.

Interpret the data. Perform the patient assessment and analyze the results in light of your previous assessment and care experience. Form a field diagnosis.

Apply the principles. With the field diagnosis in mind, devise a management plan to care for the patient according to your protocols, standing orders, and patient care algorithms.

©2004 Pearson Education, Inc.
Intermediate Emergency Care: Principles & Practice

Evaluate. Through frequent ongoing assessments, reassess the patient's condition and the effects of your interventions.

Reflect. After the call, critique your call with the emergency department staff and your crew to determine what steps might be improved and add this call to your experience base.

7. Summarize the "six Rs" of putting it all together. p. 540

Read the scene. Observe the scene or general environment for clues to the mechanism of injury or nature of the illness.

Read the patient. Observe, palpate, auscultate, smell, and listen to the patient for signs and symptoms. Assure the ABCs and obtain a set of vital signs.

React. Address the priorities of care from the ABCs to other critical, then serious, then minor problems and care priorities.

Reevaluate. Conduct frequent ongoing assessments to identify any changes caused either by the disease or by your interventions.

Revise the management plan. Based on the ongoing assessments, revise your management plan to best serve your patient's changing condition.

Review performance. At the end of every response, critique the performance of your crew and identify ways to improve future responses.

CASE STUDY REVIEW

This case study describes a typical trauma patient. The EMT-I's initial assessment suggests serious impact, but the patient at first demonstrates no signs or symptoms of serious internal injury. As assessment, care, and transport proceed, however, the patient deteriorates, requiring the EMT-I to employ critical clinical decision-making skills.

Sue responds to a routine minor trauma call. After performing an initial assessment and a rapid trauma assessment, Sue decides that the patient does not meet the criteria for rapid transport to a trauma center. Sues's rapid trauma assessment suggests that Marcie has experienced only minor facial trauma and signs and symptoms supportive of that determination. The only point of possible concern is Marcie's inability to remember what happened. However, her hemodynamic status and vital signs support the field diagnosis of minor facial injuries. Her patient acuity is determined to be non-life-threatening. Sue decides the closest community hospital is a good choice to assure quick care for Marcie's injuries and cancels the county medevac helicopter.

En route to the community hospital, Sue performs an ongoing assessment (every 15 minutes for a minor injury patient). She discovers that Marcie is showing some signs of a CNS deficit. This causes Sue to reevaluate her original patient acuity and field diagnosis. The degeneration of Marcie's level of responsiveness alarms Sue. Through divergent thinking, looking for other causes of Marcie's presentation, she changes the patient acuity to life-threatening and her field diagnosis to increasing intracranial pressure. She will no doubt now monitor Marcie every 5 minutes and focus her attention on the signs of increasing intracranial pressure, diminishing level of consciousness and orientation, as well as a slowing pulse rate and rising systolic blood pressure. If oxygen has not already been applied, Sue administers it, the urgency of transport increases, and the destination is changed to a trauma center.

Because Sue carefully monitored her patient and employed good critical decision-making skills, Marcie did not go to a community hospital. If she had, she likely would have been stabilized and then transported to a trauma or neuro-center, delaying her time to critical surgery. Such ongoing monitoring of a patient along with the anticipation of possible responses will help you provide the best care possible for your patients. As this call ends, Sue and her crew will critique their actions and search for ways to improve the care they give for patients with similar presentations.

CONTENT SELF-EVALUATION

MULTIPLE CHOICE

_A_ 1. Which of the following terms best describes the first ALS providers of the 1970s?
   A. field technician
   B. prehospital emergency care practitioner
   C. orderly
   D. field attendant
   E. field aide

_D_ 2. The term describing the severity of a patient's condition is:
   A. multiparity.
   B. epiphysis.
   C. tonicity.
   D. acuity.
   E. declivity.

_A_ 3. The EMT-I's final determination of the patient's most likely primary problem is know as the:
   A. field diagnosis.
   B. differential field diagnosis.
   C. chief complaint.
   D. improvisation.
   E. standing order.

_C_ 4. Which of the following is NOT a level of patient acuity?
   A. life-threatening condition
   B. non-life-threatening condition
   C. potential non-life-threatening condition
   D. potential life-threatening condition
   E. both A and B

_A_ 5. Which patient acuity level presents the greatest challenge to the EMT-I's critical-thinking skills?
   A. life-threatening condition
   B. non-life-threatening condition
   C. potential non-life-threatening condition
   D. potential life-threatening condition
   E. B and C equally

_C_ 6. Which of the following terms represents a flowchart of patient care procedures?
   A. protocol
   B. standing order
   C. algorithm
   D. special care enhancement
   E. proviso

_B_ 7. A policy of administering nitroglycerin to a cardiac chest pain patient is an example of a(n):
   A. protocol.
   B. standing order.
   C. algorithm.
   D. special care enhancement.
   E. proviso.

_A_ 8. A policy by which nitroglycerin can be administered to a cardiac chest pain patient without a physician's order is an example of a(n):
   A. protocol.
   B. standing order.
   C. algorithm.
   D. special enhancement.
   E. proviso.

_A_ 9. The major disadvantage to the use of protocols and standing orders is that they:
   A. apply only to atypical patients.
   B. often do not permit the EMT-I to adapt to a patient's unique presentation.
   C. only cover multiple disease etiologies.
   D. address only patients with vague presentations.
   E. none of the above

©2004 Pearson Education, Inc.
Intermediate Emergency Care: Principles & Practice

___A___ 10. In the case where a particular protocol does not seem to fit the patient presentation, you should contact the medical direction physician for advice and direction regarding your patient's care.
   A. True
   B. False

___D___ 11. The data-processing style that focuses on the most important aspect of a critical situation is:
   A. reflective.   D. convergent.
   B. impulsive.   E. anticipatory.
   C. divergent.

___B___ 12. The style of situation analysis that causes you to respond instinctively to a situation rather than to think about it is:
   A. reflective.   D. convergent.
   B. impulsive.   E. anticipatory.
   C. divergent.

___A___ 13. One way to remain in control in otherwise extremely stressful situations is to learn to perform technical skills at a pseudo-instinctive level.
   A. True
   B. False

___B___ 14. Which of the following is NOT a step in the critical decision-making process?
   A. forming a concept   D. summarizing the result
   B. interpreting the data   E. evaluating the interventions
   C. applying the principles

___B___ 15. Which of the following is NOT an element of the six "Rs" of critical decision making?
   A. reading the scene   D. reading the patient
   B. researching the management plan   E. reevaluating
   C. reacting

MATCHING

Write the letter of the step in the critical decision-making process in the space provided next to the emergency response action appropriate for that step.

A. Form a concept.
B. Interpret the data.
C. Apply the principles.
D. Evaluate.
E. Reflect.

___B___ 16. Field diagnosis

___D___ 17. Provide ongoing assessment

___A___ 18. Perform the focused physical exam

___A___ 19. Pulse oximetry

___C___ 20. Follow standing orders

___B___ 21. Differential diagnosis

___A___ 22. Assess MS-ABCs

___C___ 23. Employ protocols

___A___ 24. Determine the initial vital signs

___D___ 25. Determine if treatment is improving the patient's condition

CHAPTER 10

*

Communications

Review of Chapter Objectives

After reading this chapter, you should be able to:

1. **Identify the role and importance of verbal, written, and electronic communications in the provision of EMS.** pp. 543–549

   EMS is a team endeavor that requires effective communications among the various participants in the response and patient care. This communication is between you and the emergency dispatcher, the patient, his family, bystanders, other emergency response personnel, such as police, fire, and rescue personnel, and health-care professionals from physicians' offices, clinics, and emergency departments, and finally with the medical direction physician. These communications, be they oral, written, or electronic, establish the key links that assure the best patient outcome.

2. **Describe the phases of communications necessary to complete a typical EMS response.** pp. 546–549

   Detection and citizen access
   This marks the initial entry point into the emergency service system at which a party identifies that an emergency exists and then requests EMS assistance through a universal entry number such as 911 or some other mechanism.

   Call taking
   This is the stage of EMS response in which a call taker questions the caller about the reported emergency in order to identify its exact location, determine the nature of the call, and initiate an appropriate response.

   Emergency response
   This phase includes the activities occurring from the moment a dispatcher requests a response by an EMS unit until the call concludes with the unit back in service. It includes various radio, face-to-face, and written communications among the dispatcher, emergency response crews, the patient, family and bystanders, and health-care professionals, including the medical direction physician.

   Prearrival instructions
   These are a series of predetermined, medically approved instructions given by the dispatcher to the caller to help the caller provide some patient support until EMS personnel arrive.

   Call coordination and incident recording
   These terms refer to the interactions between the dispatcher and the responding units that assure an efficient and appropriate response. Call coordinating, for example, might involve changing the mode of response and the number and type of responding units. Incident recording refers to the logging of times associated with various response activities and the tape recording of communications associated with the call.

©2004 Pearson Education, Inc.
Intermediate Emergency Care: Principles & Practice

Discussion with medical direction

This is the opportunity for the care provider to describe the patient he or she is caring for and to obtain approval from the medical direction physician to initiate invasive or advanced life support procedures. Communication with medical direction also permits the emergency department to prepare for the patient's arrival.

Transfer communications

These are the communications that occur between the first responder and the EMT-I or as the patient is delivered to the emergency department. They are intended to communicate the results of the assessment, the care given, and the patient's response to care prior to the arrival of the EMT-I or arrival at the emergency department.

3. Identify the importance of proper verbal communications and terminology during an EMS response. pp. 543–544

Communication requires mutual language where the receiver can decode what the sender is saying. Without a mutual understanding of the words used, a patient can receive inadequate care. The same principle applies to technology. Your equipment must be reliable and designed to afford clear communication among all agencies within the system.

4. List factors that impede and enhance effective verbal and written communications. pp. 543–546

The factors impacting effective or ineffective verbal or written communications are either semantic (dealing with the meaning of words) or technical (hardware).

In the area of semantics, the use of standard codes and plain English in verbal communications enhances good and clear communications, while use of nonstandard codes and jargon may confuse it. The same holds true for written communication. Nonstandard abbreviations and subjective, sloppy, incomplete, or illegible documentation leads to confusion and miscommunication. Complete, objective, legible, and efficient documentation leads to an efficient transfer of information. A well-designed prehospital care report makes written communication easier.

In the technical area, a well-designed and maintained radio or phone communications system will go a long way in assuring good and dependable communications. Improperly maintained or operated radios will, on the other hand, likely provide only intermittent and poor quality communication.

5. Explain the value of data collection during an EMS response. p. 545

The written call report is a record that includes the patient's name and address, scene location, agency responding, crew on board, and the times associated with response, arrival, and transport to a care facility. It also contains the results of the assessment and care of the patient. This administrative information can be used to bill for services and improve EMS system efficiency, by quality assurance/improvement committees to improve system performance, and by educators and researchers to identify what the system is doing and the impacts of its interventions. Finally, the call report becomes a legal record of the incident and the EMS care provided or offered.

6. Recognize the legal status of verbal, written, and electronic communications related to an EMS response. pp. 554–555, 557

The legal guidelines that apply to verbal and written communication in emergency medical service also apply to electronic communications. The information in these communications is considered confidential and must only be released in approved circumstances. The reports must be objective and not demean, libel, or slander another person. Any such action is accountable in a court of law.

Patient Assessment

7. Identify current and new technology used to collect and exchange patient and/or scene information electronically. pp. 549–553

Cellular phones today provide duplex communications directly from the patient's side to the emergency department. These lightweight and versatile devices enhance EMS-to-physician communications and permit excellent ECG transmission. The only disadvantages to cell phones are user fees and unreliability at peak times.

Another electronic aid to dispatch is the facsimile or fax machine. It permits dispatch to send hard copy to the responding unit's station, assuring that elements of the address and nature of the dispatch are communicated accurately.

Computers are also increasing the efficiency of the dispatch system by recording times and system action in real time and making data recovery and research much easier.

Other new technologies that may affect prehospital care include: the electronic touch pad, which allows rapid recording of patient information; the handheld computer, which uses a pen-based system to log patient information and times associated with the emergency response and care; electronic transmission of diagnostic information (including pulse oximetry, 12-lead ECG, blood sugar, and end-expiratory CO_2 monitoring) provided directly to the emergency department, which may change the degree and number of field interventions permitted. In the future, voice recognition software may make real-time narrative recording of patient evaluation and interventions at the emergency scene and during transport a reality.

8. Identify the various components of the EMS communications system and describe their function and use. pp. 543, 546–549

The emergency medical dispatcher (EMD) is the person who takes the call for assistance, dispatches the appropriate units, monitors the call's progress, and assures that the pertinent response data is recorded. He or she may guide the caller through initial emergency care using prearrival instructions.

The patient, his family, and bystanders are responsible for detecting the emergency, accessing the emergency response system, and relaying information about the cause and nature of the emergency to EMS system personnel. Since they are not trained in emergency medical communication, the responsibility of assuring good communications falls on the members of the EMS system.

Personnel from other responding agencies such as the police, fire service, rescue, and other ambulance services are also individuals who provide information important to assuring proper EMS response, and their input must be taken into account to assure scene coordination and optimum utilization of resources.

Health-care professionals (aides, nurses, physician assistants, nurse practitioners, and physicians) at clinics, physicians' offices, and emergency departments are important people in the EMS system. They can provide invaluable information about the patient and the care he or she has had or should receive.

Finally, the medical director and medical direction physicians are significant resources for the prehospital emergency care provider. They are the individuals who extend their licenses to EMT-Is, thereby permitting them to practice prehospital care. These physicians also represent a body of knowledge of emergency medicine that may be tapped while EMT-Is are at the scene, en route with a patient, or at the emergency department for guidance regarding patient care.

9. Identify and differentiate among the following communications systems:

Simplex p. 550

This refers to a radio or communication system that uses only one frequency and allows only one unit to transmit at a time. With this type of communication, one party must wait until the speaking party completes his message before beginning to speak.

Multiplex p. 551

This is a duplex system with an additional capability of transmitting data, like an ECG strip, simultaneously with voice.

Duplex p. 551

©2004 Pearson Education, Inc.
Intermediate Emergency Care: Principles & Practice

This is a radio or communication system that uses two frequencies for each channel, thus permitting two units to transmit and listen at the same time. This is similar to telephone communication, where one party can interrupt the other.

Trunked   p. 551
These are computer-controlled systems that pool all radio frequencies and assign transmissions to unused frequencies to assure the most efficient use of available communications channels.

Digital communications   p. 552
These systems translate analog sounds into digital code for transmissions that are less prone to interference and are more compact than analog (normal voice) communications. This type of a system can be enhanced with devices like the mobile data terminal, which displays information such as street addresses, and can prompt the responder to send information like "arrived."

Cellular telephone   p. 552
These are part of a multiplex radio-telephone system tied to a computer that uses radio towers to transmit signals in regions called cells. The technology is inexpensive but can accrue substantial monthly charges; the transmissions may be interrupted by certain geographic features; and heavy use at peak times may limit access to the system.

Facsimile   pp. 552–553
These devices transmit and receive printed information through telephone or wireless communication systems. Such a machine might give a responding unit a print-out of the nature and street address of the call or, possibly, detailed medical information about it.

Computer   p. 553
The use of these devices in EMS is expanding rapidly. They are already helping to analyze data for review of calls and dispatches. Portable input devices, such as the touch pad and handheld computer, are being developed to permit recording of emergency response events in the field. In the future, EMT-Is may use computers with voice recognition software to complete prehospital care reports without paper.

10. **Describe the functions and responsibilities of the Federal Communications Commission.** p. 557

The Federal Communications Commission (FCC) controls and regulates all nongovernmental communications in the United States. It assigns broadcast frequencies and has set aside several frequencies within each radio bandwidth for emergency medical services. The commission also establishes technical standards for radio equipment, licenses and regulates people who repair radios, monitors frequencies for appropriate usage, and checks base stations and dispatch centers for appropriate licenses and records.

11. **Describe the role of emergency medical dispatch and the importance of prearrival instructions in a typical EMS response.** pp. 543, 547

The emergency medical dispatcher (EMD) is the first person in the EMS system who communicates with the scene and possibly the patient. He or she begins and coordinates the EMS response and communications and assures data regarding the call are recorded. He or she also provides prearrival instructions to callers—for example, how to perform mouth-to-mouth artificial ventilation on an apneic patient—so that emergency care can begin as early as possible, thus helping to maintain the victim until trained prehospital personnel can arrive.

12. **List appropriate caller information gathered by the emergency medical dispatcher.** p. 547

The information that is gathered by the EMD to determine the response priority and that is then communicated to the appropriate responding EMS service includes:
• Caller's name
• Call-back number

- Location or address of the event
- Nature of the call
- Any additional information necessary to prioritize the call

13. Describe the structure and importance of verbal patient information communication to the hospital and medical direction.   pp. 554–556

The verbal patient report to hospital personnel and the medical direction physician is essential to assure the efficient transfer and continuity of care. It consists of the following:
- Information identifying the care provider and level of training
- Patient identification information (name, age, sex, etc.)
- Subjective patient data (chief complaint, additional symptoms, past history, etc.)
- Objective patient data (vital signs, pulse oximetry readings, etc.)
- Plan for care of patient

For the trauma patient, the information and order of presentation is the same, although the subjective and objective information are modified to include mechanism of injury and suspected injuries.

14. Diagram a basic communications system.   p. 544

Basic communication is the process of exchanging information between individuals. A model for a communications system should start with an idea, followed by the encoding of that idea into useful language, sending the encoded message via a medium (direct voice, radio, or written), having another person receive and decode the message, and ultimately, receiving feedback from the original message.

15. Organize a verbal radio report for electronic transmission to medical direction.   pp. 554–556

During your classroom, clinical, and field training, you will communicate with various elements of the EMS system, including dispatchers, patients, family members, bystanders, other EMS and scene personnel, and health-care professionals, including medical direction physicians. Use the information presented in this text chapter, the information on communication presented by your instructors, and the guidance given by your clinical and field preceptors to develop good communication skills. Continue to refine these skills once your training ends and you begin your career as an EMT-I.

CASE STUDY REVIEW

This case study discusses an emergency call and the elements of communications and, specifically, the radio communications between the EMT-I and medical direction.

This case study identifies some of the common and critical elements of communication essential to the emergency response. First, someone needs to recognize an emergency exists (detection) and then they must contact the emergency response system (access). The dispatcher must then receive the call (call taking), determine its nature and seriousness, and dispatch appropriate resources to deal with the problem (emergency response). The dispatcher determines the priority of the call by asking the caller a series of medically approved questions. The dispatcher, in addition, provides the caller with basic, approved first-aid steps to perform (prearrival instructions) until EMS reaches the scene to supply more comprehensive care. The dispatcher also coordinates the responses of any fire, police, rescue, or other service units needed to the scene (call coordination). The dispatch center records the pertinent information and times associated with the call for further review by the system administrator, the medical director, the quality improvement committee, researchers, or possibly by attorneys (incident recording).

Once at the scene and actively involved in patient care, the care providers contact medical direction to communicate the patient's condition and the care they have begun. This communication paints a clear picture of the patient they are treating. It may stimulate questions from the physician regarding the findings and patient care and may elicit orders for invasive actions, such as starting an IV line or administering medications. When the EMT-I communicates with medical direction regarding orders for invasive actions, he uses the echo procedure, repeating back the physician's orders word for word to assure that both parties understand what is to be done.

The communications between the EMT-Is and medical direction also enable the emergency department staff to prepare for the arrival of the patient (transfer communications). In this case, the patient's condition is critical and time is of the essence. When the patient arrives, the hospital is ready for immediate surgery. While in this case prehospital and hospital care do not result in patient survival, support of the patient's vital signs provides organs that are used to prolong other lives.

Another factor to consider in this case study is the hardware necessary to the EMS response. The cellular phone makes communications from a bystander at the accident site possible, and the system is alerted quickly to the patient's plight. A system status management and priority dispatch system assures ambulances are close to the areas where response is needed and allows for coordinated responses. It also assures that red lights and sirens are only used for true emergencies. The enhanced 911 system uses a computer to determine the quickest route to the scene and provide the responding ambulance electronically with a printout of all the pertinent information needed to respond without taking the dispatcher away from the caller. The EMT-Is probably send an ECG to Dr. Jorol while they speak (multiplex), and Dr. Jorol can interrupt them as they deliver their report to ask questions (duplex). This hardware and a coordinated system of communication assures the best response and care for the patients of this EMS system.

CONTENT SELF-EVALUATION

MULTIPLE CHOICE

E 1. Essential participants in communications within the EMS system include:
   A. the emergency medical dispatcher.
   B. the patient, his family, or bystanders.
   C. other responders, including police, fire, and other ambulance personnel.
   D. health-care providers, including nurses, physicians, and medical direction physicians.
   E. all of the above

B 2. In general, the use of codes decreases the radio time and increases the recipient's understanding of the message, which has led many EMS systems to adopt extensive use of codes for their communications.
   A. True
   B. False

C 3. A radio band is a:
   A. series of radios that communicate one with another.
   B. pair of radio frequencies used for multiplexing.
   C. range of radio frequencies.
   D. pair of radio frequencies used for duplexing.
   E. none of the above

E 4. Use of proper terminology in both written and verbal communications will:
   A. decrease the length of communications.
   B. increase the accuracy of communications.
   C. increase the clarity of communications.
   D. reduce the ambiguity in communications.
   E. all of the above

D 5. Features of the enhanced 911 center include all of the following EXCEPT:
   A. display of the caller's location.
   B. display of the caller's phone number.
   C. immediate call-back ability.

D. a system of physician/ambulance interface.

E. both B and C

B Pg. 546 **6.** The answering center for emergency calls that then transfers them to the appropriate agency for dispatch is the:

A. enhanced 911 center.

B. PSAP.

C. GPS.

D. Emergency Routing Center.

E. none of the above

A Pg. 547 **7.** The system that uses standardized caller questioning to determine the level and type of response is:

A. priority dispatching.

B. system status management.

C. enhanced emergency medical dispatch.

D. prearrival instructions packaging.

E. dispatch triage.

E **8.** The role of the modern-day emergency medical dispatcher includes:

A. priority dispatching.

B. prearrival instructions.

C. call coordinating.

D. incident recording.

E. all of the above

E **9.** The report that occurs as you transfer patient responsibilities to the emergency department staff must include:

A. chief complaint.

B. assessment findings.

C. care rendered.

D. results of care.

E. all of the above

A **10.** A radio system that transmits and receives on the same frequency is called:

A. simplex.

B. duplex.

C. triplex.

D. multiplex.

E. none of the above

B **11.** Which radio transmission design permits the receiver to interrupt the caller while the caller is talking?

A. simplex

B. duplex

C. multiplex

D. trunking

E. none of the above

D **12.** The radio system that uses a computer to determine and assign available frequencies is called:

A. simplex.

B. duplex.

C. multiplex.

D. trunking.

E. none of the above

C Pg. 552 **13.** Advantages of cellular communications in EMS include all of the following EXCEPT:

A. duplex capability.

B. allowing direct physician/patient communication.

C. ability to handle an unlimited number of calls.

D. reduced on-line times.

E. transmission of better ECG signals.

A **14.** One of the EMT-I's most important skills is gathering essential patient information, organizing it, and communicating it to the medical direction physician.

A. True

B. False

D Pg. 554 **15.** A standard format for transmitting patient information assures all of the following EXCEPT:

A. communication efficiency.

B. physician assimilation of patient condition information.

C. completeness of medical information.

D. easier use of multiplex signals.

©2004 Pearson Education, Inc.
Intermediate Emergency Care: Principles & Practice

E. both A and C

pg. 555

__E__ 16. All of the following are appropriate for good EMS communications EXCEPT:
A. speaking close to the microphone.
B. speaking across or directly into the microphone.
C. talking in a normal tone of voice.
D. speaking without emotion.
E. taking time to explain everything in detail.

__A__ 17. It is important to press the microphone button for one second before speaking.
A. True
B. False

__D__ 18. If the portable radio you are using is unable to transmit well from your location, attempt to:
A. move to higher ground.
B. touch the antenna to something metal.
C. move towards a window or away from structural steel.
D. both A and C
E. none of the above

__A__ 19. The major difference between the medical and trauma patient reports is that the trauma format provides a description of the mechanism of injury and identifies suspected injuries.
A. True
B. False

__C__ 20. The Federal Communications Commission is responsible for all of the following below EXCEPT:
A. assigning and licensing radio frequencies.
B. establishing technical standards for radio equipment.
C. assuring the proper use of medical terminology in radio communications.
D. monitoring radio frequencies for proper use.
E. spot checking radio base stations for proper licensing and records.

SPECIAL PROJECT

Documentation: Radio Report/Prehospital Care Report

The authoring of both the radio message to the receiving hospital and the written run report are two of the most important tasks you will perform as an EMT-I. Read the following paragraphs, compose a radio message, and complete the run report for this call.

The Call:

At 1515 hours, your ambulance, Unit 89, is paged out to an unconscious person at the local baseball field on a very hot (97°F) Saturday. You are accompanied by Steve Phillips, an EMT, your partner for the day, and are en route by 1516.

You arrive on scene at 1522 to find a young male collapsed at third base. He is unarousable, perspiring heavily, and his skin is cool to the touch. The pillow under the boy's head (placed by bystanders) is removed, the patient's airway is clear, his breathing is adequate, and his pulse is rapid and bounding. One of the bystanders says the patient was playing ball and just collapsed. Another young bystander identifies himself as the patient's brother and states that "nothing like this has happened before." He says his brother is named Jim Thompson, is 13, and lives about a mile away.

The rest of the assessment reveals no signs of trauma. The assessment findings include: blood pressure 136/98; pulse 92 and strong; normal sinus rhythm as revealed by the ECG; respirations 24 and normal in depth and pattern (at 1527). The boy responds to painful stimuli, but not to verbal commands or to his name. Pupils are noted to be equal and slow to react. Oxygen is applied at 12 liters by nonrebreather mask, and the patient is moved to the shade.

Receiving Hospital is contacted, and you call in the following report:

_____

_____

_____

_____

_____

_____

_____

_____

_____

_____

_____

_____

_____

_____

Expected ETA at Receiving Hospital is 20 minutes.

Medical direction at Receiving Hospital, the closest facility, orders you to start an IV line with normal saline run just to keep open. You repeat the orders back to medical direction and then begin your care. Your first IV attempt on the right forearm is unsuccessful; the second attempt on the left forearm gets a flashback and infuses well. You retake vitals. The patient is now responding to verbal stimuli, the BP is 134/96, pulse 90, NSR via ECG, respirations 24. The patient is loaded on the stretcher at 1537 and moved to the ambulance.

©2004 Pearson Education, Inc.
Intermediate Emergency Care: Principles & Practice

You contact medical direction and provide the following update:

_____

_____

_____

_____

_____

_____

_____

_____

_____

_____

_____

_____

_____

_____

_____

_____

ETA 10 minutes.

En route, vital signs (at 1545) are BP 132/90, NSR via ECG, pulse 88, respirations at 24. The patient is now conscious and alert, though he cannot remember the incident. The trip is uneventful, and you arrive at the hospital at 1557. You transfer the responsibility for the patient to the emergency physician and restock and wipe out the ambulance. You report back into service at 1615, grab a cup of coffee, and sit down at the hospital to write the run report.

Complete the run report on the following page from the information contained in the narrative of this call.

Compare the radio communication and run report form that you prepare against the example in the Answer Key section of this Workbook. As you make the comparison, keep in mind that there are many "correct" ways to communicate this body of information. Assure that you have recorded the major points of your assessment and care and enough other material to describe the patient and his condition.

©2004 Pearson Education, Inc.
Intermediate Emergency Care: Principles & Practice

Date / /	Emergency Medical Services Run Report	Run # 911

Patient Information   Service Information   Times

Patient Information	Service Information	Times
Name:	Agency:	Rcvd :
Address:	Location:	Enrt :
City: St: Zip:	Call Origin:	Scne :
Age: Birth: / / Sex: [M][F]	Type: Emrg[ ] Non[ ] Trnsfr[ ]	LvSn :
Nature of Call:		ArHsp :
Chief Complaint:		InSv :

Description of Current Problem:

Medical Problems

Past		Present
[ ]	Cardiac	[ ]
[ ]	Stroke	[ ]
[ ]	Acute Abdomen	[ ]
[ ]	Diabetes	[ ]
[ ]	Psychiatric	[ ]
[ ]	Epilepsy	[ ]
[ ]	Drug/Alcohol	[ ]
[ ]	Poisoning	[ ]
[ ]	Allergy/Asthma	[ ]
[ ]	Syncope	[ ]
[ ]	Obstetrical	[ ]
[ ]	GYN	[ ]

Other:

Trauma Scr: Glasgow:

On Scene Care:	First Aid:
	By Whom?

02 @ L : Via	C-Collar :	S-Immob. :	Stretcher :

Allergies/Meds:	Past Med Hx:

Time	Pulse	Resp.	BP S/D	LOC	ECG
:	R: [r][i]	R: [s][l]	/	[a][v][p][u]	
Care/Comments:					
:	R: [r][i]	R: [s][l]	/	[a][v][p][u]	
Care/Comments:					
:	R: [r][i]	R: [s][l]	/	[a][v][p][u]	
Care/Comments:					
:	R: [r][i]	R: [s][l]	/	[a][v][p][u]	
Care/Comments:					

Destination:	Personnel:	Certification
Reason:[ ]pt [ ]Closest [ ]M.D. [ ]Other	1.	[P][E][O]
Contacted: [ ]Radio [ ]Tele [ ]Direct	2.	[P][E][O]
Ar Status: [ ]Better [ ]UnC [ ]Worse	3.	[P][E][O]

©2004 Pearson Education, Inc.
Intermediate Emergency Care: Principles & Practice

CHAPTER 11

✳

Documentation

Review of Chapter Objectives

After reading this chapter, you should be able to:

1. Identify the general principles regarding the importance of EMS documentation and ways in which documents are used. **pp. 560–561**

The principal EMS document, the prehospital care report (PCR), is the sole permanent written documentation of the response, assessment, care, and transport offered during an emergency call. It is a medical document conveying details of medical care and patient history that remains a part of the patient record as well as a legal document that may be reviewed in a court of law. The PCR may also be reviewed by medical direction to determine the appropriateness of your actions during the call and used by your service to bill the patient for services. Lastly, the PCR may be used by researchers to determine the effectiveness of care measures in improving patient outcomes.

2. Identify and properly use medical terminology, medical abbreviations, and acronyms. **pp. 563, 564–567**

Medical terminology is the very precise and exact wording used to describe the human body and injuries or illnesses. Proper use of this terminology turns the PCR into a medical document. However, if terms are misspelled or misused, they may distract from the document and confuse the reader about the patient's condition and the care he either has had or should receive. Carry a pocket dictionary, and only use words when you are sure of both their spelling and usage. The same holds true of medical abbreviations. They must be applied properly and have the same meaning to both the writer and reader. EMS systems should use a standardized set of abbreviations and acronyms to assure good and efficient documentation.

3. Explain the role of documentation in agency reimbursement. **p. 560**

Good documentation is essential for ambulance agencies that bill for services they provide. The PCR provides the name and address of the patient as well as the nature and circumstances of injury and illness. It also includes the care and transport provided. Without this information, the service may not be able to obtain reimbursement for services rendered and, ultimately, to afford to provide the vehicle, equipment, and personnel necessary to provide prehospital emergency care.

4. Identify and eliminate extraneous or nonprofessional information. **p. 571**

The ambulance call should be documented in a brief and professional way. The PCR describing it may be scrutinized by hospital staff, the medical direction physician, quality improvement committees, supervisors, lawyers, and the news media. Any derogatory comments, jargon, slang, biased statements, irrelevant opinions, or libelous statements will distract from the seriousness of the document and from acceptance of the preparer's professionalism.

5. **Describe the differences between subjective and objective elements of documentation.** pp. 571–573

Subjective information is information that you obtain from others or is your opinion that is not based on observable facts. It includes the patient's, family's, or bystander's description of the chief complaint and symptoms, medical history, and nature of the illness or mechanism of injury.

Objective information is information you obtain through direct observation, palpation, auscultation, percussion, or diagnostic evaluation of your patient. It includes the vital signs and the results of the physical exam, including such things as glucose level determination and ECG monitor and pulse oximeter readings.

6. **Evaluate a finished document for errors and omissions and proper use and spelling of abbreviations and acronyms.** pp. 568, 570

The PCR must contain all information obtainable and necessary for describing the patient's condition recorded in a clearly legible way. The report must be written so that another health-care provider can easily understand what is being said and can mentally picture the scene, the patient presentation, the care rendered, and the transport offered by the initial providers. In many cases, what to include in the PCR is a judgment decision made by the care provider, though the report must contain an accurate description of the patient's medical or trauma problem and an accurate and complete history. Correct spelling and use of medical terms is essential and reflects the knowledge of the care provider. Proper use of abbreviations and acronyms can help make the PCR more concise; their improper use, however, may produce ambiguity, confusion, and misunderstanding in readers. Reread the finished PCR and check it carefully before submitting it.

7. **Evaluate the confidential nature of an EMS report.** p. 580

Confidentiality is a patient right and breaching it can result in severe consequences. Do not discuss or share patient or call information with anyone not involved in the care of the patient. The only exceptions—as necessary—are administration, which may need information for billing; police agencies carrying out a criminal investigation; requests for the information under subpoena from a court; and quality assurance committees that may need the information (with the patient's name blocked out) for system review and improvement or for research.

8. **Describe the potential consequences of illegible, incomplete, or inaccurate documentation.** pp. 568, 570

A legible, complete, and accurate PCR is essential to call documentation. The information in it must be easy to read thanks to both good penmanship and conscientious attention to detail. The report must describe all the pertinent information gathered at the scene and en route to the hospital as well as all actions taken by you and others in the care of the patient. Failure to create a thorough, readable PCR reduces the information available to other care givers and may reduce their ability to provide effective care. The document you produce also reflects on your ability to provide assessment and care and your professionalism in general.

9. **Describe the special documentation considerations concerning patient refusal of care and/or transport.** pp. 576–577

Be careful in the documentation of a patient who refuses care and/or transport. While a conscious and mentally competent patient has the right to refuse care, his doing so may pose legal problems for care providers. Document the nature and severity of the patient's injuries, any care you offered, any care he refused, and document carefully the assessment criteria you used to determine the patient was capable of making the decision to refuse care or transport. Also document the patient's reasons for refusing care and your efforts to convince him to change his mind. If possible, have the refusal of care and your explanation to the patient of the consequences of care refusal signed by the patient and witnessed by family or bystanders or police. Advise the patient to seek other medical help, like his family physician, and to call EMS again if he changes his mind or his condition worsens.

©2004 Pearson Education, Inc.
Intermediate Emergency Care: Principles & Practice

10. Demonstrate how properly to record direct patient or bystander comments. p. 568

Direct statements by patients and bystanders must be recorded exactly as they were made and the key phrases placed in quotation marks. Treating the information this way is highly important because it identifies that the information is directly from the source, not an interpretation. Identify clearly the source of any quotation you include in a PCR.

11. Describe the special considerations concerning mass-casualty incident documentation. p. 578

Often a mass-casualty situation calls for an atypical EMS response and unusual documentation procedures. Care providers rarely stay with a patient from the beginning to the end of prehospital care, and the time spent at a patient's side is very much at a premium. Hence documentation must be efficient and incremental. Document your assessment findings and any interventions you perform at the patient's side quickly and clearly. Many agencies or systems have their own forms such as triage tags that simplify the documentation procedure.

12. Demonstrate proper document revision and correction. pp. 570–571

Everyone makes mistakes during a health-care career and during the process of care documentation. When this happens, it is essential to make corrections in such a way that there is no appearance of impropriety. If an error is made, draw a single line through the error and enter the correction and your initials. If the error is noted after the report is turned in, write a narrative addendum explaining both the nature of the error and the needed correction and assure that the addendum is included with all copies of the PCR. Correct errors as soon as possible after they are discovered.

13. Apply the principles of documentation to computer charting, as access to this technology becomes available. p. 580

As the technology evolves and more options become available to the EMT-I in the field such as handheld computers, pen-based input systems, digital scanners, PDAs, voice recorders, and any other options that may become available, it is important to remember the general principles of documentation must apply. Protect the patient's private records and information. There are Federal laws in which all EMS and hospital personnel must be trained to keep patient information private. Your service medical director will bring you up to date on the specific application of these laws in your state and locality. Make sure that all information obtained and charted is as accurate and complete as possible. Learn the procedure for backing up the computer system as any electrical or battery operated system is subject to failure, and your service should have a system in place for a backup of data.

14. Assume responsibility for self-assessment of all documentation. p. 580

As a well-trained medical professional and EMT-I, it is your responsibility to review all of your documentation prior to submitting it. In some cases you may be rushed to complete the call, but it is very important to note that the job is not done until the paperwork is complete. All completed paperwork must be reread and reviewed for accuracy. Failure to review your PCR at the time of its completion can result in submitting an incomplete document. Keep in mind that you may be asked to defend your actions at a later time, and your documentation should be able to outline the facts related to your decisions. It is a good habit for all the crew members who were on the call to take a look at the PCR before it is submitted to be sure they agree it represents an accurate portrayal of the incident.

CASE STUDY REVIEW

This case study identifies some of the important considerations regarding the prehospital care report and its potential to support (or incriminate) a care provider who is called into a court of law. The scenario emphasizes the importance of good documentation as described in Chapter 11.

We seldom realize the importance others may place on our prehospital documentation. In this case study, Tom Brewster is surprised when, three years after a call, he is summoned to give a legal deposition about it. While this example speaks to legal reasons for review of documentation, Tom might just as well have been asked about the quickness of the ambulance response, the time he and his crew spent on scene, or specific aspects of the care he provided. While attorneys may represent the most feared interrogators to most EMT-Is, the EMS system medical director, quality improvement personnel, or administrative personnel might also ask for details of some incident months or years in the past. For these reasons, your accurate and thorough documentation of the emergency scene and the assessment and care you provide is of great importance to you and your service.

Tom was asked about his recall of the events of the call and the comments made by the patient. His prehospital care report provided enough information to prompt Tom to remember the incident, the patient, and the care he gave. He was fortunate that his documentation provided this information and that he could piece together the events of that response. It is likely that the patient's attorney would challenge Tom's recall after three years. Documentation of the patient's statement that he "fell asleep" would be a factor critical in determining the reason for the crash (ruling out medical causes). Tom was apparently thorough in gathering the patient history and recording it on the PCR because he was able to recall that there was no history of either diabetes or heart disease. Tom further benefited from performing a routine but complete patient assessment, including glucose testing and ECG monitoring.

This case study emphasizes the importance of preparing a prehospital care report that describes exactly what happened and exactly what you did. Had Tom used sloppy penmanship or subjective statements or failed to provide complete information, the patient's attorney would have been able to challenge Tom's objectivity and accuracy. As things stood, the report supported Tom's recall and evaluation of the patient's condition.

CONTENT SELF-EVALUATION

MULTIPLE CHOICE

1. The prehospital care report is likely to be reviewed by which of the following?
   A. researchers
   B. EMS administrators
   C. lawyers
   D. medical professionals
   E. all of the above

2. Which of the following is NOT an appropriate purpose for reviewing a prehospital care report?
   A. to identify a chronological account of the patient's mental status
   B. to learn about what calls other prehospital care providers had
   C. to help detect patient improvement or deterioration
   D. to identify what bystanders and family may have said at the scene
   E. to determine baseline assessment findings

3. The prehospital care report may yield information that the quality improvement committee may use to identify problems with individual EMT-Is or with the EMS system.
   A. True
   B. False

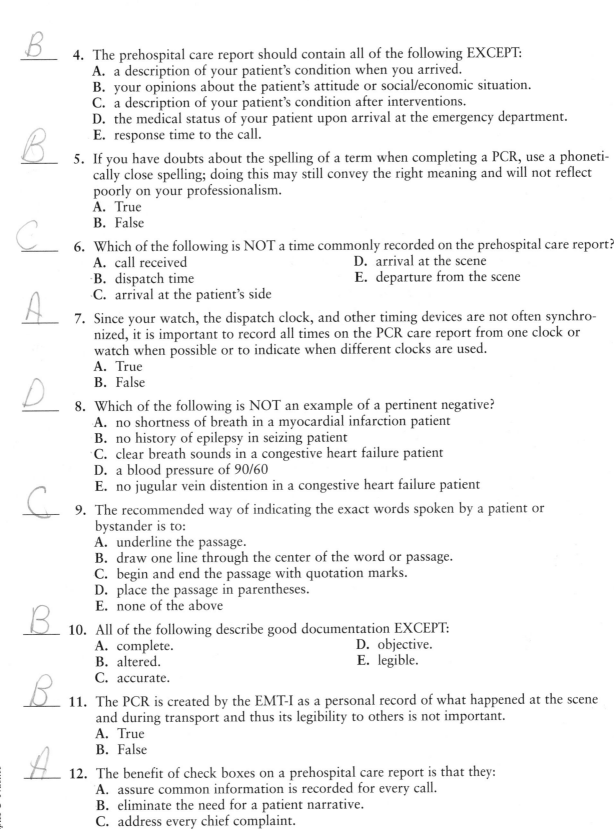

B   4. The prehospital care report should contain all of the following EXCEPT:
     A. a description of your patient's condition when you arrived.
     B. your opinions about the patient's attitude or social/economic situation.
     C. a description of your patient's condition after interventions.
     D. the medical status of your patient upon arrival at the emergency department.
     E. response time to the call.

B   5. If you have doubts about the spelling of a term when completing a PCR, use a phonetically close spelling; doing this may still convey the right meaning and will not reflect poorly on your professionalism.
     A. True
     B. False

C   6. Which of the following is NOT a time commonly recorded on the prehospital care report?
     A. call received   D. arrival at the scene
     B. dispatch time   E. departure from the scene
     C. arrival at the patient's side

A   7. Since your watch, the dispatch clock, and other timing devices are not often synchronized, it is important to record all times on the PCR care report from one clock or watch when possible or to indicate when different clocks are used.
     A. True
     B. False

D   8. Which of the following is NOT an example of a pertinent negative?
     A. no shortness of breath in a myocardial infarction patient
     B. no history of epilepsy in seizing patient
     C. clear breath sounds in a congestive heart failure patient
     D. a blood pressure of 90/60
     E. no jugular vein distention in a congestive heart failure patient

C   9. The recommended way of indicating the exact words spoken by a patient or bystander is to:
     A. underline the passage.
     B. draw one line through the center of the word or passage.
     C. begin and end the passage with quotation marks.
     D. place the passage in parentheses.
     E. none of the above

B   10. All of the following describe good documentation EXCEPT:
     A. complete.   D. objective.
     B. altered.   E. legible.
     C. accurate.

B   11. The PCR is created by the EMT-I as a personal record of what happened at the scene and during transport and thus its legibility to others is not important.
     A. True
     B. False

A   12. The benefit of check boxes on a prehospital care report is that they:
     A. assure common information is recorded for every call.
     B. eliminate the need for a patient narrative.
     C. address every chief complaint.
     D. speed the completion of the narrative.
     E. all of the above

©2004 Pearson Education, Inc.
Intermediate Emergency Care: Principles & Practice

Patient Assessment

_E_ 13. When should the prehospital care report be completed?
   A. at the end of the day
   B. at the end of your duty shift
   C. once back at quarters
   D. shortly after leaving the hospital
   E. upon or shortly after transferring patient care at the hospital

_A_ 14. Whenever possible, have all members of your crew read or reread the prehospital care report before you submit it.
   A. True
   B. False

_C_ 15. What is the best way to add additional information to the prehospital care report after it has been submitted to the hospital?
   A. Search and make changes on all copies.
   B. Change only the original report.
   C. Create an addendum and add it to all reports.
   D. Never add additional material to the report once distributed.
   E. Send a memorandum to medical direction.

_B_ 16. Use of professional jargon in the PCR is an indicator of the writer's professionalism.
   A. True
   B. False

_D_ 17. Which of the following is the best example of a subjective and possibly libelous statement?
   A. "The patient smelled of beer."
   B. "The patient walked with a staggering gait."
   C. "The patient used abusive language and spoke with slurred speech."
   D. "The patient was drunk and obnoxious."
   E. None of the above is a potentially libelous statement.

_E_ 18. Which of the following is a part of the subjective patient information?
   A. chief complaint
   B. past medical history
   C. history of the current medical problem
   D. patient description of what happened
   E. all of the above

_B_ 19. The portion of your narrative report that contains your general impression of the patient is the:
   A. subjective narrative.   D. SOAP plan.
   B. objective narrative.   E. none of the above
   C. assessment/management plan.

_A_ 20. You should document a pediatric assessment in head-to-toe order, even though you may have performed it from toe-to-head.
   A. True
   B. False

_E_ 21. Which of the following is true about the body systems method of assessment?
   A. It focuses on body systems rather than body areas.
   B. It usually addresses only the system(s) affected.
   C. It is best suited to screening and preadmission exams.
   D. It can be a comprehensive approach to documentation.
   E. all of the above

_D_ 22. The term that describes what you believe to be the patient's most likely problem is the:
   A. definitive assessment.   D. field diagnosis.
   B. clinical diagnosis.   E. none of the above
   C. assessment object.

©2004 Pearson Education, Inc.
Intermediate Emergency Care: Principles & Practice

_____ 23. The management portion of your documentation should include which of the following?
   A. any interventions
   B. the results of ongoing assessments
   C. any changes in the patient's condition
   D. the patient's condition when care is transferred at the emergency department
   E. all of the above

_____ 24. Which of the following is NOT a part of the subjective information recorded on the PCR?
   A. vital signs
   B. past medical history
   C. review of systems
   D. chief complaint
   E. none of the above

_____ 25. Which of the following are elements of the objective information recorded on the PCR?
   A. your general impression of the patient
   B. the results of any diagnostic tests
   C. the results of the physical exam
   D. vital signs
   E. all of the above

_____ 26. Which of the following formats records the chief complaint, history, assessment, treatment, and transport information in that order?
   A. SOAP format
   B. CHART format
   C. Patient Management format
   D. Call Incident format
   E. none of the above

_____ 27. The most significant feature of the patient management format of documentation is that it:
   A. documents the chronological sequence of events and actions.
   B. focuses exclusively on assessment findings.
   C. uses a free-flowing narrative style.
   D. is most frequently used for patients with minor injuries/problems.
   E. none of the above

_____ 28. The call incident format for documenting an emergency response is best suited for which type of patient?
   A. the unresponsive medical patient
   B. the responsive medical patient
   C. the trauma patient with no significant mechanism of injury
   D. the trauma patient with a significant mechanism of injury
   E. both B and C

_____ 29. In obtaining a patient refusal against medical advice, it is important to:
   A. determine that the patient is alert, oriented, and competent to make the decision.
   B. clearly explain to the patient the risks of not receiving care.
   C. try to convince the patient to obtain care.
   D. explain that if the condition worsens the patient should call for the ambulance or otherwise seek immediate care.
   E. all of the above

_____ 30. If your ambulance call is canceled en route to the scene, you should:
   A. simply return to base.
   B. write canceled on the front of the PCR.
   C. note the canceling authority and time of cancellation on the PCR.
   D. secure the name of the patient as well as any other information.
   E. none of the above

MATCHING

Write the letter of the word or phrase in the space provided next to the appropriate abbreviation.

A. shortness of breath
B. acute myocardial infarction
C. positive end-expiratory pressure
D. normal sinus rhythm
E. nausea/vomiting
F. do not resuscitate
G. breath sounds/blood sugar
H. premature ventricular contraction
I. not applicable
J. nitroglycerin
K. intraosseous
L. weight
M. sexually transmitted disease

N. against medical advice
O. congestive heart failure
P. chief complaint
Q. left lower quadrant
R. electrocardiogram
S. to keep open
T. central nervous system
U. intracranial pressure
V. jugular vein distention
W. treatment
X. motor vehicle crash
Y. year old

_____ 31. CC
_____ 32. y/o
_____ 33. wt
_____ 34. CNS
_____ 35. SOB
_____ 36. n/v
_____ 37. AMI
_____ 38. CHF
_____ 39. ICP

_____ 40. MVC
_____ 41. STD
_____ 42. NTG
_____ 43. LLQ
_____ 44. BS
_____ 45. ECG
_____ 46. JVD
_____ 47. n/a
_____ 48. AMA

_____ 49. DNR
_____ 50. PEEP
_____ 51. Tx
_____ 52. IO
_____ 53. TKO
_____ 54. NSR
_____ 55. PVC

SPECIAL PROJECTS

Documentation: Radio Report/Prehospital Care Report

The preparation of both the radio message to medical direction and the written run report are two of the most important tasks you will perform as an EMT-I. Read the following information, compose your initial and updated radio messages, and then complete the run report for this call.

The Call:

At 1832, medic rescue unit 21 is paged through dispatch and is en route to a one-car accident at the corner of Elm and Wildwood Lane. One patient is reported unconscious, and the fire department is also en route. You and your partner, Mike Grailing (an EMT-I), arrive with the ambulance at 1845 and find that there are wires down, fuel spilling from the gas tank, and window glass around the scene. Bystanders state that the car swerved wildly, then hit the power pole. You notice there are no skid marks. You stand by, awaiting arrival of the fire department and the securing of the scene.

Once the scene is safe, your partner employs a jaw thrust with cervical precautions and applies cervical stabilization, while you apply the cervical collar (1850) and begin the assessment. You notice a break in the car's windshield and a small contusion on your patient's forehead. He is unconscious, has a strong pulse, and displays some respiratory wheezing and stridor. Assessment of the neck reveals a small welt but no other apparent injuries. The pupils are equal and reactive. Oxygen is administered at 12 liters per minute via nonrebreather mask, the patient awakens, and initial vitals (including a respiratory rate of 30 with audible wheezes, BP of 110/76, a strong pulse of 90, and oxygen saturation of 94 percent) are taken at 1852. The ECG displays normal sinus rhythm.

©2004 Pearson Education, Inc.
Intermediate Emergency Care: Principles & Practice

The patient awakes and asks, "What happened?" He states that he thinks he was stung by a bee. Two years ago he had a similar sting and reaction and has a kit at home that his physician prescribed for him. He is experiencing itching, and there are noticeable hives. He says he feels like "I have a lump in my throat."

Based upon protocol, you initiate the IV run TKO with lactated Ringer's solution in the right forearm using a 16-gauge over-the-catheter needle while the patient is being immobilized and moved to a long spine board.

Medical direction is contacted and you call in the following:

_____

_____

_____

_____

_____

_____

_____

_____

_____

_____

_____

Orders for 0.3 mg epinephrine SQ (1:1,000) and 50 mg Benadryl IM are received and the medications are administered at 1855. Just prior to moving the patient to the ambulance, the patient is monitored and found to have the following vitals: BP 118/88, pulse 78 strong and regular, respirations 20 and regular with clear breath sounds, an ECG showing normal sinus rhythm, and a pulse oximetry reading of 99 percent.

The patient history, which is taken at the scene and during transport, reveals that the patient's name is William Sobeski, his age is 28, and he lives at 2145 East Brookline Drive in the city of Rochester. The patient denies any allergy, except to bee stings. He was stung by a bee two years ago and was rushed to the emergency department because he "couldn't catch his breath." He denies any headache, visual disturbances, and any numbness and tingling. He also denies taking any prescribed medications and has not eaten since noon. The patient requests Community Hospital because his sister works there. En route, vitals are BP 122/78, pulse of 68 strong and regular, respirations 22 and regular, and a pulse oximetry reading of 98 percent, all taken at 1902.

Contact medical direction and provide the following update:

_____

_____

_____

_____

_____

_____

_____

_____

Patient Assessment

ETA 10 minutes

The final vitals, taken just before arrival, are BP 122/80, pulse 86, oxygen saturation of 98 percent, and respirations 24 and regular with no wheezes. The ECG still displays normal sinus rhythm, and the patient is conscious and oriented. He states that the feeling of a lump in the throat is gone.

The trip is uneventful, and the patient is delivered to the emergency department at 1925. The patient care responsibilities are transferred to the staff, and the attending physician is given the final patient update. The vehicle is restocked, cleaned, and you are ready for service at 1955.

Using the information contained in this narrative, complete the run report on the next page.

Compare the radio communication and run report form that you prepared against the example in the Answer Key section of this Workbook. As you make this comparison, keep in mind that there are "many correct" ways to communicate this body of information. Ensure that the information you have recorded contains the major points of your assessment and care and enough other material to describe the patient and his condition to the receiving physician and anyone else who might review the form. Remember that this document may be the only record of your assessment and care for this patient. When you are done, it should be a complete account of your actions.

©2004 Pearson Education, Inc.
Intermediate Emergency Care: Principles & Practice

| Date / / | Emergency Medical Services Run Report | Run # 911 |

Patient Information

Name:		
Address:		
City:	St:	Zip:
Age:	Birth: / /	Sex: [M][F]

Nature of Call:

Chief Complaint:

Service Information

| Agency: |
| Location: |
| Call Origin: |
| Type: Emrg[ ] Non[ ] Trnsfr[ ] |

Times

Rcvd	:
Enrt	:
Scne	:
LvSn	:
ArHsp	:
InSv	:

Description of Current Problem:

Medical Problems

Past		Present
[ ]	Cardiac	[ ]
[ ]	Stroke	[ ]
[ ]	Acute Abdomen	[ ]
[ ]	Diabetes	[ ]
[ ]	Psychiatric	[ ]
[ ]	Epilepsy	[ ]
[ ]	Drug/Alcohol	[ ]
[ ]	Poisoning	[ ]
[ ]	Allergy/Asthma	[ ]
[ ]	Syncope	[ ]
[ ]	Obstetrical	[ ]
[ ]	GYN	[ ]

Other:

Trauma Scr: Glasgow:

| On Scene Care: | First Aid: |

By Whom?

| 02 @ L : Via | C-Collar : | S-Immob. : | Stretcher : |

Allergies/Meds:

Past Med Hx:

Time	Pulse		Resp.		BP S/D	LOC	ECG
:	R:	[r][i]	R:	[s][l]	/	[a][v][p][u]	

Care/Comments:

| : | R: | [r][i] | R: | [s][l] | / | [a][v][p][u] | |

Care/Comments:

| : | R: | [r][i] | R: | [s][l] | / | [a][v][p][u] | |

Care/Comments:

| : | R: | [r][i] | R: | [s][l] | / | [a][v][p][u] | |

Care/Comments:

Destination:	Personnel:	Certification
Reason:[ ]pt [ ]Closest [ ]M.D. [ ]Other	1.	[P][E][O]
Contacted: [ ]Radio [ ]Tele [ ]Direct	2.	[P][E][O]
Ar Status: [ ]Better [ ]UnC [ ]Worse	3.	[P][E][O]

Patient Assessment

Crossword Puzzle

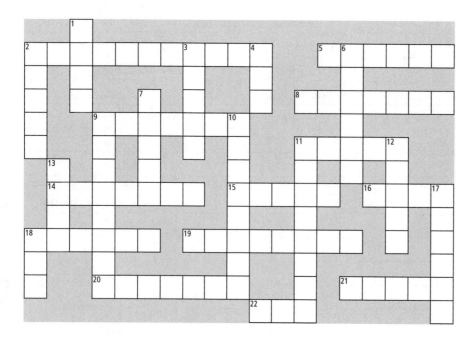

Across

2. A rapid heartbeat
5. A wound
8. High-pitched respiratory sounds
9. Related to the heart
11. _____ complaint: the reason the patient called EMS
14. Fluid build-up in the abdomen
15. Written defamation of another person
16. Type of respirator used when treating a suspected tuberculosis patient
18. Involuntary response to a stimulus
19. Acute alteration in mental function
20. Loud, high-pitched inspiratory wheeze
21. Elements of the head assessment (abbr.)
22. Advanced life support (abbr.)

Down

1. Repeat a verbal order
2. _____ volume: normal respiratory volume
3. Basic EMS communication device
4. Against medical advice (abbr.)
6. Vomitus
7. Sound indicating turbulent blood flow
9. Light, popping nonmusical inspiratory sounds
10. Type of phone service used by many EMS systems
11. Grating sensation or sound
12. _____ diagnosis; prehospital evaluation of the patient's condition and its causes
13. Questionnaire used for suspected alcoholic patients
17. Severity of an injury or illness
18. Review of the systems (abbr.)

©2004 Pearson Education, Inc.
Intermediate Emergency Care: Principles & Practice

Intermediate Emergency Care: Principles & Practice

Division 3
Trauma Emergencies

CHAPTER 12

*

Trauma and Trauma Systems

Review of Chapter Objectives

After reading this chapter, you should be able to:

1. Describe the prevalence and significance of trauma. pp. 583–584

Trauma is the fourth most common cause of mortality and the number one killer for persons under the age of 44. It accounts for about 150,000 deaths per year and may be the most expensive medical problem of society today. Traumas can be divided into those caused by blunt and penetrating injury mechanisms, with only 10 percent of all trauma patients experiencing life-threatening injuries and the need for the services of the trauma center/system.

2. List the components of a comprehensive trauma system. pp. 584–586

The trauma system consists of a state-level agency that coordinates regional trauma systems. The regional systems consist of regional, area, and community trauma centers and, in some cases, other facilities designated and dedicated to the care of trauma patients. The trauma system also consists of injury prevention, provider education, data registry, and quality assurance programs.

3. Identify the characteristics of community, area, and regional trauma centers. pp. 584–586

- **Community or Level III Trauma Center.** This is a general hospital with a commitment to provide resources and staff training specific to the care of trauma patients. Such centers are generally located in rural areas and will stabilize the more serious trauma patients, and then transport them to higher level trauma centers.
- **Area or Level II Trauma Center.** This is a facility with an increased commitment to trauma patient care including 24-hour surgery. A Level II center can handle all but the most critical and specialty trauma patients.
- **Regional or Level I Trauma Center.** This is a facility, usually a university teaching hospital, that is staffed and equipped to handle all types of serious trauma 24 hours a day and 7 days a week, as well as to support and oversee the regional trauma system.

    In some areas there is a Level IV trauma facility, which receives trauma patients and stabilizes them for transport to a higher level facility.

4. Identify the trauma triage criteria. p. 589

Trauma triage criteria include a listing of mechanisms of injury and physical findings suggestive of serious injury. The criteria identify patients likely to benefit from the care offered by the Level I or II trauma center. They include:

Mechanism of Injury

Falls greater than 20 feet (3x victim's height)
Motorcycle accidents (over 20 mph)
Severe vehicle impacts
Death of another vehicle occupant

Pedestrian/bicyclist vs. auto collisions
Ejections from vehicles
Rollovers with serious impact
Prolonged extrications

Physical Findings

Revised Trauma Score less than 11
Glasgow Coma Scale less than 14
Pulse greater than 120 or less than 50
Multiple proximal long bone fractures
Pelvic fractures
Respiratory rate greater than 29 or less than 10
Burns greater than 15% body surface area (BSA)

Pediatric Trauma Score less than 9
Systolic blood pressure less than 90
Penetrating trauma (non-extremity)
Flail chest
Limb paralysis
Airway or facial burns

5. **Describe how trauma differs from medical emergencies in the scene size-up, assessment, prehospital emergency care, and transport.** pp. 586–589

- **Scene size-up** of the trauma incident differs from that with the medical emergency in that it is usually associated with more numerous scene hazards and involves an analysis of the mechanism of injury, using the evidence of impact to suggest possible injuries (the index of suspicion).
- **Assessment** employs an initial assessment examining the risk of spinal injury, a quick mental status check, and an evaluation of airway, breathing, and circulation (ABCs), followed by a rapid trauma assessment looking to the head and torso and any sites of potential serious injury suggested by the index of suspicion or patient complaint.
- **Prehospital care and transport** of the trauma patient is designed to provide expedient and supportive care and rapid transport of the patient to the trauma center or other appropriate facility.

6. **Explain the "Golden Hour" concept and describe how it applies to prehospital emergency medical service.** p. 588

Research has demonstrated that the seriously injured trauma patient has an increasing chance for survival as the time from the injury to surgical intervention is reduced. Practically, this time should be as short as possible, ideally less than one hour. This "Golden Hour" concept directs prehospital care providers to reduce on-scene and transport times by expeditious assessment and care at the scene and by the use of air medical transport when appropriate and available.

7. **Explain the value of air medical service in trauma patient care and transport.** p. 588

Air medical transport can move the trauma patient more quickly and along a direct line from the crash scene to the trauma center, thereby reducing transport time and increasing the likelihood that the patient will reach definitive care expeditiously.

CASE STUDY REVIEW

This case study presents a good opportunity to examine the components of the trauma system and the role they fulfill in the provision of prehospital care. John's very life is dependent upon the trauma system functioning efficiently.

EMT-I Earl Antak responds to the incident alone in a vehicle with advanced life support equipment, but not designed to transport patients (sometimes called a fly car). This system configuration permits advanced life support to be more flexible and available to a larger geographic area. Less seriously injured patients may be transported by ambulance without the EMT-I, making John more quickly available for another call, or in this case available immediately after the helicopter leaves with the patient.

As Earl arrives at the scene he performs the elements of the scene survey. He assures the scene is safe and that the police are controlling traffic. Earl, in consideration of scene safety, will don gloves as there are open wounds, and he avoids the glass around the vehicle door. As he approaches the patient, Earl evaluates the mechanism of injury and notes that the bicyclist probably ran into the open car door. The mechanism of injury suggests significant impact and the probable need to enter the patient into the trauma system. Earl also notes that the rider was wearing a helmet, possibly the result of injury prevention programs in his local community, and suggesting a reduced incidence of head injuries, though not reducing the chances of spinal injury.

Earl's initial assessment reveals a well-developed young male who was unconscious but now is fully conscious and alert. Earl rules out any immediate airway, breathing, or circulation problem, applies oxygen, and ensures that the sheriff's department officer and then the ambulance crew continue to maintain immobilization of John's head and spine. As Earl moves on to the rapid trauma assessment, he notes neurologic signs that suggest a cervical spine injury. Earl also notes a likely clavicle fracture and carefully assesses for any associated respiratory injury. He also carefully watches for the early signs of shock, because clavicular injury can lacerate the subclavian artery. Vital signs are within normal limits for someone recently involved in heavy exercise and the emotional stress of trauma. Earl will, however, carefully record the vital signs and the results of his rapid trauma assessment during the ongoing assessments (every 5 minutes for this patient) and compare them to detect any trends in the patient's condition.

Earl contacts medical direction and is assigned a transport destination. This communication ensures that John is transported to an appropriate center and one that has the resources to care for his injuries. Should a particular center be overcrowded with patients or have essential services unavailable (as, for example, no surgeon immediately on hand), Earl would be directed to transport John to another facility. As time is a critical factor in caring for John, Earl quickly performs the skills necessary to protect John's spine, then moves to transport him quickly. Earl also requests air medical services because the ground transport time is in excess of 30 minutes. He does not, however, await the helicopter but intercepts it at a predesignated landing zone. His intercept with the helicopter will likely reduce the transport time by minutes, an important factor with a seriously injured trauma patient. In this case, it is clearly to John's benefit to get to the trauma center as quickly as possible. The interactions between Earl and the police officer, the responding EMTs in the ambulance, the medical direction physician, the trauma triage nurse, and the flight crew ensure that the system works in a coordinated way and to the benefit of its patient, John.

CONTENT SELF-EVALUATION

MULTIPLE CHOICE

 1. Auto accidents account for how many deaths each year?
   A. 12,000   D. 68,000
   B. 24,000   E. 150,000
   C. 44,000

 2. Although trauma poses a serious threat to life, its presentation often masks the patient's true condition.
   A. True
   B. False

 3. Some 90 percent of all trauma patients do not have serious, life-endangering injuries.
   A. True
   B. False

 4. Trauma triage criteria are mechanisms of injury or physical signs exhibited by the patient that suggest serious injury.
   A. True
   B. False

 5. The legislation that led to the development of today's Emergency Medical Services system was the:
   A. Trauma Care Systems Planning and Development Act of 1970.
   B. Consolidated Emergency Services Act of 1971.
   C. Highway Safety Act of 1966.
   D. Trauma Systems Act of 1963.
   E. National Readiness Act of 1960.

_D_ 6. The trauma system is predicated on the principle that serious trauma is:
   A. a frequent occurrence.
   B. usually a medical emergency.
   C. inevitable.
   D. a surgical disease.
   E. fatal if the patient is not seen by a qualified physician in less than 30 minutes.

_B_ 7. A Level I trauma center is usually a(n):
   A. community hospital.
   B. teaching hospital with resources available full-time for emergency cases.
   C. emergency department with 24-hour service.
   D. non-emergency health-care facility.
   E. stabilizing and transport facility.

_D_ 8. The small community hospital or health-care facility in a remote area, designated as a receiving facility for trauma, is Level:
   A. I.   D. IV.
   B. II.   E. V.
   C. III.

_E_ 9. Trauma centers may also be designated for provision of which of the following special services?
   A. pediatric trauma center   D. hyperbaric center
   B. burn center   E. all of the above
   C. neurocenter

_B_ 10. The period of time between the occurrence of serious injury and surgery suggested as a goal for prehospital care providers is the:
   A. platinum 10 minutes.   D. bleed-out equation.
   B. golden hour.   E. critical differential.
   C. trauma time differential.

_A_ 11. In applying trauma triage criteria, it is best to err on the side of precaution.
   A. True
   B. False

_A_ 12. Trauma triage criteria are designed to over-triage trauma patients to ensure those with more subtle injuries are not missed.
   A. True
   B. False

_E_ 13. The reduction in the incidence and seriousness of trauma in recent years can be credited to:
   A. better highway design.
   B. better auto design.
   C. use of auto restraint systems.
   D. development of injury prevention programs.
   E. all of the above

_D_ 14. The standardized data retrieval system used to evaluate and improve the trauma system is the:
   A. prehospital care report system.   D. trauma quality improvement program.
   B. trauma triage system.   E. CISD.
   C. trauma registry.

_A_ 15. Quality Improvement is a significant method of assessing system quality and providing for its improvement.
   A. True
   B. False

CHAPTER 13
✳
Blunt Trauma

Review of Chapter Objectives

After reading this chapter, you should be able to:

1. **Identify, and explain by example, the laws of inertia and conservation of energy.**　　**p. 594**

   - **Inertia** is the tendency for objects at rest or in motion to remain so unless acted upon by an outside force. In some cases, that force is the energy exchange that causes trauma. For example, a bullet will continue its travel until it exchanges all its energy with the tissue it strikes.
   - **Conservation of energy** is the physical law explaining that energy is not lost but changes form in the auto or other impact. An example is the deformity in the auto when it impacts a tree.

2. **Define kinetic energy and force as they relate to trauma.**　　**pp. 594–595**

   - **Kinetic energy** is the energy any moving object possesses. This energy is the potential to do harm if it is distributed to a victim.
   - **Force** is the exchange of energy from one object to another. It is determined by an object's mass (weight) and the velocity of rate change (acceleration or deceleration). This force induces injury.

3. **Describe the organ collisions that occur with blunt trauma in vehicle crashes.**　　**pp. 597–598**

   As an aspect of the human anatomy contacts the interior of the slowed vehicle, the exterior of the body begins to slow. Internal organs then impact that slowed tissue compressing, twisting, and stretching it. Since organs within the body differ in density and structure (hollow versus solid), this compression, twisting, and stretching may result in contusions, tears, and ruptures. Organs may also tear at their attachments or tear blood vessels as they decelerate.

4. **Describe the effects of restraint systems—including seat belts, airbags, and child safety seats—on injury patterns in vehicle crashes.**　　**pp. 598–601**

   Personal restraint systems clearly reduce death and disability associated with an auto crash. The lap belt alone prevents the passenger from sliding forward into the dash, steering wheel, or other interior aspects of the slowed vehicle. It does not, however, prevent the body from pivoting or the head from striking the dash or steering wheel. The shoulder belt prevents this motion and the expected injury but may cause minor chest and neck injury. The shoulder belt must be worn in conjunction with the lap belt because alone it may lead to serious neck and chest injury.

   The airbag cushions the impact as the passenger moves toward the slowed vehicle's interior. The result is a slower deceleration, less kinetic forces, and fewer and less serious injuries.

   A child safety seat provides the same protection for the child as the lap belt and shoulder strap do for the adult. The seat, however, must be rear-facing for the infant and small child and must also be located in the rear seat (or the front seat with the airbag disabled). Otherwise, rapid air bag inflation may displace the seat rearward and cause serious injury to the child. It is also imperative that the seat be properly sized for the child and properly and firmly secured.

5. Compare and contrast the types of vehicle impacts and their expected injuries.

pp. 601–613

There are basically five types of vehicle impacts—frontal, lateral, rotational, rear-end, or rollover impacts. There are four events within each impact. First, the vehicle impacts the object and quickly comes to rest. Then, the vehicle occupant impacts the vehicle interior and comes to rest. Meanwhile, various organs and structures within the occupant's body collide with one another causing compression and stretching and injury. In the fourth event, objects within the vehicle may continue their forward motion until they impact the slowed or stopped occupant. In some instances, secondary vehicle impacts occur; these are impacts that may subject the injured occupant to additional acceleration, deceleration, and injury.

Frontal impact is the most common type of auto collision, although it also offers the most structural protection for the occupant. The front crumple zones of the auto absorb energy and the restraints—seat belts and airbags—provide additional protection. The anterior surface of the victim impacts the steering wheel, dash, windshield and/or firewall resulting in chest, abdominal, head, and neck injuries as well as knee, femur, and hip fractures.

Lateral impacts occur without the benefit of the front crumple zones, thereby permitting transmission of more energy directly to the occupant. The occupant is turned 90 degrees to the impact, resulting in fractures of the hip, femur, shoulder girdle, clavicle, and lateral ribs. Internal injury may result to the aorta and spleen on the driver's side or liver on the passenger's side. An unbelted occupant may impact the other occupant, causing further injury.

Rotational impacts result from oblique contact between vehicles, spinning as well as slowing the autos. This mediates the deceleration and reduces the expected injury. Injury patterns resemble a mix of those associated with frontal and lateral patterns though the severity is generally reduced.

Rear-end impacts push the auto, auto seat, and finally the occupant forward. The body is well protected, though the head may remain stationary while the shoulders move rapidly forward. The result may be hyperextension of the head and neck and cervical spine injury. Once the vehicle begins deceleration, other injuries may occur as the body contacts the dash, steering wheel, or windshield if the occupant is unbelted.

Rollovers occur as the roadway elevation changes or a vehicle with a high center of gravity becomes unstable around a turn. The vehicle impacts the ground as it turns, exposing the occupants to multiple impacts in places where the vehicle interior may be not designed to absorb such impacts. The result may be serious injuries to anywhere on the body or ejection of the occupants. Restraints greatly reduce the incidence of injury and ejection, while ejection greatly increases the chance of occupant death.

6. Discuss the benefits of auto restraints and motorcycle helmet use.

pp. 601–605, 610–612

Lap belts and shoulder straps control the deceleration of the vehicle occupant during a crash, slowing them with the auto. The result is a great reduction in injuries and deaths. However, when improperly worn, serious injuries may result. Shoulder straps alone may account for serious neck injury while the lap belt worn too high may injure the spine and abdomen.

Airbags inflate explosively during an impact and provide a cushion of gas as the occupant impacts the steering wheel, dash, or vehicle side. This slows the impact, reduces the deceleration rate, and reduces injuries. The airbag may entrap the driver's fingers and result in fractures or may impact a small driver or passenger who is seated close to the device and result in facial injury.

Child safety seats provide much needed protection for infants and small children for whom normal restraints do not work adequately by themselves because of the children's rapidly changing anatomical dimensions. The seat faces rearward for infants and very small children, then should be turned to face forward as the child grows. This positioning permits the seat belt to provide restraint, similar to that provided for the adult. Child safety seats should not be positioned in front of airbag restraint systems because inflation of those devices may push the rear-facing child forcibly into the seat.

Motorcycle helmet use can significantly reduce the incidence and severity of head injury, the greatest cause of motorcycle crash death. Helmets do not, however, reduce the incidence of spinal injury.

©2004 Pearson Education, Inc.
Intermediate Emergency Care: Principles & Practice

7. **Describe the mechanisms of injury associated with falls, crush injuries, and sports injuries.** pp. 619–622

Falls are a release of stored gravitational energy resulting in an impact between the body and the ground or other surface. Injuries occur at the point of impact and along the pathway of transmitted energy, resulting in soft tissue, skeletal, and internal trauma.

Crush injuries are injuries caused by heavy objects or machinery entrapping and damaging an extremity. The resulting wound restricts blood flow and allows the accumulation of toxins. When the pressure is removed, blood flow may move the toxins into the central circulation and hemorrhage from many disrupted blood vessels at the wound site may be hard to control.

Sports injuries are commonly the result of direct trauma, fatigue, or exertion. They often result in injury to muscles, ligaments, and tendons and to the long bones. Special consideration must be given to protecting such an injury from further aggravation until it can be seen by a physician.

8. **Identify the common blast injuries and any special considerations regarding their assessment and proper care.** pp. 613–619

The blast injury process results in five distinct mechanisms of injury—pressure injury, penetrating objects, personnel displacement, structural collapse, and burns.

Pressure injury occurs as the pressure wave moves outward, rapidly compressing, then decompressing anything in its path. A victim is impacted by the wave and air-filled body spaces such as the lungs, auditory canals, and bowels may be damaged. Hearing loss is the most frequent result of pressure injury, though lung injury is most serious and life threatening. The pressure change may damage or rupture alveoli resulting in dyspnea, pulmonary edema, pneumothorax, or air embolism. Care includes provision of high-flow oxygen, gentle positive-pressure ventilation, and rapid transport. The hearing loss patient needs careful reassurance and simple instruction.

Penetrating objects may be the bomb casing or debris put in motion by the pressure of the explosion. They may impale or enter the body, resulting in hemorrhage and internal injury. Care specific to the resulting injury should be provided, and any hemorrhage controlled by direct pressure. Any impaled object should be immobilized and the patient given rapid transport to the trauma center.

Personnel displacement occurs as the pressure wave and blast wind propel the victim through the air and he or she then impacts the ground or other surface. Blunt and penetrating trauma may result, and such injuries are cared for following standard procedures.

Collapse of a structure after a blast may entrap victims under debris and result in crush and pressure injuries. The collapse may make victims hard to locate and then extricate. Further, the nature of the crush-type wounds may make control of hemorrhage difficult, while the release of a long-entrapped extremity may be dangerous as the toxins that accumulated when circulation is disrupted are distributed to the central circulation.

Burns may result directly from the explosion or as a result of secondary combustion of debris or clothing. Generally the initial explosion will cause only superficial damage because of the short duration of the heat release and the fluid nature of the body. However, incendiary agents and burning debris or clothing may result in severe full-thickness burns.

9. **Identify and explain any special assessment and care considerations for patients with blunt trauma.** pp. 593–622

Blunt injury patients must be carefully assessed because the signs of serious internal injury may be hidden or absent. Careful analysis of the mechanism of injury and the development of an index of suspicion for serious injury may be the only way to anticipate the true seriousness of the injuries.

10. **Given several preprogrammed and moulaged blunt trauma patients, provide the appropriate scene size-up, initial assessment, rapid trauma or focused physical exam and history, detailed exam, and ongoing assessment, and provide appropriate patient care and transportation.** pp. 593–622

During your training as an EMT-I, you will participate in many classroom practice sessions involving simulated patients. You will also spend some time in the emergency departments of local hospitals as well as in advanced-level ambulances gaining clinical experience. During these times, use your knowledge of the mechanisms of blunt trauma to help you assess and care for the simulated or real patients you attend.

CASE STUDY REVIEW

This scenario represents a typical serious auto collision in which knowledge of the kinetics of trauma assists in analyzing the mechanism of injury and helps guide assessment and care. Using this approach results in a better understanding of the potential injuries. It also provides for an orderly scene approach in which the patients are quickly assessed, prioritized, immediately stabilized, and then quickly transported. The incident is evaluated carefully, using an analysis of the mechanism of injury to anticipate both the nature and severity of patient injuries. This information is then used in combination with the data gathered through the patient assessments to develop a clear picture of what happened to the auto passengers and to determine what resources will be distributed to each patient.

The information given by the dispatcher allows Kris and Bob to begin planning for arrival at the scene. The dispatch information describes a severe accident with the potential for several seriously injured patients. While still en route, Kris and Bob locate equipment in the ambulance and set it out on the stretcher for quick transport to their patients' side. Lactated Ringer's solution in 1,000 mL bags might be readied in the ambulance with trauma tubing, pressure infusers, and large-bore catheters readied, just in case the decision is made to rapidly transport the patient. Kris and Bob may also use this time to review their responsibilities, which begin with arrival at the scene.

Given the police update, the team begins thinking about the kinetic energy associated with the collision and the injuries that it is likely to cause. One auto was stopped and was hit from behind by a vehicle at "highway speed." In the auto hit, the suspected injuries should include cervical spine injury, with the rest of the body well protected except for secondary impacts. Kris and Bob should anticipate the need for spinal precautions and ready a collar, vest-type immobilization device, and long spine board.

The auto traveling at highway speed most likely impacted the other frontally. If the occupants were unrestrained, they may have traveled either through the down-and-under or up-and-over pathway. If they were restrained, the lap, lap and shoulder, or airbag restraint systems may have protected them. (Remember that the airbag restraint system is beneficial only for the initial frontal impact.) Internal head injuries, chest trauma, and shock are the leading trauma killers. The team will anticipate these types of injuries and treat their patients accordingly.

Kris and Bob gain a great deal of information quickly during the scene size-up. Potential hazards, the number of patients, the resources needed, and the mechanism of injury all are identified. From analysis of the mechanism of injury, they anticipate the nature and extent of injuries for each of the three expected patients. By examining what happened, how badly the autos are damaged, and from what direction the impacts came, the team can garner enough information to anticipate which patient is likely to be the most seriously injured.

In this collision, the green car struck the red one from behind. The red car sustained severe rear-end damage, reflecting a strong impact. The passenger would have been pushed forward with great acceleration by the auto seat, while the unsupported head rotated backward, extending the cervical spine. An important observation was that the headrest was in the "up" position. This positioning probably limited the forceful hyperextension of the head and neck and reduced the potential for injury. The seatbelt also limited the danger of secondary impact, assuring the driver came to rest with the vehicle, not afterward.

©2004 Pearson Education, Inc.
Intermediate Emergency Care: Principles & Practice

The second car (the green one) sustained front-end damage and two spider-web cracks in the windshield. This suggests an unrestrained driver and passenger, the up-and-over pathway, and a potential for severe head, neck, thoracic, and abdominal injuries. The deformed steering wheel also provides evidence that the driver may have sustained a chest injury. Using the analysis of the mechanism of injury, Kris and Bob have a good preliminary picture of the collision process and the likely injuries it produced. As they leave their vehicle and approach the scene, they don gloves and assure the scene is safe for them, their patients, fellow rescuers, and bystanders. They also request anticipated resources (another ambulance) to handle the multiple patients they expect. Because the mechanism of injury analysis suggests the most serious patients will be found in the green car, Kris and Bob head there first.

Assessment confirms the injuries anticipated by review of the impact and the degree of auto damage. As reported by the police officer, the driver of the red car appears only shaken up with a possible spine injury. His vitals are within normal limits, given the circumstances. The choice is made to leave him with a First Responder while Kris and Bob remain with the patients in the green car. While it would be more preferable to have an ALS provider by the side of each patient, this decision is justified based upon the findings at the scene. Bob and Kris will have another First Responder hold spinal immobilization for the driver of the green car as they attend to the unconscious passenger.

The initial assessment reveals that the occupants of the green auto are in serious condition. The driver has sustained chest trauma and is experiencing dyspnea, though her breath sounds are clear at this time. She is stable for now. However, she has the potential to deteriorate rapidly at any time. Her passenger is moving rapidly into hypovolemic shock, presumably due to pelvic and femur fractures and internal hemorrhage. She is also unconscious either due to the hypovolemia or the head impact. The passenger is critical and a candidate for immediate transport. The driver, though more stable, is a candidate for immediate transport also.

This case study demonstrates the value a good scene analysis can have in triaging, in anticipating the findings of assessment, and in determining the care needed by the patient or patients. While the mechanism of injury analysis does not give definitive information regarding the nature and extent of patient injuries, it can complement the overall assessment of both the scene and each individual patient.

CONTENT SELF-EVALUATION

MULTIPLE CHOICE

_____ 1. The study of trauma is related to a branch of physics called:
   A. kinetics.
   B. velocity.
   C. ballistics.
   D. inertia.
   E. heuristics.

_____ 2. The anticipation of injuries based upon the analysis of the collision mechanism is referred to as the:
   A. mechanism of injury.
   B. index of suspicion.
   C. trauma triage criteria.
   D. mortality potential.
   E. RTS.

_____ 3. Penetrating trauma is the most common type of trauma associated with patient mortality.
   A. True
   B. False

_____ 4. The tendency of an object to remain at rest or remain in motion unless acted upon by an external force is:
   A. kinetics.
   B. velocity.
   C. ballistics.
   D. inertia.
   E. deceleration.

_____ 5. Two autos accelerate from a stop sign to a speed of 30 mph, the first one by normal acceleration and the second when it was struck from behind by another vehicle. Assuming that both vehicles have the same weight, which vehicle gained the most kinetic energy?
A. the vehicle in normal acceleration
B. the vehicle struck from behind
C. both vehicles gained the same kinetic energy
D. cannot be determined since the kinetic energy is not known
E. cannot be determined since the force is not known

_____ 6. Which of the following is an example of energy dissipation from an auto accident?
A. sound of the impact
B. bending of the structural steel
C. heating of the compressed steel
D. internal injury to the occupant
E. all of the above

_____ 7. Which of the following increases the kinetic energy of a collision most quickly?
A. the temperature of the object
B. increasing object speed
C. decreasing object speed
D. increasing object mass
E. decreasing object mass

_____ 8. Blunt trauma may cause:
A. rupture of the bowel.
B. bursting of the alveoli.
C. crushing of blood vessels.
D. contusion of the liver or kidneys.
E. all of the above.

_____ 9. Which of the following is a common cause of blunt trauma?
A. auto collisions
B. falls
C. sports injuries
D. pedestrian impacts
E. all of the above

_____ 10. In which order do the events of an auto collision usually occur?
A. body collision, vehicle collision, organ collision, secondary collisions
B. organ collision, vehicle collision, body collision, secondary collisions
C. vehicle collision, secondary collisions, body collision, organ collision
D. vehicle collision, body collision, organ collision, secondary collisions
E. body collision, vehicle collision, secondary collisions, organ collision

_____ 11. The major effect of the seat belt during the auto collision is to slow the passenger with the auto.
A. True
B. False

_____ 12. A supplemental restraint system (SRS) refers to which of the following?
A. shoulder belts
B. airbags
C. lap belts
D. child seats
E. all of the above

_____ 13. Which of the following restraint systems is likely to induce hand fractures?
A. shoulder belts
B. passenger airbags
C. driver-side airbags
D. child seats
E. lap belts

_____ 14. While less convenient than a child carrier, holding a child in the arms is relatively safe except in the most severe of crashes.
A. True
B. False

_____ 15. The type of auto impact that occurs most frequently in rural areas is:
A. lateral.
B. rotational.
C. frontal.
D. rear-end.
E. rollover.

©2004 Pearson Education, Inc.
Intermediate Emergency Care: Principles & Practice

_____ 16. Which type of auto impact occurs most frequently in the urban setting?
   A. lateral
   B. rotational
   C. frontal
   D. rear-end
   E. rollover

_____ 17. The down-and-under pathway is most commonly associated with which type of auto collision?
   A. lateral
   B. rotational
   C. frontal
   D. rear-end
   E. rollover

_____ 18. When analyzing the lateral impact injury mechanism, you must assign a higher index of suspicion for serious life-threatening injury than with other types of impact.
   A. True
   B. False

_____ 19. Which of the following injuries are associated with significant lateral impact?
   A. aortic aneurysms
   B. clavicular fractures
   C. pelvic fractures
   D. vertebral fractures
   E. all of the above

_____ 20. With rotational impacts, the seriousness of injury is often less than vehicle damage would suggest.
   A. True
   B. False

_____ 21. The most common injury associated with the rear-end impact is to the:
   A. abdomen.
   B. pelvis.
   C. aorta.
   D. femur.
   E. head and neck.

_____ 22. Which of the following is a hazard commonly associated with auto collisions?
   A. hot liquids
   B. caustic substances
   C. downed power lines
   D. sharp glass or metal edges
   E. all of the above

_____ 23. With modern vehicle construction that incorporates crumple zones, you can dependably use the amount of vehicular damage to approximate the patient injuries inside.
   A. True
   B. False

_____ 24. In fatal collisions, about what percentage of the drivers are legally intoxicated?
   A. 10 percent
   B. 20 percent
   C. 35 percent
   D. 50 percent
   E. 83 percent

_____ 25. The most common body area associated with vehicular mortality is the:
   A. head.
   B. chest.
   C. abdomen.
   D. extremities.
   E. spine.

_____ 26. In motorcycle accidents, the highest index of suspicion for injury should be directed at the:
   A. neck.
   B. head.
   C. extremities.
   D. pelvis.
   E. femurs.

_____ 27. Use of a helmet in a motorcycle crash reduces the incidence of neck injury by about:
   A. 25 percent.
   B. 35 percent.
   C. 58 percent.
   D. 75 percent.
   E. 85 percent.

_____ 28. In an auto vs. child pedestrian accident, you would expect the victim to turn toward the impact.
    A. True
    B. False

_____ 29. In addition to the danger of trauma, the boating collision patient is also likely to suffer possible hypothermia and near-drowning.
    A. True
    B. False

_____ 30. Which of the mechanisms below can cause patient injury in a blast?
    A. the pressure wave
    B. flying debris
    C. the patient being thrown into objects
    D. heat
    E. all of the above

_____ 31. Underwater detonation of an explosive generally increases its lethal range by:
    A. 10 percent.   D. 300 percent.
    B. 25 percent.   E. 500 percent.
    C. 100 percent.

_____ 32. A victim's orientation to the blast does not effect the nature and severity of the injuries he or she sustains from an explosion.
    A. True
    B. False

_____ 33. The arrow-shaped projectiles in military-type explosives that are designed to extend the injury power of a bomb are called:
    A. ordinance.   D. oatmeal.
    B. casing material.   E. granulation.
    C. flechettes.

_____ 34. When victims are within a structure that contains an explosion, like a building, the effects of the blast are concentrated and the severity of the expected injuries increases.
    A. True
    B. False

_____ 35. Which of the following are secondary blast injuries?
    A. heat injuries   D. injuries caused by structural collapse
    B. pressure injuries   E. both A and B
    C. projectile injuries

_____ 36. If you suspect that a blast was a terrorist act, you should be cautious of secondary explosive devices intended to injure rescue personnel.
    A. True
    B. False

_____ 37. The most serious and common traumas associated with explosions affect the:
    A. heart.   D. lungs.
    B. bowel.   E. brain.
    C. auditory canal.

_____ 38. When ventilating the victim of a severe blast, you should use forceful deep ventilations with the bag-valve mask as doing this will ensure good chest expansion.
    A. True
    B. False

_____ 39. Severe injury is generally associated with a fall from:
    A. three times the patient's own height.   D. more than 6 feet.
    B. twice the patient's own height.   E. none of the above
    C. greater than 12 feet.

©2004 Pearson Education, Inc.
Intermediate Emergency Care: Principles & Practice

_____ **40.** Sports injuries are frequently associated with:

    A. fatigue.   **D.** rotation.

    B. extreme exertion.   **E.** all of the above

    C. compression.

SPECIAL PROJECTS

Mechanism of Injury Analysis

Study the photographs of each accident scene below and on the next page. For each photo, identify the type of impact that has occurred and list at least three injuries that you would expect to have occurred.

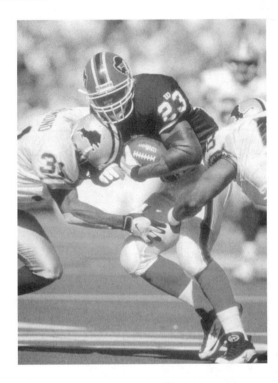

A. Mechanism of injury _____

Anticipated injuries

_____

_____

_____

_____

_____

_____

_____

_____

_____

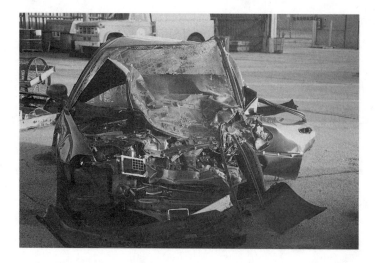

B. Mechanism of injury _____

Anticipated injuries

_____

_____

_____

_____

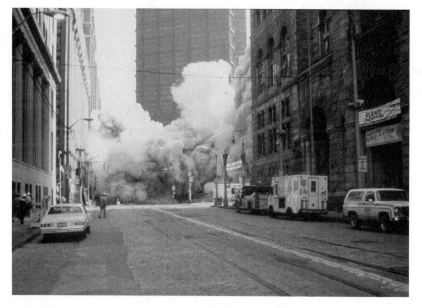

C. Mechanism of injury _____

Anticipated injuries

_____

_____

_____

_____

Personal Benchmarking—Analyzing Mechanisms of Injury

Next time you are in a vehicle for some time, take a look at your position with regard to the interior of the auto in relation to your anatomy. Visualize the forces of impact and what your body will strike during that impact. Identify protections offered by crumple zones and the likely injuries resulting from serious impact, and then determine what effect restraints will have on injury patterns (nature and seriousness).

Frontal Impact

Lateral Impact

Rear-end Impact

Rotational Impact

Rollover Impact

The next time you go to an auto collision, use this information to help you "relive" the auto impact and anticipate patient injuries.

Trauma Emergencies

CHAPTER 14

Penetrating Trauma

Review of Chapter Objectives

After reading this chapter, you should be able to:

1. **Explain the energy exchange process between a penetrating object or projectile and the object it strikes.** pp. 625–628

   The kinetic energy of a bullet is dependent upon its mass and even more so on its velocity according to the kinetic energy formula ($KE = \frac{M \times V^2}{2}$). This energy is distributed to the body tissues in the form of damage as the bullet slows. Due to the semifluid nature of body tissue, the passage of a bullet causes injury as the bullet directly strikes tissue and contuses and tears it and as it sets the tissue in motion outward and away from the bullet's path (cavitation). The faster the bullet and the larger its presenting surface (profile), the more rapid the exchange of energy and the resulting injury.

2. **Determine the effects profile, yaw, tumble, expansion, and fragmentation have on projectile energy transfer.** pp. 626–628

   The rate of projectile energy exchange and the seriousness of resulting injury are dependent upon the rate of energy exchange. That rate is directly related to the bullet's presenting surface or profile. The larger the bullet's caliber (diameter), the greater its profile, the more rapid its exchange of energy with body tissue, and the greater the damage it causes. Yaw (swinging around the axis of the projectile's travel), tumble, expansion, and fragmentation all lead to a greater area of the bullet striking tissue than simply its profile, and hence these factors increase the damaging power of a bullet.

3. **Describe elements of the ballistic injury process including direct injury, cavitation, temporary cavity, permanent cavity, and zone of injury.** pp. 626–628, 630–633

   As a penetrating object enters the body it disrupts the tissue it contacts by tearing it, displacing it from its path, and causing *direct injury*. As the object's velocity increases, the rate of energy exchange increases and the rate of displacement increases. A bullet's speed is so great that the bullet's passage sets the semifluid body tissue in motion away from the bullet's path. This creates a cavity behind and to the side of the projectile pathway. This *cavitation* further stretches and tears tissue as it creates a *temporary cavity*. The natural elasticity of injured tissue and the adjoining tissue closes the cavity, but an area of disrupted tissue remains (the *permanent cavity*). The *zone of injury* is the region along and surrounding the bullet track where tissue has been disrupted due to direct injury or to the stretching and tearing of cavitation.

4. **Identify the relative effects a penetrating object or projectile has when striking various body regions and tissues.** pp. 633–637

   The passage of a bullet (and its cavitational wave) has varying effects depending on the elasticity (resiliency) and density of the tissue the bullet strikes. Connective tissue is very resilient, stretches easily, and will somewhat resist cavitational injury. Solid organs are generally very dense and much less resilient than connective tissue. They do not withstand the force generated by the cavitational wave as well as connective tissue, and the resulting injury can be expected to be much greater. Hollow organs are resilient when not distended with fluid; if an organ is full, however, the cavitational wave may cause the organ to rupture. Direct injury can also perforate an organ and permit spillage of its contents into surrounding tissue. Lung tissue is both very resilient and air filled. The tiny air pockets (the alveoli) absorb the energy of the bullet's passage and limit lung injury. On the other hand, bone is extremely dense and inelastic. Direct contact with a bullet or, in some cases, just the cavitational wave may shatter the bone and drive fragments into surrounding tissue. Slow-moving penetrating objects do not produce a cavitational wave, and injury from them is limited to the pathway of the object.

The passage of a bullet and its associated injury are related to the bullet's path of travel and, specifically, to the body region it passes through. Extremity wounds are by far the most common, yet due to the limited major body structures in the extremities, they rarely result in life-threatening injury. If the projectile strikes the bone, however, the dramatic exchange of energy may cause great tissue disruption and vascular injury, which can result in severe hemorrhage. Abdominal penetration most commonly affects the bowel, which is reasonably tolerant of the cavitational wave. However, the upper abdomen contains the liver, pancreas, and spleen, solid organs that are subject to severe injury from direct injury and cavitation. Penetrating chest trauma may affect the lungs, heart and great vessels, esophagus, trachea, and diaphragm. The lung is rather resilient to penetrating injury, while the heart and great vessels may perforate or rupture with rapid exsanguination ensuing. Tracheal tears may result in airway compromise, while esophageal tears may release gastric contents into the mediastinum with potentially deadly results. Large penetrations of the thoracic wall may permit air to move in and out (sucking or open pneumothorax) or may open the airway internally to permit air to enter the pleural space (closed pneumothorax). Neck injuries may permit severe hemorrhage, disrupt the trachea, or allow air to enter the jugular veins and embolize the lungs. Head injuries may disrupt the airway or may penetrate the cranium and cause extensive, rarely survivable, injury to the brain.

5. **Anticipate the injury types and extent of damage associated with high-velocity/high-energy projectiles, such as rifle bullets; with medium velocity/medium-energy projectiles, such as handgun and shotgun bullets, slugs, or pellets; and with low-energy/low-velocity penetrating objects, such as knives and arrows.** pp. 628–630

- **High-velocity/high-energy projectiles** (rifle bullets) are likely to cause the most extensive injury because they have the potential to impart the most kinetic energy to the patient. Their rapid energy exchange causes the greatest cavitational wave and is most likely to produce bullet deformity and fragmentation. These characteristics cause more severe tissue damage to a greater area. The effects of these projectiles can be further enhanced if the bullet hits bone and causes it to shatter, creating additional projectiles that are driven into adjoining tissue.
- **Medium-velocity/medium-energy projectiles** (from handguns) are likely to cause only moderate injury beyond the direct pathway of the bullet as their reduced energy does not usually cause the bullet deformity, fragmentation, and extensive cavitation waves seen with rifle projectiles. The shotgun is a particularly lethal weapon at close range because its medium-energy projectiles are numerous and their numbers cause many direct injury pathways.
- **Low-velocity/low-energy penetrating objects** are commonly knives, arrows, ice picks, and other objects traveling at low speeds. They generally cause only direct injury along the path of their travel. They may, however, be moved about, once inserted and either left in place or withdrawn.

6. **Identify important elements of the scene size-up associated with shootings or stabbings.** p. 638

Penetrating trauma, especially when associated with shootings or stabbings, presents the danger of violence directed toward others (other rescuers, bystanders, your patient, and you). It is essential that you approach the scene with great caution and ensure that the police have secured it before you approach or enter. Penetrating trauma also calls for gloves as minimum BSI precaution, with goggles and gown required for spurting hemorrhage, airway management, or massive blood contamination. During the scene size-up, you should evaluate the mechanism of injury including the type of weapon, caliber, distance, and angle between the shooter and the victim, and the number of shots fired and patient impacts.

7. Identify and explain any special assessment and care considerations for patients with penetrating trauma. pp. 638–640

In assessing the patient with penetrating trauma you must anticipate the projectile or penetrating object's pathway and the structures it is likely to have injured. The exit wound from a projectile may help you better approximate the wounding potential, and remember that the bullet may have been deflected along its course and damaged or completely missed critical structures. Always suspect and treat for the worst-case scenario. Be especially wary of injuries to the head, chest, and abdomen as wounds to these regions often have lethal outcomes. Cover all open wounds that enter the thorax or neck with occlusive dressings and be watchful for the development of dyspnea due to pneumothorax, tension pneumothorax, or pulmonary emboli. Be prepared to provide aggressive fluid resuscitation, but understand that doing so may dislodge forming clots and increase the rate of internal hemorrhage. Stabilize any impaled objects and only remove them when it is required to ensure a patent airway, to perform CPR, or to transport the patient.

8. Given several preprogrammed and moulaged penetrating trauma patients, provide the appropriate scene size-up, initial assessment, rapid trauma or focused physical exam and history, detailed exam, and ongoing assessment, and provide appropriate patient care and transportation. pp. 625–640

During your training as an EMT-I you will participate in many classroom practice sessions involving simulated patients. You will also spend some time in the emergency departments of local hospitals as well as in advanced-level ambulances gaining clinical experience. During these times, use your knowledge of the mechanisms of penetrating trauma to help you assess and care for the simulated or real patients you attend.

CASE STUDY REVIEW

This scenario involves a patient who has sustained a serious penetrating injury to the chest and provides the opportunity to apply an understanding of the kinetics of trauma to the wounding process. The case also allows us to review scene considerations that should be followed when violence is involved.

Weapon use in modern society represents violence and a danger to rescuers, bystanders, the patient, and the responding EMS team. Sandy is somewhat reassured by the dispatch information, which states that the victim is in custody, and more so as she arrives at the scene and notes the police officers surrounding the patient. However, she remains cautious and ensures that the victim is free of weapons before she begins her care.

In assessing the patient, Sandy anticipates a serious injury, as police are generally equipped with relatively powerful handguns. She recognizes that the bullet delivered significant wounding energy to the thorax and may have fragmented as it hit the ribs and drove rib fragments into tissue as it passed. She anticipates lung damage along the bullet's path, probably more related to the damage seen at the exit, rather than at the entrance, wound. Sandy is also concerned about the penetration of the chest wall and the pleura caused by the bullet's passage. Such a wound may permit air to enter the pleural space and cause the lung to collapse (an open pneumothorax). She seals both the entrance and exit wounds on three sides to allow any building air pressure (tension pneumothorax) to escape. She also carefully monitors breath sounds and respiratory effort to assure an unrecognized closed tension pneumothorax does not develop. Sandy anticipates that this patient's respirations will worsen as the edema associated with the injured lung tissue gets worse and with the continued loss of blood from the internal wound.

Due to the proximity of the wound to the heart, Sandy applies the ECG electrodes and constantly monitors the patient's heart rate and rhythm. She also trends both the patient's level of consciousness and vital signs to assure that the earliest signs of hypovolemia, shock, and decreased tissue perfusion are noted. This patient is clearly a candidate for rapid transport to the closest trauma center.

©2004 Pearson Education, Inc.
Intermediate Emergency Care: Principles & Practice

CONTENT SELF-EVALUATION

MULTIPLE CHOICE

_____ 1. Approximately what number of deaths are attributable to shootings each year?
   A. 25,000
   B. 38,000
   C. 44,000
   D. 50,000
   E. 100,000

_____ 2. An object traveling at twice the speed of another object of the same weight has:
   A. twice the kinetic energy.
   B. three times the kinetic energy.
   C. four times the kinetic energy.
   D. eight times the kinetic energy.
   E. ten times the kinetic energy.

_____ 3. Wounds from rifle bullets are considered two to four times more lethal than handgun bullets.
   A. True
   B. False

_____ 4. The curved tract a bullet follows during flight is called its:
   A. ballistics.
   B. cavitation.
   C. trajectory.
   D. yaw.
   E. parabola.

_____ 5. The surface of a projectile that exchanges energy with the object struck is its:
   A. caliber.
   B. profile.
   C. drag.
   D. yaw.
   E. expansion factor.

_____ 6. When a rifle bullet hits tissue, normally it will:
   A. continue without tumbling.
   B. tumble once then travel nose first.
   C. tumble quickly, the slowly rotate.
   D. wobble but not tumble.
   E. tumble 180 degrees then continue.

_____ 7. While handgun bullets are made of relatively soft lead, their kinetic energy is generally not sufficient to cause significant deformity.
   A. True
   B. False

_____ 8. Civilian hunting ammunition is designed to deform and will frequently fragment when striking soft tissue.
   A. True
   B. False

_____ 9. Which of the following statements accurately describes a rifle bullet in contrast to a handgun bullet?
   A. It is a heavier projectile.
   B. It travels at a greater velocity.
   C. It is more likely to deform.
   D. It is more likely to fragment.
   E. all of the above

_____ 10. The shotgun is limited in range and accuracy; however, injuries it inflicts at close range can be very severe or lethal.
   A. True
   B. False

_____ 11. Which element of the projectile injury process is related to the actual damage caused as the bullet contacts tissue?
   A. direct injury
   B. pressure wave
   C. temporary cavity
   D. permanent cavity
   E. zone of injury

Trauma Emergencies

_____ 12. The movement of tissue away from the bullet's path as it passes through the body results in:
A. direct injury.
B. the pressure wave.
C. a temporary cavity.
D. fragmentation.
E. referred injury.

_____ 13. The passage of a projectile through the body results in a region where tissues are disrupted and not functioning normally that is known as the:
A. direct injury.
B. pressure wave.
C. temporary cavity.
D. permanent cavity.
E. zone of injury.

_____ 14. The temporary cavity formed as a high-velocity/high-energy bullet passes may be how large?
A. 12 times the projectile's profile
B. 14 times the projectile's profile
C. 16 times the projectile's profile
D. 100 times the projectile's profile
E. rarely more than the projectile's profile

_____ 15. The tissue structure that is very resilient, yet dense, and usually sustains limited damage with the passage of a projectile is:
A. a solid organ.
B. a hollow organ.
C. connective tissue.
D. bone.
E. a lung.

_____ 16. The tissue structure that is likely to rupture and spill its contents when struck by a projectile is:
A. a solid organ.
B. a hollow organ.
C. connective tissue.
D. bone.
E. a lung.

_____ 17. Penetrating wounds to the extremities account for about 70 percent of all penetrating wounds yet account for less than 10 percent of fatalities related to this injury mechanism.
A. True
B. False

_____ 18. The abdominal organ most tolerant to the passage of a projectile is the:
A. bowel.
B. liver.
C. spleen.
D. kidney.
E. pancreas.

_____ 19. Because of the pressure-driven dynamics of respiration, any large wound to the chest may compromise breathing.
A. True
B. False

_____ 20. The body region in which a penetrating wound has the greatest likelihood of drawing air into the venous system is the:
A. abdomen.
B. thorax.
C. head.
D. neck.
E. none of the above

_____ 21. Which of the following is NOT associated with an entrance wound?
A. tattooing
B. a small ridge of discoloration around the wound
C. a blown outward appearance
D. subcutaneous emphysema
E. propellant residue on the surrounding tissue

©2004 Pearson Education, Inc.
Intermediate Emergency Care: Principles & Practice

_____ 22. The entrance wound is more likely to reflect the actual damaging potential of the projectile than the exit wound.
A. True
B. False

_____ 23. Which of the following information should you gain through the scene size-up, if possible?
A. the gun caliber
B. the angle of the gun to the victim
C. the type of gun used
D. assurance that no other weapons are involved
E. all of the above

_____ 24. As you care for a patient at a potential crime scene, actions you take to help preserve evidence should include:
A. cutting through, not around bullet or knife holes in clothing.
B. moving what you can away from the patient.
C. removing obviously dead patients from the scene as quickly as possible.
D. disturbing only the items necessary to provide patient care.
E. all of the above

_____ 25. Frothy blood at a bullet exit or entrance wound suggests a(n):
A. simple pneumothorax.
B. open pneumothorax.
C. tension pneumothorax.
D. pericardial tamponade.
E. mediastinum injury.

CHAPTER 15

Hemorrhage and Shock

Review of Chapter Objectives

After reading this chapter, you should be able to:

1. **Describe the epidemiology, including the morbidity/mortality and prevention strategies, for shock and hemorrhage.** pp. 643–644

Shock is the transitional stage between normal physiologic function of the body and death. It is the underlying killer of all trauma patients and is prevented using the strategies described for each of the types of trauma addressed in this and the the following trauma chapters. Hemorrhage is loss of the body's precious medium, blood, and is a common cause of shock and death in the trauma patient. Strategies to prevent hemorrhage are those designed to prevent trauma.

2. **Discuss the pathophysiology of hemorrhage and shock.** pp. 644–652, 659–622 (see Chapter 2)

The cardiovascular system is a closed system of interconnected tubes (blood vessels) that direct blood to the essential organs and tissues of the body. Arteries distribute blood to the various organs and tissues of the body. Arterioles determine the amount of blood perfusing the tissue of an organ and together constrict and increase peripheral vascular resistance or dilate and reduce peripheral vascular resistance. Progressive vasoconstriction can help maintain blood pressure and circulation to the most critical organs as the body loses blood during hemorrhage or fluid during other forms of shock. The venous system collects blood and returns it to the heart. It contains about 60 percent of the total blood volume and, when constricted, can return a relatively great volume (up to 1 liter) to the active circulation.

The cardiovascular system is powered by the central pump, the heart. It circulates the blood and, against the peripheral vascular resistance, drives the blood pressure. Its output is a factor of preload (the blood delivered to it by the venous system), stroke volume (the amount of blood ejected into the aorta with each contraction), rate, and afterload (the peripheral vascular resistance). The heart can help compensate for blood loss by attempting to maintain cardiac output by increasing its stroke volume (which is hard to do in hypovolemic states) or by increasing its rate.

Finally, the cardiovascular system contains the precious fluid, blood. Blood provides oxygen and nutrients to the body cells and removes carbon dioxide and waste products of metabolism. Blood also contains clotting factors that will occlude blood vessels if they are torn or disrupted.

The central nervous system provides control of the cardiovascular system using baroreceptors in the carotid arteries and aortic arch to sense fluctuations in blood pressure. It will maintain blood pressure by increasing heart rate, cardiac preload, and peripheral vascular resistance. Hormones from the kidneys and elsewhere help control blood volume and electrolytes as well as the production of erythrocytes.

3. **Describe the body's physiologic response to changes in blood volume, blood pressure, and perfusion.**   pp. 659–662

Increased peripheral resistance is caused by the constriction of the arterioles and provides two mechanisms that combat shock. The arterioles constrict and maintain the blood pressure, and they divert blood to only the critical organs. This reduction in perfusion to the less critical organs results in the increased capillary refill time and the cool, clammy, and ashen skin often associated with shock states. It also results in reduced pulse pressure and weak pulses.

Venous constriction compensates for some blood loss and helps maintain cardiac preload. Since the veins account for about 60 percent of the blood volume, this is reasonably effective in minor to moderate blood loss.

As the cardiac preload drops, the heart rate increases in an attempt to maintain cardiac output and blood pressure. In the presence of significantly reduced preload, this may not be effective.

Peripheral vascular shunting directs the blood away from the skin, conserves body heat, and reduces fluid loss through evaporation. It also redirects blood to more critical areas.

Fluid shifts are the result of drawing fluid from the interstitial and cellular spaces. Fluid moves into the vascular space. While this is a slow mechanism, it can provide the vascular system with several liters of fluid.

4. **Describe the effects of decreased perfusion at the capillary level.**   pp. 659–661

Decreased capillary perfusion limits the amount of oxygen and nutrients delivered to the body cells. It usually causes the release of histamine that, in turn, causes precapillary sphincter dilation and an increase in perfusion. However, in shock states this is not effective, and the cells must revert to anaerobic metabolism while the byproducts of metabolism accumulate and the available oxygen is exhausted. Carbon dioxide, metabolic acids, and other waste products accumulate while body cells begin to die.

5. **Discuss the cellular ischemic, capillary stagnation, and capillary washout phases related to hemorrhagic shock.**   pp. 659–661

- **Cellular ischemia.** As shock ensues, decreased perfusion, first to the non-critical organs, then to all organs, diminishes blood flow through the microcirculation. At the cellular level this diminishes the supply of oxygen and nutrients to the cells and restricts the removal of carbon dioxide and the waste products of metabolism. The cells quickly exhaust their supply of oxygen and begin to use anaerobic metabolism as their sole source of energy to remain alive. This produces an accumulation of pyruvic acid, which in turn, converts to lactic acid and the cells become more acidotic. As cells begin to die, their decomposition releases even more toxins that then begin to affect other cells.
- **Capillary stagnation.** With diminished capillary flow, coupled with the increasingly hypoxic and acidic environment caused by the ischemic cells, the red blood cells become sticky and clump together. They form columns of coagulated erythrocytes called rouleaux that either block the capillary to further flow of blood or will wash out and cause microemboli.
- **Capillary washout.** The toxic environment of the ischemic tissue associated with severe shock finally causes the post-capillary sphincters to dilate and release the hypoxic and acidotic blood as well as the rouleaux into the venous circulation. As this washout becomes extensive, it further reduces the effectiveness of the cardiovascular system and the body moves quickly toward irreversible shock.

6. **Discuss the various types and degrees of shock and hemorrhage.**   pp. 650–652, 661–662

Hemorrhage can be divided into four stages as a patient moves through compensated, decompensated, and irreversible shock.

Stage 1 blood loss is a loss of up to 15 percent of the patient's blood volume. It generally presents with some nervousness, cool skin, and slight pallor. It is difficult to detect as the body compensates well for blood loss in this range.

Stage 2 blood loss is a loss of up to 25 percent of the patient's blood volume. Signs and symptoms become more apparent as the body finds it more difficult to compensate for the loss. The patient may display thirst, anxiety, restlessness, and cool and clammy skin.

Stage 3 blood loss is a loss of up to 35 percent of the patient's blood volume. It presents with the signs of stage 2 blood loss and air hunger, dyspnea, and severe thirst. Survival is unlikely without immediate intervention.

Stage 4 blood loss is a blood loss in excess of 35 percent of the patient's blood volume. The patient begins to display a deathlike appearance with pulses disappearing and respirations becoming very shallow and ineffective. The patient becomes very lethargic and then unconscious and survival becomes unlikely.

7. Predict shock and hemorrhage based on mechanism of injury.   pp. 652–655

Shock due to internal blood loss can be a very silent killer if not recognized and the patient brought to definitive care (surgery) quickly. Severe blunt and deep penetrating trauma can induce internal hemorrhage that is both difficult to identify and treat. If you wait until the frank signs of shock appear, too much time may have passed for care to be effective. Hence it is very important to both analyze the mechanism of injury to anticipate shock and to recognize the very early signs of shock.

A large hematoma may account for up to 500 mL of blood loss, while fractures of the humerus or tibia/fibula may account for 500 to 750 mL. Femoral fractures may account for up to 1,500 mL of blood, while pelvic fractures often involve hemorrhage of up to 2,000 mL. Internal hemorrhage into the chest or abdomen may contribute even greater losses. In penetrating or severe blunt trauma to the chest or abdomen, suspect the development of shock. Also suspect the rapid development of shock in the patient who begins to display the early signs of shock (an increasing pulse rate, decreasing pulse pressure, and anxiety and restlessness) very quickly after the trauma event.

8. Identify the need for intervention and transport of the patient with hemorrhage or shock.   pp. 656-658, 665–670

Hemorrhage and shock are progressive pathologies that eventually become irreversible. To be effective in care, we must carefully assess our patients for the earliest of signs and intervene with rapid transport to a facility that can rapidly provide surgical intervention (to halt the internal bleeding). We also must immediately halt any external hemorrhage and provide supplemental high-flow oxygen. Intravenous fluids may be run to replace volume, but care must be used to prevent increased internal hemorrhage and hemodilution.

9. Discuss the assessment findings and management of internal and external hemorrhage and shock.   pp. 662–670

Tachycardia is a compensatory cardiac action to maintain cardiac output when a reduced preload is present. A weak pulse reflects a narrowing pulse pressure and increasing peripheral vascular resistance to maintain systolic blood pressure. Cool, clammy skin is due to the redirection of blood to more critical organs than the skin. Ashen, pale skin may present due to hypoxia and peripheral vasoconstriction. Agitation, restlessness, and reduced level of consciousness occurs as the brain receives a reduced flow of oxygenated blood. The hypoxia causes the defense mechanisms of agitation and restlessness, followed by a noticeable reduction in the level of consciousness. Dull, lackluster eyes occur secondary to low perfusion and hypoxic states. Rapid, shallow respiration may occur as shock progresses, the respiratory muscles tire in the hypoxic state, and respiratory effort becomes less efficient. Dropping oxygen saturation may also provide evidence to support developing shock. As the peripheral circulation slows, the readings may drop or become erratic. Falling blood pressure heralds the progression from compensated to decompensated shock. As a late sign, it should not be used to determine the presence of shock.

External hemorrhage must be controlled by direct pressure. If direct pressure alone does not work, use elevation, pressure points or, as a last resort, the tourniquet, to stop the hemorrhage. If all sites of hemorrhage are controlled and you can rule out internal hemorrhage, provide fluid resuscitation to return the blood pressure and vital signs to normal.

©2004 Pearson Education, Inc.
Intermediate Emergency Care: Principles & Practice

Should the mechanism of injury or any early development of shock signs or symptoms suggest internal hemorrhage, or external hemorrhage cannot be controlled, transport should be expedited and care initiated immediately. Provide high-flow oxygen and ventalitory support as needed and infuse fluids to maintain the blood pressure just below 100 mmHg, ensuring it does not drop below 50 mmHg.

10. Differentiate between the administration rate and volume of IV fluid in patients with controlled versus uncontrolled hemorrhage.   pp. 665–667

If hemorrhage has been controlled (as with external hemorrhage) then fluid resuscitation can be aimed at returning the blood pressure and other vital signs toward normal. However, if the hemorrhage is internal, and especially if it involves the chest, abdomen, or pelvis, great care must be exercised not to enhance the hemorrhage or excessively dilute the remaining blood. Resuscitation is generally aimed at stabilizing the blood pressure somewhere just below 100 mmHg and preventing it from dropping below 50 mmHg. To maintain these parameters, lactated Ringer's solution (preferred) or normal saline should be run rapidly through trauma or blood tubing and large-bore short catheters. Pressure infusers may be necessary as the blood pressure begins to fall below 50 mmHg. Usually prehospital care is limited to between 1 and 3 liters of crystalloid.

11. Relate pulse pressure and orthostatic vital sign changes to perfusion status.   pp. 650–656

Pulse pressure is the difference between the systolic and diastolic blood pressures and is responsible for the pulse. It is a relative measure of the effectiveness of cardiac output against peripheral vascular resistance. One of the early signs of shock is a decreasing pulse pressure, occurring as cardiac output begins to fall and the body increases peripheral vascular resistance in an attempt to maintain blood pressure.

Normally the body can maintain blood pressure and perfusion despite rapid changes from one position to another. However, in hypovolemia the body is already in a state of compensation so it becomes more difficult to maintain the pulse rate and blood pressure as someone moves from a supine to a seated or a standing position. If hypovolemic compensation exists, this movement will cause an increase in pulse rate and a drop in systolic blood pressure (usually by 20 points or more).

12. Define and differentiate between compensated and decompensated hemorrhagic shock.   pp. 661–662

- **Compensated shock** is a state in which the body is effectively compensating for fluid loss, or other shock-inducing pathology, and is able to maintain blood pressure and critical organ perfusion. If the original problem is not corrected or reversed, compensated shock may progress to decompensated shock.
- **Decompensated shock** is a state in which the cardiovascular system cannot maintain critical circulation and begins to fail. Hypoxia affects the blood vessels and heart so they cannot maintain blood pressure and circulation.
- **Irreversible shock** is a state of shock in which the human system is so damaged that it cannot be resuscitated. Once this stage of shock sets in the patient will die, even if resuscitation efforts restore a pulse and blood pressure.

13. Discuss the pathophysiological changes, assessment findings, and management associated with compensated and decompensated shock.   pp. 661–670

As the body experiences a stressor that induces shock, the cardiovascular system is quick to compensate. The venous system constricts to maintain a full vascular system and preload. The heart rate increases to maintain cardiac output, and the arterioles constrict, increasing peripheral vascular resistance to maintain blood pressure (the pressure of perfusion). As these actions become significant, the patient becomes anxious and slightly tachycardic, and the skin becomes cool and pale (circulation is shunted from the skin to more vital organs). With increasing blood loss, the compensation becomes more significant, and thirst, a rapid, weak pulse, and restlessness become apparent. These signs become more apparent as greater compensation is required to maintain the blood pressure. When the body reaches the limits of its compensation and it can no longer maintain the blood pressure, BP drops precipitously, circulation all but stops, and the patient moves very quickly into irreversible shock.

Care for the shock patient includes high-flow oxygen, hemorrhage control, and fluid resuscitation to maintain vital signs when hemorrhage is controlled, with a stable blood pressure just below 100 mmHg (88 mmHg may be optimal with continuing hemorrhage), or use aggressive fluid resuscitation if the blood pressure drops below 50 mmHg.

14. Identify the need for intervention and transport of patients with compensated and decompensated shock.   pp. 662–670

The body's ability to compensate for shock is limited. While it can maintain blood pressure, the compensation is not without cost. As the arterioles constrict, they deny blood flow to some organs and themselves use energy and tire. The venous vessels tire as they constrict to reduce the volume of the vascular system. If compensation is significant or prolonged, the body may move into decompensation, especially if the hemorrhage is not controlled. Most serious internal hemorrhage can only be halted with surgical intervention, most commonly at a trauma center. In the time between our recognition of shock and arrival at the trauma center, we can help the body with its compensation by providing oxygen and fluid resuscitation.

15. Differentiate among normotensive, hypotensive, or profoundly hypotensive patients.   pp. 653–656, 659–662

A normotensive patient is one who has a systolic blood pressure of at least 100 mmHg. Hypotension is the patient with a blood pressure of less than 100 mmHg, while a blood pressure of less than 50 mmHg is considered profound hypotension. However, these figures apply to the young healthy adult and must be adjusted to the norms for the patient you are treating. (For example, a small young female may normally have a blood pressure below 100 mmHg and may not need fluid resuscitation.)

16. Describe the differences in administration of intravenous fluid in normotensive, hypotensive, or profoundly hypotensive patients.   pp. 665–667

Administration of intravenous fluids in the normotensive patient without hypovolemia permits the rapid administration of medications and may be indicated when hypovolemia is anticipated (the burn patient). In the patient who is in compensated shock and maintains a relatively normal systolic blood pressure, fluid resuscitation is indicated if hemorrhage is controlled. If the hemorrhage is internal and cannot be controlled in the field, aggressive fluid resuscitation may lead to increased internal hemorrhage and hemodilution making perfusion and clotting less effective. Generally, the administration of intravenous fluids in the normotensive patient is limited.

In the patient who is hypotensive (BP <100 mmHg), intravenous fluids are administered to maintain, not increase, the blood pressure. Here again aggressive fluid resuscitation would dilute the blood and decrease the effectiveness of perfusion and clotting. An increase in blood pressure would also likely break apart clots that are reducing the internal hemorrhage.

In the patient who is profoundly hypotensive (absent pulses and you are unable to determine a blood pressure, or it is < 50 mmHg), aggressive fluid resuscitation is indicated. Here the consequences of severe hypoperfusion outweigh the risks of further hemorrhage.

17. Discuss the physiologic changes associated with application and inflation of the pneumatic anti-shock garment (PASG).   pp. 667–668, 669

The pneumatic anti-shock garment (PASG) is an air bladder that circumferentially applies pressure to the lower extremities and abdomen. In theory, it compresses the venous blood vessels, returning some blood to the critical circulation, and compresses the arteries, increasing peripheral vascular resistance. These actions increase circulating blood volume and blood pressure, which should help the patient in shock. However, in some cases of shock, this may increase the rate of internal hemorrhage and may disrupt the clotting mechanisms that are restricting blood loss associated with internal injury.

18. **Discuss the indications and contraindications for the application and inflation of the PASG.** pp. 667–668

The PASG is indicated for any patient who displays internal or external hemorrhage in the lower abdomen, pelvis, or lower extremities. It is recommended for the stabilization of any pelvic fracture and may be helpful with bilateral femoral fractures with the signs and symptoms of shock.

The PASG should not be used in the patient who is experiencing pulmonary edema or has a head or penetrating chest injury. It should be used with caution on any patient who is experiencing dyspnea as it may increase intra-abdominal pressure and restrict the movement of the diaphragm. The abdominal section should not be employed if the patient is in the third trimester of pregnancy, has an abdominal evisceration, or an impaled object in the abdomen.

Prior to application of the PASG, the patient's blood pressure, pulse rate and strength, and level of consciousness should be assessed and recorded. The abdomen, lower back, and lower extremities should be visualized to ensure that no sharp debris that could harm either the patient or the garment is present.

19. **Differentiate between the management of compensated and decompensated shock.** pp. 665–667

The management for compensated shock is directed at preventing decompensated shock through patient support. The care involves hemorrhage control, high-flow/high concentrations of oxygen, fluid administration, maintenance of body temperature, body positioning, and general patient support. Once decompensation occurs, as recognized by dropping blood pressure and the lowering of the level of consciousness, aggressive fluid resuscitation and the use of PASG may be indicated. In both cases, however, the patient must be transported immediately to the emergency department.

20. **Given several preprogrammed and moulaged hemorrhage and shock patients, provide the appropriate scene size-up, initial assessment, rapid trauma or focused physical exam and history, detailed exam, and ongoing assessment, and provide appropriate patient care and transportation.** pp. 644–670

During your training as an EMT-I you will participate in many classroom practice sessions involving simulated patients. You will also spend some time in the emergency departments of local hospitals as well as in advanced-level ambulances gaining clinical experience. During these times, use your knowledge of hemorrhage and shock to help you assess and care for the simulated or real patients you attend.

CASE STUDY REVIEW

This case study presents an example of aggressive and appropriate care for a patient who, by mechanism of injury alone, is suspected of advancing into shock. It highlights both the elements of shock assessment and care.

Arriving on the scene, Dave is presented with a situation that presents with no noticeable hazards and one patient with a mechanism of injury that indicates the potential for serious internal bleeding. The overturned bulldozer trapped the patient's legs and pelvis and may have fractured the pelvis and femurs. These injuries are frequently associated with severe internal blood loss and shock.

Dave suspects, as the vehicle is lifted off Ken, internal bleeding will occur more rapidly. In preparation, he ensures good oxygenation and assesses the visible portion of the patient. He gathers a baseline set of vital signs (all of which indicate that the patient is not yet in decompensated shock), including a pulse oximeter reading. He starts two IV lines using normal saline, one infusing wide open. He places pressure infusers over the bags, just in case they are needed. The PASG is set out on the long spine board so the patient can be moved in one step to the board and immediately have the PASG applied. Dave and his fellow rescuers converse with Ken not only to calm and reassure him, but also to maintain a continuous assessment of Ken's level of consciousness and determine a patient history. Dave requests air medical service for this patient as it may reduce the patient transport time, but since

Trauma Emergencies

they do not arrive on scene when Ken is ready for transport, they move him by ground to the hospital. If it would save time, they might consider an intercept at a predesignated landing zone but must assure that the intercept results in a time savings.

As the bulldozer is removed, Ken is quickly assessed and then moved to the awaiting spine board. The pelvic, femoral, and tibial fractures suggest shock will develop quickly, so the PASG is inflated immediately, not only to stabilize the fractured pelvis and femurs but to tamponade the internal hemorrhage expected with these injuries. Both IVs are run wide open, and the patient is prepared for rapid transport.

Normally, fellow care providers would slow the IVs en route to the hospital; however, Ken is becoming restless, his pulse rate is increasing, and the oximetry reading is dropping. These signs herald the progression of shock and require continued aggressive care. The hospital is updated on the patient's condition so they can be ready with O-negative blood. Whole blood or packed red cells are required because the replacement of blood lost through hemorrhage with crystalloid dilutes the number of red blood cells and clotting factors available.

The hospital personnel are ready and waiting for the patient as the ambulance backs into the emergency department bay. The blood is hung and connected, and infusion is begun. The trauma surgeon makes his quick assessment, and the patient is en route to surgery in minutes.

If any one of a number of critical steps in the care of this patient had not been completed, this patient probably would not have survived the trip to the hospital. Dave moved quickly and decisively, performing the skills that stabilized his patient, yet omitting care that would have been provided had the patient not been critical. The EMT-I must, through experience, be quickly able to distinguish the patient who needs rapid transport and aggressive care from the patient who will best benefit from meticulous care at the scene and during transport.

CONTENT SELF-EVALUATION

MULTIPLE CHOICE

_D_ 1. Which of the following types of hemorrhage is characterized by bright red blood?
  A. capillary bleeding
  B. venous bleeding
  C. arterial bleeding
  D. both A and C
  E. both A and B

_B_ 2. Which of the following types of hemorrhage is characterized by dark red blood?
  A. capillary bleeding
  B. venous bleeding
  C. arterial bleeding
  D. both A and C
  E. none of the above

_A_ 3. Which of the following is NOT a stage in the clotting process?
  A. intrinsic phase
  B. vascular phase
  C. platelet phase
  D. coagulation phase
  E. All of the above are phases in the clotting process.

_D_ 4. Which of the following represents the phase of clotting where blood cells are trapped in fibrin strands?
  A. intrinsic phase
  B. vascular phase
  C. platelet phase
  D. coagulation phase
  E. marrow phase

_D_ 5. The clotting process normally takes about what length of time?
  A. 1 to 2 minutes
  B. 3 to 4 minutes
  C. 4 to 6 minutes
  D. 7 to 10 minutes
  E. 10 to 12 minutes

©2004 Pearson Education, Inc.
Intermediate Emergency Care: Principles & Practice

_B_ 6. Cleanly and transversely cut blood vessels tend to bleed very heavily.
  A. True
  B. False

_E_ 7. Which of the following is likely to adversely affect the clotting process?
  A. aggressive fluid resuscitation   D. drugs such as aspirin
  B. hypothermia   E. all of the above
  C. movement at the site of injury

_A_ 8. Bleeding from capillary or venous wounds is easy to halt because the pressure driving the hemorrhage is limited.
  A. True
  B. False

_B_ 9. Fractures of the femur can account for a blood loss:
  A. from 500 to 750 mL.   D. less than 500 mL.
  B. up to 1,500 mL.   E. in excess of 2,500 mL.
  C. in excess of 2,000 mL.

_D_ 10. In which stage of hemorrhage does the patient first display ineffective respiration?
  A. the first stage   D. the fourth stage
  B. the second stage   E. the terminal stage
  C. the third stage

_A_ 11. The intravascular fluid accounts for what percentage of the total body water?
  A. 7 percent   D. 45 percent
  B. 15 percent   E. 75 percent
  C. 35 percent

_B_ 12 In which stage of hemorrhage does the patient first display thirst?
  A. the first stage   D. the fourth stage
  B. the second stage   E. none of the above
  C. the third stage

_C_ 13. In which stage of hemorrhage does the patient first display air-hunger?
  A. the first stage   D. the fourth stage
  B. the second stage   E. none of the above
  C. the third stage

_E_ 14. Which of the following react differently to blood loss than the normal, healthy adult?
  A. pregnant women   D. children
  B. athletes   E. all of the above
  C. the elderly

_D_ 15. The late pregnancy female is likely to have a blood volume:
  A. much less than normal.
  B. slightly less than normal.
  C. slightly greater than normal.
  D. much greater than normal.
  E. that is normal and does not change with pregnancy.

_A_ 16. Obese patients are likely to have a blood volume:
  A. much less than normal.   D. much greater than normal.
  B. slightly less than normal.   E. none of the above
  C. slightly greater than normal.

_A_ 17. The risk of transmitting disease to your trauma patient is probably much greater than the risk of obtaining a disease from him.
  A. True
  B. False

Trauma Emergencies

_A_ 18. The sooner the signs and symptoms of shock appear in your patient, the greater the hemorrhage rate and the likelihood that the patient will move into the later stages of shock.
   A. True
   B. False

_C_ 19. Fractures of the pelvis can account for a blood loss:
   A. from 500 to 750 mL.
   B. up to 1,500 mL.
   C. in excess of 2,000 mL.
   D. up to 500 mL.
   E. of none because the pelvis does not bleed.

_B_ 20. A black, tarry stool is called:
   A. hemoptysis.
   B. melena.
   C. hematuria.
   D. hematochezia.
   E. ebony stool.

_E_ 21. A positive tilt test demonstrating orthostatic hypotension is positive when:
   A. the blood pressure rises by at least 20 mmHg.
   B. the blood pressure falls by at least 20 mmHg.
   C. the pulse rate rises by at least 20 beats per minute.
   D. the pulse rate falls by at least 20 beats per minute.
   E. both B and C

_E_ 22. For the patient in compensated shock, you should perform an ongoing assessment:
   A. every five minutes.
   B. every fifteen minutes.
   C. after every major intervention.
   D. after noting any change in signs or symptoms.
   E. all except B

_E_ 23. Which of the following is a technique used to help control hemorrhage?
   A. direct pressure
   B. elevation
   C. pressure points
   D. limb splinting
   E. all of the above

_D_ 24. When applying a tourniquet, you should inflate the cuff:
   A. until the bleeding slows.
   B. to the diastolic blood pressure.
   C. to the systolic blood pressure.
   D. to 30 mmHg above the systolic blood pressure.
   E. none of the above

_B_ 25. Which of the following is NOT a pulse pressure point?
   A. the brachial artery
   B. the carotid artery
   C. the femoral artery
   D. the popliteal artery
   E. the radial artery

_B_ 26. The column of coagulated erythrocytes caused by capillary stagnation is called:
   A. ischemia.
   B. rouleaux.
   C. capillary washout.
   D. hydrostatic reflux.
   E. compensated reflux.

_B_ 27. Which list places the stages of shock in the order of their occurrence.
   A. irreversible, decompensated, compensated
   B. compensated, decompensated, irreversible
   C. compensated, irreversible, decompensated
   D. decompensated, irreversible, compensated
   E. decompensated, compensated, irreversible

©2004 Pearson Education, Inc.
Intermediate Emergency Care: Principles & Practice

_B_ 28. Which stage of shock ends with a precipitous drop in blood pressure?
A. compensatory
B. decompensatory
C. irreversible
D. hypovolemic
E. none of the above

_C_ 29. Which of the following does NOT occur during the compensated stage of shock?
A. increasing pulse rate
B. decreasing pulse strength
C. decreasing systolic blood pressure
D. skin becomes cool and clammy
E. the patient experiences thirst and weakness

_B_ 30. Once the patient becomes profoundly unconscious and loses his vital signs, he moves into irreversible shock.
A. True
B. False

_E_ 31. Which of the following suggests shock?
A. a pulse rate above 100 in the adult
B. a pulse rate above 140 in the school-age child
C. a pulse rate above 160 in the preschooler
D. a pulse rate above 180 in the infant
E. all of the above

_D_ 32. When using a pulse oximeter, you should use oxygen and ventilation to keep the reading above which oxygen saturation value?
A. 45 percent
B. 80 percent
C. 85 percent
D. 95 percent
E. 99 percent

_A_ 33. The color, temperature, and general appearance of the skin can indicate shock before there are changes in the blood pressure.
A. True
B. False

_B_ 34. During assessment you note that the patient's lower extremities and lower abdomen are warm and pink while the upper extremities, thorax, and upper abdomen are cool and clammy. This presentation is consistent with which type of shock?
A. hypovolemic
B. neurogenic
C. obstructive
D. cardiogenic
E. respiratory

_E_ 35. Which of the following may be an indication to employ overdrive respiration?
A. severe rib fractures
B. flail chest
C. diaphragmatic respirations
D. head injury
E. all of the above

_C_ 36. Which of these fluid replacement choices would be most desirable for the patient who is losing blood through internal bleeding?
A. packed red blood cells
B. fresh frozen plasma
C. whole blood
D. colloids
E. crystalloids

_E_ 37. Most of the solutions used in prehospital care for infusion are:
A. hypotonic colloids.
B. isotonic colloids.
C. hypertonic colloids.
D. hypotonic crystalloids.
E. isotonic crystalloids.

Trauma Emergencies

_B_ 38. Which of the following characteristics of a catheter will ensure that fluids run rapidly through it?
   A. short length, small lumen
   B. short length, large lumen
   C. long length, small lumen
   D. long length, large lumen
   E. large lumen and either long or short length

_E_ 39. In the patient that has internal bleeding and hypovolemia, the objective blood pressure to maintain by PASG and fluid infusions is:
   A. 120 mmHg.   D. below 50 mmHg.
   B. 100 mmHg.   E. at a steady level.
   C. 50 mmHg.

_A_ 40. The PASG may return what volume of blood to the central circulation?
   A. 250 mL   D. 1,000 mL
   B. 500 mL   E. none at all
   C. 750 mL

SPECIAL PROJECT

Drip Math Worksheet 2

Formulas
Rate = Volume/Time   mL/min = gtts per min/gtts per mL
Volume = Rate × Time   gtts/min = mL per min × gtts per mL
Time = Volume/Rate   mL = gtts/gtts per mL

Please complete the following drug and drip math problems:

1. Upon arriving at the emergency department the physician asks how much fluid you infused into your trauma patient. Your on-scene and transport time was 35 minutes, and you ran normal saline at a rate of 120 gtts/minute through a 10 gtts/mL administration set. What would you report?

2. Protocol calls for a drug to be hung and administered by drip at 45 gtts per minute based upon a 60 gtts/mL administration set. You find that the set you have administers 45 gtts/mL. How many drops per second should you set your chamber for?

3. The transferring physician requests that you infuse 100 mL of a drug during your transport. Anticipated transport time is 1 hour and 55 minutes. At what rate would you set a 60 gtts/mL administration set?

©2004 Pearson Education, Inc.
Intermediate Emergency Care: Principles & Practice

4. You are allowed to administer a drug by IV drip at a rate of between 45 and 100 mL per hour. What drip rate range can you use with a

60 gtts/mL set?

45 gtts/mL set?

10 gtts/mL set?

5. After a call, you can't remember at what rate you ran a fluid. You do know that 350 mL are left in the 500 mL bag and that the IV was running for 1 hour and 5 minutes. What would you record?

CHAPTER 16
*
Burns

Review of Chapter Objectives

After reading this chapter, you should be able to:

1. **Describe the anatomy and physiology of the skin and remaining human anatomy as they pertain to thermal burn injuries.** (see Chapter 2)

   The skin or integumentary system is the largest organ of the body and consists of three layers, the epidermis, the dermis, and the subcutaneous layer. It functions as the outer barrier of the body and protects it against environmental extremes and pathogens. The outer-most layer is the epidermis, a layer of dead or dying cells that provides a barrier to fluid loss, absorption, and the entrance of pathogens. The dermis is the true skin. It houses the sensory nerve endings, many of the specialized skin cells that produce sweat, oil, etc., and the upper-level capillary beds that allow for the conduction of heat to the body's surface. The subcutaneous layer, although not a true part of the skin, works in concert with the skin to insulate the body from heat loss and the effects of trauma.

2. **Describe the epidemiology, including incidence, mortality/morbidity, and risk factors for thermal burn injuries as well as strategies to prevent such injuries.** pp. 672–673

   The incidence of burn injury has been declining over the past few decades but still accounts for over 1 million burn injuries and over 50,000 hospitalizations each year. Those at greatest risk are the very young, the elderly, the infirm, and those exposed to occupational risk (firefighters, chemical workers, etc.). Burns are the second leading cause of death for children under 12 and the fourth leading cause of trauma death.

   Much of the decline in burn injury and death is attributable to better building codes, improved construction techniques, and the use of smoke detectors. Educational programs that teach children not to play with matches or lighters and that instruct the family to turn the water heater down to below 130°F have also helped reduce burn morbidity and mortality.

3. **Describe the local and systemic complications of a thermal burn injury.** pp. 673–676, 684–686

   Thermal burn injury results as the rate of molecular movement in a cell increases, causing the cell membranes and proteins to denature. This causes a progressive injury as the heat penetrates deeper and deeper through the skin and into the body's interior. At the local level, the injury disrupts the envelope of the body, permitting fluid to leak from the capillaries into the tissue and evaporate, resulting in dehydration and cooling. Serious circumferential burns may form an eschar and constrict, restricting ventilation or circulation to a distal extremity.

   The systemic effects of serious burns include severe dehydration and infection. Fluid is drawn to the injured tissue as it becomes edematous and then may evaporate in great quantities as the skin loses its ability to contain fluids. Infection can be massive and can quickly and easily overwhelm the body's immune system. The products of cell destruction from the burn process may enter the bloodstream and damage the tubules of the kidneys, resulting in failure. Organ failure

©2004 Pearson Education, Inc.
Intermediate Emergency Care: Principles & Practice

due to burn byproducts may also affect the liver and the heart's electrical system. Lastly, the burn injury and the associated evaporation of fluid may cool the body more rapidly than it can create heat. The result is a lowering of body temperature, hypothermia.

4. Identify and describe the depth classifications of burn injuries, including superficial burns, partial-thickness burns, and full-thickness burns.   pp. 681–682

- **Superficial (first-degree) burns** involve only the upper layers of the epidermis and dermis. The effects are limited to an irritation of the upper sensory tissues with some pain, minor edema, and erythema.
- **Partial-thickness (second-degree) burns** penetrate slightly deeper than first-degree burns and cause blistering, erythema, swelling, and pain. Since the cells that reproduce the skin's upper layers are still alive, complete regeneration is expected.
- **Full-thickness (third-degree) burns** penetrate the entire dermis, causing extensive destruction. The burned area may display a variety of appearances and colors, the site is anesthetic, and healing is prolonged. Third-degree burns may involve not only the skin, but also underlying tissues and organs. (Organ and other tissue involvement is sometimes called fourth-degree burn.)

5. Describe and apply the "rule of nines," and the "rule of palms" methods for determining body surface area percentage of a burn injury.   pp. 682–683

The "rule of nines" approximates the body surface area burned by assigning each body region nine percent of the total. These regions include: each upper extremity, the anterior of each lower extremity, the posterior of each lower extremity, the anterior of the abdomen, the anterior thorax, the upper back, the lower back, and the entire head and neck. The remaining one percent is assigned to the genitalia. For children, the head is given 18 percent, and the lower extremities are assigned $13^{1}/2$ percent.

    The "rule of palms" method of approximating burn surface area assumes the victim's palm surface is equivalent to one percent of the total body surface area. The care provider then estimates the burn surface area by determining the number of palmar surfaces it would take to cover the wound.

6. Identify and describe the severity of a burn including a minor burn, a moderate burn, and a critical burn.   pp. 688–691

- **Minor burns** are those that are superficial and cover less than 50 percent of the body surface area (BSA), partial-thickness burns covering less than 15 percent of the BSA, or full-thickness burns involving less than two percent of the body surface area.
- **Moderate burns** are classified as superficial burns over more than 50 percent of the BSA, partial-thickness burns covering less then 30 percent of the BSA, or full-thickness burns covering less than 10 percent of the BSA.
- **Critical burns** are those partial-thickness burns covering more than 30 percent of the BSA, full-thickness burns over 10 percent of the BSA, and any significant inhalation injury. Critical burns also include any burns that involve any partial or full-thickness burn to the hands, feet, genitalia, joints, or face.

7. Describe the effects age and pre-existing conditions have on burn severity and a patient's prognosis.   pp. 685, 690

Burn patients who are very young, very old, or have a significant pre-existing disease are at increased risk for the systemic problems associated with burn injury. They cannot tolerate massive fluid losses often associated with burns because they have smaller fluid reserves and they cannot effectively fight the ensuing massive infection commonly associated with large burns. They should be considered one step closer to critical than consideration of their burn type and BSA would normally place them.

8. **Discuss complications of burn injuries caused by trauma, blast injuries, airway compromise, respiratory compromise, and child abuse.** pp. 680–681, 685–691

Traumatic injury, in the presence of burn injury, is a complicating factor that interferes with the burn healing process and may exacerbate hypovolemia. Any time these injuries coexist, the patient should be considered a higher priority than either injury would suggest, and the paramedic must care for both conditions.

Blast mechanisms produce injury through thermal burns, the pressure wave, projectile impact, and structural collapse (crush) mechanisms. When burns coexist with these other injuries, the patient priority for care and transport must be elevated at least one priority level and all injuries must be cared for. Again, the patient will have to heal from multiple injuries, making the recovery process more difficult.

Airway and respiratory compromise associated with burn injury is an extremely serious complication. The airway must be secured early, possibly with rapid sequence intubation, and adequate ventilation with supplemental oxygen ensured. Swelling of the upper or lower airway may rapidly occlude it, preventing both ventilation and intubation. Also be watchful for carbon monoxide poisoning as it can reduce the effectiveness of oxygen transport without overt signs.

Burns associated with child abuse often result from scalding water immersion, open flame burns, or cigarette-type injuries. The child presents with a history of a burn that does not make sense, such as stove burns when he or she cannot yet reach the stove, multiple circular burns (cigarettes), or burns isolated to the buttocks, which occur as the child lifts his or her legs during attempts at immersion in hot water.

9. **Describe burn management including considerations for airway and ventilation, circulation, pharmacological and nonpharmacological measures, transport decisions, and psychological support/communication strategies.** pp. 691–694

The management of the burn patient is a rather complicated, multifaceted process. The first consideration is to extinguish the fire to ensure the burn does not continue. If necessary, use water from a low-pressure hose and remove all jewelry, leather, nylon, or other material that may continue to smolder or hold heat and continue to burn the patient. Also consider removing any restrictive jewelry or clothing, as such an item may act as tourniquet, restricting distal blood flow as the burn region swells.

Then assess and ensure that the airway remains adequate. With any history suggestive of an inhalation burn or injury, carefully assess and monitor the airway for any signs of restriction. If they are found, move to protect the airway with rapid sequence intubation early, before the progressive airway swelling prevents intubation or significantly restricts the size of the endotracheal tube you can introduce. Small and painful burns may be covered with wet dressings to occlude airflow and reduce the pain; however, any extensive burn should be covered with a sterile dry dressing to prevent body cooling and the introduction of pathogens through the dressing.

Resuscitation for extensive burns must include large volumes of prehospital fluid (0.5 mL/kg × BSA) as burns often account for massive fluid loss into and through the burn. The patient must also be kept warm because by their nature burns account for rapid heat loss.

Any burns on opposing tissue, such as between the fingers and toes, should be separated by nonadherent dressings, as the burned surfaces are likely to adhere firmly together and cause further damage as they are pulled apart. In painful burns consider morphine, in 2 mg increments, for pain relief as long as there is no evidence of hypotension or respiratory depression.

Watch for any constriction from eschar formation that may reduce or halt distal circulation or restrict respiration. Medical direction may request a surgical incision to relieve the pressure (an escharotomy).

Any burn patient with serious injury should be transported to the burn center where he or she can receive the specialized treatment needed. Also ensure that the burn patient receives therapeutic communication while you are at the scene and during transport. The burn injury is very painful and the appearance can be very frightening. Constantly talk with the patient. Try to distract him or her from the injury, and monitor level of consciousness and anxiety level throughout your care and transport.

©2004 Pearson Education, Inc.
Intermediate Emergency Care: Principles & Practice

10. **Describe special considerations for a pediatric patient with a burn injury and describe the criteria for determining pediatric burn severity.** pp. 683, 685, 690

To determine the severity of a burn for a pediatric patient, you must first examine the depth of burn (superficial, partial, or full thickness) and then determine the BSA affected. With children the head is given a greater percentage of BSA (18%) and the legs are given less (13 1/2%). (Please note that there are several more specific methods to determine BSA for children that better take into account their changing anatomy, but they are more complicated and age- and size-specific and harder to use.) Once the BSA and depth of burn are determined, the pediatric patient is assigned a level of severity one place higher than that for the adult. Any serious burn to the airway, face, joint, hand, foot, or any circumferential burn is considered serious or critical as is the pediatric burn patient with another pre-existing disease or traumatic injury.

11. **Describe the specific epidemiologies, mechanisms of injury, pathophysiologies, and severity assessments for inhalation, chemical, and electrical burn injuries and for radiation exposure.** pp. 694–700

- **Inhalation injuries** are commonly associated with burn injuries and endanger the airway. They are caused by the inhalation of hot air or flame, which cause limited damage, by superheated steam, which results in much more significant thermal damage, or by the inhalation of toxic products of combustion, which results in chemical burns. Inhalation injury can also involve carbon monoxide poisoning and the absorption of chemicals through the alveoli and systemic poisoning. Any sign of respiratory involvement during the burn assessment process is reason to consider early and aggressive airway care and rapid transport.
- **Chemical burn injury** is most frequently found in the industrial setting and is frequently associated with the effects of strong acids or alkalis. Both mechanisms destroy cell membranes as they penetrate deeper and deeper. The nature of the wounding process is somewhat self-limiting, though alkali burns tend to penetrate more deeply. Any chemical burn that disrupts the skin should be considered serious.
- **Electrical burn injuries** are infrequent but can be very serious. As electricity passes through body tissue, resistance creates heat energy and damage to the cell membranes. The blood vessels and nerve pathways are especially sensitive to electrical injury. The heat produced can be extremely high and cause severe and deeply internal burn injury, depending upon the voltage and current levels involved. Any electrical burn that causes external injury or any passage of significant electrical current through the body is reason to consider the patient a high priority for transport, even if no overt signs of injury exist. Electrical injury can also affect the muscles of respiration and induce hypoxia or anoxia if the current remains. Electrical disturbances can also affect the heart, producing dysrhythmias. A special electrical injury is the lightning strike. Extremely high voltage can cause extensive internal injury, though often the current passes over the exterior of the body, resulting in limited damage. Resuscitation of the patient struck by lightning should be prolonged as this mechanism of injury may permit survival after lengthy resuscitation.
- **Radiation exposure** is a relatively rare injury process caused by the passage of radiation energy through body cells. The radiation changes the structure of molecules and may cause cells to die, dysfunction, or reproduce dysfunctional cells. Radiation hazards cannot be seen, heard, or felt, yet they can cause both immediate and long-term health problems and death. The objective of rescue and care is to limit the exposure for both the patient and rescuer. Radiation exposure is cumulative. The less time in an area of hazard, the less effect radiation will have on the human body. The greater the distance from a radiation source, the less strength and potential it has to cause damage. Radiation levels are diminished as the particles travel through dense objects. By placing more mass between the source and patient and rescuers, the exposure is reduced. Since it is very difficult to determine the extent of exposure, gather what information you can and transport the patient for further evaluation.

12. **Discuss special considerations that impact the assessment, management, and prognosis of patients with inhalation, chemical, and electrical burn injuries and with exposure to radiation.** pp. 694–700

When assessing an inhalation injury, you should examine the mechanism of injury to identify any unconsciousness or confinement during fire or any history of explosive stream expansion and inhalation. Study the patient carefully for signs of facial burns, carbonaceous sputum, or any hoarseness. Should there be any reason to suspect inhalation injury, monitor the airway very carefully and consider oxygen therapy and early intubation as needed. The airway tissues can swell quickly and result in serious airway restriction or complete obstruction.

Chemical burn injury is indicated by the signs or history of such exposure and should begin with an identification of the agent and type of exposure. Remove contaminated clothing and dispose of it properly. The site of exposure should be irrigated with copious amounts of cool water and, once the chemical is completely removed, covered with a dry sterile dressing. Special consideration should be given to contact with phenol (soluble in alcohol), dry lime (brush off before irrigation), sodium metal (cover with oil to prevent combustion), and riot control agents (emotional support). The prognosis for a serious chemical burn is related to the agent, length of exposure to it, and depth of damage. These injuries are often severe and will leave damaged or scar tissue behind.

With an electrical burn injury, direct your assessment to seeking out and examining entrance and exit wounds and to trying to determine the voltage and current of the source. The wounds should be covered with dry sterile dressings and the patient monitored for dysrhythmias. Even if the entrance and exit wounds seem minor, consider this patient for rapid transport as the internal injury may be extensive.

Radiation is invisible and otherwise undetectable by human senses. When radiation exposure is suspected, ensure that you and the patient remain as remote from the source (distance) with as much matter as possible between you and the source (shielding) and that you spend as little time close to the source as possible. Attention to these factors will reduce the amount of radiologic exposure for both you and the patient. Assessment of the patient exposed to a radiation source is very difficult because the signs of injury are delayed except in cases of extreme exposure. Any suggestion of exposure to radiation merits examination at the emergency department and assessment of the risk by specially trained experts in the field. Limited radiation exposure does not often result in medical problems, but more severe doses may cause sterility or, later in life, cancer. Extensive exposure may cause severe illness or death.

13. **Differentiate between supraglottic and infraglottic inhalation burn injuries.** p. 681

A **supraglottic inhalation burn** is a thermal injury to the mucosa above the glottic opening. It is a significant burn because the tissue is very vascular and will swell very quickly and extensively. Because of the moist environment and the vascular nature of the tissue, it takes great heat energy to cause burn injury. When such injury occurs, however, the associated swelling can quickly threaten the airway.

Infraglottic (or subglottic) inhalation burns occur much less frequently because the moist supraglottic tissue absorbs the heat energy and the glottis will likely close to prevent the injury from penetrating more deeply. However, superheated steam, as is produced when a stream of water hits a particularly hot portion of a fire, has the heat energy to carry the burning process to the subglottic region. There, airway burns are extremely critical, as even slight tissue swelling will restrict the airway.

Special consideration should also be given to the toxic nature of the hot gasses inhaled during the inhalation burn. Modern construction materials and the widespread use of synthetics are products that release toxic agents when they burn (cyanide, arsenic, hydrogen sulfide, and others). Often these agents will combine with the moisture of the airway and form caustic compounds that induce chemical burns of the airway, or they may be absorbed into the bloodstream, causing systemic poisoning. The risk for inhalation injury increases with a history of unconsciousness or with being within a confined space during a fire.

©2004 Pearson Education, Inc.
Intermediate Emergency Care: Principles & Practice

14. **Describe the special considerations for a chemical burn injury to the eye.** pp. 696–698

Chemicals introduced onto the surface of the eye threaten to damage the delicate corneal surface. It is imperative that you consider these injuries when chemicals are splashed and that the eye is irrigated for up to 20 minutes. Irrigation may be accomplished by running normal saline through an administration set into the corner of the eye and directed away from the other eye if it is not affected. If both eyes are involved, a nasal cannula may be helpful in directing fluid flow to both eyes simultaneously. Be alert for contact lenses, as they may trap chemicals under their surface and prevent effective irrigation.

15. **Given several preprogrammed, simulated thermal, inhalation, electrical, and chemical burn injury and radiation exposure patients, provide the appropriate scene size-up, initial assessment, rapid trauma or focused physical exam and history, detailed exam, and ongoing assessment, and provide appropriate patient care and transportation.** pp. 673–700

During your training as an EMT-I you will participate in many classroom practice sessions involving simulated patients. You will also spend some time in the emergency departments of local hospitals as well as in advanced-level ambulances gaining clinical experience. During these times, use your knowledge of burn trauma to help you assess and care for the simulated or real patients you attend.

CASE STUDY REVIEW

The scenario presented in this case study illustrates the dangers associated with the fire-ground and with inhalation injuries. It also identifies the difficulty you might have in recognizing respiratory injury and the importance of treating it early.

The scene observed by Ben and Ronny demonstrates the dangers associated with a working fire and a real-time assessment of the mechanism of injury. As Fire Rescue EMT-Is, they are wearing turnout gear, boots, and heavy gloves as they approach the injured firefighter. They ensure that the scene is safe and recognize that hazards can include debris, still energized electrical lines, leaking gas, further structural collapse, and much more. They will work quickly to move their fellow firefighter to a safe location and continue care. Once at a safe location, Ben and Ronny remove the firefighter's clothing as they begin their initial assessment. They replace their work gloves with sterile latex or plastic ones because they well know that infection is a common and serious consequence of the types of burns this patient received. They will do all they can to protect the wounds from further contamination by quickly covering them with dry sterile dressings.

The firefighter they assess in this incident experiences the classic evolution of the burn and inhalation injury. He was initially found to be stable with signs, symptoms, and vital signs suggestive of minor injury. The major concern for this patient might well be the fractured forearm. However, the EMT-Is are wary because of the significant area burned and the patient's history, hoarseness, and the sooty sputum. They anticipate serious fluid loss through the burn and infection risk as well as airway injury that will likely worsen during their care.

Ben must be careful regarding any articles of clothing or jewelry that could continue to burn or contain the swelling that often accompanies burn injury. His initial action should be to stop any further burning. This calls for complete inspection of the burn area and the surrounding clothing. Once the burn area is exposed, the depth and area involved can be assessed. In this case, the patient has a fracture, possible inhalation injury, and a serious burn. The area burned, the posterior chest and abdomen and the upper left extremity, represent a body surface area of about 22½ percent. The combination of traumatic injury, burn, and inhalation injury are reasons to consider the patient to have critical injuries.

The EMT-Is initiate an IV with a large-bore catheter and begin running normal saline. A 1,000 mL bag is hung with a non-flow-restrictive (trauma or blood tubing) administration set just in case the signs of shock appear. Fluids are run rapidly to get ahead of the loss normally associated with severe burns. If this were a 125 kg man with the burns identified (22½% by the rule of nines), the

Trauma Emergencies

needed fluid would be 4 mL × 22½ (percent of burn area) × 125 kg or a total of 11,250 mL in the first 24 hours (Parkland formula). Half of this is needed in the first 8 hours. That's more than 700 mL per hour.

The signs of respiratory involvement, though subtle, are even more significant than the burn or fracture. Inhalation injury is likely due either to the chemical burning caused by the products of combustion reacting with the soft tissue of the respiratory tract or to thermal burns caused by superheated steam created when the water extinguished the flames. In either case, respiratory damage can be extensive. Patients with respiratory burns usually display progressive dyspnea, as in this case. The only effective way to treat this problem is to anticipate that progression and be aggressive in airway care. Intubation equipment should be readied and used when any sign of developing airway compromise appears. Ken should also be considered for immediate transport because of the difficulty in managing the airway.

Ben and Ronny must also be prepared for the worst. If the firefighter had experienced severe dyspnea and airway restriction while 20 to 30 minutes from the hospital, a needle or surgical cricothyrotomy might have been necessary. Likewise, had they waited on the scene to splint, bandage, and care for the patient, the time spent on those tasks would have permitted the airway and patient to deteriorate. This case study clearly identifies the need for rapid recognition and transport of the patient with developing airway compromise.

CONTENT SELF-EVALUATION

MULTIPLE CHOICE

_____ 1. The incidence of burn injury has been on the decline over the past decade.
   A. True
   B. False

_____ 2. A preventative action that will reduce the incidence of scalding injuries is:
   A. use of child-proof faucets.
   B. education of children on the dangers of hot water.
   C. placing caution stickers on water faucets.
   D. lowering the water heater temperature to 130°F.
   E. none of the above

_____ 3. Burns result from the disruption of the proteins found in cell membranes.
   A. True
   B. False

_____ 4. The area of a burn that suffers the most damage is generally the:
   A. the zone of hyperemia.   D. the zone of coagulation.
   B. the zone of denaturing.   E. the zone of most resistance.
   C. the zone of stasis.

_____ 5. The theory of burns that explains the burning process is:
   A. the thermal hypothesis.
   B. Jackson's theory of thermal wounds.
   C. the Phaseal discussion of burns.
   D. the Hypermetabolism dynamic.
   E. none of the above

_____ 6. The order in which the phases of the body's response to a burn would normally be expected to occur is:
   A. emergent, fluid shift, hypermetabolic
   B. fluid shift, hypermetabolic, emergent
   C. fluid shift, emergent, hypermetabolic
   D. hypermetabolic, fluid shift, emergent
   E. emergent, hypermetabolic, fluid shift

_____ 7. Which of the following skin types has the greatest resistance to the passage of electrical current?
  A. mucous membranes
  B. wet skin
  C. calluses
  D. the skin on the inside of the arm
  E. the skin on the inside of the thigh

_____ 8. Electrical injury is likely to cause which of the following?
  A. serious injury where the electricity enters the body
  B. serious injury where the electricity exits the body
  C. damage to nerves
  D. damage to blood vessels
  E. all of the above

_____ 9. Prolonged contact with alternating current may result in respiratory paralysis.
  A. True
  B. False

_____ 10. Chemical burns involving strong alkalis are likely to be deep due to coagulation necrosis.
  A. True
  B. False

_____ 11. Burns due to strong acids are likely to be less deep than burns due to strong alkalis because they produce liquefaction necrosis.
  A. True
  B. False

_____ 12. Which of the following radiation types is least powerful?
  A. neutron
  B. alpha
  C. gamma
  D. beta
  E. delta

_____ 13. Which of the following radiation types is the most powerful type of ionizing radiation?
  A. lambda
  B. alpha
  C. gamma
  D. beta
  E. delta

_____ 14. Which of the following is a type of radiation present only inside nuclear reactors and bombs?
  A. neutron
  B. alpha
  C. gamma
  D. beta
  E. delta

_____ 15. To protect themselves from radiation exposure, EMS personnel should:
  A. limit the duration of exposure.
  B. increase the shielding from exposure.
  C. increase the distance from the source.
  D. ensure that the patient is decontaminated.
  E. all of the above

_____ 16. The radiation dose that is lethal to about 50 percent of those exposed is:
  A. 0.2 Gray.
  B. 100 rads.
  C. 1 Gray.
  D. 4.5 Grays.
  E. 200 rads.

_____ 17. As radiation exposure increases, the signs of exposure become less evident and only reappear later in the course of the disease.
  A. True
  B. False

Trauma Emergencies

18. Which of the following is commonly associated with inhalation injury?
    A. carbon monoxide poisoning
    B. toxic inhalation
    C. supraglottic injury
    D. subglottic injury
    E. all of the above

19. Which type of circumstance is most likely to cause subglottic thermal burn injury?
    A. inhalation of hot air
    B. inhalation of flame
    C. inhalation of superheated steam
    D. standing in a burn environment
    E. inhalation of toxic substances

20. What percentage of burn patients who die have associated airway burn injury?
    A. 20 percent
    B. 35 percent
    C. 50 percent
    D. 60 percent
    E. 80 percent

21. The burn characterized by erythema, pain, and blistering is the:
    A. superficial burn.
    B. partial-thickness burn.
    C. full-thickness burn.
    D. electrical burn.
    E. chemical burn.

22. The burn characterized by discoloration and lack of pain is the:
    A. superficial burn.
    B. partial-thickness burn.
    C. full-thickness burn.
    D. electrical burn.
    E. chemical burn.

23. An adult has received burns to the entire anterior chest and to the entire left upper extremity, circumferentially. Using the rule of nines, the percentage of body surface (BSA) area involved is:
    A. 9 percent.
    B. 18 percent.
    C. 27 percent.
    D. 36 percent.
    E. 48 percent.

24. A child has received burns to the entire left lower extremity and the genitals. Using the rule of nines, the percentage of the body surface area involved is:
    A. 9 percent.
    B. 10 percent.
    C. 14¹/2 percent.
    D. 19 percent.
    E. 21¹/2 percent.

25. An adult has received burns to the entire left lower extremity and the genitals. Using the rule of nines, the percentage of the body surface area involved is:
    A. 9 percent.
    B. 10 percent.
    C. 18 percent.
    D. 19 percent.
    E. 21 percent.

26. A child receives burns to his entire head and neck and upper back. What percentage of body surface area is involved?
    A. 9 percent
    B. 10 percent
    C. 18 percent
    D. 19 percent
    E. 27 percent

27. Which of the following systemic complications should you suspect with all serious burns?
    A. hypothermia
    B. hypovolemia
    C. infection
    D. eschar formation
    E. all of the above

28. Which of the following conditions would increase the impact a burn has on a patient?
    A. being very young
    B. being very old
    C. having the flu
    D. emphysema
    E. all of the above

©2004 Pearson Education, Inc.
Intermediate Emergency Care: Principles & Practice

_____ 29. Which of the following should NOT be removed from any burned area of a patient?
   A. nylon clothing such as a windbreaker
   B. small pieces of burned fabric lodged in the wound
   C. shoes and socks
   D. rings, watches, and other articles of jewelry
   E. leather belts

_____ 30. When considering intubation of the patient with suspected airway injury due to inhalation of the byproducts of combustion, you should have a supply of several smaller than normal endotracheal tubes ready.
   A. True
   B. False

_____ 31. Severe inhalation injury due to airway burns may be so extensive as to induce complete respiratory obstruction and arrest.
   A. True
   B. False

_____ 32. High-flow oxygen therapy is very helpful in cases of carbon monoxide poisoning because it will then be carried in sufficient quantities in the plasma to maintain life.
   A. True
   B. False

_____ 33. Your assessment reveals an area of burn that is reddened, painful, and just beginning to display blisters. What burn classification would you give this burn?
   A. superficial burn   D. first degree burn
   B. partial-thickness burn   E. A or D
   C. full-thickness burn

_____ 34. The patient you are attending has her entire left upper extremity seriously burned. The forearm and hand are very painful and reddened, while the upper arm is relatively painless and a dark red color. What percentage of the BSA and burn depth would you assign this patient?
   A. 9 percent full-thickness burn
   B. 9 percent partial-thickness burn
   C. 4 1/2 percent full-thickness burn
   D. 4 1/2 percent partial-thickness burn
   E. 4 1/2 percent partial-thickness and 4 1/2 percent full-thickness burn

_____ 35. Your assessment reveals a burn patient with superficial burns to 27 percent of the body. To which classification of burn severity would you assign her?
   A. minor   D. critical
   B. moderate   E. none of the above
   C. serious

_____ 36. Your assessment reveals a burn patient with full-thickness burns to the entire left thigh and calf. What classification of burn severity would you assign him?
   A. minor   D. critical
   B. moderate   E. none of the above
   C. serious

_____ 37. Your assessment reveals a burn patient with partial-thickness burns to all of both lower extremities. What classification of burn severity would you assign her?
   A. minor   D. critical
   B. moderate   E. none of the above
   C. serious

Trauma Emergencies

_____ 38. Your assessment reveals a burn patient with partial-thickness burns to her entire lower extremities and a suspected femur fracture. What classification of burn severity would you assign her?
   A. minor
   B. moderate
   C. serious
   D. critical
   E. none of the above

_____ 39. Cool water immersion may reduce the depth and significance of small burns if applied within:
   A. 1 to 2 minutes.
   B. 2 to 4 minutes.
   C. 4 to 5 minutes.
   D. 10 minutes.
   E. 20 minutes.

_____ 40. The patient with any full-thickness burn should be considered for administration of tetanus toxoid as the wound is an open one.
   A. True
   B. False

_____ 41. In general, moderate to severe burns should be covered with:
   A. moist occlusive dressings.
   B. dry sterile dressings.
   C. cool water immersion.
   D. plastic wrap covered by a soft dressing.
   E. warm water immersion.

_____ 42. Adjacent full-thickness burns, such as those affecting the fingers and toes, should be held together without dressings to ensure rapid healing.
   A. True
   B. False

_____ 43. The Parkland formula for fluid administration calls for administration of 4 mL of fluid to a patient multiplied by the patient's BSA involved. What other factor(s) determines the total fluid administered in the first 24 hours?
   A. patient's age
   B. patient's weight
   C. depth of burns
   D. age of the patient
   E. all of the above

_____ 44. Which of the following is the preferred fluid for resuscitation of the severely burned patient?
   A. normal saline
   B. 1/2 normal saline
   C. dextrose 5 percent in water
   D. lactated Ringer's solution
   E. dextrose 5 percent in normal saline

_____ 45. Which of the following drugs may be given to the patient with severe burns in the prehospital setting?
   A. ipratropium
   B. morphine
   C. epinephrine
   D. furosemide
   E. haloperidol

_____ 46. Which of the following may be appropriate when a forming eschar is restricting distal blood flow to an extremity?
   A. elevating the extremity
   B. incising the eschar to relieve the pressure
   C. wrapping the extremity in dry sterile dressings
   D. administering morphine
   E. immersing the limb in cold water

_____ 47. A patient was found unconscious in a burning mobile home. Your assessment discovers severe dyspnea, no airway restriction, chest pain, altered mental status, and some seizure activity. What condition would you suspect?
   A. carbon monoxide poisoning
   B. cyanide poisoning
   C. chemical burns to the lungs
   D. hypoxia due to inhalation of oxygen-deprived air
   E. superheated steam inhalation

©2004 Pearson Education, Inc.
Intermediate Emergency Care: Principles & Practice

_____ **48.** If an IV line is not yet established in a patient with suspected cyanide poisoning you should administer which of the following?
  A. amyl nitrate
  B. sodium nitrate
  C. sodium thiosulfide
  D. haloperidol
  E. ipratropium

_____ **49.** In addition to the entrance and exit wounds normally expected with the passage of electrical current through the human body, the EMT-I should expect:
  A. ventricular fibrillation.
  B. cardiac irritability.
  C. internal damage.
  D. smoldering clothing.
  E. all of the above

_____ **50.** In the United States, lightning strikes hit about how many people per year?
  A. 25
  B. 50
  C. 100
  D. 300
  E. 500

_____ **51.** The patient who is unresponsive, apneic, and pulseless due to a lightning strike is not a likely candidate for successful resuscitation.
  A. True
  B. False

_____ **52.** In general, caustic chemical contamination should be cared for by:
  A. dry sterile dressings.
  B. chemical antidotes.
  C. rigorous scrubbing.
  D. cool water irrigation.
  E. rapid transport.

_____ **53.** The chemical phenol is soluble in:
  A. water.
  B. dry lime.
  C. normal saline.
  D. ammonia.
  E. none of the above

_____ **54.** Which chemical agent reacts vigorously with water?
  A. phenol
  B. bleach
  C. sodium
  D. riot control agents
  E. ammonia

_____ **55.** Known antidotes and neutralizers for chemical contamination and burns will reduce the injury caused by the agent if administered immediately.
  A. True
  B. False

_____ **56.** How long should you irrigate a patient's eye contaminated with chemicals of an unknown nature?
  A. less than 2 minutes
  B. up to 5 minutes
  C. up to 15 minutes
  D. up to 20 minutes
  E. none of the above

_____ **57.** When chemicals are splashed into the eye of the patient wearing contact lenses, the contact should be removed to ensure irrigation will remove all of the agent.
  A. True
  B. False

_____ **58.** If the source of radiation cannot be contained or moved away from the patient:
  A. the patient should be brought to you.
  B. care should be offered by you in protective gear.
  C. care should be offered by specialists in protective gear.
  D. care should be offered by the highest ranking officer.
  E. A or C

_____ 59. Which action can be used reduce rescuer exposure to a radiation source?
  A. increase the distance from the source
  B. decrease the time exposed to the source
  C. increase the shielding between the rescuer and source
  D. protect against inhalation of contaminated dust
  E. all of the above

_____ 60. Once exposed to a significant radiation source, the patient will become a source of radiation that the rescuer must then protect him- or herself against. No amount of decontamination will reduce this danger.
  A. True
  B. False

SPECIAL PROJECT

Drip Math Worksheet 3

Formulas
Rate = Volume/Time   mL/min = gtts per min/gtts per mL
Volume = Rate × Time   gtts/min = mL per min × gtts per mL
Time = Volume/Rate   mL = gtts/gtts per mL

Please complete the following drip math problems:

1. You are asked to administer a 250 mL solution to a patient over 2 hours. What drip rate would you use with a:

A. 10 gtts per mL administration set

B. 15 gtts per mL administration set

C. 60 gtts per mL administration set

2. Your protocol directs that an IV drip is to be run at 30 gtts per minute with a 60 gtts per mL administration set. How long will it take to infuse:

A. 200 ml

B. 350 ml

3. How much fluid would you administer to a patient over 15 minutes with a macrodrip (15 gtts/mL) administration set, running at 1 gtt per second?

4. Your protocol requires you to administer a drug at 15 gtts per minute with a 60 gtts per mL administration set. You only have a 45 gtts per mL set available. What drip rate would you run it at?

Trauma Emergencies

CHAPTER 17

Thoracic Trauma

Review of Chapter Objectives

After reading this chapter, you should be able to:

1. **Describe the incidence, morbidity, and mortality of thoracic injuries in the trauma patient.**   **pp. 703–704**

Chest trauma accounts for about 25 percent of vehicular mortality and is second only to head trauma as a reason for death in the auto accident. Heart and great vessel injuries are the most common cause of death from blunt trauma. Penetrating trauma to the chest also results in significant mortality with heart and great vessel injuries, again, accounting for the greatest mortality. Modern auto and highway design, the speed at which the chest trauma patient arrives at the trauma center, and newer surgical techniques have significantly reduced chest trauma mortality in the last decade.

2. **Discuss the anatomy and physiology of the organs and structures related to thoracic injuries.**   **(see Chapter 2)**

The ribs, thoracic spine, sternum, and diaphragm define the structure of the thoracic cage. The skeletal components allow the cage to expand as the ribs are lifted upward and outward by contraction of the intercostal muscles, and the intrathoracic volume further expands as the diaphragm contracts and moves downward. The net action of this muscle movement is to increase the volume of the thoracic cage and to reduce its internal pressure. Air from the environment moves through the airway into the alveoli to equalize this pressure, and inspiration occurs. The intercostal muscles relax and the thorax settles, while the diaphragm rises back into the thorax and the volume of the cavity decreases. This increases the intrathoracic pressure, and air rushes out to equalize with the environment. This is expiration. The pleura, two serous membranes, seal the lungs to the interior of the thoracic cage during this action and ensure that the lungs expand and contract with the changing volume of the thoracic cavity. The lungs have exceptional circulation, with capillary beds surrounding the alveoli to ensure a free exchange of oxygen and carbon dioxide between the alveolar air and the bloodstream.

The lungs fill all but the central portion of the chest cavity and are found on either side of the central structure, called the mediastinum. The mediastinum contains the heart, trachea, esophagus, major blood vessels, and several nerve pathways. The heart is located in the left central chest and is the major pumping element of the cardiovascular system. The inferior and superior vena cavae collect blood from the lower extremities and abdomen and the upper extremities, head, and neck, respectively, and return it to the heart. The pulmonary arteries and veins carry blood to and from the lungs respectively, and the aorta distributes the cardiac output to the systemic circulation. The trachea enters the mediastinum just beneath the manubrium and bifurcates at the carina into the left and right mainstem bronchi. The esophagus enters the mediastinum just behind the trachea and exits through the diaphragm.

©2004 Pearson Education, Inc.
Intermediate Emergency Care: Principles & Practice

3. **Discuss types of thoracic injuries and predict them based on mechanism of injury.** pp. 704–707

As in other regions of the body, thoracic trauma results from either blunt or penetrating mechanisms of injury. Blunt trauma may result from deceleration (as in an auto crash), crushing mechanism (as in a building collapse), or pressure injury (as with an explosion). Deceleration frequently causes the "paper bag" syndrome, lung and cardiac contusions, rib fractures, and vascular injuries. Crushing mechanisms may cause traumatic asphyxia and vascular damage and restrict respiratory excursion. Blast mechanisms may cause lung injuries or vascular tears.

Penetrating trauma may involve any structure within the thorax, although injury to the heart and great vessels is most likely to be lethal. Lung tissue is rather resilient and suffers limited injury with a bullet's passage, while the heart and great vessels are damaged explosively, especially if engorged with blood at the time of the bullet's impact. Slower velocity penetrating objects result in damage that is limited to the actual pathway of the object.

4. **Discuss the epidemiology, pathophysiology, assessment findings, and management—including the need for rapid intervention and transport—of the patient with chest wall injuries, including:** pp. 708–710, 729

   a. **Rib fracture**

   Blunt or penetrating trauma induces a fracture and possible associated injury underneath. The fracture itself is of only limited concern; however, the pain from an such injury may limit chest excursion and suggests more serious injury beneath. Care is directed to administering oxygen, considering the possibility of underlying injury, and supplying pain medication to ensure respirations are not limited by pain. These injuries do not by themselves require immediate intervention or transport.

   b. **Flail segment**

   A flail segment is the result of several ribs (three or more) broken in numerous (two or more) places. This creates a rib segment that is free to move independently from the rest of the thorax. This paradoxical motion greatly decreases the efficiency of respiration as air that would be exhaled moves to the region under the flail segment and then returns to the unaffected lung with inspiration. Care includes seeing that the section is stabilized, the patient is given oxygen, possibly using overdrive ventilation. Consider the flail chest patient a candidate for rapid transport. Because of the severity of forces required to compromise the chest wall with this injury and the likelihood of serious underlying injury, this patient is given a high priority for care and transport.

   c. **Sternal fracture**

   As with the flail chest patient, suspect the patient with sternal fracture of having serious internal injury. The kinetic forces necessary to fracture the sternum are likely to injure and contuse the heart and other structures of the mediastinum. The patient will have a history of blunt chest trauma and may complain of chest pain similar to that of a myocardial infarction. Administer oxygen, monitor the heart with an ECG, and watch the patient very carefully for any signs of myocardial or great vessel injury. This patient is a candidate for rapid transport.

5. **Discuss the pathophysiology, assessment findings, and management—including the need for rapid intervention and transport—of the patient with injury to the lung, including:** pp. 711–716, 728–730

   a. **Simple pneumothorax**

   A simple or closed pneumothorax is an injury caused by either blunt or penetrating trauma that opens the airway to the pleural space. Air accumulates within the space and displaces the lung, resulting in less effective respirations and reduced oxygenation of the blood. This patient has a history of trauma and progressive dyspnea. Oxygen is administered and the patient is observed for progression to tension pneumothorax.

Trauma Emergencies

b. Open pneumothorax

Open pneumothorax is like simple pneumothorax, though in this case the injury penetrates the thoracic wall. The injury must be significantly large in order for air to move preferentially through the wound. The patient will have an open chest wound and dyspnea. Care includes sealing the wound on three sides to prevent further progress of the pneumothorax, provision of oxygen, and monitoring the patient for the development of tension pneumothorax.

c. Tension pneumothorax

Tension pneumothorax is a pneumothorax created under the mechanisms associated with simple or open pneumothorax that progresses because of a valve-like injury site. The valve permits air to enter the pleural space but not exit. This results in a progressive lung collapse, followed by increasing pressure that displaces the mediastinum and restricts venous return to the heart. The patient has a trauma history and progressive dyspnea that becomes very severe. The patient may also display subcutaneous emphysema and distended jugular veins. Care is directed at decompressing the thorax with the insertion of a catheter into the 2nd intercostal space, providing oxygen, and monitoring the patient for a recurring tension pneumothorax.

d. Hemothorax

A hemothorax is a collection of blood in the pleural space. It may occur with or without pneumothorax. Hemothorax will generally become a hypovolemic problem before it seriously endangers respiration because the amount of fluid loss necessary to restrict respiration is great. The patient may experience dyspnea and the signs and symptoms of hypovolemic compensation (shock). Provide the patient with shock care, oxygen, fluid replacement, and rapid transport.

e. Hemopneumothorax

A hemopneumothorax is simply the existence of blood loss into the pleura and an accumulation of air there. Its presentation includes the signs and symptoms associated with both these pathologies. Care is directed at oxygen administration and rapid transport.

f. Pulmonary contusion

Pulmonary contusion is a blunt trauma injury to the tissue of the lung resulting in edema and stiffening of the lung tissue. This reduces the efficiency of air exchange and causes an increased workload associated with respiration. If the region involved is limited, the patient may only experience very mild dyspnea. If the area is extensive, the patient may experience severe dyspnea. Care is centered around ensuring good oxygenation, including overdrive ventilation when indicated, and rapid transport.

6. **Discuss the pathophysiology, findings of assessment, and management— including the need for rapid intervention and transport—of the patient with myocardial injuries, including:**   pp. 716–719, 731–732

a. Myocardial contusion

Myocardial contusion is simply a contusion to the myocardium, usually related to blunt anterior chest trauma. The patient will present with myocardial-infarction-like pain and possible dysrhythmias. Care is directed at oxygen therapy, cardiac medications as indicated, and rapid transport.

b. Pericardial tamponade

Pericardial tamponade is usually related to penetrating trauma in which a wound permits blood from within the heart to enter the pericardium. It progressively fills the pericardium and restricts ventricular filling. The cardiac output drops and circulation is severely restricted. The patient will present with a penetrating trauma mechanism and will move quickly into shock, and possibly, sudden death. Care is insertion of a needle into the pericardial sac and the withdrawal of fluid. Any patient suspected of this injury requires immediate transport to the closest hospital.

c. Myocardial rupture

Myocardial rupture is often associated with high-velocity penetrating trauma. The bullet's passage through the engorged heart causes the blood to move outward from the bullet's path (cavitation) explosively. The heart wall tears, and the patient hemorrhages extensively as cardiac output ceases. The patient will display the signs of sudden death and no resuscitation efforts will be successful.

7. **Discuss the pathophysiology, findings of assessment, and management—including the need for rapid intervention and transport—of the patient with vascular injuries, including injuries to:** pp. 719–720, 732

a. Aorta

Aortic aneurysm is a ballooning of the aorta as blunt trauma shears open the tunica intima and tunica media. Blood under systolic pressure enters the injury site and begins to dissect the vessel, causing it to balloon like a tire's inner tube. The patient will have a history of blunt trauma and complain of a tearing central chest pain that may radiate into the back. Care is centered around gentle but rapid transport to the trauma center. Oxygen is administered and fluid infusion should be very minimal.

A rupture or penetrating injury to the aorta results in almost immediate death as the vessel is very large and contains great pressure. The patient will have a history of penetrating or severe blunt chest trauma and display the signs of shock and move quickly to decompensation and death. Care is directed to oxygen administration, shock management, and rapid transport to the trauma center.

b. Vena cava

Injury to the vena cava is only slightly less severe than aortic injury since the vessels carry the same volume of fluid, but under different pressures (less for the vena cava). The progression of injury is just slightly slower with injury to the vena cava, though the result of injury is probably the same. In the field, it may be difficult to determine the exact blood vessel involved in a penetrating injury to the chest.

c. Pulmonary arteries/veins

As with aortic and vena caval injuries, the patient will have a history of penetrating or severe blunt trauma and the signs and symptoms of hypovolemia and shock. Care is directed at helping the body compensate for shock, some fluid resuscitation, and rapid transport.

8. **Discuss the pathophysiology, findings of assessment, and management—including the need for rapid intervention and transport—of patients with diaphragmatic, esophageal, and tracheobronchial injuries.** pp. 720–721, 732

Diaphragmatic injury is usually due to severe compression of the diaphragm during blunt abdominal trauma or due to penetrating trauma along the border of the rib cage. Remember that the diaphragm is a dynamic muscle that moves up and down with respiration. Injury may result in less effective respiration and/or the movement of abdominal organs into the chest cavity, most commonly the bowel. The injury may present similarly to tension pneumothorax as the abdominal contents displace the lung tissue. Bowel sounds may also be heard in the chest, though it usually takes too much time to decipher these sounds. Care is directed at treating shock and dyspnea with rapid transport indicated.

Esophageal injury does not usually present with acute symptoms other than a history of penetrating trauma to the central chest. Perforation may permit food, drink, or gastric contents to enter the mediastinum, where it either forms an excellent medium for infection (with gastric contents) or damages some of the structures within. The result is serious damage to some of the most important structures within the chest and a significant mortality rate. The patient with such injury will present with penetrating injury to the region and care is directed toward other, more immediately important pathologies. Nevertheless, suspect esophageal injury and communicate that suspicion to the attending physician.

Tracheobronchial injuries are usually related to penetrating trauma to the upper mediastinum, and they open the major airways to the mediastinum. The injuries permit air to enter the mediastinum and possibly the neck. The patient will have dyspnea (possibly severe) and may have subcutaneous emphysema. Positive-pressure ventilation may make matters worse as air is then actively "pushed" into the mediastinal space. The patient may also experience pneumothorax and tension pneumothorax.

9. **Discuss the pathophysiology, findings of assessment, and management—including the need for rapid intervention and transport—of the patient with traumatic asphyxia.** pp. 721, 732

Traumatic asphyxia is a crushing-type injury in which the crushing mechanism remains in place and restricts both respiration and venous return to the central circulation. The patient may display bulging eyes, petechial hemorrhage, and red or blue skin above the level of compression. The injury may damage many internal blood vessels but tamponades hemorrhage because of the continuing compression. Once the compression is released, profound hypovolemia may occur and the patient may demonstrate the signs and symptoms of serious internal injury. Care is directed at oxygen administration, ventilation, fluid resuscitation, and rapid transport to the trauma center.

10. **Differentiate between thoracic injuries based on the assessment and history.** pp. 722–726

Anterior blunt trauma is most likely to cause rib fracture, pulmonary contusion, closed pneumothorax ("paper bag" syndrome) (possibly progressing to tension pneumothorax), and myocardial contusion. Sharp pain suggests rib fracture, while dull pain suggests pulmonary or myocardial contusion. Dyspnea may be present in all circumstances but will likely be progressive and become severe with pulmonary contusion or pneumothorax. Lateral impact may cause traumatic aortic aneurysm with tearing chest pain, possibly radiating to the back. Crushing injury may cause traumatic asphyxia and display with a discolored upper body and severe shock at the pressure release.

Penetrating trauma may induce an open pneumothorax but is more likely to cause closed pneumothorax unless there is a very large entrance wound. Injury to the great vessels and heart may cause immediate exsanguination, while heart injury may lead to pericardial tamponade. Penetrating trauma to the central chest may perforate any mediastinal structure, including the trachea or esophagus. Rapid hypovolemia and shock suggest great vessel or heart injury, while progressively increasing dyspnea suggests tension pneumothorax. Severe dyspnea, absent breath sounds on the ipsilateral side, and distended jugular veins confirm a probable diagnosis of tension pneumothorax. Any penetration of the thorax with possible entry into the mediastinum should suggest esophageal or tracheal injury.

11. **Given several preprogrammed and moulaged thoracic trauma patients, provide the appropriate scene size-up, initial assessment, rapid trauma or focused physical exam and history, detailed exam, and ongoing assessment, and provide appropriate patient care and transportation.** pp. 704–732

During your training as an EMT-I you will participate in many classroom practice sessions involving simulated patients. You will also spend some time in the emergency departments of local hospitals as well as in advanced-level ambulances gaining clinical experience. During these times, use your knowledge of thoracic trauma to help you assess and care for the simulated or real patients you attend.

CASE STUDY REVIEW

This case study presents many of the important elements of assessment and care for the patient who has suffered penetrating injury to the chest. It identifies the need to recognize and aggressively manage the patient. It also highlights the value of rapid transport, when called for.

The EMT-Is on Medic 101, Victoria and Christian, use the time during their response to identify their duties, the equipment that will likely by needed, and procedures they may perform. Of primary concern is scene safety for the EMT-Is, fellow rescuers, bystanders, and the patient, especially since shots have been fired. The EMT-Is are also concerned about the severity of the injuries that may have resulted. They mentally review the steps of assessment and management of both chest and abdominal injuries. As the rescue unit arrives, it is apparent that the police have secured the scene and concern can be directed to the patient.

The initial assessment of the patient presents only minor signs of injury. The wounds are small and not bleeding severely. The patient does not appear to be in much pain. Victoria and Christian do notice that the patient's level of consciousness and color suggest shock, as do the labored, rapid, and shallow breathing and the patient's ability to speak only in short phrases. Their quick initial assessment reveals reasons to be concerned about the airway (reduced level of consciousness) and breathing (speaking in short phrases and poor color). Circulation is deficient, as the EMT-Is note the distal pulses are absent and the carotid pulse is rapid and weak. This patient is clearly one who merits a rapid trauma assessment and rapid transport to the trauma center.

The rapid trauma assessment reveals that the patient was struck by four bullets, increasing the likelihood that critical structures were injured. Even though the wounds are small in nature, the EMT-Is remember the severe injuries a bullet can produce. They also note powder burns and residue on Conrad's shirt due to the proximity of the gun barrel to his chest when it was fired. They carefully remove the shirt without cutting it. (If cutting was required, they would have cut without cutting through the bullet holes.) Their actions help maintain the integrity of the evidence as it may be used in court.

Victoria and Christian quickly cover each wound with an occlusive dressing, sealed on three sides to prevent entry of air into the chest and to permit any air under pressure to escape (as with the development of tension pneumothorax). Their assessment finds full jugular veins, a normal finding in a normovolemic patient in the supine position. The slightly diminished breath sounds on the right side suggest some pneumothorax and reason to perform frequent ongoing assessments evaluating the right side for breath sounds.

Conrad receives care in anticipation of shock including high-flow oxygen and IVs started in each upper extremity with large-bore catheters and macrodrip or trauma tubing. The EMT-Is also employ spinal precautions with him, just in case one of the bullets has damaged the vertebral column and endangered the spinal cord.

Careful ongoing assessments reveal a continuing degeneration in the patient's condition. This prompts Victoria and Christian to search for a possible cause of the deterioration. Increasingly quieter breath sounds on the right side, hyperinflation of the right side, tracheal deviation (a late and infrequent sign of tension pneumothorax), increasing dyspnea, and overall patient degeneration together suggest a developing pneumothorax, possibly a tension pneumothorax. The team first tries to relieve the condition by unsealing the dressings covering the wound sites. These actions are unsuccessful, so medical direction is contacted and the EMT-Is receive authorization to perform a needle decompression of the thorax at the second intercostal space, midclavicular line. Victoria places a large-bore (14-gauge) catheter just above the third rib (into the 2nd intercostal space) until she feels a "pop" and hears air rush out. The attempt is successful, as demonstrated by the escaping air. The bullet wound dressings are reapplied and a valve assembly (a cut glove finger) is applied to the needle hub. Then Christian and Victoria watch their patient very carefully during transport for the redevelopment of the tension pneumothorax because they know that the catheter inserted in the chest may kink or clog with blood or other fluid.

CONTENT SELF-EVALUATION

MULTIPLE CHOICE

_____ 1. Which of the following is NOT likely to be associated with blunt trauma?
   A. pericardial tamponade
   B. pneumothorax (paper bag syndrome)
   C. traumatic asphyxia
   D. aortic aneurysm
   E. myocardial contusion

_____ 2. Which of the following is NOT likely to be associated with penetrating trauma?
   A. open pneumothorax   D. cavitational lung injury
   B. esophageal disruption   E. comminuted fracture of the ribs
   C. traumatic asphyxia

Trauma Emergencies

_____ 3. Rib fracture is found in about what percent of significant chest trauma?
  A. 10 percent   D. 50 percent
  B. 25 percent   E. 65 percent
  C. 35 percent

_____ 4. Which ribs are fractured the most frequently?
  A. ribs 1 and 3   D. ribs 8 through 11
  B. ribs 4 through 8   E. ribs 9 through 12
  C. ribs 7 through 9

_____ 5. Which rib group results in mortality up to 30 percent when they are fractured?
  A. ribs 1 and 3   D. ribs 8 through 11
  B. ribs 4 through 8   E. ribs 9 through 12
  C. ribs 7 through 9

_____ 6. Which of the following groups is more likely to experience internal injury without rib fracture?
  A. the pediatric patient   D. the elderly female patient
  B. the adult male patient   E. the elderly male patient
  C. the adult female patient

_____ 7. Which of the following is a sign or symptom of rib fracture?
  A. local pain   D. hemothorax
  B. crepitus   E. all of the above
  C. limited chest excursion

_____ 8. Which of the following is most frequently associated with sternal fracture?
  A. hemothorax   D. simple pneumothorax
  B. myocardial contusion   E. open pneumothorax
  C. esophageal injury

_____ 9. Air from under the flail segment in flail chest does which of the following?
  A. moves out from under the segment during expiration
  B. moves toward the segment during expiration
  C. does not move with the segment
  D. moves out from under the segment during inspiration
  E. none of the above

_____ 10. As the pain of the flail chest increases with time, the amount of paradoxical movement will decrease due to muscular splinting.
  A. True
  B. False

_____ 11. Simple pneumothorax is associated with what percent of serious thoracic trauma?
  A. 5   D. 60
  B. 10 to 30   E. more than 75
  C. 25 to 50

_____ 12. The condition in which a part of the chest wall moves in opposition to the rest of the chest due to numerous rib fractures is called:
  A. pneumothorax.   D. atelectasis.
  B. tension pneumothorax.   E. none of the above
  C. hemothorax.

_____ 13. The chest injury that causes the patient to experience increasing dyspnea because of an open or closed pneumothorax that has a valve-like function and allows intrathoracic pressure to increase is referred to as:
  A. subcutaneous emphysema.
  B. traumatic asphyxia.
  C. hyperbaric mediastinal displacement.
  D. tension pneumothorax.
  E. flail chest.

©2004 Pearson Education, Inc.
Intermediate Emergency Care: Principles & Practice

_____ 14. For air to move through an open wound to create an open pneumothorax, the wound opening must be:
A. just large enough to permit air passage.
B. two-thirds the size of the tracheal opening.
C. the size of the trachea.
D. about the size of a hunting rifle bullet.
E. larger than the trachea.

_____ 15. Which of the following is a very late sign of tension pneumothorax?
A. head and neck petechiae
B. intercostal bulging
C. a narrowing pulse pressure
D. tracheal deviation away from the injury
E. distended jugular veins

_____ 16. Each hemithorax can hold up to what volume of blood from a hemothorax?
A. 500 mL
B. 750 mL
C. 1,500 mL
D. 3,000 mL
E. 4,500 mL

_____ 17. Which of the following statements is NOT true regarding hemothorax?
A. Hemorrhage into the thorax is more severe due to decreased pressure there.
B. Serious hemothorax may displace an entire lung and has a 75 percent mortality rate.
C. Hemothorax often occurs with pneumothorax.
D. Hemothorax rarely occurs with simple rib fractures.
E. none of the above

_____ 18. Distant or absent breath sounds heard during auscultation of the chest and the signs of shock are suggestive of which pathology?
A. pneumothorax
B. tension pneumothorax
C. aortic aneurysm
D. pulmonary contusion
E. hemothorax

_____ 19. Which of the following problems would most likely result in a chest area that was dull to percussion?
A. pneumothorax
B. tension pneumothorax
C. hemothorax
D. subcutaneous pneumothorax
E. pericardial tamponade

_____ 20. Your patient has received chest trauma yet did not initially present with crackles. However, as the assessment continues, they are heard in both the lower lung fields. This condition is most likely a result of which of the following?
A. pulmonary contusion
B. hemothorax
C. pneumothorax
D. aortic aneurysm
E. pericardial tamponade

_____ 21. Extensive pulmonary contusions may account for blood losses up to 1,500 mL.
A. True
B. False

_____ 22. The most common cause of myocardial contusion is:
A. blunt anterior chest trauma.
B. blunt lateral chest trauma.
C. penetrating anterior chest trauma.
D. blunt posterior chest trauma.
E. the pressure wave of an explosion.

_____ 23. A patient presents with the signs of shock, jugular vein distention, distant heart sounds, and a narrowing pulse pressure. The lung fields are clear. Which condition is most likely the cause?
A. tension pneumothorax
B. hemothorax
C. traumatic asphyxia
D. pericardial tamponade
E. atelectasis

_____ 24. Pericardial tamponade occurs with what frequency in serious chest trauma patients?
A. less than 2 percent of the time
B. 10 percent of the time
C. 20 percent of the time
D. 25 percent of the time
E. 30 to 45 percent of the time

_____ 25. Which of the following is a sign of pericardial tamponade?
A. pulsus paradoxus
B. a narrowing pulse pressure
C. distended jugular veins
D. hypotension
E. all of the above

_____ 26. The patient with pericardial tamponade may be in hypovolemic shock due to the volume of blood lost into the pericardial sac.
A. True
B. False

_____ 27. A decrease in jugular vein distention during inspiration is known as:
A. Beck's triad.
B. pulsus paradoxus.
C. Cushing's reflex.
D. Kussmaul's sign.
E. electrical alternans.

_____ 28. If the chamber of the heart is significantly damaged yet does not rupture immediately, it is likely to rupture in around two weeks.
A. True
B. False

_____ 29. Your patient was involved in a lateral impact auto accident. The car is greatly deformed, though the patient does not have many signs of injury. During your assessment, he complains of a tearing sensation in his central chest and numbness in his left upper extremity. Your highest index of suspicion of injury is for:
A. traumatic asphyxia.
B. pulmonary contusion.
C. aortic aneurysm.
D. myocardial contusion.
E. pericardial tamponade.

_____ 30. What percentage of patients with traumatic aortic aneurysm survive the initial impact and injury?
A. as high as 10 percent
B. as high as 20 percent
C. 50 percent
D. 70 percent
E. 73 percent

_____ 31. In a patient with a history of blunt lateral trauma and a suspected traumatic aortic aneurysm, which signs or symptoms would you expect to find?
A. severe tearing chest pain
B. pulse deficit between extremities
C. reduced pulse strength in the lower extremities
D. hypertension
E. all of the above

_____ 32. A harsh systolic murmur is heard over the central chest. This is suggestive of which pathology?
A. pneumothorax
B. tension pneumothorax
C. traumatic aortic aneurysm
D. pulmonary contusion
E. hemothorax

_____ 33. The right side is the site of most diaphragmatic ruptures as most assailants are right-handed.
A. True
B. False

_____ 34. The traumatic diaphragmatic rupture is likely to present like which of the following thoracic injuries?
    A. tension pneumothorax
    B. pulmonary contusion
    C. aortic aneurysm
    D. pericardial tamponade
    E. esophageal injury

_____ 35. The two major problems associated with traumatic asphyxia are restriction of chest excursion and:
    A. distortion of the airway.
    B. restriction of venous return.
    C. atelectasis.
    D. hemorrhage during the compression.
    E. massive strokes.

_____ 36. The classic signs of traumatic asphyxia include which of the following?
    A. bulging eyes
    B. conjunctival hemorrhage
    C. petechiae of the head and neck
    D. dark red or purple appearance of the head and neck
    E. all of the above

_____ 37. Serious penetrating trauma will likely require which of the following body substance isolation procedures?
    A. gloves
    B. face shield
    C. gown
    D. mask
    E. all of the above

_____ 38. During your assessment of a supine patient with blunt chest trauma, you notice slight jugular vein distention. With no other signs of injury, this suggests which of the following?
    A. a normal patient
    B. pericardial tamponade
    C. tension pneumothorax
    D. traumatic asphyxia
    E. B, C, and D

_____ 39. Crackles heard during auscultation of the chest are suggestive of which pathology?
    A. pneumothorax
    B. tension pneumothorax
    C. aortic aneurysm
    D. pulmonary contusion
    E. hemothorax

_____ 40. Hyperresonance heard during percussion of the chest is suggestive of which pathology?
    A. pneumothorax
    B. tension pneumothorax
    C. hemothorax
    D. pulmonary contusion
    E. both A and B

_____ 41. Which of the following thoracic structures takes the least energy to fracture and often results in a more common, yet less serious, thoracic injury?
    A. ribs 1 through 3
    B. ribs 4 through 9
    C. ribs 10 through 12
    D. the sternum
    E. the manubrium

_____ 42. A patient who displays subcutaneous emphysema is most likely to have which of the conditions listed below?
    A. traumatic asphyxia
    B. tension pneumothorax
    C. the paper bag syndrome
    D. pulmonary contusion
    E. cardiac contusion

_____ 43. Overdrive ventilation (bag-valve masking) of the patient with flail chest will cause the flail segment to move with, rather than in opposition to, the chest wall.
    A. True
    B. False

_____ 44. Which of the following is an indication for the use of PASG?
  A. diaphragmatic rupture
  B. penetrating chest injury
  C. blunt chest trauma with a blood pressure below 100
  D. blunt chest trauma with a blood pressure below 60
  E. suspected pericardial tamponade

_____ 45. Meperidine, diazepam, or morphine sulfate may be given to the minor rib fracture patient to reduce pain and increase respiratory excursion.
  A. True
  B. False

_____ 46. The patient who is suspected of a flail chest or other thoracic cage injury, without suspected spine injury, should be positioned:
  A. on the uninjured side.
  B. on the injured side.
  C. supine with legs elevated.
  D. on the left lateral side.
  E. on the right lateral side.

_____ 47. The open pneumothorax should be cared for using which of the following techniques?
  A. Pack the wound with a sterile dressing.
  B. Cover the wound an occlusive dressing and tape securely.
  C. Cover the wound with an occlusive dressing, taped on three sides.
  D. Attempt to close the wound with a hemostat and then cover with a sterile dressing.
  E. Cover the wound loosely with a sterile dressing.

_____ 48. Which location is recommended for prehospital pleural decompression?
  A. 2nd intercostal space, midclavicular line
  B. 5th intercostal space, midclavicular line
  C. 5th intercostal space, midaxillary line
  D. A and B
  E. A and C

_____ 49. A few minutes after you have inserted a needle and decompressed a tension pneumothorax, you notice that a patient's dyspnea is getting worse and breath sounds on the injured side are becoming diminished. Which action would you take?
  A. Insert a second needle.
  B. Remove the dressing.
  C. Provide overdrive ventilation.
  D. Consider nitrous oxide administration.
  E. all of the above

_____ 50. A patient is trapped in a wrecked auto for about half an hour and is suspected of having traumatic asphyxia. Care should include which of the following?
  A. two large-bore IVs
  B. normal saline or lactated Ringer's solution
  C. fluids run rapidly
  D. consideration of sodium bicarbonate
  E. all of the above

SPECIAL PROJECT

Labeling the Diagram

Write the names of the organs and structures of the thorax marked A, B, C, D, E, F, G, and H in the figure below.

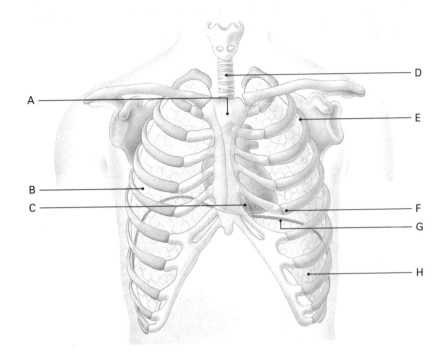

A. _____

B. _____

C. _____

D. _____

E. _____

F. _____

G. _____

H. _____

Trauma Emergencies

CHAPTER 18

Trauma Management Skills

Review of Chapter Objectives

The asterisked objectives for this chapter are in addition to the DOT EMT-Intermediate curriculum.

After reading this chapter, you should be able to:

*1. Explain the elements of trauma assessment. pp. 735–748

The assessment of the trauma patient follows the standard format for assessment including the special components that relate to trauma. The assessment progresses through the scene size-up, initial assessment, rapid trauma assessment (for the serious or critical patient) or the focused assessment and history, detailed physical exam (in rare cases), and finally, ongoing assessments.

During the scene size-up, you evaluate the scene to investigate and determine the mechanism of injury and, from that, identify an index of suspicion for specific injuries. You also analyze the potential hazards of the scene, including the need for body substance isolation procedures. You should search out and identify all patients. And, finally, you identify and summon all resources needed to manage the patients and scene.

In the initial assessment, you quickly apply spinal precautions and form a general patient impression and then determine the patient's mental status. Then, evaluate the patient's airway and breathing and perform any needed interventions (oxygen, oral or nasal airway or endotracheal intubation, and ventilation). Evaluate the circulation, control external hemorrhage, and, if hypovolemia and shock are possible, then initiate a large-bore IV. At the conclusion of the initial assessment, the patient is categorized as needing the rapid trauma assessment (emergency patients) or the focused trauma assessment.

During the rapid trauma assessment, you examine areas where significant injury is expected either from the mechanism of injury analysis or the initial assessment. It is also a time to examine the patient's chief and minor complaints, as time and priority permit. In general, during this assessment you should look in detail at the head, neck, chest, abdomen, and pelvis, as these are the areas likely to produce life-threatening injury. Take a quick set of vital signs and an abbreviated patient history. At the end of the rapid trauma assessment, decide the priority of the patient for transport. That decision is made by comparing the assessment findings against the trauma triage criteria used in your system.

The focused trauma assessment is used for the patient with limited mechanism of injury and expected, isolated, and moderate to minor injuries. During the focused assessment, you direct consideration to the likely injuries and the specific patient complaints. It usually concludes with slow transport to a nearby emergency department, or in some cases, treatment and release.

The detailed physical exam is a head-to-toe assessment of the patient while you search for signs and symptoms of injury. This procedure is useful for the unconscious patient for whom all other known or suspected life threats have been attended to, and it is then provided only during transport. However, portions of the techniques and process of the detailed assessment are used for elements of the initial and focused assessments.

During the ongoing assessment, you retake the vital signs, make a mental status assessment, reevaluate chief or serious patient complaints and significant signs of injury, and recheck any intervention you have performed. Perform an ongoing assessment every 5 minutes with seriously injured patients and every 15 minutes with other patients. Also perform the ongoing assessment after every major intervention or any sign that the patient's condition has changed or is changing.

*2. Explain the management of head, facial, and neck injury patients.
pp. 749–756

Direct management of the patient with injury to the head, face, and neck focuses first on the potential for brain injury, airway compromise, injury to the sense organs, and hemorrhage control. Assure the airway with proper patient positioning while employing the proper spinal precautions. Use suctioning and intubation as needed. Control any hemorrhage with direct pressure but be careful of any unstable fracture of the skull. If instability is possible, apply gentle pressure around the wound to help control hemorrhage. Hemorrhage can be especially severe from neck wounds, and circumferential pressure is not indicated. Also be aware that some neck wounds may aspirate air and cause life-threatening air emboli. Cover any open neck wound with an occlusive dressing held in place with gentle direct pressure. Allow blood and possibly cerebral spinal fluid to drain from the ears and protect an injured eye with a paper cup and cover the uninjured eye. Monitor and record any changes in the patient's vital signs and level of consciousness.

*3. Explain the management of spinal injury patients.
pp. 756–768

Whenever you encounter a patient who could be a spinal injury patient, treat him as though he has an injury. Gently bring the spine into alignment by bringing the nose, belly button, and toes into one plane, the shoulders and buttocks against a firm flat surface, the knees bent, and the head (of the adult) 1 1/2 to 2 inches above the flat surface. Assure that all movement and immobilization maintains this position and does not cause either axial loading or distraction. Once a potential for injury is recognized, have a rescuer apply manual immobilization of the head and neck. Once the neck is assessed during the initial assessment, apply a properly sized cervical collar. Frequently, the short spine board, KED, or other similar device is needed to bring the patient from a seated position to a full supine position. In an emergency (clear need for rapid extrication) you (and two other rescuers) may manually support the patient as he or she is brought from a seated or other position to the supine position. If the patient is found supine or prone, log roll him or her, using spinal precautions, to the long spine board. Once the patient is supine on a spine board, secure the shoulders, hips, legs, and head to the board.

*4. Explain the management of abdominal injury patients.
pp. 768–770

The care for a patient with abdominal injuries is for the most part supportive. If you suspect serious internal hemorrhage, then provide fluid therapy and rapid transport. Give high-flow, high-concentration oxygen, keep the patient warm and monitor vital signs and level of consciousness. Immobilize objects impaled within the abdomen in place and dress open wounds and cover eviscerations with occlusive dressings.

*5. Explain the management of musculoskeletal injury patients.
pp. 770–785

Musculoskeletal injuries are usually a lower priority for the serious injured trauma patient and are attended to only after the patient's serious injuries are stabilized, and then, only during transport. The first priority in caring for the patient with a musculoskeletal injury is to assure distal circulation and innervation. Then immobilize the injury using a splinting device. Assure that the device firmly immobilizes the joint above and the joint below the injury (be it a sprain, strain, dislocation, or fracture). There are many splinting devices to choose from including the traction splint (for the femur fracture), padded board splints, air splints, vacuum splints, ladder splints, and specialized splints. Choose one that is easy to apply and will firmly stabilize the wound site. Be sure to assess the distal pulse and nervous function distal to the injury before, during, and after the splinting process. If the pulse is absent after splinting, move the splint and limb around slightly to re-establish circulation or innervation.

*6. Explain the management of soft-tissue injury patients. pp. 786–798

Soft-tissue injury care is generally a lower priority in trauma patient management and is often deferred until you care for serious injury. The management of soft-tissue injuries is directed at three objectives: stop any hemorrhage, keep the wound clean, and immobilize the wound site. As needed, employ direct pressure, elevation (where indicated), arterial pressure points and, only as a last resort, a tourniquet to control any serious blood loss. Then apply a sterile, properly sized dressing, secured firmly in place, with bandaging material. Assure that the wound site is properly immobilized to assist the coagulation and wound repair processes are unimpeded.

CASE STUDY REVIEW

The patient presented in this case study has the typical signs and symptoms of shock and is cared for with the aggressiveness required if shock resuscitation is to be successful.

Peter presents with the classic signs and symptoms of shock very early in assessment and care, suggesting that blood loss is rapid and already significant. The carotid pulse is rapid and weak, reflective of volume depletion and the heart's attempt to compensate with a rapid rate. The patient has a reduced level of consciousness, is not able to remember what happened, and is both anxious and combative. These signs reflect cerebral hypoxia. Breathing is also affected. Peter's breaths are shallow and rapid, thus less efficient than slower and deeper respirations. The absence of distal pulses suggests both reduced blood pressure and peripheral vasoconstriction. This is supported by the cool, clammy skin and capillary refill time of over 4 seconds (normal being less than 3 seconds). The pulse oximetry reading is low, reflecting poor oxygenation. It is surprising that a reading was obtained at all. In low-flow states, the oximeter often provides an erratic reading, if one can be obtained at all (suggesting low flow and very weak distal arterial pulsation).

This patient is certainly a candidate for rapid transport with aggressive shock care en route. Because of the entrapment, rapid transport is not an immediately available option and aggressive field care is employed. The aggressive care offered by Alex includes two IVs begun with 14- or 16-gauge short catheters. This will allow the greatest infusion rates. The catheters are connected to trauma tubing for the rapid infusion of crystalloids and, eventually, blood in the emergency department. Alex uses one 1,000 mL bag of lactated Ringer's solution and one of normal saline. The normal saline is hung because there is an incompatibility between blood and lactated Ringer's solution. This arrangement will allow the hospital to immediately infuse the blood through the saline line, if they wish to do so.

The PASG provides a double benefit in this patient scenario. The pressure of the garment over the dressings is an effective application of direct pressure and hemorrhage control. The garment also effectively supports the body's compensatory mechanisms against shock.

Alex awaits the arrival of the medical helicopter, probably because they are moments from arriving when Peter is extricated and transport to a pre-designated landing zone might increase the transfer time. It will be important for Alex to have this patient firmly secured to the spine board and the IV lines secured as well. The patient report must be abbreviated and specific to pertinent elements of Alex's initial, rapid trauma assessment and ongoing assessments because time is a precious element in this response and Peter's chances for survival. Pressure infusers are applied to the fluid bags by the flight team and pressurized to increase fluid flow. The flight crew's care benefits Peter because they have available and can administer O-negative blood, which helps replace lost plasma and red blood cells.

The only action on the part of the paramedic team that might have improved patient care would have been to draw blood at the scene and have a police officer transport it to the emergency department. This would allow the ED staff to type and crossmatch whole blood for the patient much earlier than would otherwise be possible. Instead, O-negative blood was given, which might not be the ideal blood type for this patient.

©2004 Pearson Education, Inc.
Intermediate Emergency Care: Principles & Practice

CONTENT SELF-EVALUATION

MULTIPLE CHOICE

_____ 1. The scene size-up includes four elements. They include all of the following EXCEPT:
   A. analysis of the mechanism of injury.
   B. identifying scene hazards.
   C. locating all patients.
   D. evaluating the ABCs.
   E. requesting additional resources.

_____ 2. Employ spinal precautions when you note the patient has experienced extremes of:
   A. flexion.
   B. axial loading.
   C. rotation.
   D. distraction.
   E. all of the above

_____ 3. A person who does not recognize friends and family is NOT:
   A. oriented to time.
   B. oriented to place.
   C. oriented to persons.
   D. oriented to one's own person.
   E. none of the above

_____ 4. Which examination technique should be performed first?
   A. inspection
   B. palpation
   C. percussion
   D. auscultation
   E. questioning

_____ 5. At what angle should the normo-tensive patient display jugular vein distention?
   A. 10 degrees
   B. 15 degrees
   C. 25 degrees
   D. 35 degrees
   E. 45 degrees

_____ 6. Which of the following is NOT a part of the ongoing assessment?
   A. mental status check
   B. vital sign assessment
   C. rapid trauma assessment
   D. circulation check
   E. breathing check

_____ 7. The maneuver that displaces the cricoid ring posteriorly to help an EMT-I visualize the landmarks for intubation is:
   A. digital intubation.
   B. Anthony's maneuver.
   C. tracheal stabilization.
   D. rapid sequence intubation.
   E. Sellick's maneuver.

_____ 8. The first line drug for the patient with a head injury is:
   A. oxygen.
   B. epinephrine.
   C. mannitol.
   D. furosemide.
   E. thiamine.

_____ 9. The head of an adult should be displaced anteriorly about what distance above a flat surface the patient is lying on?
   A. flat with the surface
   B. slightly below the surface level
   C. 1 to 2 inches above the surface level
   D. 2 to 4 inches above the surface level
   E. the positioning of the head is not critical

_____ 10. A protective helmet must be removed from the patient when the helmet:
   A. does not immobilize the head within.
   B. cannot be securely immobilized to the spine board.
   C. obstructs airway care.
   D. prevents assessment of anticipated injuries.
   E. all of the above

_____ 11. The rescuer BEST positioned to coordinate the movement of a patient with a spinal injury is the one at the:
A. head.
B. neck.
C. chest.
D. abdomen.
E. feet.

_____ 12. When coordinating the movement of the spinal injured patient a four count gives the participants the best opportunity to coordinate the move together.
A. True
B. False

_____ 13. The vest-type device for the movement of the spinal injured patient is well suited for lifting the patient.
A. True
B. False

_____ 14. Which of the following is an appropriate reason to employ rapid extrication instead of normal spinal precautions?
A. the needed procedure is time consuming
B. the needed procedure is complicated
C. scene safety requires immediate movement
D. the patient condition requires immediate transport
E. both C and D

_____ 15. The recommended fluid volume for a fluid challenge in the patient with hypovolemia from neurogenic shock is:
A. 100 mL.
B. 250 mL.
C. 500 mL.
D. 1,000 mL.
E. only that which will raise the blood pressure 15 mmHg.

_____ 16. The major emphasis of abdominal injury care in the prehospital setting is:
A. stopping internal hemorrhage.
B. assuring patient comfort.
C. bringing the patient to surgery as rapidly as possible.
D. identifying the exact injuries and providing essential care.
E. none of the above

_____ 17. When caring for the late-term pregnant patient, which position is recommended for transport?
A. right lateral recumbent
B. left lateral recumbent
C. supine
D. prone
E. full seated

_____ 18. Which of the following is an objective of musculoskeletal injury care?
A. reduce the possibility of further injury during transport
B. protect open wounds
C. immobilize the injured extremity
D. reduce patient discomfort
E. all of the above

_____ 19. Proper limb positioning is important for maintaining distal circulation, sensation and increasing patient comfort.
A. True
B. False

_____ 20. Which of the following should halt the movement of an angulated limb to an aligned position.
  A. a significant increase in patient discomfort
  B. a strong distal pulse
  C. regaining distal sensation
  D. significant resistance to movement
  E. both A and D

_____ 21. The patient with an atraumatic fracture of the femur and limited discomfort requires which of the following care approaches?
  A. immediate traction splinting
  B. a long spine board and padding
  C. rapid transport
  D. careful limb repositioning and fluid resuscitation
  E. aggressive shock management

_____ 22. The anterior dislocation of the hip is most common and presents with which of the following?
  I. the knee flexed
  II. the knee extended
  III. the foot internally rotated
  IV. the foot externally rotated

  Select the proper grouping.
  A. I, III
  B. I, IV
  C. II, III
  D. II, IV
  E. none of the above

_____ 23. Which of the following devices is acceptable for immobilizing a foot injury?
  A. vacuum splint
  B. pillow splint
  C. ladder splint
  D. air splint
  E. all of the above

_____ 24. The major objectives for dressing and bandaging a soft-tissue wound include which of the following:
  A. hemorrhage control.
  B. immobilization.
  C. neat appearance.
  D. keep the wound site clean.
  E. all of the above

_____ 25. Which of the following intravenous solutions is NOT recommended for the crush syndrome patient?
  A. normal saline
  B. lactated Ringer's solution
  C. D_5W in 1/2 normal saline
  D. D_5W
  E. All of the above are acceptable.

Trauma Emergencies

Intermediate Emergency Care: Principles & Practice

Division 4

Medical Emergencies

CHAPTER 19
*
Respiratory Emergencies

Review of Chapter Objectives

After reading this chapter, you should be able to:

1. Identify and describe the function of the structures located in the upper and lower airway. (see Chapter 2)

The airway is functionally divided into the upper airway and the lower airway. The upper airway is comprised of the nasal cavity, pharynx, and larynx. The lower airway is comprised of the trachea, bronchi, alveoli, and lungs. The ability to take in oxygen and excrete carbon dioxide via the airway is essential to life. Therefore, it is critical that you be able to identify and understand the function of each structure of the airway and of the airway as a whole.

2. Discuss the physiology of ventilation and respiration. pp. 802–804; see Chapter 2

The major function of the respiratory system is the exchange of gases between the person and the environment. Three processes allow the gas exchange to take place: ventilation, diffusion, and perfusion. Ventilation is the movement of air in and out of the lungs. Diffusion is the movement of gases between the lungs and the pulmonary capillaries (oxygen from the lungs into the bloodstream; waste carbon dioxide from the bloodstream into the lungs) as well as between the systemic capillaries and the body tissues (oxygen from the bloodstream into the cells; waste carbon dioxide from the cells into the bloodstream). Perfusion is the circulation of blood through the capillaries. Adequate perfusion is critical to adequate gas exchange in the lungs and body tissues. These three processes—ventilation, diffusion, and perfusion—together provide for respiration.

3. Identify common pathological events that affect the pulmonary system. pp. 804–807

Any disease state that affects the pulmonary system will ultimately disrupt ventilation, diffusion, or perfusion, or a combination of these processes. Ventilation may be disrupted by diseases that cause obstruction of any part of the airway, disrupt the normal function of the chest wall, or impair nervous system control of breathing. Diffusion can be disrupted by a change in concentration of atmospheric oxygen or by any disease that affects the structure or patency of alveoli, the thickness of the respiratory membrane, or the permeability of the capillaries. Perfusion will be affected by any disease that limits blood flow through the lungs and the body or reduces the volume of the oxygen-carrying red blood cells or hemoglobin. Understanding how different diseases and conditions may affect the processes of respiration is important to your ability to choose appropriate emergency care for a respiratory emergency.

4. Discuss abnormal assessment findings and compare various airway and ventilation techniques used in the management of pulmonary diseases. pp. 816–835

Two principles govern the overall management of respiratory emergencies. (1) Give first priority to the airway. (2) Always provide oxygen to patients with respiratory distress or the possibility of hypoxia, including those with chronic obstructive pulmonary disease (COPD).

Medical Emergencies

5. Review the use of equipment utilized during the physical examination of patients with complaints associated with respiratory diseases and conditions.   pp. 812–814

You should be familiar with the use of equipment that is available for physical examination of patients with respiratory complaints. Equipment includes the stethoscope, the pulse oximeter, hand-held devices for measuring peak expiratory flow rate (PEFR), and end-tidal carbon dioxide detection devices.

6. Identify the epidemiology, anatomy, physiology, pathophysiology, assessment findings, and management (including prehospital medications) for the following respiratory diseases and conditions:

a. Bronchial asthma   pp. 819–820, 823–825

Asthma is an obstructive lung disease that causes abnormal ventilation. While deaths from other respiratory diseases are decreasing, deaths from asthma have been on the increase, with 50 percent of those deaths occurring before the patient reaches the hospital. Asthma is thought to be caused by a combination of genetic predisposition and environmental triggers that differ from individual to individual. These include allergens, cold air, exercise, stress, and certain medications. Exposure to a trigger causes release of histamine which, in turn, causes both bronchial constriction and capillary leakage that leads to bronchial edema. The result is a significant decrease in expiratory airflow, which is the essence of an "asthma attack." In the early phase of an attack, inhaled bronchodilator medications such as albuterol will help. In the late phase, inflammation sets in and anti-inflammatory drugs are required to alleviate the condition. Assessment must focus first on evaluation and support of the airway and breathing. Most patients will report a history of asthma. The physical exam should focus on the chest and neck to assess breathing effort. The respiratory rate is the most critical of the vital signs. EMS systems should also be able to measure the peak expiratory flow rate. Treatment is aimed at correction of hypoxia (oxygen administration) and relief of bronchospasm and inflammation. A special case is status asthmaticus—a severe, prolonged attack that does not respond to bronchodilators. It is a serious emergency requiring prompt recognition, treatment, and transport. Another special case is asthma in children, which is treated much as for adults but with altered medication dosages and some special medications.

b. Chronic bronchitis   pp. 822–823

Chronic bronchitis is classified, along with emphysema, as a chronic obstructive pulmonary disease (COPD). COPD affects 25 percent of adults, with chronic bronchitis affecting one in five adult males. Chronic bronchitis reduces ventilation as a result of increased mucus production that blocks airway passages. It is often caused by cigarette smoking but also occurs in nonsmokers. There may be a history of frequent respiratory infections. Chronic bronchitis is usually associated with a productive cough and copious sputum. Patients tend to be overweight and often become cyanotic, so they are sometimes called "blue bloaters." Auscultation of the airway often reveals rhonchi due to mucus occlusion. The goals of treatment are relief of hypoxia and reversal of bronchoconstriction. Because these patients may be dependent on a hypoxic respiratory drive (low oxygen levels stimulate respiration), respiratory effort may become depressed when oxygen is administered. Needed oxygen should not be withheld, but the patient's respirations must be carefully monitored. IV fluids may help loosen mucous congestion. Medical direction may also order administration of a bronchodilator, such as albuterol, metaproterenol, or ipratropium bromide, and may also recommend corticosteroid administration.

c. Emphysema   pp. 819–822

Like chronic bronchitis, emphysema is classified as a chronic obstructive pulmonary disease (COPD). Alveolar walls are destroyed by exposure to noxious substances such as cigarette smoke or other environmental toxins. The disease also causes destruction of the walls of the small bronchioles, which contributes to a trapping of air in the lungs. The result is a decrease in both ventilation and diffusion. Patients tend to breathe through pursed lips, which creates a positive pressure that helps to prevent alveolar collapse. A developing decrease in PaO_2 leads to a compensatory increase in red blood cell production (polycythemia). Emphysema patients are more susceptible to acute respiratory infections and cardiac dysrhythmias. They become dependant on bronchodilators and corticosteroids and, in the final stages, supplemental oxygen. In contrast to chronic bronchitis sufferers, emphysema patients often lose weight and seldom have a cough except early in the morning. Because of the habit of breathing through pursed lips and the color produced by polycythemia, they are sometimes called "pink puffers." Clubbed fingers are common. Auscultation may reveal diminished breath sounds and, at times, wheezes and rhonchi. There may also be signs of right-sided heart disease. As a result of severe respiratory impairment, COPD patients may exhibit confusion, agitation, somnolence, 1-to-2-word dyspnea, and use of accessory muscles to assist respiration.

d. Pneumonia   pp. 827–829

Pneumonia, or lung infection, is a leading cause of death in the elderly and those with HIV infection and is the fifth leading cause of death in the U.S. overall. It is an infection most commonly caused by bacterial or viral infection, rarely by fungal and other infections. Risk factors center on conditions that cause a defect in mucus production or ciliary action that weaken the body's natural defenses against invaders of the respiratory system. Common signs and symptoms include an ill appearance, fever and shaking chills, a productive cough, and sputum. Many cases involve pleuritic chest pain. Auscultation usually reveals crackles in the involved lung segments, or sometimes wheezes or rhonchi, and occasionally egophony (change in spoken "E" sound to "A"). Percussion produces dullness over the affected areas. Some forms of pneumonia do not produce these distinctive symptoms, presenting instead with systemic complaints such as headache, malaise, fatigue, muscle aches, sore throat, nausea, vomiting, and diarrhea. Diagnosis in the field is unlikely and treatment is supportive. Place the patient in a comfortable position and administer high-flow, high-concentration oxygen. In severe cases, ventilatory assistance and possibly endotracheal intubation may be necessary. Medical direction may recommend administration of a beta agonist. Antipyretics may be given to reduce a high fever.

e. Pulmonary edema   pp. 817–819

Pulmonary edema (fluid in the interstitial spaces of the lungs) is often associated with ineffective cardiac pumping action, as in left-sided ventricular heart disease. (Pulmonary edema associated with heart disease is discussed in Chapter 20, "Cardiovascular Emergencies.")

f. Pulmonary thromboembolism   pp. 830–832

A pulmonary embolism is a blood clot (thrombus) that lodges in an artery in the lungs. One in five cases of sudden death is caused by pulmonary thromboembolism. It is a life-threatening condition because it can significantly reduce pulmonary blood flow (perfusion), causing hypoxemia (lack of oxygen in the blood). Immobilization, such as recent surgery, a long bone fracture, or being bedridden, increases the risk of developing an embolism. Other risk factors for clot formation include pregnancy, oral birth control medications, cancer, and sickle cell anemia. The classic symptom of pulmonary embolism is a sudden onset of severe dyspnea, which may or may not be accompanied by pleuritic pain. The physical exam may reveal other signs including labored breathing, tachypnea, and tachycardia. In severe cases, there may be signs of right-sided heart failure, including jugular vein distention and possibly falling blood pressure. Auscultation may reveal no significant findings. In 50 percent of cases, examination of the extremities will reveal signs suggesting deep venous thrombosis (warm, swollen extremity with thick cord palpated along the medial thigh and pain on palpation or when extending the calf). Because a large embolism may cause cardiac arrest, be prepared to perform resuscitation. Primary care is aimed at support of the airway, breathing, and circulation. As necessary, assist ventilations and provide supplemental oxygen. Endotracheal intubation may be required. Establish IV access, monitor vital signs and cardiac rhythms, and transport expeditiously to a facility that can care for the patient's critical needs.

g. Spontaneous pneumothorax   p. 832

Spontaneous pneumothorax, which occurs in the absence of trauma, is a relatively common condition, occurring in roughly 18 persons per 100,000 population. It is relatively likely to recur as well (with 50% recurrence rate at two years). Significant risk factors include male

Medical Emergencies

gender, age 20 to 40 years, tall, thin stature, and history of cigarette smoking. Presentation is marked by sudden onset pleuritic chest or shoulder pain, often precipitated by a bout of coughing or by heavy lifting. The loss of negative pressure in the affected hemithorax prevents proper chest expansion, and the patient may report dyspnea. In individuals who do NOT have significant underlying pulmonary disease, a pneumothorax of up to 15 to 20% of the chest cavity can be tolerated fairly well. Monitor symptoms and pulse oximetry readings during transport. Be especially attentive in your ongoing assessment of patients who require positive-pressure ventilation. These patients are at higher risk for development of tension pneumothorax, which is marked by increasing resistance to ventilation, along with hypoxia, cyanosis, and possible hypotension. Examination will reveal tracheal deviation away from the affected side of the chest and distention of the jugular vein. Needle decompression of a tension pneumothorax may be required.

h. Hyperventilation syndrome   p. 833

Hyperventilation, with rapid breathing, chest pain, and numbness in the extremities, is often associated with anxiety, and it is called hyperventilation syndrome in this setting. However, you should remember that a number of significant and common medical conditions can cause hyperventilation, including cardiovascular and pulmonary conditions such as acute myocardial infarction and pulmonary thromboembolism, sepsis, pregnancy, liver failure, and several metabolic and neurologic disorders. Be conservative and consider hyperventilation to be a sign of a serious medical problem until proven otherwise. Management centers on reassurance and assisting the patient to consciously decrease the rate and depth of breathing (maneuvers that will increase PCO_2).

7. Given several preprogrammed patients with nontraumatic pulmonary problems, provide the appropriate assessment, prehospital care, and transport.   pp. 802–835

The airway is functionally divided into the upper airway and the lower airway. The upper airway is comprised of the nasal cavity, pharynx, and larynx. The lower airway is comprised of the trachea, bronchi, alveoli, and lungs. The ability to take in oxygen and excrete carbon dioxide via the airway is essential to life. Therefore, it is critical that you be able to identify and understand the function of each structure of the airway and of the airway as a whole.

CASE STUDY REVIEW

This case study demonstrates how EMT-Is can reach a field diagnosis and choose appropriate emergency treatment in a respiratory emergency. On this call, Tony and Lee gather critical information from the patient history.

All Tony and Lee know from the dispatch is that their patient is a male who is having difficulty breathing. They learn slightly more from the First Responder on the scene: The patient is 55 years old and is already being given oxygen.

They grab the equipment they think they may need, enter the house (checking for safety), and approach the patient, who is seated at the kitchen table, obviously short of breath. They avoid leaping to conclusions and begin their systematic assessment. The initial assessment confirms that the patient has a patent airway, is moving a little air, and has a strong pulse. They replace the nasal cannula the First Responder had provided with a nonrebreather mask and continue the assessment.

The physical exam reveals diminished breath sounds, rhonchi, use of accessory muscles of respiration, and cyanosis around the mouth. These findings confirm the original complaint: breathing difficulty. But since this is a medical patient (no mechanism of injury was noted during the scene size-up), Tony and Lee know that the most critical information is likely to come from the history.

In fact, they learn that the patient has been diagnosed with emphysema (and has an ongoing 60 pack/year smoking history), and some worsening or exacerbation of this condition is the most likely cause of the patient's current emergency.

©2004 Pearson Education, Inc.
Intermediate Emergency Care: Principles & Practice

Tony and Lee know that emphysema results in bronchoconstriction, alveolar collapse, and a decrease in pulmonary capillaries, which interfere with ventilation and diffusion. The constricted bronchi and destruction of the walls of the small bronchioles make exhalation difficult, causing the rhonchi heard on auscultation of this patient, and also prevent oxygen from reaching the alveoli. The patient no longer has enough healthy alveoli nor pulmonary capillaries to provide for adequate oxygen diffusion into the bloodstream. This, they understand, is why the patient's pulse oximetry reading is only 90 percent, even though he is receiving supplemental oxygen.

The two EMT-Is know that emergency treatment must be aimed at relief of the patient's hypoxia and bronchoconstriction. They continue administration of supplemental oxygen to compensate for the decreased diffusion the patient's diseased alveoli and capillaries are providing. In consultation with medical direction, they start an IV of normal saline, knowing that the fluid may counter any dehydration present and may help to loosen any excess mucus that may be blocking the bronchioles. Additionally, medical direction orders nebulizer administration of albuterol to relieve bronchoconstriction.

Monitoring of the patient en route to the hospital shows the effectiveness of these interventions. The patient's respirations slow to a normal rate and his oxygen saturation increases to 94 percent.

CONTENT SELF-EVALUATION

MULTIPLE CHOICE

_C_ 1. Which of the following is considered an intrinsic risk factor for respiratory disease?
A. smokestack pollutants   D. cigarette smoking
B. polluted water   E. stress
C. genetic predisposition

_A_ 2. The three processes that allow gas exchange to occur in the lungs and body tissues are:
A. ventilation, diffusion, perfusion.
B. inspiration, expiration, ventilation.
C. resistance, compliance, perfusion.
D. ventilation, inspiration, expiration.
E. inspiration, compliance, diffusion.

_A_ 3. The mechanical process of moving air in and out of the lungs is:
A. ventilation.   D. inspiration.
B. diffusion.   E. inhalation.
C. perfusion.

_D_ 4. The process by which gases move between the alveoli and the pulmonary capillaries is:
A. infusion.   D. diffusion.
B. perfusion.   E. permeation.
C. respiration.

_E_ 5. Lung perfusion is dependent on three factors—adequate blood volume, efficient pumping by the heart, and intact:
A. alveoli.   D. goblet cells.
B. respiratory membrane.   E. pulmonary ~~capillaries.~~ *arteries*
C. bronchioles.

_C_ 6. Any of the following can disrupt ventilation EXCEPT:
A. obstruction of the upper airway.
B. obstruction of the lower airway.
C. blockage of the pulmonary arteries.
D. impairment of normal function of the chest wall.
E. abnormalities of the nervous system's control of breathing.

_D_   **7.** Which of the following abnormal breathing patterns is characterized by long, deep breaths that are stopped during the inspiratory phase and separated by periods of apnea?
- **A.** ataxic (Biot's) respirations (seen with increased intracranial pressure)
- **B.** central neurogenic hyperventilation (seen with stroke or brainstem injury)
- **C.** Kussmaul's respirations (seen with metabolic acidosis)
- **D.** apneustic respirations (seen with stroke or severe central nervous system disease)
- **E.** Cheyne-Stokes respirations (seen with terminal illness or brain injury)

_B_   **8.** Which of the following is NOT likely to cause hypoxia (a supply of oxygen inadequate to meet the needs of the body's cells)?
- **A.** ascension to a high altitude
- **B.** esophageal ulceration
- **C.** black lung disease
- **D.** left-sided heart failure
- **E.** asbestos inhalation

_B_   **9.** Pulmonary shunting results from:
- **A.** alveolar collapse.
- **B.** blockage of pulmonary capillaries.
- **C.** bronchoconstriction.
- **D.** excess mucus production.
- **E.** airway obstruction.

_E_   **10.** The most important action when you arrive on scene and discover that a hazardous material is present is to:
- **A.** have supplemental oxygen available.
- **B.** remove the patient from the environment.
- **C.** search for additional patients.
- **D.** put on self-contained breathing apparatus.
- **E.** call for a hazardous materials team.

_B_   **11.** You are dispatched to a patient with difficulty breathing. Which of the following should be part of the scene size-up?
- **A.** Establish a patent airway.
- **B.** Look for clues to the possible cause.
- **C.** Evaluate AVPU mental status.
- **D.** Determine respiration rate.
- **E.** Ready the oxygenation equipment.

_A_   **12.** During the initial assessment, your general impression of the patient's respiratory status should include all of the following elements EXCEPT:
- **A.** pulse.
- **B.** position.
- **C.** color.
- **D.** mental status.
- **E.** ability to speak.

_C_   **13.** Which of the following is NOT a classic sign of respiratory distress?
- **A.** pursed lips
- **B.** tracheal tugging
- **C.** diaphoresis
- **D.** nasal flaring
- **E.** cyanosis

_B_   **14.** Which of the following is TRUE with regard to assessing the airway?
- **A.** Noisy breathing usually indicates a complete obstruction.
- **B.** Obstructed breathing is not always noisy breathing.
- **C.** If the airway is blocked, artificial respiration must be started immediately.
- **D.** If the airway is blocked, endotracheal intubation must be established.
- **E.** If the airway is open, the patient is breathing.

_A_   **15.** Which of the following is the MOST ominous sign of possible life-threatening respiratory distress?
- **A.** altered mental status
- **B.** audible stridor
- **C.** 1- to 2-word dyspnea
- **D.** tachycardia
- **E.** use of accessory muscles

©2004 Pearson Education, Inc.
Intermediate Emergency Care: Principles & Practice

_B_ 16. Orthopnea is:
   A. dizziness when rising from a supine position.
   B. dyspnea that occurs while lying supine.
   C. short attacks of dyspnea that interrupt sleep.
   D. apnea that occurs while in an upright position.
   E. pleuritic pain that occurs during breathing.

_A_ 17. Many respiratory complaints result from worsening of a long-standing disease the patient knows he has and can tell you about during the history. All of the following are such long-term respiratory diseases EXCEPT:
   A. pneumonia.   D. asthma.
   B. emphysema.   E. lung cancer.
   C. chronic bronchitis.

_C_ 18. Which of the following medications would be of LEAST significance if found in the home of a patient with a respiratory complaint?
   A. oxygen   D. corticosteroid
   B. bronchodilator   E. antibiotic
   C. vitamin C tablets

_A_ 19. Allergic reaction to a medication may be the cause of a respiratory complaint.
   A. True
   B. False

_E_ 20. A patient with significant respiratory distress may breathe through pursed lips. Breathing through pursed lips helps to:
   A. prevent tracheal collapse.
   B. force air past a bronchial obstruction.
   C. bring up excess mucus.
   D. close the epiglottis.
   E. keep the alveoli open.

_D_ 21. Pink or bloody sputum is commonly seen with any of the following EXCEPT:
   A. pulmonary edema.   D. allergic reaction.
   B. lung cancer.   E. bronchial infection.
   C. tuberculosis.

_D_ 22. Asymmetrical chest movement is most likely to be found during:
   A. auscultation.   D. inspection.
   B. capnometry.   E. percussion.
   C. oximetry.

_D_ 23. Subcutaneous emphysema is most likely to be found during:
   A. oximetry.   D. palpation.
   B. percussion.   E. inspection.
   C. capnometry.

_B_ 24. Wheezing is most likely to be detected during:
   A. oximetry.   D. capnometry.
   B. auscultation.   E. palpation.
   C. percussion.

_E_ 25. Rattling sounds in the larger airways associated with excess mucus are called:
   A. stridor.   D. snoring.
   B. wheezing.   E. rhonchi.
   C. crackles.

_B_ 26. A harsh, high-pitched sound heard on inspiration, associated with upper airway obstruction, is called:
   A. snoring.   D. rhonchi.
   B. stridor.   E. rales.
   C. crackles.

Medical Emergencies

_E_ 27. In general, tachycardia is a nonspecific finding seen, for example, with fear, anxiety, or fever. In a patient with a respiratory complaint, however, tachycardia may also indicate:
   A. hypothermia.   D. hyperopia.
   B. hypertrophy.   E. hypoxia.
   C. hypotension.

_D_ 28. Drugs that may cause an elevation in both heart rate and blood pressure include:
   A. diuretics such as furosemide.
   B. analgesics such as morphine sulfate.
   C. tranquilizers such as diazepam.
   D. sympathomimetics such as albuterol.
   E. beta blockers such as labetalol.

_C_ 29. An elevated respiratory rate in a patient with dyspnea is most likely caused by:
   A. bradycardia.   D. anemia.
   B. dysuria.   E. tachycardia.
   C. hypoxia.

_C_ 30. Which of the following measures end-expiratory carbon dioxide?
   A. spirometry   D. oximetry
   B. sphygmomanometry   E. tomography
   C. capnometry

_E_ 31. Two conditions in which respiration is frequently dependent on hypoxic respiratory drive and use of supplemental oxygen may induce respiratory depression are:
   A. asthma and pneumonia.
   B. spontaneous pneumothorax and pneumonia.
   C. asthma and emphysema.
   D. asthma and adult respiratory distress syndrome.
   E. chronic bronchitis and emphysema.

_C_ 32. The pulmonary edema characteristic of adult respiratory distress syndrome (ARDS) is caused by:
   A. left-sided cardiac ventricular failure.
   B. right-sided cardiac ventricular failure.
   C. accumulation of fluid in the pulmonary interstitial spaces.
   D. obstruction of pulmonary capillaries by thrombi.
   E. chronic constriction of terminal airways and alveoli.

_A_ 33. Factors that commonly cause acute aggravation of symptoms due to chronic obstructive pulmonary disease (COPD) include all of the following EXCEPT:
   A. progression of lung cancer.
   B. exertion, including heavy lifting and exercise.
   C. allergens such as foods and dust.
   D. tobacco smoke.
   E. occupational airborne pollutants such as chemical fumes.

_A_ 34. Common physical attributes of a person with emphysema include all of the following EXCEPT:
   A. chronic cough.   D. pinkish tone to skin.
   B. barrel chest.   E. thin build.
   C. clubbing of the fingers.

_B_ 35. Common physical attributes of a person with chronic bronchitis include all of the following EXCEPT:
   A. chronic cough.
   B. thin build.
   C. bluish, cyanotic tone to skin.
   D. cough producing large amounts of sputum.
   E. ankle edema.

©2004 Pearson Education, Inc.
Intermediate Emergency Care: Principles & Practice

_B_ 36. The epidemiology of asthma includes all of the following EXCEPT:
   A. an increase in mortality rate over the past decade.
   B. a death rate in whites that is roughly twice that in blacks.
   C. the fact that it is a common disorder in both males and females.
   D. mortality change seen mostly in persons over age 45 years.
   E. the fact that half of asthma deaths occur in the prehospital setting.

_B_ 37. Medications commonly used by persons with asthma include all of the following EXCEPT:
   A. beta agonists administered via inhaler.
   B. oral doses of aspirin.
   C. anticholinergics administered via inhaler.
   D. oral doses of corticosteroid.
   E. cromolyn sodium administered via inhaler.

_D_ 38. The chief management goals for an acute asthma attack involve improvement in:
   A. blood pH (acidosis), hypoxia, and wheezing.
   B. hypoxia, bronchospasm, and wheezing.
   C. blood pH (acidosis), hypoxia, and local inflammation.
   D. hypoxia, bronchospasm, and local inflammation.
   E. hypoxia, wheezing, and local inflammation.

_D_ 39. Be prepared for which of the following when caring for a patient with status asthmaticus?
   A. respiratory acidosis with electrolyte imbalance
   B. dehydration with early signs of renal failure
   C. respiratory depression when administered supplemental oxygen
   D. respiratory arrest requiring endotracheal intubation
   E. tracheal inflammation causing airway obstruction

_B_ 40. Upper respiratory infections can affect all of the following EXCEPT:
   A. the sinuses.   D. the nose.
   B. the lungs.   E. the pharynx.
   C. the middle ear.

_B_ 41. Pleuritic chest pain associated with pneumonia is:
   A. dull and aching in character.
   B. sharp or tearing in character.
   C. cramplike and hard to localize.
   D. likely to radiate to the jaw or left arm.
   E. only present on deep inspiration.

_A_ 42. Major risk factors for pneumonia are HIV infection, very young or very old, and immunosuppressive therapy.
   A. True
   B. False

_B_ 43. Standard management of lung cancer includes all of the following EXCEPT:
   A. checking for instructions such as DNR (do not resuscitate) orders.
   B. placement of ECG leads for cardiac monitoring.
   C. administration of supplemental oxygen.
   D. airway and ventilatory support as needed.
   E. emotional support of patient and family.

_A_ 44. Roughly one in five cases of sudden death is due to pulmonary emboli.
   A. True
   B. False

_B_ 45. The mortality rate for pulmonary emboli is greater than 50%.
   A. True
   B. False

Medical Emergencies

_A_ 46. Risk factors for pulmonary emboli include all of the following EXCEPT:
   A. obesity.
   B. pregnancy.
   C. prolonged immobilization.
   D. deep vein thrombophlebitis.
   E. use of oral contraceptives, especially in smokers.

_A_ 47. The ventilation-perfusion mismatch characteristic of pulmonary embolism is due to loss of blood flow to a ventilated segment of lung tissue.
   A. True
   B. False

_B_ 48. Common physical findings in pulmonary embolism include all of the following EXCEPT:
   A. evidence suggestive of deep venous thrombosis.
   B. labored, painful breathing.
   C. tachypnea and tachycardia.
   D. cardiac dysrhythmias.
   E. normal chest auscultation.

_C_ 49. Which of the following statements about spontaneous pneumothorax is FALSE?
   A. Most patients have acute onset pain in the chest or shoulder region.
   B. Onset of pain often follows coughing or heavy lifting.
   C. Spontaneous pneumothorax is much more common in women than in men.
   D. Spontaneous pneumothorax is more common among smokers and persons with COPD.
   E. Supplemental oxygen is sufficient therapy for the majority of patients with spontaneous pneumothorax.

_A_ 50. The respiratory alkalosis of hyperventilation syndrome often results in:
   A. cramping of the muscles of the hands and feet.
   B. slowing of cardiac electrical conduction, causing bradycardia.
   C. cramping of facial muscles causing characteristic grimace.
   D. one of several cardiac dysrhythmias.
   E. altered mental status, specifically, lethargy and depression.

_A_ 51. Respiratory emergencies due to central nervous system (CNS) dysfunction are relatively rare.
   A. True
   B. False

_A_ 52. Numerous peripheral nervous system conditions can cause respiratory compromise, including the diseases of polio and amyotrophic lateral sclerosis, as well as Guillian-Barré syndrome.
   A. True
   B. False

_C_ 53. The processes of ventilation, diffusion, and perfusion allow gas exchange to occur efficiently in the lungs and other body tissues. The derangement in pulmonary embolism is principally of:
   A. ventilation.
   B. diffusion.
   C. perfusion.
   D. a combination of ventilation and diffusion.
   E. a combination of diffusion and perfusion.

_B_ 54. Carbon monoxide exposure is potentially life threatening because carbon monoxide displaces oxygen from hemoglobin in red blood cells.
   ✳ A. True
   B. False

©2004 Pearson Education, Inc.
Intermediate Emergency Care: Principles & Practice

_D_ 55. The most common auscultation finding in a patient with pneumonia is:
   A. stridor over the involved segment.
   B. decreased or absent breath sounds over the involved segment.
   C. expiratory wheezing over the involved segment.
   D. crackles (rales) over the involved segment.
   E. pleural friction rub over the involved segment.

MATCHING

Match each respiratory emergency with its key prehospital management steps by writing the letter of the steps in the space provided next to the emergency.

_C_ 56. adult respiratory distress syndrome (ARDS)

_F_ 57. chronic obstructive pulmonary disease (COPD), either emphysema or chronic bronchitis

_A_ 58. asthma

_E_ 59. childhood epiglottitis

_G_ 60. lung cancer

_B_ 61. inhalation of a toxic substance

_D_ 62. pulmonary embolism

A. correct hypoxia, reverse bronchospasm, and reduce inflammation
B. ensure safety of rescue personnel, remove patient for transport, maintain open airway, and deliver humidified, high-concentration oxygen
C. maintain airway and ventilation as needed, deliver oxygen, establish IV access, cardiac monitoring, and pulse oximetry, and transport to facility for care of underlying condition
D. maintain airway, ventilation, and circulation as needed, deliver oxygen, establish IV access, cardiac monitoring, and pulse oximetry, and check extremities during transport to appropriate facility
E. maintain airway and ventilation as needed with exception that examination of the throat should be avoided
F. relieve hypoxia, reverse bronchoconstriction, assist ventilations as needed
G. deliver oxygen, support ventilation as allowed by orders or advance directive, correct hypoxia as possible, and provide emotional support

Medical Emergencies

LABEL THE DIAGRAMS

Supply the missing labels for the drawing of the upper airway by writing the appropriate letters in the spaces provided.

A. Cricoid cartilage
B. Cricothyroid membrane
C. Epiglottis
D. Esophagus
E. Glottic opening
F. Thyroid cartilage
G. Tongue
H. Tonsils and adenoids

I. Trachea
J. Turbinates
K. LARYNGOPHARYNX
L. LARYNX
M. NASAL CAVITY
N. NASOPHARYNX
O. OROPHARYNX

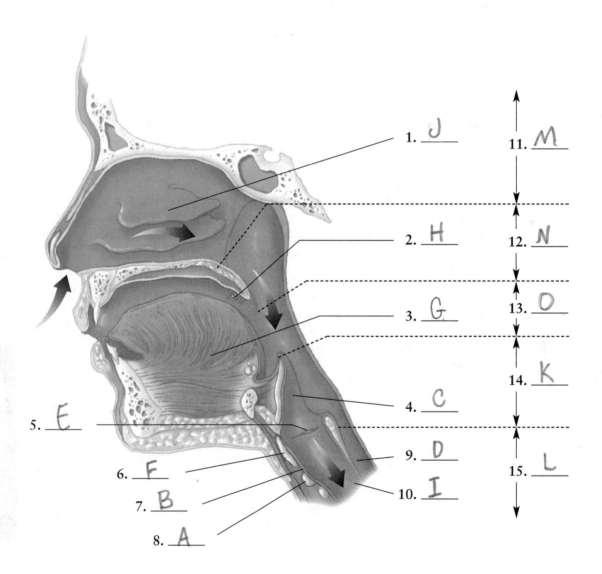

1. _J_   11. _M_

2. _H_   12. _N_

3. _G_   13. _O_

4. _C_   14. _K_

5. _E_

6. _F_   9. _D_   15. _L_

7. _B_   10. _I_

8. _A_

page 201

Supply the missing labels for the drawing of the lower airway by writing the appropriate letters in the spaces provided.

A. Carina
B. Larynx
C. Left mainstem bronchus
D. Right mainstem bronchus
E. Trachea

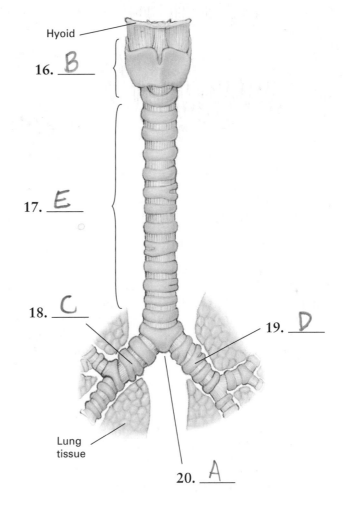

Hyoid

16. __B__

17. __E__

18. __C__

19. __D__

Lung tissue

20. __A__

SPECIAL PROJECT

Evaluating Abnormal Breathing Patterns

On the line provided, write the name of each abnormal breathing pattern illustrated below.

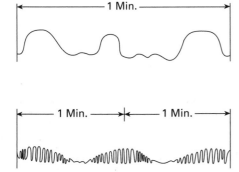

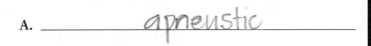

A. _____ apneustic

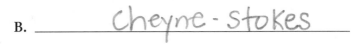

B. _____ Cheyne-stokes

C. _cnh_

D. _kussmals_

E. _Biot's_

Read the following three scenarios about patients who present with abnormal breathing patterns. On the lines—on the basis of the brief information given—write the name of the breathing pattern the patient seems to display and the condition (or conditions, if you think there is more than one possibility) you think is most likely causing the abnormal breathing pattern. (You must decide which three of the five patterns illustrated above are represented in the scenarios.) Review the text, pages 805–807, for help in completing your answers.

Scenario 1: You are called to the home of an elderly woman who is unresponsive. Her family tells you she had her ninetieth birthday last month but has been bedridden for two weeks and has "not been doing very well." Today, they have not been able to rouse her. On assessment, you find that the patient is breathing in a pattern of progressively increasing tidal volume, followed by progressively declining volume, separated by periods of apnea.

Breathing pattern: _Cheyne-Stokes_   **Probable cause:** _terminal disease_

Scenario 2: You are called to a local fitness center where a middle-aged man who was participating in an exercise class suddenly complained of a terrible headache. He lurched sideways, then sat down hard on the exercise mat. By the time you arrive, he has lost consciousness. When you assess his breathing, you find repeated sets of gasping ventilations separated by periods of apnea.

Breathing pattern: _biots_   **Probable cause:** _Stroke_

Scenario 3: You are dispatched to a downtown office where the billing manager has fallen ill. You find her slumped on a sofa in the women's restroom. She has an altered mental status and is barely coherent. A medical ID bracelet identifies her as a diabetic. A co-worker says that she has been diabetic since childhood and takes insulin by injection but has lately been neglecting to take her injections regularly. Her respirations are deep and rapid.

Breathing pattern: _kussmaul's_   **Probable cause:** _DKA_

©2004 Pearson Education, Inc.
Intermediate Emergency Care: Principles & Practice

CHAPTER 20

*

Cardiovascular Emergencies

Part 1: Cardiovascular Anatomy and Physiology, ECG Monitoring, and Dysrhythmia Analysis

Review of Chapter Objectives

Because Chapter 20 is lengthy, it has been divided into two parts to aid in your study. Read the assigned text pages, then progress through the objectives and self-evaluation materials as you would with other chapters. When you feel secure in your grasp of the content, proceed to the next part.

After reading this part of the chapter, you should be able to:

1. **Describe the incidence, morbidity, and mortality of cardiovascular disease.**   pp. 838–839

   Cardiovascular disease (CVD) is serious and extremely common, with more than 60 million Americans affected. Morbidity is considerable: An American has a nonfatal heart attack (myocardial infarction, MI) roughly every 29 seconds. Coronary heart disease (CHD), one type of CVD, is the single largest killer of Americans and Canadians. Roughly 466,000 Americans die annually from CHD, half of them before reaching a hospital. Many deaths from CHD are sudden and involve lethal cardiac dysrhythmias. Many deaths from MI occur within the first 24 hours, frequently within the first hour.

2. **Review cardiovascular anatomy and physiology.**   pp. 839–843; see Chapter 2

   Cardiac anatomy and physiology were discussed in detail in Chapter 2. The adult heart is the size of a clenched fist and lies in the center of the mediastinum posterior to the sternum and anterior to the spine. It is a muscular organ, with three tissue layers: endocardium, or innermost layer that lines the chambers; the myocardium, or middle layer with its unique ability to generate and conduct electrical impulses causing the heart to contract; and the pericardium, which is a protective sac surrounding the heart. Normally, about 25 mL of pericardial fluid is contained between the two layers of pericardium, and the heart can move freely within the pericardial sac.

   The heart contains four chambers, two superior, the atria, and two inferior, the ventricles. Valves control the flow of blood through the heart. The mitral valve is between the left atrium and ventricle; the tricuspid valve is between the left ventricle and aorta and the pulmonary valve between the right ventricle and the pulmonary artery.

   The right atrium receives deoxygenated blood from the body via the superior and inferior venae cava. The right ventricle sends the deoxygenated blood to the lungs via the pulmonary artery. Oxygenated blood is returned from the lungs to the left atrium via the pulmonary veins. The left ventricle pumps the oxygenated blood to the body via the aorta. Oxygenated blood is pumped from the heart to the tissues via the arteries, and deoxygenated blood is transported from the tissues back to the heart via the veins. The capillaries connect arteries and veins. The exchange of oxygen and carbon dioxide with the body tissues takes place through the very thin capillary walls.

The heart receives its nutrients from the coronary arteries that originate in the aorta and spread over the heart. The left coronary artery supplies the left ventricles, interventricular septum, part of the right ventricle, and the conduction system. Its two main branches are the anterior descending artery and circumflex artery. The right coronary artery supplies a portion of the right atrium and right ventricle and part of the conduction system. Its two major branches are the posterior descending artery and marginal artery.

The cardiac cycle consists of diastole, the relaxation phase that takes place at the end of a cardiac contraction, and systole, the contraction phase. Normally when the heart contracts, each ventricle ejects about two thirds of its blood, which is about 70 mL. This volume is known as the ejection fraction or the stroke volume and it depends on three factors: preload, cardiac contractility, and afterload. Preload is the end-diastolic volume and influences the force of the next contraction because of the stretch it exerts. Frank Starling's law of the heart states that the more myocardial muscle is stretched, the greater its force of contraction will be. Afterload is the resistance against which the heart muscle must pump. An increase in peripheral vascular resistance will decrease stroke volume.

Cardiac output is calculated as stroke volume times the heart rate. Since the normal heart rate is 60–100 beats per minute and the average stroke volume is 70 mL, the average cardiac output is about 5 liters per minute (70 mL $\times$ 70 bpm = 4,900 mL/min).

The heart function is regulated by the sympathetic and parasympathetic nervous components of the autonomic nervous system, working in opposition to one another to maintain a balance. During stress, the sympathetic system dominates to raise the heart rate and increase contractile force. During sleep, the parasympathetic system dominates to decrease heart rate and contractile force. The autonomic control of the heart is defined by three terms: chronotropy or rate, inotropy or contractile strength, and dromotropy or rate of impulse conduction. Lastly, the cardiac function depends heavily on electrolyte balances. Electrolytes that affect cardiac function include sodium, potassium, chloride, and magnesium.

3. **Discuss prevention strategies that may reduce the morbidity and mortality of cardiovascular disease.** pp. 838–839

There are two public health prevention strategies. The first is to educate people about the risk factors for CVD and encourage lifestyle modifications to minimize the potential impact of risk factors. The second strategy is to teach signs and symptoms of a heart attack so patients can receive medical intervention as soon as possible. As you will see, the likelihood of success with thrombolytic therapy for a heart attack in evolution (treatment with a clot-buster drug to dissolve the clot causing myocardial ischemia/hypoxia) is highest when care is instituted very early in the course of the attack.

4. **Identify the risk factors most predisposing to coronary artery disease.** pp. 838–839

Factors proven to increase the risk of CVD include (1) smoking, (2) older age, (3) family history of cardiac disease, (4) hypertension, (5) hypercholesterolemia, (6) diabetes mellitus, (7) cocaine use, and (8) male gender. Factors that are thought to increase risk include (1) diet, (2) obesity, (3) oral contraceptives, (4) sedentary lifestyle, (5) Type A personality (competitive and aggressive), and (6) psychosocial tension (stress).

5. **Explain the purpose of ECG monitoring and its limitations.** pp. 843–855

The electrocardiogram (*electro* = electrical, *cardio* = heart, *gram* = record) visualizes the heart's electrical activity as recorded from skin-surface electrodes. The heart is the largest generator of electrical energy in the body, and this is conducted through the body to the skin. An ECG machine records changes in current as a positive impulse (shown on the machine or on a paper printout as an upward deflection), a negative impulse (shown as a downward deflection), or no change (a flat, isoelectric line). The pattern shown over time is a chronological record of the heart's electrical activity, and it is called a rhythm strip.

The ECG in no way assesses the contractility of the myocardium or the pumping ability of the left ventricle, only the electrical activity in the different regions of the heart. There are other limitations of ECG monitoring. Artifacts may occur on the tracing, deflections that do NOT reflect the electrical activity of the heart. Artifacts may be due to a variety of causes, including muscle tremor, shivering, movements by the patient, loose electrodes, interference at the 60-hertz range, and machine malfunction. It is important that you be able to recognize artifacts and try to eliminate them from the tracing.

6. Describe how ECG wave forms are produced and correlate the electrophysiological and hemodynamic events occurring throughout the entire cardiac cycle with the various ECG wave forms, segments, and intervals. pp. 843–855

The components of an ECG tracing reflect the electrical changes in the heart with each impulse conducted through the heart:

- *P wave.* This first component of the ECG reflects atrial depolarization. On Lead II, it appears as a positive, rounded wave that comes before the QRS complex. Normally, this correlates hemodynamically with the opening of the AV valves and atrial contraction, which completes the filling of the ventricles with blood.
- *QRS complex.* This second component of the ECG reflects ventricular depolarization. The Q wave is the initial negative deflection after the P wave; the R wave is the first positive deflection after the P wave; and the S wave is the first negative deflection after the R wave. You should note that not all three waves need be present, and the shape of the QRS complex can vary among individuals. Normally, this correlates hemodynamically with the opening of the semilunar valves and ventricular contraction, pumping blood into the pulmonary arteries and aorta.
- *T wave.* The T wave, which follows the QRS complex, reflects repolarization of the ventricles. It is normally positive in Lead II, rounded, and moves in the same direction as the QRS complex. This is the correlate of ventricular relaxation after contraction.
- *U wave.* A U wave is an occasional finding; when it occurs, it follows the T wave and is usually positive in deflection. U waves are normal in some individuals. You should note that it reflects electrolyte abnormalities in other patients.

In addition, three time intervals and a segment of the ECG reading also have clinical significance:

- *P-R interval (called PRI or P-Q interval, PQI).* The P-R interval is the distance from the beginning of the P wave (the beginning of atrial depolarization) to the beginning of the QRS complex (the beginning of ventricular depolarization). It represents the time taken to send the impulse from the atria to the ventricles (the delay at the AV junction and node). The R wave is absent in some individuals, and in these patients you will see a P-Q interval instead. The terms PRI and PQI are used interchangeably.
- *QRS interval.* The QRS interval is the distance from the first deflection of the QRS complex to the last, and it represents the time necessary for ventricular depolarization and onset of ventricular contraction.
- *Q-T interval.* This is the distance from the beginning of the Q wave to the beginning of the T wave, and it represents the total duration of ventricular depolarization. The duration of the Q-T interval normally has an inverse relationship with heart rate. At increased heart rates (tachycardia), the Q-T interval is generally shortened. With bradycardia, Q-T interval is generally lengthened.
- *S-T segment.* This is the distance from the S wave to the beginning of the T wave, and generally it is isoelectric. In some states such as myocardial ischemia, this segment may be either elevated or depressed.

7. Identify how heart rates may be determined from ECG recordings. pp. 844–846

ECG graph paper is standardized such that paper always moves across the recording stylus at 22 mm/sec. (Each small box represents 0.04 second, and each large box is equivalent to five small boxes, or 0.20 second.) ECG paper also has time interval markings at the top of the paper, with marks placed at 3-second intervals (or 15 large boxes, 15 × 0.20 = 3.0 seconds).

Three methods exist for quickly establishing heart rate. First, if a patient has a regular rhythm, you can take the number of heartbeats in 6 seconds, multiply by 10, and get rate in beats per minute (bpm). Second, you can measure the R-R interval (also in a patient with a regular rhythm) in seconds, divide into 60, and you have heart rate per minute. If the R-R interval is 0.65 second, 60 ÷ 0.65 = 92 bpm. (Other methods using the R-R interval are described on text page 854) The triplicate method, also useful only in the case of a regular rhythm, requires you to find an R wave that falls on a dark line bordering a large box. You can then assign numbers corresponding to heart rate to the next six dark lines to the right: This equates to 300, 150, 100, 75, 60, and 50 bpm. The number corresponding to the dark line closest to the peak of the next R wave is a rough estimate of heart rate. Last, you can use a commercial heart rate calculator ruler. If you prefer this method, make sure you are comfortable with at least one alternative method that does not require a physical aid!

8. Describe a systematic approach to the analysis and interpretation of cardiac dysrhythmias. pp. 855–897

The following characterize normal sinus rhythm: (1) heart rate between 60 and 100 bpm; (2) regular rhythm, with constant P-P and R-R intervals; (3) P waves that are normal in shape, upright, and appear only before each QRS complex; (4) P-R interval that is constant and lasting 0.12–0.20 second; and (5) QRS complex with normal shape and duration less than 0.12 second. Any deviation from the normal electrical rhythm constitutes a dysrhythmia. The term arrhythmia is properly reserved for states in which there is no cardiac electrical activity.

Dysrhythmias can be approached in a number of ways, including nature of origin (namely, changes in automaticity versus disturbances in conduction), magnitude (major versus minor), severity (life-threatening versus non-life-threatening), and site (or location) of origin. This book classifies dysrhythmias into six categories by origin: (1) dysrhythmias originating in the SA node; (2) dysrhythmias originating in the atria; (3) dysrhythmias originating within the AV junction; (4) dysrhythmias sustained or originating in the AV junction; (5) dysrhythmias originating in the ventricles; (6) dysrhythmias resulting from disorders of conduction.

9. Explain how to confirm asystole using more than one-lead. pp. 890–891

On each lead, you should see an absence of all cardiac electrical activity: There will be no discernible components of the ECG sequence (no P waves, QRS complexes, or T waves).

10. List the clinical indications for defibrillation pp. 890–891

Asystole (cardiac standstill) is the absence of all cardiac electrical activity, usually associated with massive myocardial infraction, ischemia, and necrosis. Treat asystole with CPR, airway management, oxygenation, and medications. If you have any doubt about underlying rhythm, attempt defibrillation. Always check for evidence that you should not attempt resuscitation (e.g., DNAR order, signs of death?).

11. Identify the specific mechanical, pharmacological, and electrical therapeutic interventions for patients with dysrhythmias causing compromise. pp. 855–897

- *Sinus bradycardia.* The overall goal of treatment is satisfactory heart rate, with subsequently adequate cardiac output and blood pressure and decreased risk of more dangerous dysrhythmias. Thus, treatment is based on symptoms, and no treatment may be needed unless hypotension or ventricular irritability is present. If treatment is needed, give a 0.5 mg bolus atropine sulfate, and repeat every 3–5 minutes until rate is satisfactory or you have given 0.04 mg/kg atropine. If atropine fails, consider transcutaneous cardiac pacing (TCP), if available.
- *Sinus tachycardia.* Treatment is directed at the underlying cause. Hypovolemia, fever, anemia, or other cause should be corrected. The overall goal is to reduce heart rate to a level compatible with adequate ventricular filling time, with supports in place to maintain an adequate stroke volume.
- *Sinus dysrhythmia.* Sinus dysrhythmia is a normal variant, particularly in the young and aged. Treatment is thus typically not required.
- *Sinus arrest.* If the patient is extremely bradycardic or symptomatic, give a 0.5 mg bolus atropine sulfate. The goal of pharmacologic therapy is to bring rate up to a level where symptoms are eliminated because cardiac output is adequate.

- *First-degree AV block.* Treatment is generally restricted to observation unless heart rate drops significantly. If possible, avoid administration of any drug that will further slow AV conduction, such as lidocaine and procainamide. The goal of treatment, if needed, is to preserve or improve AV conduction, eliminating the risk of development of a higher degree of heart block. When necessary, treatment may be needed to increase heart rate to a level compatible with adequate cardiac output.
- *Type I second-degree AV block* (also termed *second-degree Mobitz I* or *Wenckebach*). Treatment is generally restricted to observation. If possible, you want to avoid administration of any drug that will further slow AV conduction, such as lidocaine and procainamide. If heart rate falls and the patient becomes symptomatic, give 0.5 mg atropine IV. Repeat every 3–5 minutes until rate is satisfactory or you have given 0.04 mg/kg of atropine. If atropine fails, consider TCP if available. Overall goal is preservation or improvement of AV conduction and maintenance of a heart rate associated with adequate cardiac output.
- *Type II second-degree AV block* (also called *second-degree Mobitz II* or *infranodal block*). Definitive treatment is pacemaker insertion to preserve a normal rhythm and adequate cardiac output. In the prehospital setting, give medications if needed to stabilize the patient. Use caution in giving atropine to patients with second-degree Mobitz II blocks because the atropine may increase atrial rate but also worsen the AV nodal block. Consider TCP if available. If the patient remains symptomatic, do not delay application of TCP while waiting for IV access or time for atropine to take affect.
- *Third-degree AV block.* Definitive treatment is pacemaker insertion to preserve adequate cardiac output. In the prehospital setting, give medications if needed to stabilize patient. Use caution in giving atropine to patients with third-degree blocks because the atropine may increase atrial rate but also worsen the AV nodal block. Consider TCP if available. If the patient remains symptomatic, do not delay application of TCP while waiting for IV access or time for atropine to take affect. NEVER use lidocaine to treat third-degree block with ventricular escape beats.
- *Premature junctional contractions (PJCs).* Treatment is restricted to observation if the patient is asymptomatic.
- *Junctional escape rhythm.* Treatment in the field is generally restricted to observation (as patients are asymptomatic); however, care is needed if hypotension or ventricular irritability is present. If needed, give 0.5 mg bolus atropine, and repeat every 3–5 minutes until rate is satisfactory or you've given 0.04 mg/kg atropine. If atropine fails, consider TCP if available. Overall goal is preservation of cardiac output and blood pressure and prevention of more dangerous ventricular dysrhythmias.
- *Accelerated junctional rhythm.* Treatment goal is to correct ischemia.
- *Paroxysmal junctional tachycardia (PJT).* Treatment in the patient who is not tolerating PJT, as evidenced by hemodynamic instability, consists of the following sequence of steps. (1) Vagal maneuvers. (2) Therapy with adenosine (Adenocard), followed by verapamil if rate does not respond and there are no contraindications to verapamil. Verapamil should not be used with beta blockers. Verapamil-induced hypotension can often be reversed with 0.5–1.0 gm calcium chloride IV. (3) Electrical therapy with synchronized cardioversion if ventricular rate is higher than 150 bpm or patient is hemodynamically unstable. If time allows, use presedation. Apply synchronized DC countershock of 100 joules. Remember that DC countershock is contraindicated if digitalis toxicity is suspected. The overall goal is to reach a heart rate compatible with adequate ventricular filling time and good cardiac output, as well as to ensure adequate coronary artery perfusion.
- *Atrial tachycardia.* Treatment options for symptomatic patients include consideration of adenosine or verapamil to lower heart rate and prevent other dysrhythmias, including atrial fibrillation.
- *Multifocal atrial tachycardia.* Treatment of the underlying medical condition usually resolves the dysrhythmia. Specific antidysrhythmic therapy is usually not needed.
- *Premature atrial contractions (PACs).* Treatment for the symptomatic patient is oxygen via nonrebreather mask and establishment of IV access, along with consultation with medical direction. Field goal is to maintain tissue oxygenation and prepare for possible development of other, more clinically significant dysrhythmias.

Medical Emergencies

- *Paroxysmal supraventricular tachycardia (PSVT)*. Treatment for patients who are not tolerating the rapid heart rate, as evidenced by hemodynamic instability, should consist of the following series of techniques: (1) Vagal maneuvers. Note that carotid sinus massage should not be done in patients with carotid bruits or known cerebrovascular or carotid artery disease. (2) Pharmacological therapy with adenosine IV. If this fails and patient has normal blood pressure and a narrow QRS complex, consider use of verapamil if no contraindications exist. (3) Electrical therapy with synchronized cardioversion. DC countershock is contraindicated when digitalis toxicity is suspected. The overall goal is attainment of heart rate compatible with adequate cardiac output and coronary perfusion.
- *Atrial flutter*. Treatment is indicated for cases with rapid ventricular rates and hemodynamic compromise. Immediate cardioversion is indicated in unstable patients. Occasionally, you may use pharmacological therapy with stable patients, especially if the rapid ventricular rate is causing congestive heart failure. Several medications slow ventricular rate, including diltiazem (Cardizem), verapamil, digitalis, beta blockers, procainamide, and quinidine. Procainamide and quinidine are often used to convert back to sinus rhythm. Consult local medical direction for protocol specifics.
- *Atrial fibrillation*. Prehospital treatment is necessary when rapid ventricular rates with hemodynamic instability occur. Electrical therapy with immediate cardioversion is required in unstable patients—persons with heart rates greater than 150 bpm and associated chest pain, dyspnea, decreased level of consciousness, or hypotension. Pharmacological therapy may be useful, especially when rapid heart rate is causing congestive heart failure. Drugs that may be used include diltiazem, verapamil, digitalis, beta blockers, procainamide, and quinidine. Atrial fibrillation is a documented risk factor for stroke because atrial dilation allows for stagnation of blood and development of clots. You may wish to consider administration of an anticoagulant. Consult medical direction for specifics of possible pharmacological options. Immediate treatment goal is improvement of cardiac output. (Ultimate goal is adjustment of digitalis level, if toxicity is cause.)

    Patients with accessory pathways such as those with Wolff-Parkinson-White who develop atrial flutter or atrial fibrillation present special concerns. Verapamil, which decreases conduction through the AV node and may shorten the refractory period of the accessory path, may precipitate either ventricular tachycardia or ventricular fibrillation.
- *Ventricular escape rhythms*. Treatment depends on whether the rhythm is perfusing or not. If perfusing, the goal is to increase heart rate with atropine or, if it fails, TCP if available. With a nonperfusing rhythm, follow your pulseless electrical activity (PEA) protocol, including airway stabilization and CPR and IV epinephrine. Direct treatment is aimed at the primary problem, such as hypovolemia, hypoxia, cardiac tamponade, acidosis, or other. Consider a fluid challenge.
- *Accelerated idioventricular rhythm*. This is a subtype of ventricular escape rhythm and is an abnormally wide ventricular dysrhythmia typically associated with an acute MI. The rate is usually 60–110 bpm, and the patient does not require treatment unless hemodynamic instability is present, in which case the ventricular focus should be treated with atropine or overdrive pacing. The principal goal is treatment of the underlying MI.
- *Premature ventricular contractions (PVCs)*. Treatment is indicated for patients with a prior history of heart disease or symptoms or if the PVCs are malignant. Administer oxygen and establish IV access. If the patient is symptomatic, give lidocaine at a dose of 1.0–1.5 mg/kg body weight. Give an additional bolus of 0.5–0.75 mg/kg every 5–10 minutes as needed until a total of 3.0 mg/kg has been reached. If PVCs are effectively suppressed, start a lidocaine drip at a rate of 2–4 mg/minute. Reduce dose in appropriate patients, and consider procainamide or bretylium if the ceiling dose of lidocaine has been reached or the patient is allergic to lidocaine. Overall goal is adequate ventricular filling and cardiac output and prevention of ventricular tachycardia or ventricular fibrillation.
- *Ventricular tachycardia (VT)*. Treatment type depends on whether VT is perfusing or nonperfusing. If there is a pulse (perfusing VT), give oxygen and place an IV line. Give lidocaine IV at 1.0–1.5 mg/kg and additional doses of 0.5–0.75 mg/kg up to a total of 3.0 mg/kg. If unsuccessful, try procainamide or amiodarone as a second-line agent. Instability (namely, chest pain, dyspnea, or systolic BP less than 90 mmHg) calls for synchronized cardioversion. If you note

©2004 Pearson Education, Inc.
Intermediate Emergency Care: Principles & Practice

instability at the outset of treatment, such as falling blood pressure or altered level of consciousness, initiate cardioversion immediately after starting oxygen and an IV. If there is no pulse (nonperfusing VT), treat as for ventricular fibrillation. Treatment goals are to maintain adequacy of cardiac output and coronary artery perfusion and to prevent ventricular fibrillation.

- *Ventricular fibrillation.* Treatment of ventricular fibrillation and nonperfusing VT is the same: Initiate CPR and follow with DC countershock at 200 joules. If unsuccessful, repeat at 200–300 joules; if still unsuccessful, try at 360 joules. Subsequent to countershock, control airway and establish IV access. Epinephrine 1:10,000 is the drug of first choice; give every 3–5 minutes as needed. If unsuccessful, consider second-line agents such as lidocaine, bretylium, amiodarone, procainamide, or even magnesium sulfate.
- *Asystole* (or *cardiac standstill*). Treatment is CPR, airway management, oxygenation, and medication. If there is any doubt of an underlying rhythm, attempt defibrillation.

CASE STUDY REVIEW

This case study demonstrates how EMT-Is react to a typical medical emergency involving chest pain. In addition to observing how the team conducts the patient's initial assessment, note how they respond as the situation quickly changes into a more complex and urgent one.

David and Bart are called to a nursing home to evaluate a man with chest pain. You aren't told if they are given any additional information or if any sense of urgency is conveyed, but a call for chest pain in an adult should always bring differential diagnoses to mind. Cardiac conditions, including angina and acute MI, are at the top of the list.

They find an 80-year-old man who has been in the emotionally stressful situation of a large family gathering and who has developed substernal chest pain that radiates to the left arm. Staff who are present immediately add some useful information: Mr. Henry has a history of this type of pain, but it typically resolves with nitroglycerin. Pain has not subsided today, and so the staff activated EMS. At this point, the possibility of an acute MI becomes quite marked.

The EMT-Is immediately place Mr. Henry on supplementary oxygen, connect him to a cardiac monitor, and establish IV access. They take the time to do a focused history and begin an exam when Mr. Henry screams and collapses. You don't know if Bart had a chance to take a peripheral pulse or listen to Mr. Henry's heart, so you don't have any information about the patient's heart rate or rhythm when the team came, but the change in condition is unmistakable. After his collapse, Mr. Henry is unresponsive, apneic, and pulseless. The monitor shows coarse ventricular fibrillation. He is in cardiac arrest.

The protocol for cardiac arrest is immediately begun. David charges the defibrillator (note that it was on-scene and ready) and delivers a 200-joule charge. The rhythm does not change, and a second charge of 300 joules is delivered. Because the patient remains in ventricular fibrillation, a third charge of 360 joules is delivered. You aren't told whether CPR is performed between defibrillation attempts, but you can assume this was done because a note is made that CPR is continued when the additional crew arrives within 2 minutes of the time Mr. Henry went down.

At this time, with more people and (probably) more equipment at the ready, management can become more comprehensive, and it does. An endotracheal tube (ET) is placed for airway control, and the patient is ventilated with 100% oxygen. The clear bilateral lung sounds and end-tidal CO_2 detector not only confirm ET placement but also indicate pulmonary function is adequate. (There is no evidence of pulmonary edema.) Epinephrine is given IV and a fourth shock is delivered. After this, the patient's heart assumes a slow idioventricular rhythm that improves to sinus tachycardia with a weak but palpable peripheral pulse. As the pulse becomes stronger, chest compressions are stopped. The patient's condition continues to spontaneously improve as systolic blood pressure rises to 110 mmHg.

The complication for which you always need to be ready in the setting of an acute MI or resuscitation from a cardiac arrest is dysrhythmia, and this is seen with Mr. Henry. Even as his clinical condition improves, the ongoing scan of the cardiac monitor shows ectopy: a few premature ventricular contractions (PVCs). This is promptly addressed by administration of a lidocaine bolus followed by IV drip. Mechanical ventilation continues, and the patient is readied for transport.

Medical Emergencies

During transport, the patient's condition continues to improve. Not only does he have an acceptable heart rhythm without PVCs, but he begins to breathe on his own as well. At this point, he has moved from complete loss of airway, breathing, and circulation (the state at the outset of his cardiac arrest) to a controlled airway and spontaneous breathing and circulation. You don't know what report is given to the receiving team, but you do know it will include the following information: the minimal down time between collapse and institution of resuscitation, details about the duration of ventricular fibrillation, and the history of vitals (including cardiac rhythm) from time of cardioconversion to arrival at the emergency department.

You should note one other thing about this case study. The team was able to provide appropriate care in timely fashion and with good result without actually treating the underlying cause, the acute MI. This case study serves as a reminder that you should always treat life-threatening problems as they occur and defer other matters such as field diagnosis until the patient is stable or the emergency department is reached. Familiarity with the algorithms for care of various cardiac emergencies, including cardiac arrest, will help you to reflexively do the correct thing in emergency situations such as the one with Mr. Henry.

CONTENT SELF-EVALUATION

MULTIPLE CHOICE

A   1. From innermost to outermost, the three tissue layers of the heart are:
  A. the endocardium, the pericardium, and the myocardium.
  B. the endocardium, the myocardium, and the syncytium.
  C. the endocardium, the myocardium, and the pericardium.
  D. the myocardium, the epicardium, and the pericardium.
  E. the epicardium, the myocardium, and the endocardium.

D   2. The blood supply to the left ventricle, interventricular septum, part of the right ventricle, and the heart's conduction system comes from the two branches of the left coronary artery, which are the:
  A. anterior descending artery and the circumflex artery.
  B. anterior descending artery and the posterior descending artery.
  C. circumflex artery and the posterior descending artery.
  D. circumflex artery and the marginal artery.
  E. marginal artery and the posterior descending artery.

E   3. Stimulation of the heart by the sympathetic nervous system results in:
  A. negative inotropic and chronotropic effects.
  B. negative chronotropic and dromotropic effects.
  C. positive chronotropic and dromotropic effects.
  D. positive inotropic and chronotropic effects.
  E. positive inotropic and dromotropic effects.

B   4. The cardiac conductive cells have which of the following properties?
  A. excitability   D. contractility
  B. conductivity   E. all of the above
  C. automaticity

B   5. All of the following can cause an artifact on ECG EXCEPT:
  A. an artificial pacemaker.   D. shivering by the patient.
  B. an enlarged heart.   E. loose electrodes.
  C. movement by the patient.

A   6. A prolonged QT interval is longer than 0.38 second.
  A. True
  B. False

©2004 Pearson Education, Inc.
Intermediate Emergency Care: Principles & Practice

_____ 7. Common causes of dysrhythmias include all of the following EXCEPT:
A. myocardial ischemia or infarction.
B. electrolyte and pH disturbances.
C. CNS or autonomic nervous system damage.
D. drug effects.
E. hyperthermia.

_____ 8. In the bradycardia algorithm, the first drug in the intervention sequence is:
A. procainamide.
B. epinephrine.
C. atropine.
D. isoproterenol.
E. dopamine.

_____ 9. Of the atrial dysrhythmias listed below, which is often an indication of serious underlying medical disease?
A. atrial tachycardia
B. atrial flutter
C. premature atrial contractions (PACs)
D. multifocal atrial tachycardia (MAT)
E. paroxysmal supraventricular tachycardia (PSVT)

_____ 10. The diagnostic finding for first-degree AV block on the ECG is:
A. the presence of some QRS complexes not preceded by a P wave.
B. a P-R interval longer than 0.20 second.
C. a QRS complex widened to longer than 0.12 second.
D. an R-T interval widened for those beats with an initial P wave.
E. the presence of some P waves without following QRS complexes.

_____ 11. The chief difference between Type I and Type II second-degree AV block is the pattern of lengthening P-R interval before the blocked impulse in Type I second-degree AV block.
A. True
B. False

_____ 12. All of the following statements about third-degree AV block are true EXCEPT:
A. the atrial rate is unaffected, and ventricular rate depends on site of ventricular pacemaker.
B. P waves are normal but show no relationship to the QRS complex.
C. there is an absence of conduction between the atria and the ventricles.
D. both atrial and ventricular rhythms are usually regular.
E. QRS complexes are normal in length.

_____ 13. Never use lidocaine to treat third-degree heart block in patients with ventricular escape beats.
A. True
B. False

_____ 14. All of the following statements about ECG findings for dysrhythmias originating in the AV junction are true EXCEPT:
A. P-R interval is less than 0.12 second.
B. P waves are inverted in Lead II.
C. T waves are blunted and widened.
D. QRS complexes are normal in duration.
E. P waves are masked if atrial depolarization occurs during ventricular depolarization.

_____ 15. Caffeine, tobacco, alcohol, and sympathomimetic drugs are common causes of:
A. junctional escape rhythms.
B. accelerated junctional rhythm.
C. paroxysmal junctional tachycardia.
D. premature junctional contractions.
E. junctional bradycardia.

_____ 16. All of the following statements about dysrhythmias originating in the ventricles are true EXCEPT:
A. ischemia, hypoxia, and drug effects are common causes.
B. T waves are blunted and widened.
C. P waves are absent.
D. the pacemaker site determines QRS morphology.
E. QRS complexes are 0.12 second or longer in duration.

_____ 17. *Torsades de pointes* varies in both cause and ECG appearance from other forms of:
A. ventricular escape rhythm.
B. accelerated idioventricular rhythm.
C. ventricular fibrillation.
D. premature ventricular contraction.
E. ventricular tachycardia.

_____ 18. Possible characteristics of malignant PVCs include all EXCEPT:
A. R on T phenomenon.
B. couplets or longer runs of ventricular tachycardia.
C. more than eight PVCs per minute.
D. multifocal origin within the ventricles.
E. accompanying chest pain.

_____ 19. Nonperfusing ventricular tachycardia and ventricular fibrillation are treated identically, including initiation of CPR followed by:
A. epinephrine 1:10,000 IV bolus.
B. adenosine IV bolus.
C. transcutaneous cardiac pacing (TCP).
D. DC countershock at 200 joules.
E. atropine IV bolus.

_____ 20. Causes of asystole include all of the following EXCEPT:
A. pre-existing alkalosis (respiratory or metabolic).
B. hyperkalemia.
C. hypokalemia.
D. drug overdose.
E. hypothermia.

MATCHING

Write the letter of the definition or description regarding cardiac function in the space provided next to the term to which it applies. The same description or definition may be used more than once or not at all.

_____ 21. cardiac cycle

_____ 22. diastole

_____ 23. systole

_____ 24. ejection fraction

_____ 25. preload

_____ 26. afterload

_____ 27. cardiac output

_____ 28. stroke volume

A. the ratio of blood pumped from the ventricle compared with the amount contained at the end of diastole
B. the series of events between the end of a cardiac contraction to the end of the next
C. the resistance against which the heart must pump
D. the phase of the cardiac cycle during which the heart contracts
E. the amount of blood pumped by the ventricle during one cardiac contraction
F. the amount of blood pumped by the ventricle during one minute
G. the phase of the cardiac cycle during which the heart muscle is relaxed
H. the end-diastolic volume in the ventricle
I. the phase of the cardiac cycle during which blood enters the coronary arteries

©2004 Pearson Education, Inc.
Intermediate Emergency Care: Principles & Practice

Write the letter of innate rate of impulse discharge in beats per minute (bpm) in the space provided next to the part of the cardiac conduction system to which it applies.

_____ 29. Purkinje system

_____ 30. AV node

_____ 31. SA node

A. 60–100 bpm
B. 15–40 bpm
C. 40–60 bpm

LABEL THE DIAGRAMS

Supply the missing labels for the drawing showing the chambers of the heart by writing the appropriate letters in the spaces provided for Figure 1.

A. right ventricle
B. interatrial septum
C. left atrium
D. right atrium
E. interventricular septum
F. left ventricle

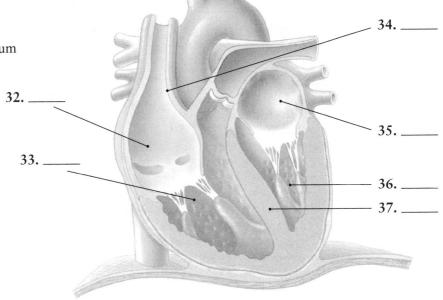

32. _____

33. _____

34. _____

35. _____

36. _____

37. _____

Figure 1

Supply the missing labels for the drawing showing the cardiac conductive system by writing the appropriate letters in the spaces provided for Figure 2.

A. Purkinje fibers
B. left bundle branch
C. SA node
D. AV node
E. bundle of His
F. Internodal atrial pathway
G. AV junction

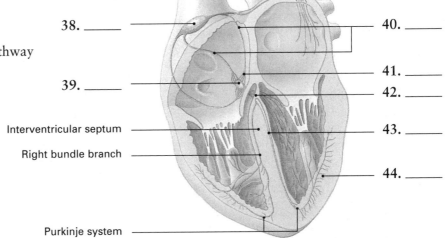

38. _____

39. _____

Interventricular septum

Right bundle branch

Purkinje system

40. _____

41. _____

42. _____

43. _____

44. _____

Figure 2

Medical Emergencies

Use the terms below to fill in the missing labels for Figure 3 in the spaces provided.

A. QRS complex
B. Ventricular depolarization
C. Atrial depolarization
D. T wave
E. Ventricular repolarization
F. P wave

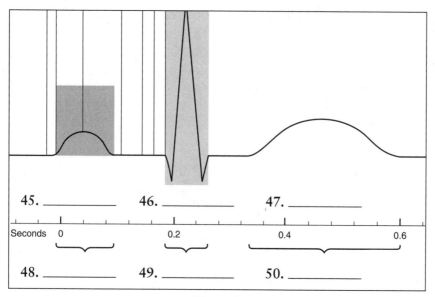

45. _____   46. _____   47. _____

Seconds   0   0.2   0.4   0.6

48. _____   49. _____   50. _____

Figure 3

SPECIAL PROJECT

ECG Interpretation

The chapter introduces a five-step procedure for analyzing ECG strips: (1) analysis of rate; (2) analysis of rhythm; (3) analysis of P waves; (4) analysis of P-R interval; and (5) analysis of QRS complexes.
Look at each of the five ECG tracings shown and complete the information grid asked for below each tracing.

ECG #1

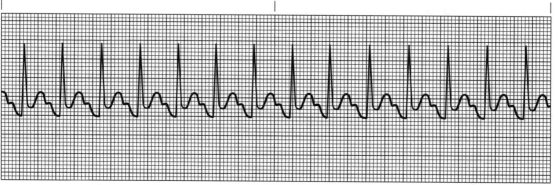

Rate: _____

Rhythm: _____

P waves: _____

P-R interval: _____

QRS complexes: _____

Overall rhythm (or Dysrhythmia): _____

ECG #2

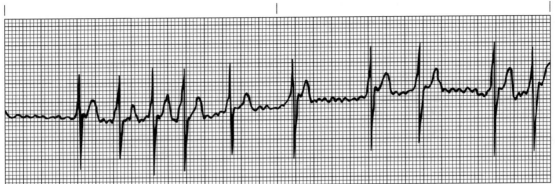

Rate: _____

Rhythm: _____

P waves: _____

P-R interval: _____

QRS complexes: _____

Overall rhythm (or Dysrhythmia): _____

ECG #3

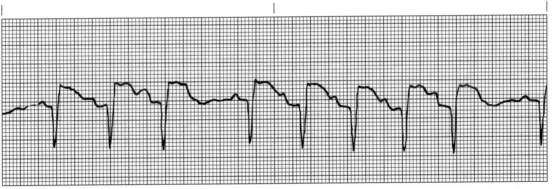

Rate: _____

Rhythm: _____

P waves: _____

P-R interval: _____

QRS complexes: _____

Overall rhythm (or Dysrhythmia): _____

ECG #4

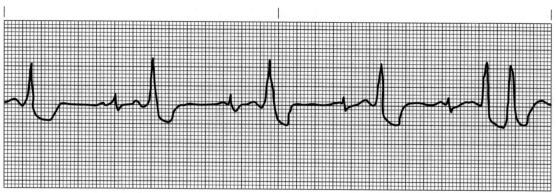

Rate: _____

Rhythm: _____

P waves: _____

P-R interval: _____

QRS complexes: _____

_____

Overall rhythm (or Dysrhythmia): _____

_____

ECG #5

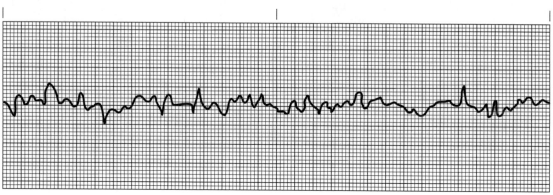

Rate: _____

Rhythm: _____

P waves: _____

P-R interval: _____

QRS complexes: _____

Overall rhythm (or Dysrhythmia): _____

©2004 Pearson Education, Inc.
Intermediate Emergency Care: Principles & Practice

CHAPTER 20

✳

Cardiovascular Emergencies

Part 2: Assessment and Management of the Cardiovascular Patient

Review of Chapter Objectives

After reading this part of the chapter, you should be able to:

1. **Identify and describe the components of assessment as it relates to the patient with cardiovascular compromise.** **pp. 897–905**

   The focused history for cardiac situations uses the same format you learned for pulmonology, the SAMPLE format: Signs/Symptoms, Allergies, Medications, Past medical history, Last oral intake, and Events preceding the incident.

   - *Signs/Symptoms.* The most common symptoms of cardiac disease/compromise include chest pain or discomfort, dyspnea, cough, syncope, and palpitations.

     Use the OPQRST format (also something you encountered with pulmonology) to assess chest pain or discomfort: Onset of pain, Provocation/Palliation of pain, Quality of pain, Region where felt/Radiation, Severity, and Timing (duration). (See also objective 7 for full detail.) Questions concerning dyspnea are similar: You want to know how long it has lasted and whether it is continuous or intermittent. Was onset rapid or gradual? Does anything specific either worsen or palliate the dyspnea, and is it exertional or not? Last, be sure to see if orthopnea exists: Does sitting upright give any relief? Questions about cough center on whether it is chronic or acute and whether it suggests congestive heart failure (dry or productive, presence of any wheezing with cough, etc.).

     In addition, observe and question for these possible signs/symptoms: level of consciousness, diaphoresis, restlessness/anxiety, feeling of impending doom, nausea/vomiting, fatigue, palpitations, edema of extremities or positional (sacral), headache, syncope, behavioral change, facial expression, limitation of activity, signs of recent trauma. Many signs/symptoms of cardiovascular disease and compromise can be subtle or change (either rapidly or gradually) over time.
   - *Allergies.* Check for allergies to medication (prescription and over-the-counter) or X-ray contrast dyes. Try to distinguish between details suggestive of side effect (such as GI upset) and those of allergy (rash, hives, anaphylactic shock).
   - *Medications.* Check both for current medications (again, prescription and over-the-counter) and recent medication changes. If there has been a recent change, ask why. Look for use of cardiovascular drugs such as nitroglycerin, propranolol or other beta blockers, digitalis (digoxin, Lanoxin), diuretics (Lasix, Dyazide), antihypertensives (Capoten, Prinivil, Vasotec), antidysrhythmics (Quinaglute, Mexitil, Tambocor), and lipid-lowering agents (Mevacor, Lopid). If possible, check directly (by inspecting med tray, if there is one) or indirectly (by history) about drug compliance and bring containers to the hospital with you.

Medical Emergencies

- *Past medical history.* Ask directed questions about history of heart disease, MI, stroke, high blood pressure, as well as why suggestive drugs are taken. Specific problems you should inquire about include history of rheumatic heart disease (valvular problems), previous cardiac surgery, congenital cardiac anomalies, pericarditis or other inflammatory cardiac disease, or congestive heart failure (CHF). Relevant problems of other organ systems include pulmonary disease/ COPD, diabetes mellitus, renal disease, hypertension, atherosclerosis. Also ask whether there is any family history of illness/death (particularly early deaths before age 50) from cardiovascular disease or other relevant disorders. Last, be sure to ask whether patient smokes or smoked tobacco and whether he/she knows his/her cholesterol level.
- *Last oral intake.* Valuable as a screening question for anyone with a possible surgical condition, this also gives you the chance to ask about most recent caffeine or tobacco use, as well as whether there was a recent fatty meal. (For some patients, this may help steer you to gallbladder disorders.)
- *Events preceding incident.* Ask what the patient was doing just before onset of symptoms. Was there emotional stress or physical exertion? Was there sexual activity? If the patient is male, does he take Viagra? It is often uncomfortable to take a sexual history, but sometimes the information gained is life saving, and you can explain to the patient the possible importance of the answer.

2. List the clinical indications for an implanted defibrillation device. p. 912

Permanent artificial pacemakers are generally inserted into patients who have chronic high-grade AV block or sick sinus syndrome or who have had episodes of severe symptomatic bradycardia in the past. The pacemaker (the pulse generator) is implanted near the heart, and its discharge lead is inserted into either the right ventricle or right atrium and ventricle, depending on whether it is a ventricular-type pacemaker or a dual-chambered pacemaker. The battery packs are usually palpable in their subcutaneous position (often in the shoulder or axillary region). Permanent pacemakers are of two functional types: either they can pace continuously or they can pace when the heart's natural rate falls below a preset number of beats per minute. (The two types are called fixed-rate and demand pacemakers.) In all cases, the pacemaker should enable the patient to have a heart rate and rhythm that supports adequate cardiac output.

3. Define angina pectoris and myocardial infarction (MI). pp. 922–930

Angina pectoris, or pain in the chest, occurs when the myocardial demand for oxygen exceeds the available supply through the coronary arteries. Myocardial ischemia causes the chest pain. Usually, reduced blood flow through the coronary arteries is correlated with permanent partial obstruction by atherosclerotic lesions. Angina can also result from spasm of the coronary arteries (arterial vasospasm), temporarily reducing the diameter of the lumen and blood flow. About two-thirds of patients with vasospastic angina (commonly called Prinzmetal's angina) have atherosclerosis involving the coronaries. Epidemiologically, though, this still means roughly one-third of patients with Prinzmetal's angina do not have significant coronary atherosclerosis and thus may not fit the risk factor profile for atherosclerosis.

Each year about 466,000 Americans die from coronary heart disease (CHD), and myocardial infarction (MI) is the usual direct cause of death. In addition, an American suffers a nonfatal MI every 29 seconds. Myocardial infarction, the death of myocardial tissue, is the result of prolonged oxygen deprivation or when myocardial oxygen demand exceeds oxygen supply for an extended period. MI is most often associated with atherosclerotic heart disease (ASHD, which is the same as atherosclerotic coronary heart disease). The precipitating event is often development of a thrombus in a partially occluded artery, with the thrombus completely occluding the vessel. Other pathophysiologic bases for MI include coronary artery spasm, microemboli as can be seen with cocaine use, acute volume overload, hypotension (causing myocardial hypoperfusion), or acute respiratory failure (leading to acute hypoxia). Trauma can also cause MI, often by loosening atherosclerotic plaque in the coronary artery, blocking it.

The region of the heart affected and the size of the eventual infarcted area depend on the coronary artery involved and the specific site of the obstruction. Most infarctions involve the left ventricle. Obstruction of the left coronary artery or its branches may result in infarction of the

©2004 Pearson Education, Inc.
Intermediate Emergency Care: Principles & Practice

anterior or lateral ventricle or the interventricular septum. Right coronary artery occlusions tend to result in infarction of the inferior or posterior wall of the left ventricle or infarction of the right ventricle.

The pathophysiologic progression of events starts with ischemia, followed by cell death. The infarcted tissue becomes necrotic and eventually forms scar tissue, if the affected individual survives. Ischemic tissue at the periphery of the infarct will survive but may become the origin of dysrhythmias. Dysrhythmias are the most common complication of MI and the most common cause of death from an MI.

Infarction of myocardium can cause congestive heart failure. Heart failure implies that the heart is working poorly but adequately. If the heart cannot meet body oxygen demand, cardiogenic shock results. Last, if the damaged portion of the ventricular wall is too weakened, it may form a ventricular aneurysm and rupture, causing death.

Based on pathophysiology, the basic strategies of intervention are pain relief and reperfusion. For reperfusion to be effective, rapid, safe transport is essential.

4. List other clinical conditions that may mimic signs and symptoms of angina pectoris and myocardial infarction.   **p. 923**

Causes of chest pain fall into four categories: cardiovascular, respiratory, gastrointestinal, and musculoskeletal. You'll note that the causes range from the troublesome but benign (dyspepsia, or heartburn) to the life threatening (aortic dissection). Cardiovascular causes include coronary artery disease and angina, but also pericarditis and dissection of the thoracic aorta. Respiratory causes include pulmonary embolism, pneumothorax, pneumonia, and pleurisy (pleural inflammation). GI causes are diverse: cholecystitis (gallbladder origin), pancreatitis, hiatal hernia, esophageal disease, gastroesophageal reflux (GERD), peptic ulcer disease, and dyspepsia. Musculoskeletal causes include chest wall syndrome, costochondritis, acromioclavicular disease, herpes zoster (shingles), chest wall trauma, and chest wall tumors. You should always be prepared to treat patients with chest pain as if they may have cardiac ischemia or another major disease process. Only after you have excluded these possibilities should you consider the less critical causes.

5. List the mechanisms by which an MI may be produced by traumatic and non-traumatic events.   **pp. 923, 925**

See objectives 3 and 4 above.

6. List and describe the assessment parameters to be evaluated in a patient with chest pain.   **pp. 925–927**

Initial size-up, inspection, and vital signs may reveal a lot. Is breathing labored? Is the patient diaphoretic and pale? Are there other signs of shock? Remember that blood pressure usually elevates during an episode of ischemia and then returns to normal. Hypotension more likely suggests cardiac compromise and possible shock. Peripheral pulses should be regular and equal. Irregularities may suggest dysrhythmia.

7. Identify what is meant by the OPQRST of chest pain assessment.   **pp. 898–899**

Use the OPQRST format (also something you encountered with pulmonology) to assess chest pain or discomfort: Onset of pain, Provocation/Palliation of pain, Quality of pain, Region where felt/Radiation, Severity, and Timing (duration). Questions about onset include when pain began and what was happening at the time. Ask a patient who has had prior episodes of chest pain to compare this one with prior episodes. If it is described as similar to pain that signaled a prior heart attack, you can strongly assume the pain is cardiac in origin. Questions on provocation and palliation of pain also may point to angina or toward another cause. In particular, ask about any relationship to exertion of any type or palliation with rest. If there have been multiple episodes, ask whether it takes less to trigger an episode now than in the past. Ask a general question about the quality of the pain and let the patient describe it. Common words include sharp, tearing, pressured, or heavy. Radiation of chest pain may occur to arm(s), neck, jaw, and/or back. Again, ask if this pattern fits earlier episodes. Ask the patient to evaluate the severity of the pain on a scale

Medical Emergencies

of 1–10 (be sure you use the same scale that will be used at the hospital in order to standardize response significance): You can ask the same question later to assess efficacy of therapy. Timing questions get information on how long the pain has lasted (write down the time the patient first noted pain as this may affect decisions later regarding possible thrombolytic therapy) as well as whether pain has been constant or intermittent or has changed with time (Better? Worse?).

8. List and describe the initial assessment parameters to be evaluated in—and the anticipated presentation of—a patient with chest pain that may be myocardial in origin. pp. 898, 923–924, 926

See objective 6 in Part 2. In addition, as you move through the OPQRST mnemonic, look for these signs of MI: sudden onset chest pain that proves to be severe, constant, and unrelenting over a period longer than 30 minutes. Pain may radiate to the arms (usually the left), neck, back, or into the epigastrium. Myocardial ischemia can easily produce pain in the 8–10 range and the pain may be associated with nausea and vomiting. Unlike the situation with angina, neither rest nor nitroglycerin will palliate MI pain. Remember that patients with diabetes mellitus may NOT have this picture even when an MI is in evolution. These patients may minimize the severity of their discomfort or simply complain of feeling unwell. Typically, these patients do not have nausea and vomiting. MIs typically evolve over 48–72 hours, and so the pain seen at 24–48 hours may be very different than if you had seen the patient in the first 12–24 hours after onset of discomfort.

Emotion may suggest MI. Patients with severe chest pain often are very frightened and complain of a sense of doom or fear of death. Denial of emotional upset or severity of pain does not mean a benign episode. Denial may hide severe fear or pain.

Auscultation of the lung fields may show clear fields or congestion in the bases. Other physical findings typical of MI include pallor and diaphoresis, coldness in the extremities, and possible change in body temperature. Heart rate and rhythm may be irregular or not. Blood pressure may be baseline, high, or low.

The ECG should be checked first for underlying rhythm and any sign of dysrhythmia. If you have a 12-lead ECG, look at the S-T segment and QRS complex. Check S-T segment for height, depth, and overall contour. Note any depression or elevation. A pathological Q wave (one deeper than 5 mm and wider than 0.04 sec) can indicate infarcted tissue or extensive transient ischemia. Anticipate dysrhythmias.

Next, assess whether the patient is a likely candidate for rapid transport and reperfusion therapy with thrombolytic agents. The time window for thrombolytic therapy to be effective is generally considered to be the first 6 hours from onset of symptoms. Consult medical direction. Note that some patients will have contraindications to thrombolytic therapy, including bleeding or clotting disorders, possible blood in the stool, uncontrolled hypertension, recent trauma, recent hemorrhagic stroke, or recent surgery. Generally, signs of acute injury or pathological Q waves indicate transport for reperfusion if you are within the 6-hour window. If you are uncertain whether the patient meets criteria for reperfusion therapy, assume that he/she does. Be sure to relay information to medical direction including time of pain onset, any S-T segment change (particularly elevation), and location of ischemia or infarct according to a 12-lead ECG.

9. Describe the pharmacological agents available to the EMT-Intermediate for use in the management of dysrhythmias and cardiovascular emergencies. pp. 910, 911

The classes of drugs you are most likely to use in the setting of an MI are antidysrhythmics, sympathomimetics, and drugs specific for use in the setting of ischemia (including the thrombolytics), along with less frequently used prehospital medications.

Antidysrhythmics

Antidysrhythmics control or suppress dysrhythmias. Among the most commonly used are atropine, lidocaine, procainamide, bretylium, adenosine, amiodarone, and verapamil.

- *Atropine sulfate* is a parasympatholytic agent (one that decreases parasympathetic effect by acting as an anticholinergic) used to treat symptomatic bradycardias, especially those arising in the atria, and is sometimes used as part of a treatment regimen for asystole. Dose is 0.5–1.0 mg IV for bradycardia and 1.0 mg for asystole, repeated every 3–5 minutes as needed until a total dose of 0.04 mg/kg is reached. Endotracheal (ET) doses are 2.0–2.5 times the IV doses. Side effects include blurred vision, dilated pupils, dry mouth, tachycardia, and drowsiness. It has no contraindications in the EMS setting.

- *Lidocaine* is a first-line antidysrhythmic used to treat and prevent life-threatening ventricular dysrhythmias such as ventricular tachycardia. It suppresses abnormal irritability in the ventricles while having little effect on normal myocardial tissue. Dose is 1.0–1.5 mg/kg slow IV push (50 mg/min) for ectopy, or normal IV push in cardiac arrest. An IV drip is prepared by mixing 1 gram into 250 cc D_5W or saline. Typical maintenance dose is 2–4 mg/minute. Maximum bolus dose is 300 mg. The drug can be given IV bolus, IV drip, or through an ET tube. Side effects include drowsiness, seizures, confusion, bradycardia, heart blocks, and nausea and vomiting. Lidocaine is contraindicated by the presence of second- or third-degree AV block.

- *Procainamide* is a second-line antidysrhythmic to lidocaine, and it is used for ventricular dysrhythmias refractory to lidocaine or for patients who are allergic to lidocaine. It is administered by slow IV bolus or IV drip. IV bolus is 100 mg given over 5 minutes, with a maximum dose of 17 mg/kg. Discontinue when the dysrhythmia is suppressed, hypotension ensues, the QRS complex widens 50%, or the maximum dose is given. Drip rate is the same as for lidocaine. Side effects and contraindications are the same as for lidocaine.

- *Bretylium* is a second-line antidysrhythmic used to treat life-threatening ventricular dysrhythmias, especially ventricular fibrillation. Although its mechanism of action is poorly understood, bretylium apparently raises the ventricular fibrillation threshold. Bretylium is administered by IV bolus and IV drip. Dose is 5 mg/kg IV push with drip rate of 1–2 mg/min. A subsequent dose of 10 mg/kg is repeated if the dysrhythmia persists. Maximum dose is 30 mg/kg. Side effects include hypo- or hypertension, dizziness, syncope, seizures, and nausea and vomiting. Bretylium is now being used less frequently because of development of other agents.

- *Adenosine* is used to manage supraventricular tachydysrhythmias. It is a naturally occurring nucleoside that acts on the AV node to slow conduction and inhibit reentry pathways. It is given by IV rapid bolus through a venous site as close to the heart as possible. Flush the line with saline immediately after giving adenosine to ensure drug delivery. Initial dose is 6 mg (rapid push) followed by a 15–30 cc saline flush. If the tachydysrhythmia is not eliminated, a second dose of 12 mg and, if needed, a third dose of 12 mg may be given. Maximum dose is 30 mg. Side effects include apprehension, burning sensation, heavy sensation in the arms, hypotension, chest pressure, diaphoresis, numbness or tingling, dyspnea, tightness in the throat and/or groin pressure, headache, and nausea and vomiting. Adenosine is contraindicated in the presence of second- or third-degree AV block or in sick sinus syndrome unless a pacemaker is present.

- *Amiodarone* (Cordarone) is an antidysrhythmic used in management of recurring ventricular fibrillation and hemodynamically unstable ventricular tachycardia (nonperfusing tachycardia). Amiodarone is also being used more frequently in the prehospital setting of cardiac arrest. Although it is a second-line drug in the United States, it is a first-line agent in several Commonwealth countries. Dosage is 150–300 mg by slow IV infusion. Side effects include hypotension (the most common), bradycardia, and AV blocks. It is contraindicated in cardiogenic shock, marked sinus bradycardia, and second- or third-degree AV block.

- *Verapamil* is a calcium channel blocker that slows heart rate in symptomatic atrial tachycardias. It is used to terminate paroxysmal supraventricular tachycardia as well as to control the rapid ventricular response often seen with atrial flutter or fibrillation. It is administered by slow IV bolus with a maximum dose of 30 mg.

Sympathomimetic agents

Sympathomimetic agents are similar to the naturally occurring hormones epinephrine and norepinephrine, and they mimic sympathetic nervous system stimulation on either alpha or beta adrenergic receptors. Alpha receptor stimulation causes peripheral vasoconstriction and beta receptor stimulation increases heart rate and cardiac contractility, causes bronchodilation and peripheral vasodilation. Stimulation of dopaminergic receptors in the renal and mesenteric vascular beds causes dilation. Commonly used sympathomimetic agents include epinephrine, norepinephrine, isoproterenol, dopamine, and dobutamine.

- *Epinephrine,* which acts on alpha and beta receptors, is the mainstay of cardiac arrest resuscitation. It is used with ventricular fibrillation, asystole, and pulseless electrical activity. It is also sometimes used for bradycardia refractory to atropine. It is given as IV bolus, subcutaneously, and via ET tube. Dose is 1 mg of 1:10,000 solution given every 3–5 minutes.

- *Norepinephrine* has alpha agonist properties greater than those of epinephrine. It acts on beta receptors to a lesser degree. It is used occasionally in hemodynamically significant hypotension and cardiogenic shock, although dopamine is the first-line agent for these conditions. Norepinephrine may be effective if total peripheral resistance is low, such as in neurogenic shock. It is administered by IV infusion via drip by placing 4 mg into 1000 cc of D_5W (ONLY) to give a concentration of 4 µg/cc. Initial loading dose is 8–12 µg/min to give blood pressure of 80–100 mmHg systolic. Maintenance dose is 2–4 µg/min. Side effects include anxiety, trembling, headache, dizziness, and nausea and vomiting. It can also cause bradycardia. DO NOT use norepinephrine in patients with hypotension from hypovolemia.
- *Isoproterenol* is rarely used with the advent of TCP, but it is a potent beta agonist that increases heart rate and cardiac contractility. It is used in bradycardia refractory to atropine and to manage asystole. Isoproterenol is given via IV infusion. Add 1 mg to 250 cc D_5W or saline to give 4 µg/cc. The drip rate is 2–20 µg/min. Common procedure is to start with a low dose and titrate upward until a satisfactory rate is achieved. TCP is preferred to use of isoproterenol.
- *Dopamine* (Intropin) is a vasopressor that increases cardiac output. It stimulates both alpha and beta receptors. It has the advantage over other drugs of preserving renal perfusion at recommended doses. Dose is given via IV drip by mixing 800 mg into 500 cc D_5W or saline to give a concentration of 1600 µg/cc (400 mg into 250 cc also works). Dopamine's effects are dose-related: At 1–2 µg/kg/min, renal artery dilation occurs; at 2–10 µg/kg/min, beta receptors are primarily stimulated; at 10–15 µg/kg/min, both beta and alpha receptors are stimulated; and at 15–20 µg/kg/min, alpha receptors are primarily stimulated. Side effects include nervousness, headache, dysrhythmias, palpitations, chest pain, dyspnea, and nausea and vomiting. Note: Dopamine is contraindicated for hypovolemic shock until fluid resuscitation has been completed.
- *Dobutamine* (Dobutrex), like dopamine, increases cardiac output and increases stroke volume. It has little effect on heart rate and is occasionally used in isolated left heart failure until medications such as digitalis can take effect. Dobutamine is given by IV infusion by mixing 250 mg into 250 cc D_5W or saline to give a concentration of 1000 µg/cc. Dose is 2–10 µg/kg/min titrated to effect. Its side effects are the same as dopamine's. Do not use dobutamine as the sole agent in hypovolemic shock unless fluid resuscitation is complete. Dopamine is preferred over dobutamine to increase cardiac output in cardiogenic shock.

Drugs used for myocardial ischemia

Drugs used to treat myocardial ischemia and relieve its pain include oxygen, nitrous oxide, nitroglycerin, morphine, and nalbuphine.

- *Oxygen* is important because it increases the blood's oxygen content and aids oxygenation of peripheral and cardiac tissues. It is indicated in any situation where hypoxia or ischemia is possible.
- *Nitrous oxide* (Nitronox) is purely an analgesic with no significant hemodynamic effects. However, delivery in fixed combination with 50% oxygen can increase myocardial oxygen supply. Nitrous oxide is self-administered by inhalation via a modified demand valve to the desired effect. Its effects subside within 2–5 minutes. Side effects include CNS depression and potential respiratory depression. Do not give nitrous oxide to patients who cannot comprehend verbal instructions or who are intoxicated with alcohol or other drugs.
- *Nitroglycerin* is an organic nitrate that dilates peripheral arteries and veins, reducing preload and afterload and myocardial oxygen demand. It may cause some coronary artery dilation, thus increasing blood flow through the collateral circulation. Nitroglycerin use often helps to distinguish the pain of angina from that of an MI. Nitroglycerin does not relieve the pain of an MI, but it should be given before morphine because it works in conjunction with morphine in an MI. Dosage is one tablet sublingually repeated every 5 minutes up to a total of three tablets. Monitor blood pressure before each dose. Its side effects include headache, dizziness, weakness, hypotension, and tachycardia. Note that nitroglycerin loses potency as soon as the bottle is opened to the air. Always use the nitroglycerin provided on the medical intensive care unit and check the date before administration.

- *Morphine sulfate* is a narcotic drug that is important in managing MI. It reduces myocardial oxygen demand by reducing both preload and afterload. It also acts directly on the CNS to relieve pain, and it reduces sympathetic discharge, which can further decrease myocardial oxygen demand. Dosage is in 1–2 mg increments via slow IV push, titrated to pain relief. Monitor blood pressure before each dose. Side effects include nausea and vomiting, abdominal cramping, respiratory depression, hypotension, and potential altered mental status. Toxic effects are apnea and severe hypotension. Check for drug allergy before administration.
- *Nalbuphine* (Nubain) is used in some EMS systems instead of morphine. Nalbuphine is an analgesic, but it lacks the desirable hemodynamic effects of morphine. Dose is 10–20 mg IV, IM, or subcutaneously. Side effects include sedation, clammy skin, dizziness, dry mouth, hypotension, hypertension, and nausea and vomiting. It is contraindicated in patients who have taken depressants or alcohol.

Thrombolytic agents

The use of thrombolytic agents as a definitive treatment for myocardial ischemia is one of the most important recent advances in medicine. In some instances, thrombolytic therapy may even have benefit in the field, and this is especially true in areas with a long transit time to a definitive care facility. Thrombolytic agents are generally very expensive, and their use requires a 12-lead ECG. Alteplase (tPA, Activase) and reteplase (Retavase) are thrombolytic agents. Although aspirin is not a thrombolytic agent, it merits discussion in this section.

- *Aspirin* is important in treatment of cardiac ischemia because it inhibits platelet aggregation and thus is effective in treating coronary ischemia and stroke secondary to thrombus development. The standard dosage is 325 mg by mouth, although some physicians prefer smaller doses. Baby aspirin may be useful because it can be chewed, thus more quickly reaching a therapeutic blood level. Its most common side effect is GI upset, although bleeding can be a problem in certain patients.
- *Alteplase* (Activase, tPA). Alteplase, or tPA (tissue plasminogen activator) is a potent thrombolytic agent that is manufactured through recombinant technology, which means it is the same as the biological compound. This minimizes chances of allergic reaction. TPA is effective if given within 6 hours of onset of coronary ischemia. It is given as a bolus dose followed by infusion. The typical dose is 100 mg given over 1.5–2 hours. Complications of tPA include hemorrhage, which can be fatal. Also, when reperfusion occurs, potentially life-threatening dysrhythmias can develop.
- *Reteplase* (Retavase) is another human plasminogen activator. It functions in a manner similar to tPA and has the same basic side effects and complications. It is administered as a single 10-unit bolus by IV push over 2 minutes. A second 10-unit bolus is given 30 minutes afterward. This dosing regimen makes reteplase attractive for prehospital care.

Other prehospital drugs

Less frequently used agents you may administer in the prehospital setting include furosemide, diazepam, promethazine, and sodium nitroprusside.

- *Furosemide* (Lasix) is a potent loop diuretic that also relaxes the venous system with effects seen within 5 minutes. Its diuretic effect decreases intravascular fluid volume. Dose is 40 mg slow IV push (40 mg/min). If the patient takes furosemide or another diuretic, you may need to double the dosage. Side effects include hypotension, ECG changes, chest pain, dry mouth, hypokalemia, hypochloremia, hyponatremia, and hyperglycemia. Furosemide should only be used in life-threatening emergencies during pregnancy because it can cause fetal abnormalities.
- *Diazepam* (Valium) is not an analgesic but rather an anti-anxiety drug, and it may be given to patients who are extremely apprehensive or agitated. Dose is 2–5 mg IV or deep IM.
- *Promethazine* (Phenergan) has sedative, antihistamine, antiemetic, and anticholinergic properties. It also potentiates narcotics, making it useful in the MI setting by reducing the nausea associated with morphine while enhancing its effects. Dosage is 12.5–25.0 mg given slow IV push or deep IM (25.0 mg/min). Its side effects are drowsiness, sedation, blurred vision, tachycardia, bradycardia, and dizziness. Promethazine is contraindicated in unresponsive patients or

those taking large doses of depressants. Extrapyramidal symptoms (namely, dystonia) have been reported with promethazine.

- *Sodium nitroprusside* (Nipride) is a potent arterial and venous vasodilator, making it popular for use in hypertensive crisis. It is given as an IV infusion, which makes administration more controlled and the patient's response more predictable.

Drugs infrequently used in the prehospital setting

Lastly, certain medications commonly associated with in-hospital use or long-term patient use are included in this discussion. You are most likely to use these often if you work in an emergency department. Drugs in this group include digitalis, beta blockers, calcium channel blockers, and alkalinizing agents.

- *Digitalis* (digoxin, Lanoxin) is a cardiac glycoside that increases cardiac contractility and cardiac output. It slows impulse conduction through the AV node and decreases the ventricular response to certain supraventricular dysrhythmias such as atrial flutter or fibrillation and paroxysmal supraventricular tachycardia. It is also used long term to treat heart failure. The dose is 8–12 µg/kg slow IV push over 15–20 minutes. If possible, obtain the patient's digitalis level beforehand (if the patient is on digoxin) before administering any cardiac glycoside. Most patients taking digitalis will remain therapeutic at 10–15 µg/kg over a 24-hour period. Giving digitalis to patients who already take a cardiac glycoside involves complicated calculations, which makes it impractical for prehospital use in most settings. Its side effects include fatigue, muscle weakness, agitation, hallucinations, headache, malaise, dizziness, vertigo, stupor, blurred vision and yellow-green halo vision, photophobia, diplopia, and nausea and vomiting. Digitalis toxicity, which is not uncommon in some patients, can cause almost any dysrhythmia, including some of the same dysrhythmias it is used to treat, and these will often be refractory to traditional antidysrhythmic drugs. Digitalis is contraindicated in any digitalis-induced toxicity, ventricular fibrillation, or ventricular tachycardia not caused by CHF.
- *Beta blockers* are frequently used to control dysrhythmias, hypertension, and angina. Many beta blockers such as propranolol (Inderal) are non-selective; other beta blockers such as metoprolol are selective for either B_1 or B_2 receptors. Beta blockers may precipitate CHF, heart block, or asthma in patients predisposed to them. The beta-blocker labetalol (Trandate, Normodyne) effectively decreases blood pressure. It is given by IV bolus and infusion. The IV bolus is 20 mg over 20 minutes and may be repeated at 40–80 mg over 10 minutes. Maximum bolus is 300 mg. Drip is established by mixing 200 mg into 160 cc D_5W, and the drip dose is 2 cc/min.
- *Calcium channel blockers* are a relatively new class of antihypertensive medication that include verapamil (Isoptin, Calan), diltiazem (Cardizem), and nifedipine (Procardia). Nifedipine is now being used in addition to nitroglycerin to treat angina. Like nitroglycerin, it is a vasodilator but with a different mechanism. It is given orally. Calcium channel blockers are being used increasingly for angina, dysrhythmias, and other cardiovascular problems.
- *Alkalinizing agents* such as sodium bicarbonate are used late in the management of cardiac arrest, if at all. Occasionally, metabolic acidosis from another disorder may cause pulseless electrical activity, asystole, ventricular tachycardia, or ventricular fibrillation. In these cases, sodium bicarbonate may aid in converting to a perfusing rhythm. Adequate CPR, prompt defibrillation, and appropriate drug administration should always precede the use of bicarbonate. Sodium bicarbonate has few side effects and no contraindications in the emergency setting. Dose is initially 1 mEq/kg followed by 0.5 mEq/kg every 10 minutes. When possible, doses should be based on arterial blood gas (ABG) results.

10. **Develop, execute, and evaluate a treatment plan based on the field impression for the patient with chest pain that may be indicative of angina or myocardial infarction.** pp. 924, 927–930

Act expediently and calmly and keep the patient in as much physical and emotional rest as possible. Provide supplemental oxygen to decrease myocardial oxygen demand and increase available oxygen. Always have good IV access (possibly more than one IV line). Be sure to ask about medication allergies (especially to any that may have been used previously in a cardiac setting)

©2004 Pearson Education, Inc.
Intermediate Emergency Care: Principles & Practice

before the patient or family may become unable to give you this information. Transport as rapidly as possible with no lights or sirens if possible. Delay in transport, however, is preferable to a patient's refusal to leave the scene.

Management includes placing the patient at physical and emotional rest to decrease myocardial oxygen demand: Give oxygen, generally at high-flow rate. Establish IV access on scene or en route to the hospital. Conduct the ECG; do not, however, delay transport to perform it. You can give nitroglycerin sublingually as a tablet or spray. If symptoms persist after 1–2 doses, raise your suspicion for a more serious condition such as acute MI. Nifedipine and other calcium channel blockers can also be used for relief of anginal pain: Morphine may be used for nonresponsive chest pain.

Patients with an initial episode of angina or an episode that does not respond to medication are usually admitted for observation. Immediate transport is indicated if relief does not come after oxygen and nitrates. The absence of relief may signal the beginning of infarction, and in this case reperfusion is crucial. Hypotension may occur, especially if nitroglycerin has been given. It indicates transport as well because it can lead to or worsen hypoperfusion of myocardial tissue. S-T segment changes, particularly elevation, also indicate the need for rapid, efficient transport: Transport should be WITHOUT lights or siren, if possible, in order to minimize patient anxiety.

If the patient refuses transport, be sure you clearly explain that immediate evaluation is vital because of the potential for problems such as MI. If you can't reverse the patient's decision, be sure the patient reads and signs the refusal and understands the potential risks. Ask that they contact their cardiologist or other physician for follow-up as soon as possible.

11. Define the terms "congestive heart failure" and "pulmonary edema" and the cardiac and non-cardiac causes and terminology associated with them.   pp. 930–931

Congestive heart failure (CHF) is a general term for ventricular failure (left, right, or both) that causes excess fluid to accumulate in body tissues (hence, congestion). The excess fluid is manifest as edema, which may be pulmonary, peripheral, sacral, or within the abdomen as ascites. You may find it in the acute setting of MI, pulmonary edema, or pulmonary hypertension. In the chronic setting, it can reflect cardiac enlargement.

Manage a patient with severe CHF by assessing in an ongoing manner for life-threatening symptoms and intervene promptly while readying the patient for rapid transport. Do not allow the patient to exert in any way, including standing up. Positioning in a seated position with feet dangling promotes venous pooling and, consequently, reduced preload. Administer high-flow oxygen. If necessary, provide positive-pressure ventilations with either a demand valve or a bag-valve-mask device. Establish an IV line at a keep-vein-open rate or place a saline or heparin lock. Place ECG electrodes. If the patient is extremely diaphoretic, apply tincture of Benzoin first so electrodes will adhere tightly to skin. Record a baseline ECG and continue monitoring.

Medication use will be according to your local protocols or the order of medical direction. Always remember to ask about drug allergies or reactions to any medication.

Transport as a nonemergency unless clinical conditions say otherwise. Indications for emergency transport include hypertension or hypotension, severe respiratory distress or pending respiratory failure, or life-threatening dysrhythmias. If you feel nonemergency transport will compromise the patient's condition, use lights and siren.

As the left ventricle's pumping ability falls, it cannot pump out all of the blood delivered to it from the lungs. Consequently, left atrial pressure rises and is transmitted to the pulmonary veins and the pulmonary capillary beds. When pulmonary capillary pressure increases sufficiently, blood plasma is forced into the alveoli and interstitial spaces; this is pulmonary edema (swelling of the lungs). Progressive fluid accumulation in the alveoli decreases the lungs' oxygenation capacity and can cause hypoxia that can be fatal.

For left ventricular failure, the cardinal symptom is dyspnea due to pulmonary edema. Signs include cyanosis, tachycardia, noisy, labored breathing, rales, cough, blood-tinged, frothy sputum, and a gallop rhythm of the heart. The major signs of right ventricular failure: neck veins engorged and pulsating, edema of body and extremities, engorged liver and spleen, abdominal distention with ascites (fluid), as well as tachycardia.

Medical Emergencies

12. Describe the early and late signs and symptoms of pulmonary edema. pp. 931–932

Pulmonary edema reflects backup of fluid into the pulmonary alveoli and interstitium, but it does not necessarily imply etiology. Left ventricular failure, however, is probably the best known and most common cause, and you should look for other signs of congestive heart failure in a patient who presents with signs of pulmonary edema. If pulmonary edema seems to be very acute in onset, look for precipitating causes, such as cardiac dysrhythmia or acute MI. Dependent edema represents edema in the gravity-dependent portions of the body. For a bedridden patient, this often manifests as sacral edema. Sometimes edema will be so severe it will eliminate your ability to find a pulse in the affected area (such as a pedal pulse). If edema is severe enough to be pitting edema (a situation in which you press firmly into the affected tissue, lift the finger, and find that the depression caused by your finger persists), you can make a semi-quantitative evaluation by scoring as 0 to 4+.

13. Explain the clinical significance of paroxysmal nocturnal dyspnea. pp. 931–932

Paroxysmal nocturnal dyspnea (PND) is an episode of waking during the night due to shortness of breath, and it reflects the presence of pulmonary edema. If these episodes become more frequent (more nights or more times/night), it suggest worsening of the underlying pathophysiologic process.

14. List and describe the pharmacological agents available to the EMT-Intermediate for use in the management of a patient with cardiac compromise. pp. 932, 933

The drugs most likely to be used in the setting of cardiac compromise include morphine sulfate, nitroglycerin, furosemide (Lasix), dopamine (Intropin), dobutamine (Dobutrex), promethazine (Phenergan), and nitrous oxide (Nitronox). Dosages and other information on these medications are given in objective 9 above.

15. Define the term "hypertensive emergency." p. 934

A hypertensive emergency is a life-threatening elevation in blood pressure. It occurs in 1% or less of patients with hypertension, usually when the hypertension is poorly controlled or left untreated. It is characterized by a rapid increase in diastolic pressure (usually 0.130 mmHg) and the patient may experience restlessness, confusion, blurred vision, nausea, and vomiting. It often occurs with hypertensive encephalopathy.

16. Describe the clinical features of the patient in a hypertensive emergency. pp. 934–935

Clinically, the emergency is usually characterized by a rapid increase in diastolic pressure (generally, to greater than 130 mmHg) accompanied by restlessness and confusion, blurred vision, and nausea and vomiting. It often occurs with hypertensive encephalopathy, a consequence of severe hypertension marked by severe headache, vomiting, visual changes including transient blindness, paralysis, seizures, and stupor or coma. With modern medications, hypertensive encephalopathy has become rare, although it is still seen in the hospital setting. Both ischemic and hemorrhagic strokes are more common results of severe hypertension and can have devastating consequences. Hypertensive emergency can also cause left ventricular failure and pulmonary edema.

The major causes of hypertensive emergency include noncompliance with antihypertensive drugs or other prescribed medications and lack of treatment for hypertension. Risk factors include age (older age) and race (hypertension is more common in blacks, and morbidity and mortality appear to be higher, too). Among pregnant women, one cause of hypertension is preeclampsia (also called toxemia of pregnancy), which can appear at any point after the 20th week of pregnancy.

17. List the interventions prescribed for the patient with a hypertensive emergency. p. 935

Assessment findings on physical exam of a patient with hypertensive emergency commonly include a chief complaint of headache accompanied by any of the following: nausea, vomiting, blurred vision, shortness of breath, epistaxis, and dizziness (vertigo). The patient may be semiconscious or unconscious and seizing. In toxemia of pregnancy, the woman usually has edema of hands or face. Photosensitivity and headache are common complaints in this group. Determine whether there is a documented history of hypertension and to what degree prescribed medications have been taken. Find out whether the patient may have borrowed someone else's medications or taken herbal or over-the-counter drugs. Skin may be pale or flushed, normal, cool, or warm. Look for edema. The patient may confirm PND, orthopnea, vertigo, epistaxis, tinnitus, or visual acuities. Look for possible motor or sensory deficits in parts of the body or on one side. ECG findings are generally inconclusive unless there is an underlying cardiac condition such as angina or MI. If left ventricular failure is present, pulmonary edema may be present. Otherwise, lungs are generally clear. The pulse is strong and may feel bounding. Hypertension is present with systolic pressure greater than 160 mmHg and/or diastolic pressure greater than 90 mmHg. Signs or symptoms of hypertensive encephalopathy in the presence of measured hypertension should be considered hypertensive emergency.

Management centers on positioning for comfort and watching for possible airway compromise if vomiting or stroke occurs. Give oxygen and decide upon transport based on clinical presentation. Attempt supportive IV therapy on-scene or en route. Place pregnant patients on their left sides and transport as smoothly and quietly as possible.

Medications that may be used in the prehospital setting have notably changed recently; know your local protocol. Medications often used include morphine, furosemide, nitroglycerin, sodium nitroprusside, and labetalol (Trandate, Normodyne).

18. Define the term "cardiogenic shock." p. 935

Cardiogenic shock is the extreme state of heart failure: Cardiac output is so low it cannot sustain minimal physiologic activity. Clinically, you will see it after existing dysrhythmias, hypovolemia, or altered vascular tone have been corrected, leaving only the possibility of endogenous pump failure. This failure of the heart and overwhelming of any compensatory mechanisms usually happens after an extensive MI, often involving more than 40% of the left ventricle, or with diffuse ischemia. Note that cardiogenic shock can occur at any age, but it is most often seen as an end-stage event in geriatric patients with underlying disease. Mortality rate is high for elderly patients following massive MI or septic shock because end-organ damage is so severe that life cannot be sustained.

19. Identify the clinical criteria for cardiogenic shock. pp. 936–938

Numerous mechanisms can lead to cardiogenic shock, and onset may be gradual or acute. Among mechanical causes are tension pneumothorax and cardiac tamponade. Interference with ventricular emptying or afterload (such as pulmonary embolism and prosthetic or natural valve dysfunction) can also cause shock. Impairment in cardiac contractility is also a general cause: examples include MI, myocarditis, and recreational drug use. Trauma is another general cause, either primarily through cardiac damage or secondarily through hypovolemia. Finally, shock can develop secondarily to underlying conditions such as neurologic, GI, renal, or metabolic disorders.

Assessment findings depend on whether the patient is in an early phase of shock or a most advanced state. Look for evidence of a possible contributing cause such as hypovolemia, sepsis, or trauma. Among direct cardiac causes, you will most often see cardiogenic shock in the setting of MI if the MI affects the anterior wall or 40% or more of the left ventricle. Information about the patient's medications may give clues about pre-existing pump compromise. Inquire about the degree of compliance with medication regiments and ask about borrowed or over-the-counter drugs, which might have unpredictable interaction effects.

The altered mental status associated with advancing shock may begin as restlessness and progress through confusion to loss of consciousness. Airway findings include dyspnea, productive cough, or labored breathing. Tachypnea is often present due to pulmonary edema. Also common is a history of paroxysmal nocturnal dyspnea. Typical ECG findings include tachycardia and atrial dysrhythmias such as atrial tachycardia. Ectopy is also common.

MI often precedes cardiogenic shock; symptoms will be compatible with those expected with MI. Expect hypotension to develop as shock progresses. Systolic pressure will often fall to less than 80 mmHg. Try to correct any discovered dysrhythmias.

Management of cardiogenic shock begins by placing the patient in a position of comfort. With pulmonary edema, this may be sitting upright. Treatment consists mostly of caring for underlying conditions (such as MI or CHF) and supportive care. Remember to treat heart rate and rhythm and transport rapidly. Medications that may be used in this setting include the vasopressors dopamine, dobutamine, and norepinephrine. Other medications include morphine, promethazine, nitroglycerin, nitrous oxide, furosemide, digitalis, and sodium bicarbonate.

20. Define the term "cardiac arrest." p. 938

Cardiac arrest and sudden death account for 60% of all deaths from coronary heart disease. Cardiac arrest is defined as the absence of ventricular contractions that immediately results in systemic circulatory failure. Sudden death is any death that occurs within one hour of the onset of symptoms. At autopsy, signs of MI are not present, and authorities generally believe lethal dysrhythmia secondary to severe atherosclerosis is the most common cause of death. The risk factors for sudden death are similar to those for ASHD and CHD. Other causes of sudden death include drowning, acid-base imbalance, electrocution, drug intoxication, electrolyte imbalance, hypoxia, hypothermia, pulmonary embolism, stroke, hyperkalemia, trauma, and end-stage renal disease.

21. Define the term "resuscitation." p. 938

Resuscitation and management start with simultaneous efforts on the ABCs. Ventilate with a bag-valve mask using 100% oxygen. Intubate or insert an airway as quickly as possible. If ECG changes indicate defibrillation or synchronized cardioversion, perform it in conjunction with CPR, stopping CPR only long enough to apply the pads or paddles and deliver the shock. If the patient has an internal pacemaker or defibrillator, be sure not to defibrillate over the device.

After starting CPR and advanced airway management, get IV access with a venous site as close to the heart as possible (for instance, the antecubital area in the arm or the external jugular vein). Follow IV medications with a 30–45 second flush to ensure complete delivery. After each flush, set the line to a keep-vein-open rate. Agents used with cardiac arrest include atropine, lidocaine, procainamide, bretylium, epinephrine, norepinephrine, isoproterenol, dopamine, dobutamine, and sodium bicarbonate.

If blood pressure and pulse return, be aware that the blood pressure itself may be low, normal, or high because of the drugs administered. Pulse may return with a bradycardic, normal, or tachycardic rate. Ventricular ectopy is the most serious concern. If the patient presented in ventricular tachycardia or ventricular fibrillation or if ectopy is seen postarrest, use an antidysrhythmic such as lidocaine.

Transport should be done as safely and smoothly as possible and with lights and siren.

22. Identify local protocol dictating circumstances and situations where resuscitation efforts would not be initiated or would be discontinued. pp. 939–942

In some situations, the patient will not survive despite resuscitation efforts, and in these cases resuscitation is contraindicated and should not be begun: These settings are rigor mortis, fixed dependent lividity (pooling of blood in gravity-dependent fashion), decapitation, and incineration. Less obvious but equally important settings include those where there is an advance directive to withhold resuscitation.

23. Identify the critical actions necessary in caring for the patient in cardiac arrest. pp. 938–939

Assessment for cardiac arrest shows an unresponsive, apneic, pulseless individual. After initiating CPR, place ECG leads and initiate monitoring. Dysrhythmias you may find include ventricular tachycardia or fibrillation, asystole, or PEA. If you find asystole, confirm it in two or more leads. Question bystanders with the goal of finding some specific, prognostic information: Did anyone witness the arrest? If CPR was begun before you arrived, try to learn as precisely as possible the length of time between arrest and initiation of effective CPR. Often, the emergency room physician will also want to know total down time from the beginning of the arrest until arrival at the emergency department. Also, try to get a list of the patient's medications as well as a past history.

©2004 Pearson Education, Inc.
Intermediate Emergency Care: Principles & Practice

24. **Synthesize patient history and assessment findings to form a field impression for the patient with chest pain and cardiac dysrhythmias that may be indicative of a cardiac emergency.** pp. 897–945

- **Cardiovascular disease.** Assessment findings are specific to the region of the vascular system affected by occlusion. Central findings such as tachypnea and change in heart rate or rhythm suggest pulmonary embolism or aortic aneurysm. Care is largely supportive unless a life-threatening problem (such as hypotension or dysrhythmia) develops.
- **Chest pain.** Chest pain can have a cardiac (pericarditis, angina, or MI) or vascular (aortic aneurysm) origin, or it can reflect problems of the respiratory system, GI tract, or musculoskeletal system. Look for pain on exertion that is relieved by rest and/or nitroglycerin as a sign of possible angina and pain that is unremitting for an MI. With both you may well see ECG changes including sinus tachycardia, S-T segment depression or elevation, ectopy, or dysrhythmias.
- **In need of a pacemaker.** A patient with a history of high-degree AV block or symptomatic bradycardia or atrial fibrillation has inadequate cardiac output for body needs during the periods of those dysrhythmias. If medications don't convert the dysrhythmia to a rhythm compatible with adequate cardiac output, a pacemaker should be considered. Other patients may have recurrent episodes of life-threatening dysrhythmias such as ventricular tachycardia or ventricular fibrillation, and they may also need a pacemaker.
- **Angina pectoris.** The typical presentation for angina is pain lasting from 3-5 minutes, or perhaps as long as 15 minutes, that is relieved by rest and/or nitroglycerin. Prinzmetal's (vasospastic) angina most often occurs at rest or without a known trigger but has similar duration. Prinzmetal's angina is often accompanied by S-T segment elevation on ECG. A patient with fixed (obstructive) angina may show S-T depression and/or T wave inversion on 12-lead ECG. Relief of pain is generally associated with resolution of ECG disturbances.
- **A suspected myocardial infarction.** The patient with an acute MI has chest pain that is severe, constant, and lasts longer than 30 minutes. Neither rest nor nitroglycerin relieves the pain, and the patient may be fearful or feel a sense of doom. On ECG, check the S-T segment for depression, which suggests ischemia, or elevation, which suggests tissue injury. A pathological Q wave (deeper than 5 mm and longer than 0.04 sec) can indicate either widespread transient ischemia or infarcted tissue. Ectopy and dysrhythmia can appear without warning.
- **Heart failure.** Heart failure, inadequacy of pumping ability to meet the body's oxygen demand, can be left-sided, right-sided, or both. Left-sided ventricular failure typically presents with dyspnea and the following additional signs: cyanosis, tachycardia, noisy, labored breathing, rales, cough, blood-tinged, often frothy sputum, and galloping heart sounds. Decreased lung sounds on exam reflect pulmonary edema. Right-sided ventricular failure typically presents with tachycardia, jugular venous distention, edema of body and extremities, engorged (palpable) liver and spleen, and abdominal distention due to ascites fluid. History will usually reflect past cardiac disease or pulmonary disease (COPD). Paroxysmal nocturnal dyspnea suggests left heart failure.
- **A hypertensive emergency.** The patient with a hypertensive emergency will have extreme hypertension (diastolic greater than 130 mmHg) and usually will show some signs of hypertensive encephalopathy such as headache, visual change, nausea and vomiting, restlessness, or seizures or coma.
- **Cardiogenic shock.** Cardiogenic shock represents shock of cardiac origin: Exam will show characteristic signs of shock (hyperperfusion to extremities, hypotension, tachycardia) but history and exam will rule out extracardiac causes such as hypovolemia or sepsis. ECG may reveal an underlying acute event such as MI.
- **Cardiac arrest.** Patients in cardiac arrest are unresponsive, apneic, and pulseless. ECG may show asystole, PEA, or ventricular tachycardia or ventricular fibrillation. Confirm arrest in two or more ECG leads before beginning management.

Medical Emergencies

25. **Given several preprogrammed patients with cardiac complaints, provide the appropriate assessment, treatment, and transport.** **pp. 897–945**

Because cardiovascular disease is so common and so serious, accounting for considerable morbidity and mortality, you will see patients who have the problems or conditions discussed in this chapter. Review objectives 3, 4, 6–20, 23, and 24 in Part 2 of the chapter in particular to familiarize yourself with care in the setting of chest pain, angina, and MI, as well as care of heart failure and acute cardiovascular emergencies.

CONTENT SELF-EVALUATION

MULTIPLE CHOICE

_____ 1. Chest pain is the most common chief complaint among patients with cardiac disease, but not all patients with cardiac disease will have chest pain.
   A. True
   B. False

_____ 2. Atropine, lidocaine, and adenosine are in which group of drugs?
   A. sympathomimetics
   B. sympatholytics
   C. thrombolytics
   D. antidysrhythmics
   E. drugs used for myocardial ischemia and its pain

_____ 3. Dopamine, dobutamine, and epinephrine are in which group of drugs?
   A. sympatholytics
   B. drugs used for myocardial ischemia and its pain
   C. antidysrhythmics
   D. parasympathomimetics
   E. sympathomimetics

_____ 4. Nitrous oxide, nitroglycerin, and morphine are in which group of drugs?
   A. sympathomimetics
   B. drugs used for myocardial ischemia and its pain
   C. antidysrhythmics
   D. antiatherosclerotics
   E. sympatholytics

_____ 5. Indications for synchronized cardioversion in an unstable patient include all of the following EXCEPT:
   A. rapid atrial fibrillation.
   B. nonperfusing ventricular tachycardia.
   C. paroxysmal supraventricular tachycardia.
   D. perfusing ventricular tachycardia.
   E. 2:1 atrial flutter.

_____ 6. Potentially urgent noncardiac causes of chest pain include all of the following EXCEPT:
   A. stroke.
   B. peptic ulcer disease.
   C. pneumothorax.
   D. pulmonary embolism.
   E. esophageal disease.

_____ 7. Always consider the possibility of cardiac tamponade when you encounter a patient:
   A. with a chest wall tumor.
   B. with muffled or distant heart and lung sounds.
   C. with a gallop rhythm (S_1, S_2, S_3, S_4 heart sounds).
   D. who has just entered ventricular fibrillation.
   E. who received CPR and later deteriorated.

_____ 8. Causes of cardiogenic shock include all of the following EXCEPT:
  A. subendocardial MI.
  B. tension pneumothorax.
  C. pulmonary embolism.
  D. diffuse myocardial ischemia.
  E. prosthetic valve malfunction.

_____ 9. Return of spontaneous circulation occurs when resuscitation results in resumption of a pulse; spontaneous breathing may or may not return.
  A. True
  B. False

_____ 10. Which of the following is NOT a possible criteria for termination of resuscitation efforts?
  A. successful and maintained endotracheal intubation
  B. patient remains in asystole after four rounds of ALS drugs
  C. on-scene ALS efforts have been sustained for 25 minutes
  D. arrest is associated with blunt trauma, hypothermia, or drug overdose
  E. ACLS standards have been applied throughout the arrest

MATCHING

Write the letter of the definition in the space provided next to the term to which it applies.

_____ 11. orthopnea

_____ 12. bruit

_____ 13. paroxysmal nocturnal dyspnea

_____ 14. pulsus paradoxus

_____ 15. pulsus alternans

_____ 16. intermittent claudication

_____ 17. thrombophlebitis

A. inflammation and clots within a vein
B. relief of dyspnea on sitting upright
C. alternation of weak and strong pulse over time
D. pain in the calf muscles secondary to local ischemia
E. episodes of being awakened at night by shortness of breath
F. murmur heard over an artery due to turbulent blood flow
G. drop of more than 10 mmHg in systolic BP with inspiration

Write the letter of the clinical setting in the space provided next to the procedure that should be carried out in that setting.

_____ 18. defibrillation

_____ 19. transcutaneous cardiac pacing

_____ 20. precordial thump

_____ 21. synchronized cardioversion

_____ 22. carotid sinus massage

A. effort made immediately after onset of ventricular fibrillation or pulseless ventricular tachycardia that may cause conversion to organized rhythm
B. passage of electrical current through the heart during a specific part of the cardiac cycle to terminate certain dysrhythmias
C. manipulation of an arterial baroreceptor in an effort to increase parasympathetic tone
D. electrical pacing of the heart with use of special skin electrodes
E. passage of electrical current through a fibrillating heart to depolarize a critical mass of myocardium, resulting in conversion to an organized rhythm

Medical Emergencies

Write the letter of the cardiac condition in the space provided next to the ECG finding that would suggest it.

_____ 23. pathological Q wave

_____ 24. S-T segment elevation

_____ 25. T wave inversion

_____ 26. S-T segment depression

A. infarcted tissue or extensive transient ischemia
B. myocardial ischemia
C. myocardial injury
D. old infarcted tissue that has formed a scar

Write the letter of the probable diagnosis in the space provided next to the appropriate description of the condition. A letter response may be used more than once or not at all.

A. pulmonary edema   E. right ventricular failure
B. heart failure   F. cardiac arrest
C. acute MI   G. cardiac tamponade
D. left ventricular failure   H. hypertensive encephalopathy

_____ 27. constant chest pain that is not relieved by rest or nitroglycerin and lasts longer than 30 minutes

_____ 28. dyspnea, tachycardia, noisy, labored breathing, gallop heart rhythm

_____ 29. syndrome in which the heart's pumping ability does not meet body needs

_____ 30. unresponsiveness with apnea and pulselessness

_____ 31. jugular venous distention, engorged liver, edema, tachycardia

_____ 32. pulsus paradoxus and pulsus alternans

_____ 33. dyspnea, orthopnea, decreased systolic BP with narrowing pulse pressures

_____ 34. severe headache, visual disturbance, seizures, stupor, diagnostic vital signs

©2004 Pearson Education, Inc.
Intermediate Emergency Care: Principles & Practice

CHAPTER 21
*
Diabetic Emergencies

Review of Chapter Objectives

After reading this chapter, you should be able to:

1. Discuss the anatomy and physiology of the endocrine system.

pp. 948–949; see Chapter 2

There are eight major structures associated with the endocrine system located throughout the body: the hypothalamus, pituitary gland, thyroid gland, parathyroid glands, thymus, pancreas, adrenal glands, and gonads. The pineal gland is also part of the endocrine system.

The hypothalamus, located deep within the cerebrum of the brain, is the junction between the endocrine system and the central nervous system. About the size of a pea, the pituitary gland is located adjacent to the hypothalamus within the cerebrum. The pineal gland is also located adjacent to the hypothalamus. The double-lobed thyroid gland is located in the neck anterior to and just below the cartilage of the larynx. The parathyroid glands are very small and are found on the posterior lateral surface of the thyroid gland. The thymus is located in the mediastinum just behind the sternum. The pancreas is located in the upper abdomen behind the stomach and between the duodenum and the spleen. The adrenal glands are somewhat triangular in shape and are located on the superior surface of the kidneys. Gonads can be found in the lower pelvis in women, with each ovary resembling an almond in size and shape. In men, the gonads are located in the scrotum.

The endocrine system is closely linked to the nervous system and plays a critical role in our ability to maintain life by regulating many bodily functions through chemical substances called hormones. The endocrine system is made up of ductless glands, which manufacture and secrete hormones that act in adjacent tissues or travel via the bloodstream to target organs or other endocrine glands to produce specific or generalized effects. Hormones regulate metabolic activity, growth and development, as well as mediate chemical reactions, maintain homeostatic balance, and initiate our adaptive response to stress.

2. Describe the pathophysiology of diabetes mellitus.

pp. 949–951

Juvenile onset or Type I diabetes mellitus is a serious disease characterized by very low production of insulin by the beta cells of the pancreas. In many cases, there is no insulin being produced. It is called juvenile onset diabetes because of the average age of the patient at the time of diagnosis. Type I diabetes is also known as insulin-dependent diabetes mellitus (IDDM) because patients require regular injections of insulin to control their disease. Heredity appears to be an important factor in determining which people will develop Type I diabetes. The cause of Type I diabetes is not clear. Other factors attributed to triggering juvenile onset diabetes are viral infection, an autoimmune response, or genetically determined premature deterioration of beta cells. The immediate cause of Type I diabetes is the destruction of pancreatic beta cells.

Type II diabetes mellitus, also known as non-insulin-dependent diabetes (NIDDM), is responsible for almost 90 percent of all cases of diabetes. Type II diabetes usually begins in later life and is often associated with obesity, so it is known as adult onset diabetes. Type II diabetes is associated with a moderate decline in insulin production accompanied by a marked decrease in the utilization of the insulin within the body. The cause is not clearly understood, although obesity is believed to play a role in its development. Increased weight, along with the increased size of fat cells, causes a relative deficiency in the number of insulin receptors, thus making the fat cells less responsive to insulin. Type II diabetes is usually managed through a combination of diet, exercise, and the administration of medications to reduce either blood glucose or enhance the efficiency of insulin. Occasionally insulin administration is required.

3. Differentiate between normal glucose metabolism and diabetic glucose metabolism.
pp. 950–953

Metabolism, which means "to change," is a term used to refer to all of the chemical and energy transformations within the body. Two kinds of change take place in the cell. One kind builds complex molecules from simple ones (anabolism), such as the synthesis of glycogen from glucose. The other kind breaks down complex molecules into simpler ones (catabolism), such as occurs with the breakdown of glucose into carbon dioxide, water, and energy (in the form of ATP). When materials are abundant after meals and the glucose is high, insulin enables cells to use glucose directly and to store energy as glycogen, protein, and fat. Insulin stimulates glucose pathways. In contrast, glucagon, the dominant hormone during periods of low blood glucose, stimulates catabolic pathways to produce usable energy from the body's stores.

The rate at which glucose can enter the cell is dependent upon insulin levels. Insulin combines with insulin receptors on the surface of the cell membrane, allowing glucose to enter the cell by increasing the permeability of the cell membrane. The rate at which glucose can be transported into the cells can be accelerated tenfold by insulin.

Sometimes the body cannot use glucose as its primary energy source, as is the case in patients with diabetes mellitus. Without insulin, the amount of glucose that can be transported into the cells is far too small to meet the body's energy demands. Without insulin, the glucose remains in the bloodstream, resulting in hyperglycemia. Carbohydrate depletion is also seen in other conditions, such as a high-fat, low-carbohydrate diet or starvation (which can be associated with some eating disorders). Under these conditions, the body slowly switches from glucose to fat as the primary energy source. Adipose cells break down fats into their component free fatty acids, and the blood concentration of these acids rises considerably.

Most of the fatty acids are used directly by the body's cells as an energy source. The liver takes in some, where the catabolism of fatty acids produces acetoacetic acid. When more acetoacetic acid is released by the liver than can be effectively utilized by body cells, it accumulates in the bloodstream along with two other closely related substances, acetone and β-hydroxybutyric acid. The three substances are collectively called ketone bodies. Their presence in excessive quantities is called ketosis.

4. Describe the mechanism of ketone body formation and its relationship to ketoacidosis.
pp. 951, 953–954

When the body's carbohydrate stores begin to become depleted, small amounts of glucose can be formed by the breakdown of protein and fat through the process of gluconeogenesis. The byproducts of amino acid breakdown include carbon dioxide and water and the formation of urea. The breakdown of fat results in the formation of carbon dioxide, water, and ketone bodies.

The normal blood ketone level in humans is low because ketones are usually metabolized as rapidly as they are formed. If there are low levels of glucose stored in the cells, the ability of the body to oxidize the ketones is soon exceeded and ketones begin to build up in the bloodstream, resulting in a condition known as ketosis. This results in an increased amount of acid in the body fluids. The resulting metabolic acidosis is often severe and can be fatal.

5. Discuss the physiology of the excretion of potassium and ketone bodies by the kidneys.
pp. 951, 953–954

Whenever the flow rate of fluid inside the tubules of the kidney rises, as in osmotic diuresis, an increase in excretion of potassium occurs. This leads to the potential for significant hypokalemia and its effects, such as potentially life-threatening cardiac dysrhythmias. In ketotic states, ketone bodies are excreted through respiration and will also spill into the urine.

©2004 Pearson Education, Inc.
Intermediate Emergency Care: Principles & Practice

6. Describe the relationship of insulin to serum glucose levels.   pp. 949–957

Insulin is a glucagon antagonist and lowers the blood glucose level by promoting energy storage. Insulin increases the rate at which various body cells take up glucose by changing the permeability of the cell membranes. These changes also make the cell more permeable to potassium, magnesium, and phosphate ions, as well as many amino acids. Because the liver rapidly breaks down insulin, the hormone must be secreted constantly.

Homeostasis of blood glucose is remarkably effective. In non-diabetics, when blood glucose is high, as after a meal, the beta cells of the pancreas release insulin. Insulin enables cells to use glucose directly as well as to store energy as glycogen, protein, and fat. If you were to draw a venous blood sample to measure fasting blood glucose levels, you'd find the level in healthy individuals is usually between 80–90 mg glucose/dL blood. In the first 60–90 minutes after a meal the level will increase to approximately 120–140 mg/dL before dropping off to near-fasting levels as insulin is released to move the glucose from the bloodstream into the cells. Conversely, when blood glucose levels are low, the alpha cells of the pancreas release glucagon to raise the blood glucose level.

7. Describe the effects of decreased levels of insulin on the body.   pp. 949–956

Insulin deficiency contributes to the development of hyperglycemia. Without insulin to facilitate the movement of large glucose molecules across cell membranes, the blood glucose level rises even as the intracellular level of glucose plummets. At the same time, the alpha cells of the pancreas release glucagon to increase blood glucose by stimulating the breakdown of glycogen, as well as stimulating the breakdown of body proteins and fats with subsequent chemical conversion to glucose (gluconeogenesis).

8. Describe the effects of increased serum glucose levels on the body.   pp. 949–956

With a rise in blood glucose levels, as is the case in Type I diabetes, the body's cells cannot take up circulating glucose. Glucose then spills into urine, leading to a large water loss, via osmotic diuresis, and significant dehydration. This can lead to significant loss of potassium and hypokalemia.

9. Discuss the pathophysiology, assessment findings, and management of the following endocrine emergencies:

a. nonketotic hyperosmolar coma   pp. 955–956

This condition is a complication of Type II diabetes due to inadequate insulin activity and is marked by high blood glucose, marked dehydration, and decreased mental function.

Development of the coma is slower than with ketoacidosis. Early signs include increased urination and thirst. Later signs may include orthostatic hypotension, dry skin, and tachycardia.

This condition is difficult to distinguish from ketoacidosis in the field. Field management focuses on maintaining ABCs and fluid resuscitation.

b. diabetic ketoacidosis   pp. 953–955

Diabetic ketoacidosis is a serious, potentially life-threatening complication of diabetes mellitus. It occurs when profound insulin deficiency is coupled with increased glucagon activity.

The onset is slow, lasting from 12 to 24 hours. In its early stages, the signs and symptoms include intensified thirst, excessive hunger, increased urination, and malaise. Increased urination results from the osmotic diuresis accompanying glucose spillage into the urine. Intensified thirst is caused by the body's attempt to replace the fluids lost by increased urination. Nausea, vomiting, marked dehydration, tachycardia, and weakness characterize diabetic ketoacidosis. The skin is usually warm and dry. Coma is not uncommon. The breath may have a sweet or acetone-like character due to the increased ketones in the blood. Very deep, rapid respirations, called Kussmaul's respirations, also occur. Kussmaul's respirations represent the body's attempt to compensate for the metabolic acidosis produced by the ketones and organic acids present in the blood. It may be complicated by several electrolyte imbalances. The most significant is decreased potassium. Decreased potassium (hypokalemia) can lead to serious dysrhythmias or even death.

The approach used with the patient suffering from diabetic ketoacidosis is essentially the same as with any unconscious patient. You should first complete your initial assessment of airway, breathing, and circulation. You will then complete your focused history and physical exam. Pay particular attention to the presence of a Medic-Alert bracelet and/or insulin in the refrigerator. Also, obtain a history from bystanders. The fruity odor of ketones occasionally can be detected on the breath. If possible, complete the rapid test for blood glucose.

It is not uncommon for patients in ketoacidosis to have blood glucose levels well in excess of 300 mg/dL. The field management of such cases is focused on maintenance of ABCs and fluid resuscitation to counteract the patient's dehydration. Treatment should include drawing a red top tube (or the tube specified by local protocols) of blood. Following this, you should administer one to two liters of normal saline per protocol. If transport time is lengthy, the medical direction physician may request intravenous or subcutaneous administration of regular insulin.

If the blood glucose level cannot be quickly determined, draw a red top tube of blood for analysis and start an IV of normal saline. Following this, administer 50 ml (25 grams) of 50 percent dextrose solution. This additional glucose load will not adversely affect the ketoacidotic patient because it is negligible compared to the total quantity present in the body. If the patient is alcoholic, consider administering 100 mg of thiamine. Transportation to an appropriate facility should be expedited.

c. hypoglycemia   pp. 956–957

Hypoglycemia, or low blood glucose, is a potentially life-threatening medical emergency. Sometimes called insulin shock, it can occur if a patient accidentally or intentionally injects too much insulin, eats an inadequate amount of food after taking insulin, or has overexercised and burned up all available glucose. Untreated, the insulin will cause the blood glucose to drop to a very low level. The longer the period of hypoglycemia persists, the greater the risk that the brain cells will be permanently damaged or even killed.

The signs and symptoms of hypoglycemia are many and varied. An abnormal mental status is the most important and often the earliest sign. In the earliest stages of hypoglycemia, the patient may appear restless or impatient or complain of hunger. As the blood sugar falls lower, he or she may display inappropriate anger or display a variety of bizarre behaviors. Physical signs may include diaphoresis and tachycardia. If the blood sugar falls to a critically low level, the patient may sustain a hypoglycemic seizure or become comatose. In contrast to diabetic ketoacidosis, hypoglycemia can develop quickly. When encountering a patient behaving bizarrely, you should always consider hypoglycemia.

In suspected cases of hypoglycemia, perform the initial assessment quickly. Inspect the patient for a Medic-Alert bracelet. If possible, determine the blood glucose level. If the blood glucose level is noted to be less than 60 mg/dL, draw a red top tube of blood and start an IV of normal saline. Next, administer 50–100 milliliters (25–50 grams) of 50 percent dextrose intravenously. If the patient is conscious and able to swallow, complete glucose administration with orange juice, sodas, or commercially available glucose pastes.

If the blood glucose cannot be obtained and if the patient is unconscious, you should start an IV of normal saline and administer 50–100 milliliters (25–50 grams) of 50 percent dextrose. Expedite transport to the nearest medical facility. If you suspect alcoholism, administer 100 mg of thiamine prior to the administration of dextrose.

d. hyperglycemia   pp. 953–957

Diabetes mellitus results from either inadequate amounts of circulating insulin or inadequate utilization of insulin. This means that there is an excess of blood glucose while there is an intracellular deficit. In diabetes, glucose builds up in the bloodstream, especially after meals. The blood glucose level rises higher and returns to normal more slowly in the diabetic than in the non-diabetic. An oral glucose tolerance test uses this phenomenon in the diagnosis of diabetes. The diabetic's inadequate insulin level and impaired glucose tolerance are partly due to the decreased entry of glucose into the cells, thus leaving more glucose in the bloodstream.

The second cause of hyperglycemia in the diabetic results from difficulties with the function of the liver. When blood glucose levels are high, insulin secretion is normally increased and the breakdown of glycogen is decreased. In the diabetic, however, insulin secretion is

©2004 Pearson Education, Inc.
Intermediate Emergency Care: Principles & Practice

decreased, and the alpha cells secrete glucagon to stimulate glycogenolysis by the liver, thus raising the blood glucose level.

In Type I diabetes the decreased insulin secretion is accompanied by a steady accumulation of glucose in the blood. Hyperglycemia acts like an osmotic diuretic and glucose "spills over" into the urine (glycosuria) pulling large amounts of water with it (polyuria). The body's attempt to dilute the concentration of glucose in the bloodstream results in intracellular dehydration and stimulates thirst (polydipsia). As the cells become glucose-depleted, they begin to use proteins and fats as an energy source resulting in weight loss and the formation of harmful byproducts, such as ketones and organic free fatty acids. The body's response to this state of cellular starvation is to trigger hunger in the patient (polyphagia). If the acids and ketones continue to collect in the blood, severe metabolic acidosis occurs and coma ensues, resulting in serious brain damage or death.

Type II diabetes does not usually result in diabetic ketoacidosis. It can, however, develop into a life-threatening emergency termed hyperglycemic hyperosmolar nonketotic (HHNK) coma. In Type II diabetes, when blood glucose levels exceed 600 mg/dL, the high osmolality of the blood causes an osmotic diuresis and marked dehydration of body cells. However, sufficient insulin is produced to prevent the manufacture of ketones and the complications of metabolic acidosis. In this respect, the condition differs from diabetic ketoacidosis.

10. Describe the actions of epinephrine as it relates to the pathophysiology of hypoglycemia.   p. 956

Hypoglycemia, or low blood sugar, reflects high insulin and low glucose levels. Regardless of the cause, when insulin levels are high, glucagon may be ineffective in raising blood glucose levels. In prolonged fasts, almost half the glucose normally produced through gluconeogenesis is of renal origin. This activity is stimulated by epinephrine.

15. Describe the compensatory mechanisms utilized by the body to promote homeostasis when hypoglycemia is present.   pp. 949, 956; see Chapter 2

When blood glucose levels fall, the alpha cells of the pancreas secrete glucagon. Glucagon stimulates the breakdown of glycogen into glucose for release into the bloodstream. This process, called glycogenolysis, takes place throughout the body but occurs primarily in the liver. In addition to stimulating the breakdown of glycogen, glucagon also stimulates the breakdown of proteins and fats with subsequent conversion to glucose. This process of producing sugar from nonsugar sources is called gluconeogenesis. Both of these processes contribute to the maintenance of homeostasis by raising blood glucose levels.

CASE STUDY REVIEW

This case study draws attention to the assessment and management of a commonly encountered patient presentation, altered mental status, which is subsequently determined to be due to the potentially life-threatening endocrine emergency, hypoglycemia.

Shauna and Steve arrive at the scene of an "unknown medical emergency." Prior to their entry into the house, they are joined on scene by two police officers. Many jurisdictions have dispatch protocols in place that specify dual dispatch of EMS and law enforcement personnel for calls of an unknown nature or those where there has been or is a potential for violence.

As is sometimes the case at emergency scenes, the patient may not have placed the call for service. Whenever possible, it is helpful in those situations where the 911 call has been placed by a third-party caller to be able to interview that individual to obtain information about the situation on your arrival on scene. In this case, Mrs. Spencer is a concerned neighbor who is able to provide a great deal of information about the usual residents of this home.

The scene size-up and bystander-provided information raise a high index of suspicion about potential dangers, and the police enter the house first to secure the scene. Only after the scene is declared safe do Shauna and Steve enter. It is important to always remember that there is no benefit to be gained by risking your own personal safety. There is truth to the adage that "fools rush in."

Shauna begins her initial assessment of the patient even as she approaches the teenager identified by Mrs. Spencer as Mark McKenzie. Although he is conscious, his responses to Shauna are incoherent. The overturned furniture and disarray on the scene, along with Mark's confusion, lead Shauna and Steve to consider hypoglycemia or drug use as possible causes for the situation. Sudden changes in mental status or bizarre behavior should always make you consider hypoglycemia. Mark's confusion and apparent violent behavior, along with his tachycardia and diaphoresis, are very typical manifestations of hypoglycemia. The decision to gently restrain Mark is based on his lack of appropriate interaction with his environment as well as concern for his own safety and the safety of all of the personnel on the scene.

Routine assessment of oxygen saturation via pulse oximetry and blood glucose level determination via a glucometer reflects the standard of care for any patient presenting with an altered mental status. Most EMS agencies also routinely obtain pre-treatment venous blood samples for analysis at the hospital when dealing with patients presenting with altered mental status.

The glucometer reading of "LOW" indicates a blood glucose level that is less than 50 mg/dL, confirming the presumptive diagnosis of hypoglycemia. Prompt and careful administration of 50 percent dextrose intravenously is the treatment of choice. It is imperative that this medication is administered into a patent IV line in a large vein. Localized venous irritation is likely when small veins are used, and if the dextrose should extravasate, tissue necrosis is common.

Mark's prompt improvement in response to the administration of dextrose is fairly typical. It is not uncommon for diabetics to have no recall of the events that transpired while they were hypoglycemic. The arrival of Mark's mother on scene allows the EMS personnel to get more information about Mark's usual health status. It is not uncommon for diabetics to have some variation in their usual level of control when their insulin dosages have been changed. Although it makes good sense for diabetics to wear some type of medical alert device on their bodies, it is not uncommon for adolescents to be non-compliant with that practice. Follow your agency's protocols regarding "refusal of transport."

CONTENT SELF-EVALUATION

MULTIPLE CHOICE

_____ 1. Which of the following is an exocrine gland?
    A. pineal   D. parathyroid
    B. thymus   E. adrenal
    C. salivary

_____ 2. The term describing the sum of cellular processes that produce energy and molecules needed for growth and repair is:
    A. anabolism.   D. homeostasis.
    B. catabolism.   E. physiology.
    C. metabolism.

_____ 3. Insulin's primary function is to:
    A. metabolize glucose at the cellular level.
    B. free glucose from muscle storage sites.
    C. transport glucose across the cell membrane.
    D. store glucose at the cellular level.
    E. enhance the function of glucagon.

_____ 4. Diabetes mellitus is caused by the inadequate production or activity of:
    A. polypeptide.   D. cortisol.
    B. glucagon.   E. insulin.
    C. somatostatin.

©2004 Pearson Education, Inc.
Intermediate Emergency Care: Principles & Practice

_____ 5. Osmotic diuresis, a characteristic of untreated diabetes, contributes to the development of:
   A. polydipsia and polyphagia.
   B. polydipsia and polyuria.
   C. polyuria and polyphagia.
   D. polyuria.
   E. polyphagia.

_____ 6. All of the following are signs and symptoms of diabetic ketoacidosis EXCEPT:
   A. abdominal pain.
   B. deep rapid respirations.
   C. decreased mental function.
   D. cold, clammy skin.
   E. tachycardia.

_____ 7. Diabetic ketoacidosis, characterized by high blood glucose and metabolic acidosis, occurs as a result of all of the following EXCEPT:
   A. profound insulin deficiency.
   B. increased glucagon activity.
   C. cessation of insulin injections.
   D. physiologic stress.
   E. overexertion.

_____ 8. Kussmaul's respirations are a primary compensatory mechanism for reducing acidosis in the patient with diabetic ketoacidosis.
   A. True
   B. False

_____ 9. Which of the following signs or symptoms will be present in the patient experiencing diabetic ketoacidosis?
   A. acetone breath odor
   B. apathy
   C. diplopia
   D. drooling
   E. diaphoresis

_____ 10. Kussmaul's respirations are seen in which of the following conditions?
   A. diabetic ketoacidosis
   B. hyperglycemic hyperosmolar nonketotic coma
   C. hypoglycemia
   D. insulin shock
   E. thyrotoxicosis

_____ 11. The most important sign or symptom associated with hypoglycemia is:
   A. tachycardia.
   B. cool, clammy skin.
   C. altered mental status.
   D. polydipsia.
   E. polyphagia.

_____ 12. Hyperglycemic hyperosmolar nonketotic acidosis differs from diabetic ketoacidosis because significant production of ketone bodies is prevented by the action of:
   A. polypeptide.
   B. glucagon.
   C. somatostatin.
   D. cortisol.
   E. insulin.

_____ 13. Even in the absence of a blood glucose level, altered mental status in a known diabetic should always be treated with 50 percent dextrose.
   A. True
   B. False

_____ 14. In contrast to hypoglycemia, diabetic ketoacidosis develops quickly and may cause a rapidly developing bizarre behavior.
   A. True
   B. False

_____ 15. You should administer 50% dextrose if the blood glucose level fall below:
   A. 200 mg/dh.
   B. 150 mg/dh.
   C. 60 mg/dh.
   D. 30 mg/dh.
   E. 10 mg/dh.

Medical Emergencies

CHAPTER 22

*

Allergic Reactions

Review of Chapter Objectives

After reading this chapter, you should be able to:

1. **Discuss the pathophysiology of allergy and anaphylaxis.** pp. 962–963

   The signs and symptoms associated with allergy and anaphylaxis are due to the physiologic changes triggered by the chemical mediators of the immune response that are released from the basophils and mast cells. Histamine is the primary mediator of all allergic reactions. It is a potent substance that causes bronchoconstriction, vasodilation and increased vascular permeability, and increased intestinal motility. Other chemical substances are also released that have effects similar to or synergistic with histamine, such as SRS-A (slow-reacting substance of anaphylaxis), which results in an asthma-like attack or asphyxia.

2. **Describe the common routes of substance entry into the body.** pp. 962–963

   Allergens can enter the body through various routes including oral ingestion, inhalation, topically, and through injection or envenomation. The vast majority of anaphylactic reactions result from injection or envenomation.

3. **Define allergic reaction, anaphylaxis, antigen, antibody, and natural and acquired immunity.** pp. 959–962

   An **allergic reaction** is an exaggerated immune response to a foreign protein or other substance, while **anaphylaxis** is an unusual or exaggerated allergic reaction to a foreign protein or other substance.

   An **antigen** is any substance that is capable, under appropriate conditions, of inducing a specific immune response. An **antibody** is a member of a unique class of chemicals that are manufactured by specialized cells of the immune system. The antibody is the principle agent of a chemical attack on an invading substance. Following exposure to an antigen, antibodies are released from cells of the immune system. The antibodies attach themselves to the invading substance so it can be removed from the body by other cells of the immune system.

   Natural immunity refers to the immunity that is present at birth; also called innate immunity, it is genetically determined. **Acquired immunity** is immunity that develops over time and results from exposure to an antigen.

4. **List common antigens most frequently associated with anaphylaxis.** pp. 959–962

   Any substance that is capable, under appropriate conditions, of inducing a specific immune response is known as an antigen. Most antigens are proteins. The following agents are among those that commonly trigger anaphylaxis: antibiotics, foods, or insect stings. Refer to Table 22-1 on text page 960 for a more complete list.

5. Describe the physical manifestations of anaphylaxis. pp. 963–965, 967

The signs and symptoms of anaphylaxis begin within 30 to 60 seconds following exposure for the vast majority of patients. The more rapid the onset, the more severe the patient presentation. Respiratory manifestations of anaphylaxis include laryngeal edema and bronchoconstriction. Cardiovascular symptoms include tachycardia plus massive vasodilation resulting in profound hypotension. The combination of respiratory and cardiovascular signs will lead to a rapid deterioration of the patient's mental status. Generalized flushing and urticaria (hives) are common, as is angioedema about the head, face, and neck. Nausea, vomiting, and diarrhea may accompany hypermotility of the gastrointestinal tract.

6. Identify and differentiate between the signs and symptoms of allergic reaction and anaphylaxis. pp. 963–965, 967–968

Allergic reactions can range from a mild skin rash to a severe life-threatening multisystem response. Allergic reaction, also known as hypersensitivity, takes two forms, delayed or immediate. Delayed hypersensitivity is the result of cellular immunity and does not involve antibodies. It may occur hours to days after exposure and is very common. Delayed hypersensitivity usually presents as a skin rash and is often due to exposure to certain drugs and chemicals, for instance, poison ivy. Other signs and symptoms may include mild bronchoconstriction, mild intestinal cramps, or diarrhea, while the patient's mental status and vital signs will remain normal.

Immediate hypersensitivity is antibody-mediated immunity and often has a genetic link. The range of clinical presentation is widely variable. Examples of these reactions include hay fever, drug and food allergies, eczema, and asthma. Allergens can enter the body by various routes, but as a rule, those that enter by injection tend to have more rapid and more severe effects. Immediate hypersensitivities may be merely annoying, like the itching eyes and runny nose of hay fever, or may pose a real and immediate life threat, as seen in the anaphylactic reaction described in the case study at the beginning of this chapter.

The signs and symptoms of anaphylaxis begin within seconds following exposure. The more rapid the onset of symptoms, the more severe the patient presentation. Respiratory manifestations of anaphylaxis include laryngeal edema and bronchoconstriction. Cardiovascular symptoms include tachycardia plus massive vasodilation resulting in profound hypotension. A rapid deterioration of the patient's mental status accompanies the cardiovascular collapse. Generalized flushing and urticaria are common, as is angioedema about the head, face, and neck. Nausea, vomiting, and diarrhea may accompany hypermotility of the gastrointestinal tract. Refer to Table 22-2 on text page 967 for a comparison of signs and symptoms of mild allergic reactions and severe allergic reactions or anaphylaxis.

7. Explain the various treatments and pharmacological interventions used in the management of allergic reactions and anaphylaxis. pp. 965–968

The first priority in the management of allergic reactions and anaphylaxis is to establish and maintain the patient's airway. Administer oxygen immediately along with ventilatory support as needed. You should be prepared to intubate, recognizing that laryngeal edema may change the size and appearance of the airway.

Establish vascular access as soon as possible and be prepared to run crystalloid solutions wide open if the patient is hypotensive.

Epinephrine is the drug of choice for severe allergic reaction and anaphylaxis. In mild to moderate cases, administer 0.3–0.5 mg of 1:1,000 epinephrine subcutaneously; while in severe reactions and anaphylaxis, administer 0.3–0.5 mg of intravenous 1:10,000 epinephrine. Remember that the effects of epinephrine wear off quickly, so be prepared to repeat boluses in 3 to 5 minutes. It may be necessary to establish a continuous epinephrine infusion.

Antihistamines, such as diphenhydramine, are widely used for the management of allergic reactions due to their ability to block histamine receptors. The usual dosage is 25–50 mg given either intravenously or intramuscularly. It may also be helpful to administer beta agonist agents via hand-held nebulizer to help reverse bronchospasm. Adult patients should receive 0.5 ml of albuterol in 3 ml of normal saline.

Medical Emergencies

As is always the case, your management approach should always be dictated by local protocols. Other medications that may be used to manage severe anaphylaxis include corticosteroids, such as SoluMedrol, to suppress the inflammatory response or vasopressors, such as dopamine, to enhance cardiac output. You'll recall that adequate fluid resuscitation prior to initiating vasopressor therapy is important.

8. Correlate abnormal findings in assessment with the clinical significance in the patient with an allergic reaction or anaphylaxis. pp. 963–965, 967–968

The central physiological action in severe allergic reaction and anaphylaxis is the massive release of histamine and other chemical mediators of the immune system. The resultant bronchospasm, airway edema, peripheral vasodilation, and increased capillary permeability can take a patient from his or her usual state of health to the brink of death in mere seconds. This chemically caused transformation is readily evident in the patient's clinical presentation: air hunger, dyspnea, angioedema, tachycardia, and hypotension. Your timely intervention is imperative to your patient's survival.

9. Given several preprogrammed and moulaged patients, provide the appropriate assessment, care, and transport for the allergic reaction and anaphylaxis patient. pp. 960–968

Throughout your classroom, clinical, and field training, you will encounter a variety of real and simulated patients with allergic reactions or anaphylaxis emergencies. Use the information provided in this chapter of your text, as well as the application of this information as demonstrated by your instructors, preceptors, and mentors to enhance your ability to assess, manage, and transport these patients.

CASE STUDY REVIEW

This case study draws attention to the typical presentation and management for a patient experiencing severe anaphylaxis.

The majority of fatal anaphylaxis cases in the United States are attributed to injections, usually of penicillin. It is for this reason that patients receiving injections in an outpatient setting are asked to remain on site for at least 20 to 30 minutes afterward to insure the availability of emergency care should the need arise. In this case, the injection was an immunization received just 15 minutes earlier. The patient's immediate response was a red rash and generalized itching that quickly progressed to marked respiratory compromise and cardiovascular collapse. The clinic staff had administered oxygen via a nasal cannula and was setting up an IV.

With the arrival of Steve and Beth on-scene, appropriate emergency care was quickly initiated; the nasal cannula was replaced with high-flow oxygen via nonrebreather mask, keeping an ET kit readily accessible. Beth established vascular access and initiated fluid resuscitation to correct massive vasodilation, while Steve administered epinephrine subcutaneously to counteract the immune system response. Although the patient showed improvement within 2 minutes of the epinephrine administration, Steve knew that the medication wears off quickly and was prepared to administer IV 1:10,000 epinephrine in case the improvement did not continue. Diphenhydramine was also administered to block the histamine receptors. All of these efforts were effective in reversing the anaphylaxis, and the patient was treated in the ER with corticosteroids to suppress the immune response and additional IV fluids and released within 2 hours.

Subsequent questioning at the hospital revealed that this patient had received a tetanus injection at the clinic and that he had a similar reaction with a prior tetanus immunization. This situation highlights the importance of patient education about the potential for repeat and possibly more severe allergic reactions. It also underscores the importance for every health-care professional to carefully question patients about allergies or untoward responses to medication prior to administering any drug.

©2004 Pearson Education, Inc.
Intermediate Emergency Care: Principles & Practice

CONTENT SELF-EVALUATION

MULTIPLE CHOICE

_____ 1. The type of immunity resulting from a direct attack of a foreign substance by specialized cells of the immune system is known as:
- A. humoral.
- B. cellular.
- C. natural.
- D. acquired.
- E. genetic.

_____ 2. The unique class of chemicals that are manufactured by specialized cells of the immune system to attack invading foreign proteins is:
- A. allergens.
- B. antigens.
- C. toxins.
- D. antibodies.
- E. pathogens.

_____ 3. Any substance that is capable, under appropriate conditions, of inducing a specific immune response is a(n):
- A. immunoglobulin.
- B. antigen.
- C. toxin.
- D. antibody.
- E. pathogen.

_____ 4. The type of immunity that is present at birth and has no relation to a previous exposure to a particular antigen is:
- A. humoral.
- B. cellular.
- C. natural.
- D. acquired.
- E. genetic.

_____ 5. The type of immunity that develops over time as a result of exposure to an antigen is:
- A. humoral.
- B. cellular.
- C. natural.
- D. acquired.
- E. genetic.

_____ 6. An allergic reaction is best defined as an exaggerated, sometimes potentially life-threatening response by the immune system to a foreign substance.
- A. True
- B. False

_____ 7. All of the following are common allergens EXCEPT:
- A. insect stings.
- B. drugs.
- C. antibodies.
- D. seafood.
- E. radiology contrast materials.

_____ 8. The vast majority of anaphylactic reactions occur as a result of:
- A. inhalation.
- B. ingestion.
- C. injection.
- D. topical exposure.
- E. genetics.

_____ 9. The antibody most commonly associated with hypersensitivity reactions is:
- A. IgA.
- B. IgD.
- C. IgE.
- D. IgG.
- E. IgM.

_____ 10. The primary chemical mediator of an allergic reaction is:
- A. heparin.
- B. histamine.
- C. SRS-A.
- D. basophil.
- E. the mast cell.

_____ 11. All of the following are physiologic effects associated with the release of the chemical mediators of anaphylaxis EXCEPT:
  A. bronchodilation.
  B. vasodilation.
  C. increased intestinal motility.
  D. increased vascular permeability.
  E. secretion of gastric acids.

_____ 12. Urticaria, a wheal and flare reaction characterized by red raised bumps that appear on the skin, is due to:
  A. bronchodilation.
  B. vasodilation.
  C. increased intestinal motility.
  D. decreased vascular permeability.
  E. secretion of gastric acids.

_____ 13. The first line parenteral drug for the management of anaphylaxis is:
  A. oxygen.
  B. diphenhydramine.
  C. epinephrine.
  D. methylprednisolone.
  E. albuterol.

_____ 14. The first priority when responding to a patient with an anaphylactic reaction is to:
  A. protect the airway.
  B. administer diphenhydramine.
  C. stabilize the cervical spine.
  D. ensure scene safety.
  E. establish vascular access.

_____ 15. Hypotension that is seen in severe anaphylaxis is due to:
  A. internal hemorrhage.
  B. inadequate oxygenation.
  C. bradycardia.
  D. vasodilation.
  E. gastrointestinal hypermotility.

©2004 Pearson Education, Inc.
Intermediate Emergency Care: Principles & Practice

CHAPTER 23

$*$

Poisoning and Overdose Emergencies

Review of Chapter Objectives

After reading this chapter, you should be able to:

1. Identify appropriate personal protective equipment and scene safety awareness concerns and situations in which additional non-EMS resources need to be contacted in dealing with toxicological emergencies. **p. 973**

Although specific protocols for managing toxicological emergencies may vary, certain basic principles apply to all situations. First and foremost your safety and that of your crew is the primary concern. This means that the scene size-up begins right from time of dispatch assuring law enforcement have been assigned as needed and the scene is safe to enter. Upon arrival assess the scene with a thorough evaluation taking note of where you are and who is around you. Be alert for any potential danger to you, the rescuer. Remember despite your natural urge to immediately assess and treat the patient, if you are incapacitated you will not be able to help anyone, and you will become a patient yourself. Be especially careful around patients who have abused drugs as they may be suicidal or have the potential for violence. They are often intoxicated, may act irrationally, and will not always be cooperative or happy to see you. Therefore look for signs of overdose such as empty pill bottles and used needles or other drug paraphernalia. Never put your hand blindly into a patient's pocket as it may contain used needles. Chemical spills and hazardous material emergencies can quickly incapacitate any individuals who are nearby. Since as an EMT-I, you will be or may be trained to the Hazardous Materials Awareness Level and as such you will be able to recognize the hazard and call for the most appropriate level of resources to handle the situation within their community. Make sure you have the proper clothing and equipment needed for the particular emergency or back out and call and wait for the appropriate rescuers who do have the proper equipment to arrive. Other resources, depending upon local protocol, that can be utilized during a toxicological emergency may include: FD hazmat team, mental health crisis team, Poison Control Center, local medical direction, and law enforcement personnel.

2. Describe the routes of entry of toxic substances into the body. **pp. 971–972**

There are four routes of entry into the body: ingestion, inhalation, surface absorption, and injection. Ingestion via the mouth is the most common route of entry for toxic exposure. Inhalation of a poison into the lungs results in rapid absorption from the alveolar air into the blood. Causative agents are in the form of gases, vapors, fumes, or aerosols. Surface absorption applies to cases in which entry is through the skin or mucous membranes. Injection applies when the toxic agent is injected under the skin, into muscle, or directly into the bloodstream.

3. Discuss the role of Poison Control Centers in the United States. **p. 971**

Poison Control Centers assist in the treatment of poison victims and provide information on new products and new treatment recommendations. They are usually based in major medical centers serving large populations, and many have computer systems that allow staff to rapidly and accurately access information. Centers are available to you 24 hours a day, 7 days a week: Take the time to memorize the telephone number of the Center serving your area. Your Center can help you determine the potential toxicity for your patient when you give them the following information: type of agent, amount and time of exposure, and physical condition of the patient. With this information, you may be able to start the current, definitive treatment in the field. The Center can notify the receiving facility before you get the patient there.

4. Discuss the pathophysiology, assessment findings, need for rapid intervention and transport, and management of toxic emergencies. pp. 970–1006

- *Pathophysiology:* With each route of entry, there is a general pattern of possible toxic effects depending on the type and amount of agent involved: Immediate effects involve the tissues exposed to the toxic agent during entry. Delayed, systemic effects are related to absorption into the bloodstream and circulation throughout the body. In ingestion, corrosive agents can cause immediate injury through burns of the lips, oral mucous membranes, tongue, throat, and esophagus. Delayed effects can arise from absorption via the small intestine into the blood with effects on distant organs and tissues. In inhalation, immediate injury can occur from irritation of the airways resulting in extensive edema and damaged tissue. Delayed, systemic effects occur when the agent travels through the bloodstream and interacts with distant organs and tissues. In surface absorption, immediate injury can occur in the involved skin or mucous membranes. Delayed effects again relate to absorption into the bloodstream. With injection, immediate injury is seen as irritation at the injection site, usually visible as red, irritated, edematous skin. Delayed, systemic effects are again due to distribution throughout the body via the bloodstream.

- *Assessment:* Certain basic principles of assessment apply to most toxicological emergencies. For instance, maintain a high index of suspicion that a poisoning or drug overdose may have occurred. During scene size-up, look for potential dangers to yourself and other rescuers, such as a threat of violence from suicidal patients and the threat of accidental injection from used needles that may be hidden on the patient's person or at the scene. In cases with chemicals and hazardous materials, it is crucial that you use the proper clothing and equipment. Be sure that such articles are distributed to team members who have been trained in their use.

    Assessment of the patient begins with a history if the patient appears to be able to give one. Critical questions include what kind of toxin the patient was exposed to and when exposure occurred (so you have clues for likelihood of immediate or delayed effects or both). Physical involves a rapid head-to-toe exam with full vital signs.

- *Time needs:* In accordance with your local protocols, relay information to Poison Control. Generally speaking, you never want to delay initiation of supportive or definitive care or transport because of delays in sending information to, or receiving information from, Poison Control. Time is of the essence, literally. Ongoing assessment is particularly important for this group of patients because they can deteriorate rapidly. Repeat initial assessment and vitals every five minutes for critical or unstable patients and every fifteen minutes for stable patients. Specific assessment findings are given for each type of agent.

- *General management:* The preliminary steps of management include securing rescuer safety and removing the patient from any toxic environment. Support ABCs as you would with any other patient, keeping in mind that damage may have occurred to the mouth, pharynx, and/or airway in inhalation injury, and to the mouth and pharynx in ingestion incidents. The direct access to the cardiovascular system that occurs with injection cases may also complicate support of the ABCs.

    The first management step specific to toxicological emergencies is decontamination, that is, minimization of toxicity by reducing the amount of toxin absorbed into the body. Decontamination involves three steps: The first is reduction of intake of toxin (steps will be route-specific, such as removal from fume-filled atmosphere in inhalation, removal of clothes and cleansing of skin in surface absorption, removal of stinger in injection, etc.).

    The second step is reduction of absorption after toxin is in the body, and this usually applies to ingestion incidents. The most common method entails use of activated charcoal to bind molecules of the toxin to it and prevent absorption into the bloodstream. Gastric lavage (stomach pumping) is of limited use as a step to reduce absorption. Lavage must be done within about one hour of exposure to be effective, and its possible complications (aspiration and perforation) are significant. Lavage is uncommon except in specific circumstances, for example, when the toxin doesn't bind to activated charcoal or when the toxin has no antidote. The third step in decontamination is enhanced elimination of toxin from the body. Cathartics enhance gastric mobility and thus may shorten the time the toxin is in the GI tract. Know the limitations in use of cathartics in your area, especially among pediatric patients, in whom they can induce severe electrolyte disturbances. Whole bowel irrigation with use of a gastric tube seems to be effective and carries few potential complications; however, its use is limited to only a few centers.

The third management step specific to toxicological emergencies is use of an antidote, a substance that neutralizes the specific toxin and counteracts its effects in the body. As you can see in Table 23-1 on text page 975, there are not many antidotes, and few are 100% effective. Your best guide is to be thoroughly knowledgeable with your local protocols, the directions given by the Poison Control Center, and by counsel given by medical direction.

5. **Differentiate among the most common poisonings, pathophysiology, assessment findings, and management of poisoning by ingestion, inhalation, absorption, injection, and overdose.** pp. 971–1006

Ingestion is the most common route of poisoning that you will see. Frequently ingested poisons include household products, petroleum-based agents such as gasoline and paint, cleaning agents such as alkalis and soaps, cosmetics, drugs (prescription, non-prescription, and illicit), plants, and foods. Some poisons can remain in the stomach for several hours, which may permit removal of the poison from the stomach and the body before systemic absorption can occur via passage through the small intestine. In at least one case, ingestion of aspirin, removal from the stomach is difficult because the ingested tablets bind together to form one large bolus. Useful questions for historical assessment include: (1) What did you ingest? (Obtain samples or containers whenever possible) (2) When did you ingest the substance? (3) How much did you ingest? (4) Did you drink any alcohol? (5) Have you attempted to treat yourself? (including induction of vomiting) (6) Have you been under mental health care, and, if so, why? (answer may indicate potential for suicide) (7) What is your weight? Physical exam is especially important because history may be unavailable or unreliable. Your exam should provide physical evidence of intoxication and discover co-morbid conditions that may affect treatment or response. Pay particular attention to skin, eyes, mouth, chest, circulation status, and abdomen (review text page 976). Be aware that a patient may have ingested multiple substances. Management centers on prevention of aspiration, intubation where necessary (RSI may be required to avoid patient's clamping down on tube), use of high-flow oxygen, and IV access for volume replacement and possible IV drug administration. Remember that it is always important to have ongoing cardiac monitoring and reassessment of vital signs.

Toxic inhalations can be self-induced or due to accidental exposure. Commonly inhaled poisons include toxic gases, carbon monoxide, ammonia, chlorine, freon, toxic vapors, fumes, or aerosols (from products such as paint and other hydrocarbons, glue, etc.), carbon tetrachloride, methyl chloride, tear gas, mustard gas, amyl nitrite, butyl nitrite, and nitrous oxide. Inhaled toxins primarily cause direct injury in the respiratory system, and these problems may be most severe in patients who inhaled a chemical or propellant concentrated in either a paper or plastic bag.

Given the pathophysiology of inhaled toxins, you should look for signs/symptoms related to three major systems: the central nervous system (dizziness, headache, confusion, hallucinations, seizures, or coma), the respiratory system (tachypnea, cough, hoarseness, stridor, dyspnea, retractions, wheezing, chest pain or tightness, rales or rhonchi), and the heart (dysrhythmias). Management starts with protecting yourself from any toxins in the atmosphere and removal of the patient from the injurious environment. Follow these guidelines: Wear protective clothing, use appropriate respiratory protection, and remove the patient's contaminated clothing. Then you can perform the initial assessment, history, and physical examination focusing on the central nervous system, respiratory, and cardiac systems. Support ABCs as you would with any other patient, keeping in mind that damage may have occurred to the mouth, pharynx, and/or airway as a direct, immediate injury. Contact medical direction and your Poison Control Center according to your particular protocols.

For **surface absorption,** the most common contacts are with poisonous plants such as poison ivy, poison sumac, and poison oak. Many toxic chemicals can be absorbed through the skin.

Organophosphates, which are used as pesticides, are easily absorbed through the skin and mucous membranes, as is cyanide. The signs and symptoms vary widely depending on the toxin involved. Whenever you suspect surface absorption, take the following general steps: (1) wear protective clothing; (2) use appropriate respiratory protection; (3) remove the patient's contaminated clothing; (4) perform initial assessment, history, and physical exam; (5) initiate supportive measures; and (6) contact Poison Control Center and medical direction.

Females in the insect class *Hymenoptera,* honeybees, hornets, yellow jackets, wasps, and fire ants, are common causes of **injection injury.** In addition, spiders, ticks, snakes, and certain marine animals are known causes of toxic exposure by injection. In addition to intentional injections, most poisonings by injection involve bites and stings from insects and animals. Be alert for the possibility of allergic reactions or anaphylaxis. Over time, beware of delayed systemic reactions. General principles of field management include the following: (1) protection of all rescue personnel because the culprit organism may still be in the area; (2) removal of the patient from danger of repeated injection (particularly in the case of yellow jackets, wasps, or hornets); (3) whenever possible and safe, obtain the injury-causing organism and bring it to the emergency department; (4) perform initial assessment and rapid physical exam; (5) prevent or delay further absorption of the poison; (6) initiate supportive measures as needed; (7) watch for anaphylaxis; (8) transport as rapidly as possible; and (9) contact Poison Control Center and medical direction per protocols.

6. **Define substance abuse and drug overdose and differentiate among the most common drugs of abuse, including alcohol, and their assessment and management.** pp. 999–1006

Substance or **drug abuse** is use of a pharmacological product for purposes other than medically defined reasons. **Drug overdose** is the over administration of a drug such that it causes unfocused effects.

The most commonly abused drugs include: (1) alcohol in its fermented and distilled forms; (2) barbiturates such as phenobarbital and thiopental; (3) cocaine (both crack and rock forms); (4) narcotics/opiates such as heroin, codeine, meperidine, morphine, hydromorphone, pentazocine, methadone, Darvon, and Darvocet; (5) marijuana and hashish (also called grass or weed on the street); (6) amphetamines such as Benzedrine, Dexedrine, and Ritalin (called speed on the street); (7) hallucinogens including LSD, STP, mescaline, psilocybin, and PCP (also called angel dust); (8) sedatives from different chemical families such as Seconal, Valium, Librium, Xanax, Halcion, Restoril, Dalmane, and phenobarbital; and (9) the benzodiazepines, Valium, Librium, Xanax, Halcion, Restoril, Dalmane, Centrax, Ativan, and Serax.

In addition to the specific drugs discussed below, it is notable that many groups of drugs produce definable toxic syndromes. Knowledge of these syndromes is useful because it helps you cluster information for compounds that produce similar clinical pictures. (1) Anticholinergic toxidrome is caused by belladonna alkaloids, atropine, scopolamine, synthetic anticholinergics, and incidental anticholinergics such as antihistamines, tricyclic antidepressants, and phenothiazines. Signs and symptoms include dry skin/mucous membranes, blurred near vision, fixed dilated pupils, tachycardia, hyperthermia and flushing, lethargy, and CNS signs, respiratory failure, and cardiovascular collapse. Management is as described for the tricyclics below. (2) Narcotic toxidrome is due to illicit drugs such as heroin and opium, prescription narcotics such as meperidine and methadone, and combination medications including narcotic agents such as hydromorphone, diphenoxylate (Lomotil), and oxycodone. Assessment findings include CNS depression, pinpoint pupils, slowed respirations, hypotension, positive response to naloxone. Note that pupils may be dilated and excitement may predominate the clinical picture. Management is described below. (3) The sympathomimetic toxidrome is caused by aminophylline, amphetamines, caffeine, cocaine, ephedrine, dopamine, methylphenidate (Ritalin), and phencyclidine. Features include CNS excitation, hypertension, seizures, tachycardia (hypotension with caffeine). Management is discussed below.

a. **Cocaine** p. 1001

Cocaine has sympathomimetic effects, and assessment findings include CNS excitation, dilated pupils, hyperactivity, hypertension, seizures, tachycardia, and hypotension if taken with caffeine. Benzodiazepines may be required for seizures or diazepam 5–10 mg can be given as a seizure precaution; beta blockers are contraindicated because their unopposed alpha receptor stimulation can cause cardiac ischemia, increased hypertension, and hyperthermia. General measures include ABCs, respiratory support and oxygenation, ECG monitoring, IV access, and treatment of any life-threatening dysrhythmia.

b. Marijuana and cannabis compounds
p. 1002

Marijuana and related compounds can be smoked (inhaled) or taken orally, and pertinent signs and symptoms include euphoria, dry mouth, dilated pupils, and altered sensation. Management centers on ABCs, reassurance and speaking in a quiet voice, and ECG monitoring if indicated.

c. Amphetamines and amphetamine-like drugs
p. 1002

Amphetamines are CNS stimulants that can be taken orally or injected. Assessment findings include exhilaration, hyperactivity, dilated pupils, hypertension, psychosis, tremors, and seizures. Management centers on ABCs, oxygenation and ECG monitoring, IV access, treatment of any life-threatening dysrhythmia, and diazepam 5–10 mg as a seizure precaution. Diazepam and haloperidol in combination may be useful in controlling hyperactivity.

d. Barbiturates
p. 1001

The barbiturates, which are CNS depressants, can be taken orally or injected. Signs and symptoms include lethargy, emotional lability, incoordination, slurred speech, nystagmus, coma, hypotension, and respiratory depression. Management focuses on ABCs and respiratory support with oxygenation, IV access, ECG monitoring, and contact with Poison Control. Alkalinization of urine and diuresis may improve elimination of barbiturates from the body.

e. Sedative-hypnotics
p. 1002

Sedative-hypnotics are generally taken orally, and they are also CNS depressants. Assessment findings include altered mental status, hypotension, slurred speech, respiratory depression, shock, bradycardia, and seizures. Management centers on ABCs with respiratory support and oxygenation, IV access, ECG monitoring, and possible use of naloxone dependent on agent taken and advice of medical direction.

f. Cyanide
pp. 978–979

Cyanide can enter the body by different routes dependent on the product in which it is found. It is present in household items such as rodenticides and silver polish, as well as in foods such as fruit pits and seeds. It can be liberated into inhalable form through burning of nitrogen-containing products such as plastics, silks, or synthetic carpets. Cyanide also forms in patients on long-term therapy with nitroprusside. Regardless of entry, cyanide acts extremely quickly as a cellular asphyxiant, inhibiting the vital process of cellular respiration. Signs and symptoms include a burning sensation in mouth and throat, headache, confusion, combative behavior, hypertension, and tachycardia, followed by hypotension and further dysrhythmias, seizures and coma, and pulmonary edema. Management relies on removal from the source, immediate supportive measures, and treatment with a cyanide antidote kit containing amyl nitrite ampules, a sodium nitrite, and a sodium thiosulfate solution. Adding nitrites to blood converts some hemoglobin to methemoglobin, which binds cyanide, removing it from its free form in the blood. Thiosulfate binds with cyanide to form a soluble nontoxic compound. Note: Cyanide is rapidly toxic, so it is crucial you be familiar with a cyanide antidote kit if your unit carries one.

g. Narcotics/opiates
p. 1001

The narcotics can be taken orally or by injection. Pertinent assessment findings include CNS depression, constricted pupils, respiratory depression, hypotension, bradycardia, pulmonary edema, and coma. General management centers on ABCs with respiratory support and oxygenation, IV access, and ECG monitoring. You may use the antidote naloxone, which can be titrated to relieve symptoms of toxicity without provoking withdrawal symptoms in addicts. General instructions involve use of 1–2 mg naloxone IV or endotracheally per medical direction until respiration improves. Larger doses (2–5 mg) may be required in the management of Darvon overdose and alcoholic coma.

h. Cardiac medications   pp. 982–983

The number of available cardiac medications grows continually, and many classes exist, including antidysrhythmics, beta blockers, calcium channel blockers, glycosides, ACE inhibitors, etc. General pharmacology includes regulation of heart function by reducing heart rate, suppressing automaticity, reducing vascular tone, or some combination of these. Although overdose can be intentional, it often is due to an error in dosage. At the level of overdose, signs and symptoms include (1) nausea and vomiting, (2) headache, dizziness, and confusion, (3) profound hypotension, (4) cardiac dysrhythmias (usually bradycardic), (5) cardiac conduction blocks, and (6) bronchospasm and pulmonary edema (especially with beta blockers). Management centers on initiating standard toxicological emergency assessment and treatment immediately. Severe bradycardia may not respond well to atropine, so you should have an external pacing device at hand. Some cardiac medications have antidotes; these include calcium for calcium channel blockers, glucagon for beta blockers, and digoxin-specific Fab (Digibind) for digoxin. Contact medical direction before giving any of these antidotes.

i. Caustics   pp. 983–984

Caustic substances can either be acids or alkalis, and such substances are common at home and in the industrial workplace. Strong caustics can cause severe burns at the site of contact; if ingested, they can cause tissue destruction at the lips, mouth, esophagus, and more distal regions of the GI tract. Strong acids by definition have a pH less than 2; they are found in plumbing solutions and bathroom cleaners. Contact usually produces immediate, severe pain due to tissue coagulation and necrosis. Often this type of burn produces an eschar over the site, which may act as a shield to protect deeper tissues from damage. Because the substance is in the stomach much longer than the esophagus, the stomach is the more likely to sustain damage. Immediate or delayed hemorrhage is possible, as is perforation. Absorption of acids into the bloodstream produces acidemia, which needs to be managed along with the local, direct effects.

Strong alkaline agents by definition have a pH greater than 12.5; they are present in solid or liquid form in household products such as drain cleaners. These agents cause local injury through liquefaction necrosis. Because of a delay in pain sensation, these agents are often present longer at the site of contact, allowing for greater tissue damage and deeper tissue injury. Solid products can stick to the oropharynx or esophagus, causing bleeding, perforation, and inflammation of central chest structures. Liquid alkalis are more likely to injure the stomach because, like the liquid strong acids, they pass quickly through the esophagus. Within 1–2 days of exposure to a strong alkali, complete loss of mucosal tissue can occur, followed either by gradual healing or further bleeding, necrosis, and stricture formation. Assessment findings include facial burns, pain in the lips, tongue, throat and/or gums, drooling and trouble swallowing, hoarseness, stridor, or shortness of breath, and shock from bleeding and vomiting. Both assessment and initiation of management must be rapid and aggressive to avoid significant morbidity and mortality.

As with other toxicological situations, protect yourself and initiate standard toxicological assessment and treatment: Pay particular attention to the airway. Injury to the oropharynx and/or larynx may make airway control and ventilation very difficult and may go so far as to require cricothyrotomy. Because caustic substances do not adhere to activated charcoal, there is no indication for it. It is controversial whether ingestion of milk or water acts effectively to coat the stomach lining or dilute the caustic. It is clear that rapid transport is essential. Hydrofluoric acid, which is used to clean glass in laboratory settings and in etching glass in art work, is a specific example of a strong acid that can be lethal in even small exposure doses. Management specific to this agent is immersion of the exposed limb in iced water with magnesium sulfate, calcium salts, or benzethonium chloride.

j. Common household substances   pp. 983–984

Many of these substances contain caustic agents (either strong acids or strong alkalis) as major ingredients; see objective 6. i above for details.

k. Drugs abused for sexual purposes/sexual gratification   p. 1003

This group includes a number of miscellaneous agents that are used to stimulate and enhance sexual experience but do not have medically approved indications for such use. MDMA,

©2004 Pearson Education, Inc.
Intermediate Emergency Care: Principles & Practice

popularly known as Ecstasy, is an example. Ecstasy is a modified form of methamphetamine and has similar, although milder, effects. Look for its use on college campuses and in nightclub settings. Initial signs and symptoms of use include anxiety, tachycardia, nausea, and hypertension, followed by relaxation, euphoria, and feelings of enhanced emotional insight. Studies indicate prolonged use may cause brain damage. Cases that can lead to death have the following assessment findings: confusion, agitation, tremor, high temperature, and diarrhea. No specific treatment exists, so supportive measures should be taken. Flunitrazepam, or Rohypnol, is illegal in the U.S. but has been used as a "date rape drug" when slipped into a woman's drink. The drug is a strong benzodiazepine that causes sedation and amnesia. When this drug is suspected, treat as for other benzodiazepines but remember to look for consequences of sexual assault and be sure to treat them as well.

l. Carbon monoxide   pp. 981–982

Carbon monoxide is a tasteless, odorless gas that is often created by incomplete combustion. Because of its chemical structure, it has an affinity for hemoglobin over 200 times greater than that of oxygen. Once carbon monoxide has bound to hemoglobin, it is very difficult to displace and it causes an effective hypoxia. Because of the variability of signs and symptoms (depending on dose and duration of exposure), many people ignore poisoning until toxic levels are in the blood. Early symptoms resemble those of the flu. Combining likely causes of carbon monoxide generation with early symptoms raises this red flag: Beware carbon monoxide poisoning in multiple patients living together in a poorly heated and ventilated space who have "flu-like" symptoms. Specific signs and symptoms include headache, nausea and vomiting, confusion or other manifestation of altered mental status, and tachypnea. Because of the difficulty of displacing carbon monoxide from hemoglobin, definitive treatment may require use of a hyperbaric chamber (in which oxygen is present at greater than atmospheric pressure). In the field, take these steps: Ensure safety of rescuing personnel, remove the patient(s) from contaminated area, begin immediate ventilation of affected area, and initiate supportive measures including high-flow oxygen via nonrebreather device (this last is critical).

m. Alcohols   pp. 1003–1006

Ethyl alcohol is the form of alcohol in beverages, and it is the single most common substance of abuse among Americans. Alcoholism, dependence on alcohol, progresses in much the same way as drug dependence discussed earlier in the chapter. The early symptoms of alcohol use, especially at low doses, include loss of inhibitions and emotionally excitatory effects, which can cause some of the aberrant behaviors associated with alcohol intoxication. Once ingested, alcohol is completely absorbed from the stomach and intestinal tract within approximately 30–120 minutes. After absorption, it is widely distributed in blood to all body tissues, and concentrations of alcohol in the brain rapidly approach the level in the blood. Alcohol's major physiologic effects are as a CNS depressant: toxicity, can include stupor, coma, and death. Because the liver is the major site of detoxification within the body, compromise of liver function increases the course and severity of alcohol intoxication. Another significant health effect is peripheral vasodilation, which results in flushing of the skin and a feeling of warmth. In cold conditions, this can increase loss of body heat and help to produce hypothermia. Alcohol-related diuresis is due to inhibition of vasopressin, a hormone responsible for homeostasis of water balance. The dry mouth associated with hangovers may in part be due to the alcohol-induced dehydration. Methanol, wood alcohol, is so toxic it is not safe for human consumption. However, methanol toxicity can occur either as an accident or because an alcoholic individual could not obtain ethyl alcohol. Methanol causes visual disturbances, abdominal pain, and nausea and vomiting even at low doses. Occasionally, methanol toxic patients complain of headache or dizziness or present with seizures and obtundation. Ethylene glycol, a related compound, can also be involved in toxic emergencies. It produces similar symptoms, but its CNS effects, including hallucinations, coma, and seizures, present at even earlier stages.

Assessment findings in an individual with chronic alcoholism include poor nutrition, alcoholic hepatitis, liver cirrhosis with subsequent esophageal varices, loss of sensation in hands and feet, loss of cerebellar function shown as poor balance and coordination, pancreatitis, upper GI hemorrhage (which is often fatal), hypoglycemia, subdural hematoma secondary to falls, and rib and extremity fractures, also secondary to falls. When you are in the field,

Medical Emergencies

keep in mind that conditions such as a subdural hematoma, sepsis, and diabetic ketoacidosis can, along with other conditions, mimic alcohol intoxication. For instance, the breath odor of ketoacidosis can resemble that of alcohol.

Abrupt discontinuance of alcohol by a dependent individual may provoke a withdrawal syndrome that can prove to be potentially lethal. Withdrawal symptoms can occur several hours after sudden abstinence and last up to 5–7 days. Common signs and symptoms include a coarse tremor of hands, tongue, and eyelids, nausea and vomiting, general weakness, increased sympathetic tone, tachycardia, sweating, hypertension, orthostatic hypotension, anxiety, irritability or depressed mood, and poor sleep. Seizures may occur, as can delirium tremens (DTs). DTs usually develop on the second or third day of withdrawal and are characterized by a decreased level of consciousness associated with hallucinations and misinterpretation of nearby events. Both seizures and delirium tremens are ominous signs.

Alcohol intoxication, whether acute or chronic, should not be underestimated as a toxic emergency. In cases of suspected alcohol abuse, manage as follows: (1) Establish and maintain the airway, (2) determine if other drugs or substances are involved, (3) start an IV with lactated Ringer's solution or normal saline, (4) use a Chemstrip and give 25 g $D_{50}W$ if the patient is hypoglycemic, (5) administer 100 mg thiamine IV or IM, (6) maintain a sympathetic and supportive attitude with the patient, and (7) transport to emergency department for further care. Note: Medical direction may suggest diazepam in severe cases of seizure or hallucination.

n. Hydrocarbons   p. 984

Numerous household substances contain hydrocarbons, organic compounds composed primarily of carbon and hydrogen. Hydrocarbons include kerosene, naphtha, turpentine, mineral oil, chloroform, toluene, and benzene, and they are found in lighter fluid, paint, glue, lubricants, solvents, and aerosol propellants. Exposure can be via ingestion, inhalation, or surface absorption. Signs and symptoms of hydrocarbon exposure vary according to agent, dose, and route of exposure, but common problems include burns due to local contact, respiratory signs (wheezing, dyspnea, hypoxia, or pneumonitis from aspiration or inhalation), CNS signs (headache, dizziness, slurred speech, ataxia, and obtundation), foot and wrist drop with numbness and tingling, and cardiac dysrhythmias. Research has shown that fewer than 1% of hydrocarbon poisonings require physician care. In cases where you know the agent in question and in which the patient is asymptomatic, medical direction may permit the patient to stay at home. On the other hand, hydrocarbon poisonings can be very serious. If the patient is symptomatic, does not know the causative agent, or has taken a specific agent (such as halogenated or aromatic hydrocarbon compounds) that requires GI decontamination, standard toxicological emergency procedures and prompt transport are indicated.

o. Psychiatric medications   pp. 985–988

The tricyclic antidepressants were standard therapy for depression for years, despite concerns that their generally narrow therapeutic window made accidental toxic-level exposure, as well as intentional overdose, potentially common. Despite the introduction of newer, safer antidepressants, a number of tricyclics are still in use for depression, as well as chronic pain syndromes and migraine prophylaxis. Agents still in use include amitriptyline (Elavil), amoxapine, clomipramine, doxepin, imipramine, and nortriptyline. Signs and symptoms on assessment include dry mouth, blurred vision, urinary retention, and constipation. Late into overdose, you may find confusion and hallucinations, hyperthermia, respiratory depression, seizures, tachycardia and hypotension, and cardiac dysrhythmias (such as heart block, wide QRS complex, and *torsade de pointes*.) In addition to standard toxicological procedures, cardiac monitoring is critical because dysrhythmias are the most common cause of death. If you suspect a mixed overdose with a benzodiazepine, DO NOT use Flumazenil because it might precipitate a seizure. If significant cardiac toxicity is evident, sodium bicarbonate may be used as an additional therapy; contact medical direction as needed.

p. Newer anti-depressants and serotonin syndromes   pp. 986–987

In the recent past, a number of new antidepressants that are not related to the tricyclics have been introduced. Because of their high safety profile in both therapeutic and overdose amounts, these drugs have virtually replaced the tricyclics in clinical practice. This group includes trazodone (Desyrel), bupropion (Wellbutrin), and the large group of drugs known as selective serotonin reuptake inhibitors (SSRIs). Drugs in this group include Prozac, Luvox, Paxil, and Zoloft. Their pharmacology, as indicated by group name, centers on prevention of reuptake of serotonin from neural synapses in the brain, theoretically raising the amount of serotonin available to modulate brain function. The usual signs and symptoms in overdose cases are generally mild, including drowsiness, tremor, nausea and vomiting, and sinus tachycardia. Occasionally trazodone and bupropion cause CNS depression and seizures, but deaths are rare, and they have been reported in situations with mixed overdoses and multiple ingestions. You should know that the SSRIs have been associated with serotonin syndrome, a constellation of signs/symptoms correlated with increased serotonin level and triggered by increasing the dose of SSRI or adding a second drug such as a narcotic or another antidepressant. Serotonin syndrome is marked by the following: (1) agitation, anxiety, confusion, and insomnia, (2) headache, drowsiness, and coma, (3) nausea, salivation, diarrhea, and abdominal cramps, (4) cutaneous piloerection and flushed skin, (5) hyperthermia and tachycardia, and (6) rigidity, shivering, incoordination, and myoclonic jerks. Because of the lower morbidity and mortality in these drugs compared with overdoses with the older antidepressants, standard toxicological emergency procedures suffice. The patient should discontinue all serotonergic drugs and you should institute supportive measures. Benzodiazepines or beta blockers are occasionally used to improve patient comfort, but they are rarely given in the field.

q. Lithium
p. 987

Lithium is the most effective drug used in the treatment of bipolar disorder (a psychiatric disorder also known as manic depression). Pharmacology is unclear. However, it is known that lithium has a narrow therapeutic index, making toxicity relatively common during normal use and in overdose situations. Assessment findings of toxicity include thirst and dry mouth, tremor, muscle twitching, increased reflexes, confusion, stupor, seizures, coma, nausea, vomiting, diarrhea, and bradycardia and dysrhythmias. Lithium overdose should be treated primarily with supportive measures. Use standard toxicological procedures but remember that activated charcoal does not bind lithium and should not be used. Alkalinization of the urine with sodium bicarbonate and diuresis with mannitol may increase elimination of lithium, but severe toxicity requires hemodialysis.

r. MAO inhibitors
pp. 985–986

Monoamine oxidase inhibitors (MAO inhibitors) have been used historically as psychiatric agents, primarily as antidepressants. Recently they have found limited use as treatment for obsessive-compulsive disorder. These drugs have always had relatively limited usage for several reasons: They have a narrow therapeutic index, multiple drug interactions, potentially serious interactions with foods rich in tyramine (for instance, red wine and cheese), and high morbidity and mortality in overdose incidents. The pharmacology of MAO inhibitors directly affects CNS neurotransmitters: The drugs inhibit the breakdown of norepinephrine and dopamine while increasing the molecular components necessary to produce more. Remember that overdose with this group of drugs is very serious, even though symptoms may not appear for up to 6 hours. Assessment findings include headache, agitation, restlessness, tremor, nausea, palpitations, tachycardia, severe hypertension, hyperthermia, and eventually bradycardia, hypotension, coma, and death. Newer MAO inhibitors have been introduced into the marketplace; they appear to be less toxic and avoid the food interactions that involved the older generation of MAO inhibitors. They are reversible in effect; however, overdose outcome data are not yet available for these drugs. Management includes reversal if the drug is in the newer class of reversible MAO inhibitors, prompt institution of standard toxicological procedures, and, if needed, symptomatic support for seizures and hyperthermia with use of benzodiazepines. If a vasopressor is needed, use norepinephrine.

s. Non-prescription pain medications: (1) nonsteroidal anti-inflammatory agents (2) salicylates (3) acetaminophen
p. 988

(1) Nonsteroidal anti-inflammatory agents (called NSAIDs) are a large, commonly used group of drugs such as naproxen sodium, indomethacin, ibuprofen, and ketorolac (Toradol). Overdose is common, and assessment findings include headache, ringing in the ears (tinnitus), nausea, vomiting, abdominal pain, swelling of the extremities, mild drowsiness, dyspnea, wheezing, pulmonary edema, and rash and itching. There is no specific antidote for NSAID

toxicity, so use general overdose procedures including supportive care and transport to the emergency department for evaluation and any necessary symptomatic treatment.

(2) Salicylates are some of the most common over-the-counter drugs taken and among the most common taken in overdose. They include aspirin, oil of wintergreen, and some prescription combination medications. About 300 mg/kg aspirin can cause toxicity. In these amounts, the salicylate inhibits normal energy production and acid buffering in the body, resulting in metabolic acidosis that further injures other organ systems. Assessment findings include tachypnea, hyperthermia, confusion, lethargy and coma, cardiac failure and dysrhythmias, abdominal pain and vomiting, and non-cardiogenic (inflammatory) pulmonary edema and adult respiratory distress syndrome. The findings of chronic overdose are somewhat less severe and tend not to include abdominal complaints. It is thus difficult to distinguish chronic overdose from early acute overdose or acute overdose that has progressed past the initial abdominal irritation stage. In all cases, management of salicylate poisoning should be treated with use of standard toxicological emergency procedures. Activated charcoal definitely reduces drug absorption and should be used. If possible, learn the time of ingestion because blood levels measured at the right interval can be indicative of the expected degree of injury. Most symptomatic patients require generous IV fluids and may need urine alkalinization with sodium bicarbonate. Severe cases may require dialysis.

(3) Acetaminophen (paracetamol, Tylenol) has few side effects in normal dosage, and it is one of the most commonly used drugs in America for fever/pain. It is also a common ingredient in combination medications and is found in some prescription combination medications. In large doses, acetaminophen can be very dangerous: A dose of 150 mg/kg is considered toxic and may result in death secondary to liver damage. A highly reactive metabolite is responsible for most adverse effects, but this is avoided in most cases by detoxification. When large amounts enter the body in overdose, this detoxification system is overloaded and gradually depleted, leaving the metabolite in the circulation to cause liver necrosis. It is important for you to learn and remember that the signs and symptoms of toxicity appear in four stages: Stage 1—0.5 to 24 hours after ingestion, marked by nausea, vomiting, weakness, and fatigue; Stage 2—24 to 48 hours, marked by abdominal pain, decreased urine, elevated liver enzymes; Stage 3—72 to 96 hours, marked by liver function disruption; and Stage 4—4 to 14 days, marked by gradual recovery or progressive liver failure. Field management relies on standard toxicological procedures. Again, it is important to find time of ingestion because this may allow blood levels to be drawn at a time appropriate to predict potential injury. An antidote (N-acetylcysteine, or NAC, Mucomyst) is available and highly effective. However, NAC is usually given based on clinical and lab studies and in the hospital setting.

t. Theophylline   p. 989

Theophylline is a member of the group of drugs called xanthines. It is generally used by patients with asthma or COPD because it has moderate bronchodilation and mild anti-inflammatory effects. It has a narrow therapeutic index and high toxicity, so it has been used less frequently recently. Thus, it is not a factor as often as it once was in overdose injuries. Assessment findings include agitation, tremors, seizures, cardiac dysrhythmias, and nausea and vomiting. Theophylline can cause significant morbidity and mortality. In an overdose setting, you must start toxicological emergency procedures immediately. Theophylline is on a short list of drugs that have significant entero-hepatic circulation. Thus, activated charcoal in multiple doses over time will continuously remove more and more theophylline from the body. Dysrhythmias should be treated according to ACLS procedures.

u. Metals   pp. 989–990

With the exception of iron, heavy metal overdose is rare. Metals that can cause toxicity include lead, arsenic, and mercury, all of which affect numerous enzyme systems in the body and thus cause a variety of symptoms. Some also have direct local effects when ingested and they accumulate in various organs.

- *Iron:* The body needs only small daily amounts of iron; excess amounts are easily obtained through non-prescription supplements and multivitamins. Children have the tendency to overdose on iron by taking too many candy-flavored chewable vitamins containing iron. Symptoms occur when more than 20 mg/kg of elemental iron are ingested. Excess iron

©2004 Pearson Education, Inc.
Intermediate Emergency Care: Principles & Practice

causes GI injury and possible hemorrhagic shock, especially if it forms concretions (lumps formed when tablets fuse together). Patients with significant iron ingestions may have visible tablets or concretions in the stomach or small intestine on X-ray. Other signs and symptoms include vomiting (often hematemesis) and diarrhea, abdominal pain, shock, liver failure, metabolic acidosis with tachypnea, and eventual bowel scarring and possible obstruction. It is essential to start standard toxicological procedures promptly. Because iron inhibits GI motility, tablets remain in the stomach for a long time and may possibly be easier to remove via gastric lavage (especially if concretions are not present). Because activated charcoal does not bind metals, it should not be used for iron overdose or for any other metal overdose. Deferoxamine, a chelating agent, may be used in iron overdose as an antidote because it binds iron such that less enters cells to cause damage.

- *Lead and mercury:* Both metals are found in varying amounts in the environment. Lead was often used in glazes and paints before its toxic potential was realized. Mercury is a contaminant from industrial processing and is also found in some thermometers and temperature-control switches in homes. Both acute and chronic overdose are possible with both metals. Signs and symptoms of heavy metal toxicity include headache, irritability, confusion, coma, memory disturbance, tremor, weakness, agitation, and abdominal pain. Chronic poisoning can result in permanent neurological injury, which makes it crucial that heavy metal levels be monitored in the environment of a patient with toxicity. You need to remember the signs and symptoms of heavy metal poisoning and promptly institute standard procedures. Although activated charcoal is not helpful, various chelating agents (such as DMSA, BAL, and CDE) are available and may be used in definitive management in the hospital.

v. Plants and mushrooms pp. 991–992

Plants, trees, and mushrooms are common contributors to accidental toxic ingestions. You should know that many decorative home plants can present a toxic danger to children. Most Poison Control Centers distribute pamphlets that list relevant household plants. In nature, it is impossible to identify all toxic plants and mushrooms. A general approach for you to take is to obtain a sample of the offending plant if possible, trying to find a complete leaf, stem, or flower. Mushrooms are very difficult to identify from small pieces. Because many ornamental plants contain irritating material, be sure to examine the patient's mouth and throat for redness, blistering, or edema. Identify other findings during the focused physical exam. Mushroom poisonings generally involve a mistake in identification of edible mushrooms or accidental ingestion by children. Mushrooms in the class *Amanita* account for over 90% of deaths; they produce a poison that is extremely toxic to the liver and carry a mortality rate of about 50%. Signs and symptoms of poisonous plant ingestion include excessive salivation, lacrimation, diaphoresis, abdominal cramps, nausea, vomiting, and diarrhea, as well as decreasing levels of consciousness, eventually progressing to coma. Contact Poison Control if at all possible for guidance on management. If contact isn't possible, follow the procedures outlined under food poisoning (text pages 990–991).

7. Discuss common causative agents or offending organisms, pharmacology, assessment findings, and management for a patient with food poisoning, a bite, or a sting. pp. 992–999

Food poisoning can be due to a variety of causes including bacteria, viruses, and bacterial-associated chemical toxins. All notoriously produce varying degrees of gastrointestinal distress. Bacterial food poisonings range in severity. Bacterial exotoxins (secreted by bacteria) and enterotoxins (exotoxins associated with GI diseases) cause nausea, vomiting, diarrhea, and abdominal pain. Food contaminated with the bacteria *Shigella, Salmonella,* or *E. coli* can produce more severe reactions, often leading to electrolyte imbalance and hypovolemia. The world's most toxic poison is produced by *Clostridium botulinum,* and exposure presents as severe respiratory distress or even arrest. Fortunately, botulism rarely occurs except in cases of improper food storage procedures such as canning. A variety of seafood poisonings result from toxins produced by dinoflagellate-contaminated shellfish such as clams, mussels, oysters, and scallops. This exposure syndrome is called paralytic shellfish poisoning and can lead to respiratory arrest in addition to the GI symptoms. Toxicological emergencies can also arise from toxins found within commonly eaten fish. Bony fish poisoning (Ciguatera poisoning) is most frequent in fish caught in the Pacific Ocean or along the tropical reefs of Florida and the West Indies. Ciguatera may have an incubation period of 2–6 hours before producing myalgia and paresthesia. Scombroid (histamine) poisoning results from bacterial contamination of mackerel, tuna, bonitos, and albacore. Both Ciguatera and scombroid poisoning cause the standard GI symptoms; scombroid poisoning also produces immediate facial flushing due to histamine-induced vasodilation.

Except for botulism, food poisoning is rarely life threatening and treatment is largely supportive. In cases of suspected food poisoning, contact Poison Control and medical direction, and take the following steps: (1) perform necessary assessment, (2) collect samples of suspected food source, (3) support ABCs with airway maintenance, high-flow oxygen, intubation or assisted ventilation as needed, and establish IV access. In addition, consider administration of antihistamines (especially in seafood poisonings) and antiemetics.

Spider and snake bites can be common and significant toxicological emergencies in certain parts of the country. The brown recluse spider lives in southern and midwestern states. It is found in large numbers in Tennessee, Arkansas, Oklahoma, and Texas. It has also been reported in Hawaii and California. The brown recluse is about 15 mm in length, generally lives in dark, dry locations, and can often be found in or around a house. The bites themselves are usually painless, and bites often occur at night while the victim is asleep. The initial, local reaction occurs within minutes and consists of a small erythematous macule surrounded by a white ring. Over the next 8 hours or so localized pain, redness, and swelling develop. Tissue necrosis develops over days to weeks. Other symptoms include fever, chills, nausea, vomiting, joint pain, and in severe cases, bleeding disorders (namely, disseminated intravascular coagulation, DIC). Treatment is largely supportive, and there is no antivenin. Antihistamines may reduce systemic reactions and surgical excision may be required for necrotic tissue. Black widow spiders live in all parts of the continental U.S. and are often found in woodpiles or brush. The female spider bites, and the venom is very potent, causing excessive neurotransmitter release at the synaptic junctions. Immediate, local reaction includes pain, redness, and swelling. Progressive muscle spasms of all large muscles can develop and are usually associated with severe pain. Other systemic symptoms are nausea, vomiting, sweating, seizures, paralysis, and decreased level of consciousness. Field treatment is largely supportive, with reassurance an important factor. IV muscle relaxants may be needed for severe spasms. If medical direction orders it, you may use diazepam or calcium gluconate. Calcium chloride is ineffective and should not be used. Because hypertensive crisis is possible, monitor BP carefully. Transport as rapidly as possible so antivenin can be given in the hospital.

There are several thousand snake bites annually in the U.S., but few deaths. The assessment findings depend on snake, location of the bite, and the type and amount of venom injected. Two families of poisonous snakes are native to the U.S.: the pit vipers (cottonmouths, rattlesnakes, and copperheads) and the coral snake, a distant relative of the cobra. Pit viper venom contains hydrolytic enzymes capable of destroying most tissue components. They can produce hemolysis, destroy of other tissue elements, and may affect the clotting ability of the blood. They produce tissue infarction and necrosis, especially at the site of the bite. A severe pit viper bite can produce death within 30 minutes. However, most fatalities occur from 6 to 30 hours after the bite, with 90% within the first 48 hours. Assessment findings for pit viper bites include fang marks (often little more than a scratch or abrasion), swelling and pain at wound site, continued oozing from wound, weakness, dizziness, or faintness, sweating and/or chills, thirst, nausea and vomiting, diarrhea, tachycardia and hypotension, bloody urine and GI hemorrhage (these are late), ecchymosis, necrosis, shallow respirations progressing to respiratory failure, and numbness and tingling around face and head. The first goal in treatment is to slow absorption of venom; remember that about 25% of bites are dry, that is, no venom is injected. Antivenin is available but should only be considered for severe cases as evidence by marked systemic signs and symptoms. Routine treatment involves keeping the patient supine, immobilizing the affected limb with a splint, maintaining the extremity in a neutral position without any constricting bands, and giving supportive care with high-flow oxygen, IV with crystalloid fluid, and rapid transport. Note: DO NOT apply ice, cold pack, or freon spray to wound, DO NOT apply an arterial tourniquet, and DO NOT apply electrical stimulation from any source in an attempt to retard or reverse venom spread. Coral snakes, which are small and with small fangs, are primarily found in the southwest. A mnemonic that you should remember is "Red touch yellow, kill a fellow; red touch black, venom lack." This indicates the stripe pattern of the coral snake: red-yellow-black-yellow-red. Coral snake venom contains some of the same enzymes as pit viper venom, but it additionally has a neurotoxin that will result in respiratory and skeletal muscle paralysis. Assessment findings include the following (noting that there may be no local or systemic effects for as long as 12–24 hours): localized numbness, weakness, and drowsiness, ataxia, slurred speech and excessive salivation, paralysis of tongue and larynx producing difficulty in swallowing and breathing, drooping of eyelids, double vision, dilated pupils, abdominal pain, nausea and vomiting, loss of consciousness, seizures, respiratory failure, and hypotension. Treatment includes the following steps: (1) wash the wound with lots of water, (2) apply a compression bandage and keep extremity at the level of the heart, (3) immobilize the limb with a splint, (4) start an IV with crystalloid fluid, and (5) transport to the emergency department for antivenin. Note: DO NOT apply ice, cold pack, or freon spray to the wound; DO NOT incise the wound; and DO NOT apply electrical stimulation from any device in an attempt to retard or reverse venom spread.

Stings (injection injuries) can come from insects and marine animals. Many people die from allergic reactions to insect stings, particularly wasps, bees, hornets, and fire ants. Only the common honeybee leaves a stinger. Wasps, hornets, yellow jackets, and fire ants sting repeatedly until removed from contact. Assessment findings include localized pain, redness, swelling, and a skin wheal. Idiosyncratic reactions are not considered allergic if they respond well to antihistamines. Signs and symptoms of an allergic reaction include localized pain, swelling, redness, and skin wheal, itching or flushing of skin or rash, tachycardia, hypotension, bronchospasm, or laryngeal edema, facial edema, and uvular swelling. General management includes washing of the sting area, gentle removal of stinger, if present (scrape, do not squeeze), application of cool compresses, and observation for allergic reaction or anaphylactic shock. Marine animal injection injuries are a threat in some coastal areas, especially in warmer, tropical waters. Toxin injection can be from jellyfish or coral stings or from punctures by the bony spines of animals such as sea urchins and stingrays. All marine venoms contain substances that produce pain that is disproportionate to the size of the injury. These toxins are unstable and heat sensitive, and heat will relieve the pain and inactivate the venom. Signs and symptoms of marine animal injection include intense local pain and swelling, weakness, nausea and vomiting, dyspnea, tachycardia, and hypotension or shock (in severe cases). In any case of suspected injection, treat by establishing and maintaining airway, application of a constriction bandage between the wound and the heart no tighter than a watchband (to occlude lymphatic flow only), application of heat or hot water, and inactivation or removal or any stingers. Because both fresh and salt water contain considerable bacterial and viral pollution, you should always be alert to possible secondary infection of a wound. In cases of marine-acquired infections, be sure to consider *Vibrio* species.

8. **Given several scenarios of poisoning or overdose, provide the appropriate assessment, treatment, and transport.**   pp. 970–1006

Remember that the basic assessment of a patient with a toxicological emergency includes careful scene size-up, protection of rescue personnel, and rapid response to any needs to support the ABCs. Treatment includes decontamination and use of antidotes, where available. Rapid transport is standard. Detailed specifics for many drugs, toxic substances, and animal bites and stings are given in other objectives for this chapter.

CASE STUDY REVIEW

This case study demonstrates how EMT-Is react to a stressful emergency involving an unconscious person who proves to be someone familiar to them as a former patient. It demonstrates many of the general challenges involved in recognition and response to a life-threatening toxicological emergency.

Kevin, Charles, and David receive one of the briefest of calls, "unconscious person." Even before the team reaches the address, they realize that the address seems familiar to them; as they see the location, they remember that they have been called here before to care for a woman with a history of chronic depression and difficulty coping with stressful situations. The study does not state how David knows that a team had been called here as recently as four days previously; it is possible that the team called for log information after realizing that the patient was well known in their service sector.

Initial scene size-up does not reveal any sign of toxicological threat to the team. The woman's boyfriend, who placed the 911 call, is apparently unharmed by any gas or other potentially invisible threat. There are a number of clues obvious to the team that indicate that the woman's unconsciousness is tied to an intentional toxicological emergency: They see an empty bottle of Tylenol (acetaminophen) and an empty bottle of nortriptyline, a tricyclic antidepressant. The nearby pharmacy receipt has the current day's date on it. In addition, the team can smell alcohol in the air and can see several empty bottles of wine. Even as one team member begins an initial assessment of the patient, the others can conclude that a multiple-ingestion overdose has occurred that involves acetaminophen, a tricyclic antidepressant, and alcohol. This is substantiated by the only history, a statement by the boyfriend that the patient had called him and said she "just couldn't take it anymore." The timing of the ingestion is unclear. Certainly the woman was able to make a telephone call and speak coherently two hours or so before the 911 call was made.

Initial assessment reveals that the woman is alive but in extremis: She is unresponsive, has slow, shallow respirations indicative of respiratory depression, and tachycardia with weak pulses. The team begins with the ABCs, intubating the patient and beginning mechanical ventilation. Although the study does not state that they are also giving supplemental oxygen, you should assume that they are doing so with high-flow, high-concentration oxygen. They quickly establish IV access and place essential monitors; again, details are not given, but ECG monitoring and pulse oximetry would be indicated. Continuous assessment of vitals is essential in this type of unstable situation.

The team checks for signs of trauma or other coexisting conditions and finds evidence of previous suicidal intent: multiple shallow scars across both wrists. Rapid transport is initiated, and the team remembers to bring all bottles of medicine found at the scene. Despite their intensive supportive care, the patient does not improve en route and has a generalized, grand mal seizure in the emergency department. Further care and transfer to the ICU are insufficient, and the patient dies in the ICU roughly 48 hours after admission due to cardiac dysrhythmias and liver failure. An autopsy, the results of which are pending, may provide further information on the details of her ingestion and her progressive organ failure.

This vignette contains many of the elements of common toxicological emergencies: a severely ill patient, little history of the immediate event besides clues apparent at the scene, and a struggle for the EMT-I team to support the woman's vital functions while transporting her to the hospital for more definitive treatment. This case study also points out something else you will see with some toxicological emergencies: It isn't possible to save every patient. Whether the emergency is accidental or intentional, some patients cannot be saved, even when everything is done correctly and promptly by the EMT-I team.

CONTENT SELF-EVALUATION

MULTIPLE CHOICE

_____ 1. Which of the following statements about the epidemiology of toxicological emergencies is NOT true?
   A. The frequency of toxicological emergencies continues to increase both in number and severity.
   B. About 70% of accidental poisonings occur among children aged 6 years or younger.
   C. Toxicological emergencies account for about 5% of emergency department visits and EMS responses.
   D. More serious poisonings, especially in older children, may represent intentional poisoning by a parent or caregiver.
   E. Adult poisonings and overdoses account for 95% of the fatalities in this category.

_____ 2. Immediate effects of toxins are often localized to the site of entry, whereas delayed effects are often systemic in nature.
   A. True
   B. False

340 DIVISION 4 *Medical Emergencies*

©2004 Pearson Education, Inc.
Intermediate Emergency Care: Principles & Practice

_____ 3. Many inhalation exposures are accidental, and leading agents include the following:
   A. carbon dioxide, carbon tetrachloride, and ammonia.
   B. toxic vapors, plants, and chlorine.
   C. carbon monoxide, nitrous oxide, and petroleum-based products such as gasoline.
   D. carbon monoxide, ammonia, and toxic vapors.
   E. chlorine, cleaners (soaps and alkalis), and carbon monoxide.

_____ 4. All of the following are guidelines to follow in cases of toxicological emergencies EXCEPT:
   A. maintaining a high index of suspicion for possible poisonings.
   B. recording everything you see or smell at the scene that might help determine cause.
   C. taking appropriate measures to protect all rescue personnel and any bystanders.
   D. centering general management on support of ABCs, decontamination of patient, and use of antidote, if there is one.
   E. removing the patient from a toxic environment as promptly as possible.

_____ 5. Never delay supportive measures or transport due to a delay in contacting Poison Control Center.
   A. True
   B. False

_____ 6. The most common route of entry for toxic substances is:
   A. inhalation.   D. injection.
   B. ingestion.   E. adsorption.
   C. surface absorption.

_____ 7. The three principles of decontamination are:
   A. removal of patient from toxic environment, reduction in intake of toxin, and increase in elimination of toxin from body.
   B. removal of patient from toxic environment, removal of patient's clothing and washing of patient's body, increase in elimination of toxin from body.
   C. removal of patient from toxic environment, reduction in intake of toxin, and use of antidote, if one.
   D. removal of patient's clothing and washing of body, reduction in intake of toxin, and reduction in absorption of toxin already in body.
   E. reduction in intake of toxin into the body, reduction of absorption of toxin already in the body, and increase in elimination of toxin from the body.

_____ 8. The most widely used means of reducing absorption of toxins in the body is:
   A. gastric lavage (stomach pumping).   D. whole bowel irrigation.
   B. activated charcoal.   E. chelating agents.
   C. syrup of ipecac.

_____ 9. Do not involve law enforcement in a possible suicide case until it is clear that suicide was intended.
   A. True
   B. False

_____ 10. Flumazenil is an antidote for which of the following ingested substances?
   A. arsenic   D. ethylene glycol
   B. benzodiazepines   E. methyl alcohol
   C. cyanide

_____ 11. Which of the following is not a question commonly asked of a poisoning patient during the focused history?
   A. How much of the agent(s) did you ingest?
   B. How long ago did you ingest the agent(s)?
   C. Were any people with you when you ingested the agent(s)?
   D. What is your weight?
   E. Have you attempted to treat yourself in any way?

_____ 12. The physical exam is crucial in toxicological emergencies, and it has two purposes: (1) documenting physical evidence of intoxication and (2) detecting any underlying illness or condition that might affect either patient's symptoms or outcome of exposure.
  A. True
  B. False

_____ 13. All of the following statements are correct when treating ingestion emergencies EXCEPT:
  A. Maintaining the ABCs is the top priority along with monitoring of all vitals.
  B. Prevention of aspiration is a major objective, and intubation may be necessary.
  C. An IV at keep-vein-open rate is recommended for all potentially dangerous ingestion incidents.
  D. Induce vomiting unless it is against local protocol or you are told not to do so by Poison Control.
  E. Follow general treatment guidelines with decontamination procedures.

_____ 14. The first priorities, in proper order, with surface-absorption exposures are to remove the patient from the toxic environment, perform the initial assessment, and then ensure your safety.
  A. True
  B. False

_____ 15. All of the following are respiratory signs or symptoms of a toxic inhalation exposure EXCEPT:
  A. bradycardia.   D. tachypnea.
  B. chest tightness.   E. dizziness.
  C. cough.

_____ 16. The typical signs and symptoms of carbon monoxide poisoning include:
  A. a burning sensation in mouth and throat, headache, and confusion.
  B. headache, seizure or coma, tachypnea.
  C. tachypnea, pulmonary edema, a burning sensation in mouth and throat.
  D. tachypnea, tachycardia, headache, and confusion.
  E. headache, nausea and vomiting, confusion or other altered mental status.

_____ 17. The narcotic toxidrome is characterized by CNS depression, whereas the sympathomimetic toxidrome is characterized by CNS excitation.
  A. True
  B. False

_____ 18. Response to poisoning with one of the cardiac medications often involves bradycardia, which may require use of:
  A. atropine.   D. digoxin.
  B. an external pacing device.   E. calcium.
  C. a beta blocker.

_____ 19. Common assessment findings for ingestion with a caustic include all of the following EXCEPT:
  A. chest and abdominal pain.   D. hoarseness and/or stridor.
  B. drooling and trouble swallowing. E. pain in the lips, tongue, throat, or gums.
  C. facial burns.

_____ 20. A patient has spilled a large quantity of an unknown acid on his skin. Treatment should consist of:
  A. contacting Poison Control for instructions.
  B. covering the area with activated charcoal.
  C. diluting the acid with bicarbonate.
  D. irrigation with copious amounts of water.
  E. irrigation with copious amounts of milk.

©2004 Pearson Education, Inc.
Intermediate Emergency Care: Principles & Practice

_____ 21. Ingestion of alkalis usually results in:
   A. immediate and intense pain.
   B. bradycardia.
   C. local burns to the mouth and throat.
   D. ulceration and perforation of the stomach lining.
   E. liquefaction necrosis.

_____ 22. Drugs with narrow therapeutic indexes are more likely to be involved in accidental toxicological emergencies. Two such drugs are:
   A. lithium and the selective serotonin reuptake inhibitors (SSRIs).
   B. tricyclic antidepressants and salicylates.
   C. tricyclic antidepressants and lithium.
   D. tricyclic antidepressants and SSRIs.
   E. salicylates and lithium.

_____ 23. It is particularly important to know time of ingestion when a blood test (timed properly) can predict degree of damage. Two drugs to which this statement especially applies are:
   A. acetaminophen and tricyclics.
   B. SSRIs and tricyclics.
   C. acetaminophen and non-steroidal anti-inflammatory drugs.
   D. salicylates and non-steroidal anti-inflammatory drugs.
   E. salicylates and acetaminophen.

_____ 24. If you suspect mixed ingestion with tricyclics and benzodiazepines, do NOT use Flumazenil because it may precipitate seizures.
   A. True
   B. False

_____ 25. Serotonin syndrome includes all of the following signs and symptoms EXCEPT:
   A. nausea, diarrhea, abdominal cramps.
   B. hypotension.
   C. agitation and confusion.
   D. hyperthermia.
   E. rigidity, incoordination, myoclonic jerks.

_____ 26. Chelating agents are often useful in cases of toxicity due to:
   A. lithium.   D. heavy metals.
   B. theophylline.   E. salicylates.
   C. some cardiac medications.

_____ 27. All of the following statements are true about MAO inhibitors EXCEPT:
   A. Overdose cases may be very serious, even though initial signs/symptoms may appear hours after ingestion.
   B. MAO inhibitors have been used to treat depression and obsessive-compulsive disorder.
   C. MAO inhibitors as a group have a narrow therapeutic index.
   D. MAO inhibitors may interact negatively with foods containing tyramine, such as cheese and wine.
   E. In overdose, death usually follows the eventual signs of tachycardia, hypertension, and coma.

_____ 28. In cases of suspected food poisoning or poisoning involving plants and mushrooms, it is important to bring samples along with the patient if possible.
   A. True
   B. False

_____ 29. In cases involving bites or stings, fatalities are most likely among patients who have an allergic reaction or anaphylaxis to insect stings.
   A. True
   B. False

Medical Emergencies

_____ 30. In common toxic drug ingestions, the use of benzodiazepines is frequently recommended with:
  A. alcohol, narcotics, and barbiturates.
  B. alcohol, hallucinogens, and barbiturates.
  C. cocaine, amphetamines, and hallucinogens.
  D. cocaine, alcohol, and amphetamines.
  E. cocaine, amphetamines, and barbiturates.

_____ 31. Alcohol is a(n):
  A. depressant.   D. stimulant.
  B. narcotic.   E. oxidant.
  C. opiate.

_____ 32. Signs and symptoms associated with amphetamine usage include all of the following EXCEPT:
  A. constricted pupils.   D. psychosis.
  B. exhilaration.   E. tremors.
  C. hypertension.

_____ 33. Altered mental status and slurred speech are signs/symptoms of Xanax overdose.
  A. True
  B. False

_____ 34. Which of the following statements about delirium tremens is NOT true?
  A. They usually develop 2–3 days after withdrawal of alcohol.
  B. They can occur in individuals who have experienced recent binge drinking.
  C. DTs are marked by decreased level of consciousness with hallucinations.
  D. Seizures and delirium tremens are ominous signs.
  E. DTs are associated with a significant mortality rate.

MATCHING

Write the letter of the definition in the space provided next to the term to which it applies.

_____ 35. injection

_____ 36. tolerance

_____ 37. toxin

_____ 38. inhalation

_____ 39. poisoning

_____ 40. substance abuse

_____ 41. therapeutic index (or window)

_____ 42. ingestion

_____ 43. delirium tremens (DTs)

_____ 44. enterotoxin

_____ 45. decontamination

_____ 46. surface absorption

_____ 47. overdose

_____ 48. toxidrome

_____ 49. withdrawal

_____ 50. addiction

A. an exposure to a nonpharmacological toxic substance
B. entry of a substance into the body via a break in the skin
C. result of drug discontinuance in which body reacts severely to absence of drug
D. group of clinical signs and symptoms consistently associated with exposure to a particular type of toxin
E. dependence on a drug, physiological, psychological, or both
F. potentially lethal syndrome found when alcohol withdrawn from chronic abusers
G. dosage range between effective and toxic dosages
H. need to progressively increase dosage to achieve same effect
I. process of minimizing toxicity by reducing amount of toxin absorbed into the body
J. entry of a substance into the body via the skin or mucous membranes
K. exposure to an amount of pharmacological substance greater than normally tolerated

©2004 Pearson Education, Inc.
Intermediate Emergency Care: Principles & Practice

L. bacterial exotoxin that produces GI symptoms and diseases such as food poisoning
M. entry of a substance into the body via the respiratory tract
N. any chemical that causes adverse effects on an organism exposed to it
O. use of pharmacological product for purposes other than those medically defined for it
P. entry of a substance into the body via the GI tract

SPECIAL PROJECT

Analyzing an Emergency Scene

Use your experience and what you have learned in this chapter to answer the questions about the following scenario.

You are called to the apartment of an elderly gentleman after his son phoned 911 to report that when he telephoned his father for a nightly check, his father had slurred speech and sounded confused. The son told dispatch that his father had felt "under the weather" with a cold recently but had otherwise been in his usual, somewhat fragile, state of health. No specifics were given.

You find the patient alone in his apartment. He is an unkempt, confused gentleman who repeatedly introduces himself and asks your names. He looks moderately uncomfortable, has nasal congestion and a mild cough, and says he has been "a bit ill" for several days. He states that he took a long nap, and then got up and took his pills. He says he doesn't need any help, he just needs to sit a bit to clear his head. When asked what pills he took, and how long ago, he says he "thinks" he just took the bedtime pills, but he may also have taken the afternoon ones because he might have slept through the normal time to take them. He doesn't know where the pharmacy bottles are because his visiting nurse makes up his pill case once a week. You note on the nightstand next to the bed a pill case, one of those that has the days of the week and several times per day marked on it with a compartment for each dosing time. You observe that several compartments for each day have tablets or capsules, often multiple.

1. What kind of toxicological emergency might this situation represent, and would you suspect accidental or intentional circumstances?

As you start your physical assessment, the patient says, "Oh, my, I'm dizzy," and sits awkwardly on the floor. His pulse is difficult to determine, but it is weak, slow, and possibly irregular.

2. What are your initial interventions?

3. What priorities do you give to calling the Poison Control Center, medical direction, and initiating transport?

4. What, if anything, do you take with you from the apartment?

CHAPTER 24

*

Neurological Emergencies

Review of Chapter Objectives

After reading this chapter, you should be able to:

1. **Define and discuss the epidemiology (including the morbidity/mortality and preventative strategies), pathophysiology, assessment findings, and management for the following neurologic problems:**

   a. Coma and altered mental status   pp. 1018–1019

   Altered mental status is extremely common, as you'll understand when you consider the wide variety of causes. Morbidity and mortality are often correlated to cause. Vigilant assessment and management on your part will optimize your patient's chances, regardless of causes. An alteration in mental status is the hallmark sign of CNS injury or illness; as such, any alteration, be it subtle or as florid as coma, requires evaluation. In coma, the patient cannot be aroused by even powerful external stimuli such as pain. The two mechanisms generally capable of causing altered mental status are structural lesions (such as tumor, trauma, degenerative disease, or another process that destroys or encroaches on the substance of the brain) and toxic-metabolic states (such as the presence of toxins including ammonia or the absence of vital substances such as oxygen, glucose, or thiamine). Causes of toxic-metabolic disturbances include anoxia, diabetic ketoacidosis, hepatic failure, hypoglycemia, renal failure, thiamine deficiency, and toxic exposure (for instance, cyanide). Some of the most common causes you'll see for altered mental status (meaning they can cause a structural lesion or a toxic-metabolic state) are the following: (1) drugs, including depressants such as alcohol, hallucinogens, and narcotics; (2) cardiovascular, including anaphylaxis, cardiac arrest, stroke, dysrhythmias, hypertensive encephalopathy, and shock; (3) respiratory, including chronic obstructive pulmonary disease (COPD), inhalation of a toxic gas such as carbon monoxide, and hypoxia; and (4) infectious, such as AIDS, encephalitis, and meningitis.

   During history taking and assessment, remember the mnemonic AEIOU-TIPS, and look for signs of these common causes: A (acidosis or alcohol), E (epilepsy), I (infection), O (overdose), U (uremia, or kidney failure), T (trauma, tumor, or toxin), I (insulin, either hypoglycemia or ketoacidosis), P (psychosis or poison), S (stroke, seizure). During physical assessment, use the AVPU method for determining level of consciousness. Unresponsive patients require especially vigilant monitoring and protection of the airway. Remember that in some cases you will not be able to determine the cause of the problem in the prehospital setting.

   Management begins with the ABCs. The initial priority is the airway; be sure to immobilize the C-spine in cases of suspected head or neck injury. Then attend to breathing, administering supplemental oxygen and assisting ventilations if needed. An unresponsive patient requires an airway adjunct. As an evaluation of circulation, check heart rate and rhythm and blood pressure. Then perform the following steps:

   - IV of normal saline or lactated Ringer's solution at a keep-vein-open rate; alternatively place a heparin lock.

- Determine blood glucose level with reagent strip or glucometer. If serum glucose is low, give 50% dextrose to mediate the hypoglycemia. Even if the patient is an uncontrolled diabetic, any transient hyperglycemia will do limited harm at most in the short prehospital period. In many cases of hypoglycemia, dextrose can be life saving, and you may see an immediate response. Glucose may also be life saving for the alcoholic patient with hypoglycemia. (See Chapter 21, "Diabetic Emergencies.)
- Administer naloxone if there is suspicion of narcotic overdose. (See Chapter 23, "Poisoning and Overdose Emergencies," for details).
- If there is suspicion of alcoholism, consider use of 100 mg thiamine (Vitamin B_1).

In chronic alcoholism, intake, absorption, and use of thiamine is impaired. Among these patients, you may see Wernicke's syndrome, a condition marked by loss of memory and disorientation that is associated with a diet deficient in thiamine. Of even greater concern is Korsakoff's psychosis, marked by memory disorder, because it may be irreversible. Thus, the of administration of thiamine as per local protocols and the judgment of medical direction may be important.

If increased intracranial pressure is possible, as in a closed head injury, hyperventilate the patient at 20 breaths per minute. The decrease in carbon dioxide causes cerebral vasoconstriction and reduces brain swelling. DO NOT over-hyperventilate, as this can decrease CO_2 to dangerously low levels. Medical direction may order use of mannitol (Osmotrol) to cause a diuresis that may shift fluid from the intravascular space through the kidneys.

b. Seizures
pp. 1025–1029

A seizure is a temporary alteration in behavior due to a massive discharge of one or more groups of neurons in the brain. Seizures can be induced in anyone under certain stressful conditions such as hypoxia or rapidly decreasing blood glucose. Febrile seizures often occur in young children with a sudden increase in body temperature. Structural diseases of the brain such as tumors, head trauma, toxic eclampsia, and vascular disorders can also cause a seizure. Recurrent seizures without such a known cause are termed epilepsy. Epilepsy affects about 2.5 million persons, who may present with a neurological emergency or have another condition complicated by their seizure disorder. Most cases of epilepsy are idiopathic, that is, without known cause, whereas others arise secondary to damage from strokes, head trauma, tumor, surgery or radiation, etc.

Assessment begins with history according to the patient or bystanders, as well as physical impression. Remember that many people think the only kind of seizure is a "grand mal," so a bystander who does not know the patient may suggest he is on drugs, or that he fainted, or give other information that is misleading. In addition, other medical conditions can present similarly to a seizure: Examples are migraine headaches, cardiac dysrhythmias, hypoglycemia, or orthostatic hypotension. Hyperventilation, as well as a number of CNS conditions, can cause stiffness in the extremities. Decerebrate movements can be caused by increased intracranial pressure. Thus, there is often more potential harm than good in administering an anticonvulsant.

The patient history should include an attempt to ascertain the following information: (1) history of seizures, and, if so, particulars of type, nature, and frequency, (2) recent history of head trauma, (3) possibility of alcohol or other drug use, (4) recent history of fever, headache, or stiff neck, (5) history of diabetes, heart disease, or stroke, and (6) current medications. During physical exam, look for evidence of head injury or injury to the tongue and for evidence of alcohol or drug abuse. Be sure to document any dysrhythmias.

Active management may not be needed for many types of seizures, including short generalized tonic-clonic seizures that have ended before you arrive. Management for most generalized seizures in process is supportive: Manage the airway, make sure the patient does not injure him- or herself, and monitor for possible hyper- or hypothermia, depending on environmental conditions. General procedures include the following: (1) assurance of scene safety, (2) maintenance of airway (DO NOT force objects between the patient's teeth or push objects into the mouth that may initiate vomiting), (3) administration of high-flow oxygen, (4) establishment of IV access, running normal saline or lactated Ringer's solution at keep-vein-open rate, (5) determination of blood glucose level, with 50% glucose given in hypoglycemia, (6) physical

©2004 Pearson Education, Inc.
Intermediate Emergency Care: Principles & Practice

protection of patient from surroundings, (7) maintenance of temperature, (8) postictal positioning on left side with suction if required, (9) monitoring of cardiac rhythm, (10) consideration of an anticonvulsant if seizure is prolonged (greater than 5 minutes), (11) transport the patient in supine or lateral recumbent position in quiet, reassuring atmosphere.

Status epilepticus, two or more generalized seizures without intervening return of consciousness, can be a life-threatening emergency. The most common cause in adults with epilepsy is failure to comply with medication regimen. Status is a major emergency because it involves a prolonged period of apnea with the possibility of CNS hypoxia. The most valuable intervention is to protect the airway and to deliver 100% oxygen, preferably by BVM device. After airway and breathing have been addressed, start an IV with normal saline at keep-vein-open rate, monitor cardiac rhythm, give 25 g 50% dextrose IV push if hypoglycemia is present, give 5–10 mg diazepam IV push for an adult, and continue to monitor airway. Note that some patients will require large doses of diazepam, and this may cause respiratory depression. Depression, if significant, can be reversed with flumazenil, although this may also result in the return of seizures.

c. Syncope
pp. 1029–1031

Syncope, or fainting, is characterized by a sudden, temporary loss of consciousness caused by insufficient blood flow to the brain, with recovery almost immediate upon supine positioning. Syncope is very common, accounting for roughly 3% of all emergency department visits. It can occur at any age. Symptoms may include prior feelings of dizziness or lightheadedness or there may be no warning at all. By definition, if return of consciousness does not occur within a few moments, the event is NOT syncope, it is something more serious. (Review Table 24-2, text page 1027, for help in distinguishing between syncope and seizure.)

There are three pathophysiologic mechanisms for syncope: cardiovascular, non-cardiovascular, and idiopathic. Cardiovascular causes include dysrhythmias or mechanical problems such as an abnormally functioning heart valve. Non-cardiovascular causes include metabolic, neurological, or psychiatric conditions. For instance, hypoglycemia, a transient ischemic attack (TIA), or an anxiety attack my all precipitate syncope. Idiopathic, as always, means there is no known cause even after careful evaluation. Management begins with an attempt to find and treat the underlying cause. If no cause is established, the patient should be transported to an appropriate emergency department for evaluation. Field management is somewhat similar to that for seizure: assure scene safety, maintain open airway, administer high-flow oxygen and assist ventilations as needed, check circulatory status (heart rate and rhythm, blood pressure), check and continue monitoring mental status, start IV with normal saline or lactated Ringer's at keep-vein-open rate, determine blood glucose level, monitor cardiac rhythm, and transport in reassuring environment.

d. Headache
pp. 1030–1031

Headaches, either acute or chronic, are a tremendously common complaint: You've probably had problems with a headache at least once. Nearly 45 million Americans suffer from chronic headaches. There three general categories of headache: vascular, tension, and organic. Headaches of vascular origin include migraines and cluster headaches. Migraines occur more commonly in women, whereas cluster headaches occur more commonly in men. Migraines are typically characterized by intense, throbbing pain, sensitivity to light or sound, nausea, vomiting, and sweating. Migraines may last from several minutes to several days. They typically present as one-sided headaches and they may be preceded by an aura. Cluster headaches usually occur as a series of one-sided headaches that are sudden in onset, intense, and continue for roughly 15 minutes to 4 hours. Symptoms may include nasal congestion, drooping eyelid, and an irritated eye. Tension headaches account for a significant percentage of headaches. Most personnel in emergency medicine, have, or will, have a tension headache. Some people experience them on a daily basis. These persons may wake with a headache that worsens over the course of the day. The typical tension headache has a dull, achy pain that feels as if forceful pressure is being applied to the neck or head. The last class of headache, organic headaches, is less common. They occur in association with tumor, infection, or other diseases of the brain, eye, or other body system.

Medical Emergencies

Because headaches can herald serious illness or precede a catastrophic event such as a ruptured aneurysm, it is always important to keep these possible underlying causes in mind when you speak with a patient complaining of headache. A continuous throbbing headache, particularly if over the occiput, accompanied by fever, confusion, and stiffness of the neck is classic for meningitis. Sudden onset pain, often described as "the worst pain of my life," or changes in pain pattern should all be considered possible signs of conditions as grave as intracranial hemorrhage. In general, any headache of acute onset or of changing pattern demands immediate attention on your part.

A complete and thorough history is important in evaluating the patient with headache. Questions that may evoke valuable information include the following: What were you doing when the pain started? Does anything make the pain worse (such as light, sound, or movement)? What is the quality of the pain, throbbing, crushing, tension? Does pain radiate to the neck, arm, back, or jaw? What is the severity of the pain on a scale of 1–10 and has severity changed? How long has the headache been present (is it acute or chronic)? You will see that the same line of questioning about pain is used in other settings, too, as with patients who complain of abdominal pain.

Management is supportive and generally includes the following: (1) assurance of scene safety, (2) protection of airway, (3) placement of patient in position of comfort (often accomplished by patients themselves), (4) high-flow oxygen with ventilation assistance as needed, (5) IV with normal saline or lactated Ringer's at keep-vein-open rate, determination of blood glucose, monitoring of cardiac rhythm, (6) transport with reassurance in an environment that is calm and quiet, (7) consideration of use of antiemetics or analgesics. Antiemetics that might be helpful for migraine include prochlorperazine (Compazine) and abortive agents such as sumatriptan (Imitrix).

e. Weakness/dizziness
pp. 1031–1032

The complaint of feeling weak and dizzy or weak all over is a common complaint which the EMT-I encounters. Although vague, the complaint it is often the symptom of many other conditions, and your assessment skills will be important to best determine the most appropriate treatment plan. Obtain a detailed history of the illness. What has changed in the past 72 hours? Does the patient complain of any GI distress or symptoms? These patients should receive a focused assessment including a neurological exam. Be alert for the presence of nystagmus (a constant, involuntary, cyclical motion of the eyeball), which can indicate a CNS or inner ear problem. Assess muscle groups to see if the weakness is localized or diffuse.

Be alert for possible causes of the weakness such as: neurological, respiratory, cardiovascular, endocrine, or infectious. Many patients with mild volume depletion (dehydration) will have these symptoms.

The management of a patient who is weak and dizzy, provided you have not isolated a specific cause, is basically supportive care. Be sure to include the following:

- Assure scene safety.
- Establish and maintain an adequate airway.
- Place the patient in a position of comfort which is usually head elevated. Avoid sudden or exaggerated movement of the head as it can exacerbate symptoms.
- Administer high-flow, high-concentration oxygen.
- Start an IV kvo (consider fluid challenge of saline or lactated Ringer's).
- Check blood sugar.
- Monitor ECG.
- Consider antiemetics per your local protocol.
- Ensure calm quiet environment.
- Reassure patient.
- Transport to the ED.

f. Stroke
pp. 1020–1025

Stroke is a general term for injury or death of brain tissue, usually due to interruption of blood flow to that region of the cerebrum. The term "brain attack" is being used more frequently because of some similarities between stroke and heart attack, the latter also being due to oxygen deprivation. You should also realize that there are more treatment similarities to heart

©2004 Pearson Education, Inc.
Intermediate Emergency Care: Principles & Practice

attacks. Strokes due to thromboembolic causes may be aborted or minimized with use of thrombolytic agents now used with heart attack (such as tissue plasminogen activator, tPA). The importance to you is that prompt recognition and transport of stroke patients is greater than ever. Stroke patients who may be candidates for thrombolytic therapy must receive definitive treatment within 3 hours of onset.

Strokes are the third most common cause of death and a frequent cause of considerable disability among middle-aged and elderly persons. Major risk factors include atherosclerosis, heart disease, hypertension, diabetes, abnormal blood lipid levels, use of oral contraceptives, and sickle cell disease. Strokes can be caused either by occlusion of an artery or by hemorrhage. Both interrupt blood flow to distal tissues. An occlusive stroke is any caused by blockage of the artery, resulting in ischemia to brain tissue that may progress to infarction if oxygen deprivation continues long enough. Infarcted brain tissue swells, further damaging nearby tissue that might have only a marginal blood supply itself. If swelling is sufficiently severe, herniation (protrusion of tissue through the foramen magnum, the opening at the base of the skull through which the spinal cord emerges from the cranium) can occur. Occlusive strokes are either thrombotic or embolic in origin.

Thrombotic strokes are due to a thrombus, or blood clot, that forms in and then obstructs a cerebral artery. Thrombosis is often related to atherosclerotic change in the artery. Unsurprisingly, the signs and symptoms of a thrombotic stroke are often gradual in onset. The stroke often occurs at night and is characterized by the patient waking with altered mental status and/or loss of speech, sensation, or motor function. An embolic stroke is caused by a solid, liquid, or gaseous mass that is carried to the site of obstruction from a remote site. The most common brain emboli are blood clots that often arise from diseased blood vessels in the neck (namely, the carotid artery) or from abnormal cardiac contraction. Atrial fibrillation often results in atrial dilation, a precursor to clot formation. Other types of emboli include air, tumor tissue, and fat. Typically, embolic strokes present with sudden onset of severe headaches. Hemorrhagic strokes are due to bleeding within brain tissue, and they can be categorized as intracerebral or subarachnoid (see Figure 24-7, text page 1022). They are discussed in detail below under intracranial hemorrhage.

Prompt and proper assessment of a stroke in progress is very important. Signs and symptoms will depend on the type of stroke and the area of the brain affected by it. Onset of symptoms may be acute, and the patient may be unconscious. You may observe stertorous breathing due to paralysis of part of the soft palate. Respiratory expirations may be puffs of air out of the cheeks and mouth. The patient's pupils may be unequal. If so, the larger pupil will be on the side of the hemorrhage. Paralysis, when present, usually involves one side of the face, one arm, or one leg. Speech disturbances may be noted, and the patient's skin may be cool and clammy.

In list form, common signs and symptoms of stroke include the following: one-sided facial drooping, headache, confusion and agitation, dysphasia (difficulty in speech), aphasia (inability to speak), dysarthria (impairment of tongue and muscles making speech difficult), vision problems such as blindness in one eye or double vision, hemiparesis (one-sided weakness), hemiplegia (one-sided paralysis), paresthesias, inability to recognize by touch, gait disturbances or uncoordinated motor movements, dizziness, incontinence, or coma.

Management of stroke emphasizes early recognition, supportive measures, prompt, rapid transport, and notification of the emergency department (see algorithm in Figure 24-8, text page 1024). Remember that aggressive airway management is vital in these patients. Other field measures include the following: (1) assurance of scene safety, including body substance isolation, (2) airway management including suction as needed, (3) ventilation assistance as needed: If the patient is apneic or breathing is inadequate, provide positive-pressure ventilation at 20/minute. Hyperventilation eliminates excessive CO_2 levels. Avoid over-hyperventilation because excessively low CO_2 levels can cause profound cerebral vasoconstriction. If breathing is adequate, give oxygen via nonrebreather mask at 15 L/minute, (4) complete a detailed patient history, (5) keep patient supine or in recovery position. If the patient has congestive heart failure, place patient in semi-upright position as needed. If patient has altered mental status and you suspect potential for airway compromise, keep him or her in left lateral recumbent, or recovery position, (6) determine blood glucose level; if hypoglycemia is present,

Medical Emergencies

consider 50% dextrose by IV push, (7) start an IV of normal saline or lactated Ringer's at a keep-vein-open rate or place a saline or heparin lock (avoiding dextrose solutions, which may increase intracranial pressure due to osmotic effect), (8) monitor cardiac rhythm, (9) protect paralyzed extremities, (10) reassure patient and explain all procedures as patient may be able to understand even if he or she cannot respond, and (11) transport without excessive movement or noise.

g. Intracranial hemorrhage
p. 1021

Hemorrhagic strokes are due to blood within brain tissue, and they can be categorized as intracerebral or subarachnoid. These intracranial hemorrhages often occur with sudden onset of a severe headache. Most intracranial hemorrhages occur in a hypertensive patient when a small vessel deep within brain tissue ruptures. Subarachnoid hemorrhages most commonly result from either congenital blood vessel anomalies or from head trauma. Congenital anomalies include aneurysms and arteriovenous malformations. Aneurysms tend to be on the brain's surface and may either hemorrhage into brain tissue or into the subarachnoid space. Hemorrhage within brain tissue may tear and separate normal brain tissue. Release of blood into the ventricles containing CSF may paralyze vital centers. If blood impairs drainage of CSF, the resultant increase in intracranial pressure may cause herniation of brain tissue.

h. Transient ischemic attack
pp. 1023–1025

A transient ischemic attack (TIA) is a temporary manifestation of the signs and/or symptoms of stroke that is due to temporary interference with blood supply to the affected part of the brain. These symptoms may persist for a few minutes or for hours, but they almost always resolve within 24 hours. After the attack (because it reflects ischemia, not infarction), there is no evidence of brain or neurological damage. The most common cause is carotid artery disease (provoking an embolic event). Other causes can be small emboli of different origin, decreased cardiac output, hypotension, overmedication with antihypertensive medications, or cerebrovascular spasm. Part of the importance of recognizing TIAs is that they may be the precursor to a stroke. One third of TIA patients suffer a stroke soon afterward. A TIA is typically sudden in onset, with specific signs and symptoms depending on the part of the brain involved.

In the prehospital setting, it is virtually impossible to distinguish a TIA from a stroke. While taking the history, try to get the following information: previous neurological symptoms, if any; initial symptoms and their progression; changes in mental status; precipitating factors, if any; dizziness; palpitations; history of hypertension, cardiac disease, sickle cell disease, or previous TIA or stroke. Because TIAs and strokes are generally indistinguishable in the field, the management is the same. (See Stroke above.)

2. Describe and differentiate the major types of seizures
pp. 1025–1027

Seizures can be clinically grouped as generalized or partial on a pathophysiologic basis. Generalized seizures begin with an electrical discharge in a small part of the brain but the abnormal activity spreads to involve the entire cerebral cortex. In contrast, partial seizures may remain confined to a small area, causing localized malfunction, or they may spread and become secondarily generalized seizures.

Generalized seizures include tonic-clonic (also commonly called grand mal) and absence seizures. A tonic-clonic seizure is a generalized motor seizure that produces a temporary loss of consciousness. Usually, it includes a tonic phase (in which muscle tone is increased) and a clonic phase (in which muscles in the extremities jerk rhythmically). In some cases, temporary paralysis of the intercostal muscles causes an interruption in breathing and cyanosis may become evident. When respirations resume, you may see copious amounts of frothy oral secretions. Incontinence is also common during a seizure, and you may note agitation or confusion, drowsiness, or even coma following a seizure, depending on the norm for that patient. Absence seizures present very differently. They are characterized by a sudden onset of a brief (typically 10- to 30-second) loss of consciousness or awareness. Loss of consciousness may be so brief that the casual observer misses it altogether. These idiopathic seizures of childhood rarely occur after age 20 years. Note that absence seizures may not respond to your normal treatment modalities.

Pseudoseizures, also called hysterical seizures, are not true electrical seizures. Rather, they represent psychiatric phenomena. The patient typically presents with sharp, bizarre movements that may be interrupted with a terse command such as "Stop it!"

Partial seizures may be either simple or complex. Simple seizures involve local motor, sensory, or autonomic dysfunction in one area of the body; there is no loss of consciousness. You should remember, however, that they may spread in area of involvement and progress to a generalized, tonic-clonic seizure. Complex seizures, which usually originate in the temporal lobe, are often characterized by an aura and focal findings such as alterations in mental status or mood. Patients in the midst of such a seizure may appear intoxicated or mentally unstable: They may be confused, stagger, have purposeless movements, or show sudden personality changes. These seizures typically last 1–2 minutes, and the patient will slowly come back to baseline after that period.

3. Describe the phases of a generalized seizure. **pp. 1025–1026**

Although patients are individuals with their own seizure patterns, many tonic-clonic seizures progress through seven phases: (1) aura, a subjective sensation that serves as a warning to those patients who experience it, (2) loss of consciousness, during the aura sensation, if there is one, (3) tonic phase, (4) hypertonic phase, during which you will see extreme muscular rigidity, including hyperextension of the back, (5) clonic phase of muscle spasms (often including the jaws) marked by rhythmic movements, (6) post-seizure, during which the patient is in a coma, and (7) postictal, during which the patient awakens.

4. Define and discuss the pathophysiology, assessment findings, and management for nontraumatic spinal injury, including:

a. Low back pain **p. 1032**

Low back pain, defined as pain felt between the lower rib cage and the gluteal muscles, often radiating to the thighs, is an extremely common complaint but only occasionally the reason for an EMS call. Men and women are equally affected, but you should keep in mind that back pain in women over 60 years may represent the first sign of osteoporosis, an important medical condition. Vertebral fractures from causes other than osteoporosis are also possible causes. Other causes of low back pain include sciatica, which is reflected as severe pain along the path of the sciatic nerve down the back of the thigh and inner leg. Sciatica may be due to compression or trauma to the sciatic nerve or its roots, perhaps from a herniated intervertebral disk or an osteoarthritic lumbosacral vertebral bone. Sciatica may also be due to inflammation of the nerve secondary to metabolic, toxic, or infectious causes. Pain at the level of L-3, L-4, L-5, and S-1 may be due to inflammation of interspinous bursae. Other causes of low back pain are inflammation or sprain of muscles and ligaments that attach to the spine. Most low back pain, though, is found to be idiopathic.

Assessment of back pain is based on chief complaint, history, and physical exam. When the complaint is low back pain, a precise diagnosis is likely to be difficult. Preliminary diagnosis may focus on occupational risk from repetitive lifting or exposure to machinery vibrations. Listen for clues in the history about the nature and timing of the pain and whether the current complaint is acute pain or exacerbation of a chronic condition. Your priorities in the field are to determine whether pain is due to a life-threatening or non-life-threatening condition. Note: The presence of any identifiable neurological deficit may point to a serious underlying cause, as may a gradual onset of pain consistent with degenerative disk disease or tumor growth. The location of the injury may be revealed on exam by a limited range of motion in the lumbar spine, point tenderness on palpation, alterations in sensation, pain, and temperature at a localized point, or pain or paresthesia below a point of injury. Always keep in mind that you are unlikely to be able to determine the cause of the pain in the field. Your primary goal is to look for signs of life-threatening problems and to gather historical and exam information that will be useful to the receiving physician. You will also need to decide, perhaps after consultation with medical direction, whether immobilization (and, if so, to what degree) is necessary during transport.

If there are no clear life-threatening problems requiring intervention, management is primarily aimed at minimizing pain and immobilizing as per local protocol. If there is no historical reason to suspect injury in the past or an underlying condition such as osteoporosis (which makes patients vulnerable to pathologic fracture), C-spine immobilization may still be recommended as a comfort measure during transport. Also remember that some patients will require parenteral analgesia and diazepam before they can lie on a stretcher. Consult medical direction if you feel your patient might fit into this category. Last, remember to provide ongoing assessment en route with special attention to the ABCs, vitals, and the possible presence or development of motor or sensory deficits that might indicate a critical condition capable of compromising ventilatory efforts.

b. Herniated intervertebral disk   pp. 1032–1033

Intervertebral disks may rupture due to injury or due to degeneration associated with aging. Degenerative disk disease is most common in patients over 50 years of age. A herniated disk occurs when the gelatinous center of the disk extrudes through a tear in the tough outer capsule, and the resulting pain is due to pressure on the spinal cord or to muscle spasm at the site. The disks themselves are not innervated. Non-injury-related herniation may also be caused by improper lifting. Men aged 30 to 50 years are more prone to herniated disks than are women. Herniation is most common at levels L-4, L-5, and S-1, but it also may occur at C-5, C-6, and C-7. Assessment and management are discussed under low back pain in objective 8a.

c. Spinal-cord tumors   p. 1033

A cyst or tumor along the spine or intruding into the spinal canal may cause pain by pressing on the spinal cord, causing degenerative changes in bone, or interrupting blood supply. The specific manifestations depend on location and type of tumor or cyst. Assessment and management are discussed under low back pain above.

5. Differentiate between neurologic emergencies based on assessment findings.   pp. 1010–1017

Because many signs and symptoms of neurologic dysfunction are subtle, you should use the observations made during scene size-up and formation of general impressions to look for evidence suggesting focus on the neurological system. Environmental clues may include medical equipment, medication bottles, Medic-Alert identification, alcohol bottles, etc. Note, for instance, if the patient is conscious, and, if so, is he confused or lucid? Are his posture and gait normal? Speech can give many clues, particularly if either the patient or a bystander can tell you if the speech you hear is normal for the patient. Skin color, temperature, and moisture are valuable, as is any evidence of facial drooping or muscle spasm. Mental status can then be quickly ascertained through the AVPU method. Assessment of higher cerebral functioning includes assessment of emotional status. Try to evaluate the patient's affect, thought patterns, perceptions, judgments, and memory and attention. ANY alteration from the patient's normal mental status or mood is considered significant and warrants further assessment. After that level of assessment is done, evaluate for the ABCs, including respiration pattern, effort of breathing, heart rate, rhythm, and ECG pattern. An unresponsive patient can be evaluated further with use of the Glasgow Coma Scale. Be aware that a midlevel GCS score (such as 5, 6, or 7) that drops on reevaluation has grim implications.

Scene size-up and initial history will usually make clear whether trauma is involved or not. Regardless of whether trauma is a factor, try to get information on the presence or severity of medical conditions that are risk factors for neurologic conditions, hypertension, heart disease, diabetes, atherosclerosis, as well as any chronic neurologic conditions such as epilepsy. In addition, history should try to establish whether current complaint is acute, an exacerbation of a chronic problem, or a chronic state.

Physical exam of a patient with a neurologic emergency includes the standard head-to-toe exam as well as a more detailed neurological evaluation. Look closely at the patient's face. The ability to smile, frown, or wrinkle the forehead gives information about the status of the facial nerve. Although slight pupillary asymmetry is normal, abnormal pupils can be an early indicator of increasing intracranial pressure. If both pupils are dilated and don't react to light, suspect brainstem injury or serious anoxia. If the pupils are dilated but still react, injury may be reversible. Most of all, remember that any patient with altered mental status and a unilaterally dilated pupil is in the "immediate transport" category. When you check the pupils, look for contact lenses. If present, they should be removed, placed in their container or saline solution, and transported with the patient.

Respiratory derangements are common with CNS illness or injury. Five abnormal breathing patterns may be commonly observed in this setting: Cheyne-Stokes respiration is a pattern marked by apnea lasting 10–60 seconds followed by gradually increasing depth and frequency of respiration. It can be seen with brain damage due to trauma or cerebral hemorrhage and with chronic hypoxia. Kussmaul's respirations are deep, rapid breaths caused by severe metabolic or CNS problems. Central neurogenic hyperventilation is caused by a lesion in the CNS and is marked by rapid, deep, noisy respirations. Ataxic respirations are poor breaths due to CNS damage causing ineffective thoracic muscular coordination. Apneustic respiration is breathing marked by prolonged inspiration unrelieved by expiration attempts and it is due to damage in the upper pons. Always remember that CO_2 has a critical effect on cerebral vessels: Increased levels cause vascular dilation, whereas low levels cause vasoconstriction. This is the basis for controlled hyperventilation in settings where some degree of vasoconstriction might minimize brain swelling.

Cardiovascular status is always important. Even if a primary cardiovascular problem is not present, CNS events are likely to cause changes to the cardiovascular system. In particular, assess heart rate, ECG rhythm, bruits over the carotid arteries, and possible presence of jugular venous distention, a sign of ineffective cardiac pumping. You should be aware that vital signs and changes in them are crucial in following the course of a neurological emergency. Note Cushing's reflex, a grouping of four characteristics in vital signs that signals increased intracranial pressure: increased blood pressure, decreased pulse, decreased respirations, and increased temperature. The earliest signs are the decrease in pulse rate and an increase in blood pressure and temperature.

The exam for neurologic system status is covered in detail on text pages 1014–1015. Note that the components of the exam include sensorimotor evaluation (if posture is abnormal, consider whether it might be decorticate or decerebrate in nature), motor system status, and cranial nerve status.

Last, be particularly aware with elderly patients and with patients with a chronic neurological condition (such as the degenerative disorders) that it is vital to know the patient's baseline values in all areas before you can put your current findings into the context of acute changes or not. Interviewing family members or caregivers may be very helpful.

6. **Given several preprogrammed nontraumatic neurological emergency patients, provide the appropriate assessment, management, and transport.**   pp. 1010–1034

The priorities for someone who is unconscious or clearly in urgent distress with neurologic difficulties are the same as for a patient who is affected by a potentially life-threatening emergency of another origin: Ensure adequate airway, breathing (ventilation), and circulation. This is particularly important for someone whose emergency may be originating in, or affecting, the CNS: The brain requires a constant supply of oxygen, glucose, and vitamins. After 10–20 seconds without blood flow, unconsciousness will occur. Significant deprivation of oxygen (anoxia) or glucose (hypoglycemia) can cause seizures or coma. You should always give high-flow oxygen to a patient with a neurologic emergency and give glucose to any one found to be hypoglycemic.

Neurologic injuries and illnesses usually require treatment as soon as possible to prevent progressive damage. In the case of thromboembolic stroke, this may be particularly true because therapies are coming into use that can minimize the region of brain tissue infarcted in the stroke or even prevent the progression of tissue ischemia to tissue infarction. Patients who show altered mental status and/or any clear neurologic impairment (pupillary dilation, especially unilateral, facial drooping, slurred speech, abnormal posturing—if these appear to be new or progressing findings) that may suggest TIA or stroke need immediate intervention and transport. Management of seizures and syncope often mandates prompt intervention and care, as well.

You will see many calls for complaints such as low back pain and headache. These conditions may be relatively minor or the signal of a serious underlying disorder. History suggesting new onset, severe pain, or clearly progressive pain indicates the need for aggressive assessment and management, whereas other patients with chronic pain of either origin also require full assessment but may need only supportive care.

Medical Emergencies

CASE STUDY REVIEW

This case study demonstrates how EMT-Is react to a relatively common neurological emergency: a "possible stroke patient." The case study demonstrates how initial impressions, assessment findings, and knowledge of the likely pathophysiology not only reveal diagnosis but directly guide the team in prioritizing transport and in identifying the appropriate receiving center.

Jack and Linda are dispatched to a bank with some important information already in hand: The patient is a man in his 60s with reported (presumably new-onset) neurological signs of right-sided weakness and inability to speak. Because possible stroke is a true emergency, one in which time can make a substantial difference to outcome, it is in the patient's favor that the team can respond within 3 minutes or so of the dispatch.

Their initial impression is of an elderly man sitting upright, with some assistance, in a chair. The neurological deficit of aphasia (inability to speak) appears to be confirmed on attempts to communicate with the patient, and the team realizes that the patient, although unable to speak, appears to be oriented and cooperative. Their attention then turns to airway and breathing as priorities. The man's airway is patent (at the moment), and his respirations are normal.

Blood pressure is measured in the unaffected arm, and it is hypertensive at 160/90. Chronic hypertension is a risk factor for stroke, so it is important for the team to ask about a history of hypertension and any associated medications when they get the opportunity to talk with the patient's family. If none of the bystanders knew the gentleman, and if he seemed lucid, the team might be able to solicit limited information from him via a Medic-Alert tag (if he wears one) and/or via requests for head nodding or for written responses to questions. Changes in his ability to comply with such requests might serve as a signal of decreasing mental status. The rest of his initial physical exam is largely benign except for confirmation of unilateral (right-sided) weakness. You are told that there is marked right-sided weakness, but you aren't told the extent: Does it involve the arm only, or does it also involve the face or the leg, or both? Extent of weakness, as well as any sign of additional extent, is an indicator of stroke progression and also signals that sudden airway compromise may be more likely.

Only at this point, after initial assessment, is oxygen started, a heparin lock placed in the unaffected arm, and ECG monitoring begun. The timing of the IV access and ECG monitoring is appropriate, but the team should have considered oxygen supplementation as soon as they knew the patient was unable to talk. Any time advantage in reversal of brain anoxia should be taken. On the other hand, it is a positive sign that pulse oximetry after initiation of oxygen administration is 99%.

You aren't told what information is elicited regarding personal medical history, but you are told that the ECG shows atrial fibrillation at a rate of 90. Atrial fibrillation is a risk factor for embolic (occlusive) stroke because small clots form in the heart and break off to enter the systemic circulation. This knowledge increases the importance of timely transport, as well as expedient consideration of appropriate facility, because current guidelines indicate that thrombolytic therapy within the first 3 hours of an embolic occlusion may well be successful in minimizing or preventing infarction of brain tissue.

Indeed, the team packages the patient carefully but expediently and transports him to a facility that can handle a "brain attack." On arrival, a hemorrhagic stroke of significant magnitude is ruled out via CT scan and the team decides to initiate therapy with tPA. The outcome is positive: The patient's aphasia resolves completely and most of his right-sided weakness reverses. The patient is discharged to a rehabilitation unit for further therapy on his hemiparesis. You don't know how or whether the man's atrial fibrillation (AF) is resolved, but you should assume that in-hospital care would have involved adjustment of medication (if he were taking any for AF) or possible electrical conversion to normal rhythm.

©2004 Pearson Education, Inc.
Intermediate Emergency Care: Principles & Practice

CONTENT SELF-EVALUATION

MULTIPLE CHOICE

_____ 1. The two mechanisms that generally cause altered mental status are:
  A. occlusive and hemorrhagic strokes.
  B. systemic diseases and drugs or toxic agents.
  C. structural lesions and toxic-metabolic states.
  D. head trauma and CNS disease.
  E. toxic-metabolic states and brain tumors.

_____ 2. If the patient is able to smile, frown, and wrinkle forehead muscles, which cranial nerve is intact?
  A. I   D. XI
  B. V   E. XII
  C. VII

_____ 3. The Glasgow Coma Scale assesses eye opening, verbal response, and motor response. Which correlation of score and likely outcome is incorrect?
  A. score or 3 or 4, 10% favorable outcome
  B. score of 8 or higher, 94% favorable outcome
  C. score of 5–7 that increases to 8 or higher, 80% favorable outcome
  D. score of 5–7, 50% favorable outcome in adults and 90% in children
  E. score of 5–7 that decreases by one point, 10% favorable outcome

_____ 4. Three interventions that may be indicated in treatment of a patient with altered mental status of unknown cause are:
  A. hyperventilation, 50% dextrose, and naloxone.
  B. mannitol (Osmotrol), 50% dextrose, and naloxone.
  C. 50% dextrose, thiamine, and naloxone.
  D. mannitol (Osmotrol), hyperventilation, and 50% dextrose.
  E. mannitol (Osmotrol), thiamine, and naloxone.

_____ 5. A condition characterized by a loss of memory and disorientation and often associated with chronic alcoholism and a diet deficient in thiamine is:
  A. Korsakoff's psychosis.   D. Esselstyne's syndrome.
  B. Wernicke's syndrome.   E. Makynen seizure.
  C. Lein's psychosis.

_____ 6. The type of stroke caused by a ruptures cerebral artery is a(n) _____ stroke.
  A. occlusive   D. hemorrhagic
  B. embolic   E. aneural
  C. thrombotic

_____ 7. If a stroke patient is apneic or breathing inadequately, controlled positive-pressure hyperventilation may be beneficial because it:
  A. causes cerebral vasoconstriction, decreasing cerebral swelling.
  B. causes a reflex increase in respiration rate.
  C. eliminates excess CO_2 levels.
  D. increases CO_2 levels toward normal range.
  E. increases the ability of brain cells to take up any available oxygen.

_____ 8. Among the many types of epileptic seizures, the most likely to require intervention on your part are:
  A. absence seizures.   D. simple partial seizures.
  B. tonic-clonic seizures.   E. complex partial seizures.
  C. petit mal seizures.

_____ 9. The phase of a seizure in which a patient experiences alternating contraction and relaxation of the muscles is the _____ phase.
   A. tonic
   B. clonic
   C. aural
   D. hypertonic
   E. postictal

_____ 10. All of the following are characteristics of a complex partial seizure EXCEPT:
   A. auditory hallucinations.
   B. a sense of deja vu.
   C. localized tonic-clonic movement of one extremity.
   D. unusual odors.
   E. strange tastes.

MATCHING

Write the two letters giving the cause and description of the abnormal breathing pattern in the space provided next to the name of the pattern.

Cause   Description

_____ _____ **11.** Cheyne-Stokes respiration

_____ _____ **12.** Central neurogenic hyperventilation

_____ _____ **13.** Kussmaul's respiration

_____ _____ **14.** ataxic respirations

_____ _____ **15.** apneustic respirations

A. rapid, deep respirations
B. brain damage due to trauma or cerebral hemorrhage and with chronic hypoxia
C. ineffective thoracic muscular coordination due to CNS damage
D. severe metabolic or CNS conditions
E. rapid, deep, noisy respirations involving hyperventilation
F. prolonged inspiration unrelieved by expiration attempts
G. brief period of apnea followed by increasing depth and frequency of respirations
H. lesion in the CNS
 I. poor respirations
J. pattern due to damage in the upper part of the pons

Write the two letters giving the major cause and characteristic of presentation in the space provided next to the type of stroke to which they apply. A letter may be used more than once.

Cause   Characteristic

_____ _____ **16.** thrombotic stroke

_____ _____ **17.** intracerebral hemorrhage

_____ _____ **18.** embolic stroke

_____ _____ **19.** subarachnoid hemorrhage

A. gradual development of signs/symptoms, often first noticed on waking during night
B. congenital blood vessel abnormalities or head trauma
C. sudden onset of severe headache
D. blood clot that forms in an area of a cerebral artery narrowed by atherosclerosis
E. rupture of a small blood vessel within brain tissue
F. lodging of a blood clot, air bubble, tumor tissue, or fat in an artery that is far from its site of origin

©2004 Pearson Education, Inc.
Intermediate Emergency Care: Principles & Practice

CHAPTER 25

Non-Traumatic Abdominal Emergencies

Review of Chapter Objectives

After reading this chapter, you should be able to:

1. **Discuss the pathophysiology of non-traumatic abdominal emergencies.** pp. 1036–1037

The most threatening non-traumatic abdominal emergency is referred to as an acute abdomen which is defined as an acute abdominal pain. Emergency surgical intervention must be considered. Common causes include: appendicitis, cholecystitis, pancreatitis, peptic ulcers, bowel obstruction, acute renal failure, chronic renal failure, kidney stones, and urinary tract infection.

- *Appendicitis* is an inflammation of the vermiform appendix and occurs in approximately 10% to 20% of the U.S. population. It is the most common surgical emergency you will encounter in the field, mostly in older children and young adults. The appendix has no known anatomic or physiologic function. It can become inflamed, and if left untreated it can rupture, spilling its contents into the peritoneal cavity and setting up peritonitis. The pathogenesis of appendicitis is most often due to obstruction of the appendiceal lumen by fecal material. This inflames the lymphoid tissue and often leads to bacterial or viral infection that ulcerates the mucosa. The inflammation also causes the appendix's internal diameter to expand, which can block the appendicular artery and cause thrombosis. With its blood supply cut off, the appendix becomes ischemic, and infarction and necrosis of tissue follows. At this point the vessel walls often weaken to the point of rupture, spilling the appendiceal contents into the peritoneal cavity.

- *Cholecystitis,* an inflammation of the gallbladder, causes gallstones and is common in 15% of the adult population in the U.S. There are two types of gallstones, cholesterol-based and bilirubin-based. Cholesterol-based stones are far more common and are associated with a specific risk profile: obese, middle-aged women with more than one biological child. Cholecystitis caused by gallstones can be chronic or acute. Gallstones can lead to acute *pancreatitis* which can lead to digestive enzymes that actually begin to digest the pancreas itself. This tissue destruction erodes to hemorrhage and intense pain in the left upper quadrant that may radiate to the back or epigastric region. The patient will appear acutely ill with diaphoresis, tachycardia, and possible hypotension if massive hemorrhaging is involved.

- *Peptic ulcers* are erosions caused by gastric acid that can occur anywhere in the GI tract. Duodenal ulcers occur in the proximal portion of the duodenum and gastric ulcers occur in the stomach. Nonsteroidal anti-inflammatory medications (aspirin, Motrin, Advil, Naprosyn), acid-stimulating products (alcohol, nicotine), or *Helicobacter pylori* bacteria are the most common causes of peptic ulcers. These irritants damage the barrier to the lining of the GI tract, exposing it to highly acidic fluid which results in the development of peptic ulcers. A blocked pancreatic duct can also contribute to duodenal ulcers. As chime passes through the pyloric sphincter from the stomach into the duodenum, the pancreas secretes an alkalotic solution laden with bicarbonate ions that neutralize the acidic hydrogen ions in the chime. If the pancreatic duct is blocked, however, the acidic chime can cause ulcerations throughout the intestine. One other cause of duodenal ulcers is Zollinger-Ellison syndrome, in which an acid-secreting tumor provokes the ulcerations.

- *Bowel obstructions* are blockages of the hollow space, or lumen, within the small and large intestines. Obstructions can be either partial or complete. An obstructed bowel segment can be catastrophic if not rapidly diagnosed and treated. Of this malady's many different causes, hernias, intersusception, volvulus, and adhesions are the four most frequent, accounting for over 70% of all reported cases. The obstruction may be chronic, as with tumor growth or adhesion progression, or its onset may be sudden and acute, as with obstruction by a foreign body. Chronic obstruction usually results in a decreased appetite, fever, malaise, nausea and vomiting, weight loss, or if rupture occurs, peritonitis. Acute onset pain may follow ingestion of a foreign body. Pain might also be due to a strangulated hernia, one that has rotated through the muscle wall of the abdomen such that blood flow is suddenly cut off and ischemia, or even infarction, of the tissue occurs.

- *Acute renal failure* is, over a period of days, a sudden drop in urine output to less than 400-500 mL per day. This condition is called oliguria. If the output is zero, the condition is called anuria. The overall mortality is roughly 50%, because the condition usually appears in significantly injured or ill persons. Normally, the kidneys receive about 20% to 25% of cardiac output. This high level of perfusion is essential to sustaining a glomerular filtration rate (GFR) sufficient to maintain blood volume and composition and to clear wastes such as urea and creatinine from the bloodstream. As GFR drops, less urine forms, and the bloodstream retains water, electrolytes, including H+ and K+. Metabolic acidosis and hyperkalemia may appear. A very significant history would be one that includes an altered level of consciousness as well as limited urine output for days and obvious development of peripheral edema.

- *Chronic renal failure* (CRF) is inadequate kidney function due to permanent loss of nephrons. Usually, at least 70% of the nephrons must be lost before significant clinical problems develop and the diagnosis is made. Metabolic instability does not occur until about 80% or more of nephrons are destroyed. When this point of dysfunction is reached, an individual is said to have developed end-stage renal failure and must have either dialysis or a kidney transplant to survive. Anuria is not necessarily present in either CRF or end-stage failure. Together, diabetes mellitus and hypertension cause more than half of all cases of end-stage renal failure. Kidney failure affects almost every organ and major function in the body.

- *Kidney stones,* or renal calculi, represent crystal aggregation in the kidney's collecting system. This condition affects about 500,000 persons a year in the U.S. Brief hospitalization is common due to the severity of pain as a stone travels from the renal pelvis, through the ureter, to the bladder, and is eliminated in urine. Stones may form in metabolic disorders such as gout or primary hyperparathyroidism, which produce excessive amounts of uric acid and calcium, respectively. More often they occur when the general balance between water conservation and dissolution of relatively insoluble substances such as mineral ions and uric acid is lost and excessive amounts of the insoluble aggregate into stones. The problem boils down to "too much insoluble stuff" and urine "too concentrated," a situation that may more likely arise with change in diet, climate, or physical activity. Stones consisting of calcium salts are by far the most common. These compounds are found in from 75% to 85% of all stones. Calcium stones are from two to three times more common in men than in women, and the average age at onset is between 20 and 30 years. Their formation frequently runs in families, and anyone who has had a calcium stone is at fairly high risk to form another within two to three years.

- *Urinary tract infection* (UTI) affects the urethra, bladder, or kidney, as well as the prostrate gland in men. They are extremely common, accounting for over 6 million office visits yearly. Almost all UTIs start with pathogenic colonization of the bladder by bacteria that enter through the urethra. Thus, females in general are at higher risk because because of their relatively short urethra. Other groups at risks for UTI are paraplegic patients or patients with nerve disruption to the bladder, including some diabetic patients. Any condition that promotes urinary stasis (incomplete urination with urine remaining in the bladder that may serve as nutrition for pathogens) places a person at higher risk. Pregnant women often have urinary stasis due to pressure from the gravid uterus. People with neurological impairment also tend to have urinary stasis, which predisposes them to infection. The use of instrumentation in patients who

©2004 Pearson Education, Inc.
Intermediate Emergency Care: Principles & Practice

require bladder catheterization places them at even higher risk of UTIs. UTIs are generally divided into those of the lower urinary tract, namely, urethritis (urethra), cystitis (bladder), and prostatitis (prostate gland), and those of the upper urinary tract, pyelonephritis (kidney).

2. Discuss the signs and symptoms of non-traumatic acute abdominal pain. pp. 1037–1050

In addition to acute abdominal pain, other signs and symptoms, such as nausea, vomiting, and/or diarrhea may be present in the patient with the acute non-traumatic abdomen. Pain is the hallmark of the acute abdominal emergency. The three main classifications of abdominal pain are: 1) Visceral, which originates in the walls of hollow organs such as the gallbladder or appendix, in the capsules of solid organs such as the kidney or liver, or in the visceral peritoneum. 2) Somatic pain is a sharp type of pain that travels along definite neural routes determined by dermatomes or tissue blocks to the spinal column. Because these routes are clearly defined, the pain can be localized to a particular region or area. Bacterial or chemical irritations of the abdomen commonly cause somatic pain such as the pain from a ruptured appendix. 3) Referred pain is not a true pain producing mechanism. As its name implies, referred pain originates in a region other than where it is felt. Many neural pathways from various organs pass through or over regions where the organ was formed during embryonic development. An example would be the appendicitis that presents with periumbilical pain or pneumonia causing pain in the lower margin of the rib cage. Specific signs and symptoms accompany each of the specific causes of non-traumatic acute abdominal pain, examples include:

- Appendicitis would have diffuse colicky pain originating in the periumbilical area and moving into the right lower quadrant as the condition worsens. This is also associated with nausea and vomiting and a low-grade fever. When the appendix actually ruptures the pain is diffuse from the peritonitis.
- Pancreatitis causes intense left upper quadrant pain that may radiate into the back or epigastric region. Most patients experience nausea followed by uncontrolled vomiting and retching that can further aggravate the hemorrhage.
- Peptic ulcer may have signs and symptoms of shock (pale, cool, clammy skin, tachycardia, alterations in level of consciousness, and hypotension). These patients often have relief of pain after eating or coating their GI tract with a liquid such as milk.
- Bowel obstruction patients have vomit that looks and smells like feces. These patients present with diffuse visceral pain, usually poorly localized to any one specific location. They may be hemodynamically unstable due to necrosis within an organ, and you may see signs and symptoms of shock (pale, cool, clammy skin, tachycardia, alterations in level of consciousness, and hypotension).
- Renal failure patients have extreme edema in all of the extremities.
- Chronic renal failure patients often show significant abnormalities on direct examination of their major organ systems. Because of the failure of vital urinary system functions, cardiovascular stress can be enormous. Either hypertension or hypotension may occur, dependent on the degree of fluid retention (detectable as either peripheral or pulmonary edema) and the level of cardiac function. Tachycardia is common with both presentations and the ECG findings may include dysrhythmias secondary to hyperkalemia. Metabolic acidosis, when present, compounds the effects of hyperkalemia. Pericarditis is also common, and a rub may be heard on chest auscultation. Neuromuscular abnormalities, in addition to impaired mentation, include muscle cramps and "restless legs syndrome," as well as muscle twitching or tonic-clonic or other forms of seizure.
- Kidney stones are generally believed to be among the most painful of human medical conditions. Typically, the patient first notes discomfort as a vague, visceral pain in one flank. Within 30 to 60 minutes it progresses to an extremely sharp pain that may remain in the flank or migrate downward and anteriorly toward the groin. Migrating pain indicates the stone has passed into the lowest third of the ureter. The physical exam will almost always reveal someone who is very uncomfortable and can find no painless position.
- Urinary tract infection patients, on physical exam, appear restless and uncomfortable. Typically, patients with pyelonephritis (which is an infectious inflammation of the renal parenchyma: nephrons, interstitial tissue, or both) appear more ill and are far more likely to

have a fever. Skin will often be pale, cool, and moist (in lower UTI) or warm and dry (in febrile upper UTI).

3. **Describe the technique for performing a comprehensive physical examination on a patient with non-traumatic abdominal pain.** pp. 1050–1052

Always start the physical examination of the patient complaining of non-traumatic abdominal pain by first assuring that the scene size-up and initial assessment has been completed and the ABCs have all been assessed and dealt with appropriately. Be sure to obtain a set of baseline vital signs before the examination. Changes in vitals along with alterations in mental status may indicate early shock due to hemorrhage or other processes. A focused assessment of the abdomen should begin with the least invasive step which is a visual inspection. This includes checking the patient appearance and positioning as well as visually inspecting the abdomen for signs of distention or discoloration. Auscultation and percussion often do not provide useful information in the field. However, if you do auscultate, be sure to do so before palpating in order to avoid perturbation in abdominal sounds. Palpation with gentle pressure should start in the least affected quadrant and move toward the area of greatest pain. Remember to immediately stop palpation if you feel any pulsation. Further palpation may cause rupture of the affected blood vessel or organ.

4. **Describe the management of the patient with non-traumatic abdominal pain.** p. 1052

Always start the physical examination of the patient complaining of non-traumatic abdominal pain by first assuring that the scene size-up and initial assessment has been completed and the ABCs have all been assessed and dealt with appropriately. General management of the patient with non-traumatic abdominal pain would include: maintaining the ABCs by providing high-flow, high-concentration oxygen, placing the patient in a position of comfort, giving psychological support, diligently managing airway to prevent aspiration since the patient may vomit, establishing IV access and providing fluid resuscitation with crystalloid as warranted if the patient appears hemodynamically unstable, and transporting to the most appropriate hospital. Monitor the patient to assure he/she remains hemodynamically stable and consult with medical direction as needed.

5. **Given several preprogrammed patients with non-traumatic abdominal pain and symptoms, provide the appropriate assessment, treatment, and transport.** pp. 1036–1052

Care of any hemorrhagic case entails close monitoring of ABCs with attention to airway (minimizing risk of aspiration of any vomitus), breathing (high-flow oxygen is often indicated), and circulation (establishment of one or two IV lines with ability for blood transfusion where appropriate, and fluid resuscitation as needed). Although there are some conditions such as Crohn's disease in which bleeding rarely leads to hypovolemic shock, you should always be prepared to treat shock. Cases that seem to represent progressive, nonhemorrhagic conditions such as appendicitis, cholecystitis, or diverticulitis should also be monitored for stability and signs of acute events such as rupture or hemorrhage. Last, be aware that GI emergencies often present in older patients with coexisting morbid conditions and monitor cardiopulmonary status and other organ function carefully. Take close note of conditions such as alcoholism, consider GI problems associated with them (such as hepatitis, pancreatitis, or esophageal varices), and adjust assessment and treatment accordingly.

CASE STUDY REVIEW

This case study demonstrates how EMT-Is react to a stressful medical emergency involving severe pain of unknown origin. In addition to noting how the team reacts to the patient's presentation and assessment, note how clues to the nephrologic origin of his condition emerge from the assessment and history.

Rachel and Jack receive a call that is nonspecific but concerning: A man has fallen and cannot get up. Jack and Rachel have almost no information before arriving at the scene. They do not know the age

©2004 Pearson Education, Inc.
Intermediate Emergency Care: Principles & Practice

of the patient, whether traumatic injury is involved, the nature of the underlying cause of the fall. In their first moments at the house they realize that they are dealing with a relatively young, apparently healthy man who is having an acute episode of severe pain and apparently is not getting up because of the pain.

Their initial actions center on historical questions about the pain and on an initial physical assessment. The patient tells them that the pain was of sudden onset and is very severe. His concerns about the possible cause of his problem give them an immediate clue: He tells them there is a family history of kidney stones, that his brother had one recently, and could he be suffering from one. At the time this information is received, a urine specimen is obtained that appears to have blood in it.

You aren't told whether there are any significant findings on physical exam, so the assumption is that the exam was largely benign. You do know that the patient's vital signs are consistent with pain and stress: a relatively high blood pressure (at least if the patient isn't chronically hypertensive), tachycardia, and brisk respirations.

The team secures IV access and starts oxygen supplementation and transports to the emergency department, where a diagnostic IVP shows complete ureteral obstruction due to an apparent radiopaque renal stone. Treatment centers on rest, gentle analgesia, and IV fluid to promote urine formation and flow. Finally, a visible stone is passed, David's pain subsides, and he can go home.

Although you aren't told about predischarge counseling, you do know that calcium-containing stones, the most common kind, tend to appear in men of approximately his age group, tend to run in families, and tend to recur in an affected individual. The patient should learn about the pathophysiology of stones and any dietary, physical, or other lifestyle modifications that might help reduce the likelihood of recurrence.

CONTENT SELF-EVALUATION

MULTIPLE CHOICE

_____ 1. Which of the following statements about non-traumatic abdominal emergencies is NOT true?
A. Non-traumatic abdominal emergencies account for about 5% of all annual visits to the emergency department.
B. The majority of non-traumatic abdominal emergencies entail GI hemorrhage.
C. The number of non-traumatic abdominal emergencies is expected to rise, in part due to aging of the population.
D. The risk factors for non-traumatic abdominal emergencies are well known, and most (such as familial predisposition to non-traumatic abdominal conditions) are out of control of the patient.
E. The number of non-traumatic abdominal emergencies is expected to rise, in part due to delays in seeking treatment by patients who treat themselves as long as symptoms allow.

_____ 2. Risk factors for non-traumatic abdominal emergencies include excessive use of alcohol and tobacco, stress, ingestion of caustic substances, and poor bowel habits.
A. True
B. False

_____ 3. All of the following statements about physical examination of the abdomen are true EXCEPT:
A. Visual inspection should always be done first.
B. Palpation should always precede auscultation.
C. Of auscultation, percussion, palpation, and visual inspection, palpation may be most likely to produce a lot of useful information.
D. Discoloration of the skin (specifically, ecchymosis) may indicate where hemorrhage has occurred into the abdominal cavity.
E. Abdominal distention may be an ominous sign, suggesting either free air in the abdomen or loss of a large amount of circulating volume.

_____ 4. Three organs intimately associated with the GI tract are the:
   A. teeth, tongue, and epiglottis.
   B. appendix, gallbladder, and parotid gland.
   C. cystic duct, the bile duct, and the common bile duct.
   D. appendix, the rectum, and the anus.
   E. liver, pancreas, and gallbladder.

_____ 5. Patients who have abdominal pain lasting more than 6 hours should always be evaluated by a physician.
   A. True
   B. False

MATCHING

Write the letter of the type of pain in the space provided next to the appropriate description of the pain.

   A. somatic   D. radiated
   B. peritonitis   E. referred
   C. visceral

_____ 6. pain originating in the walls of hollow organs that is typically produced by the processes of inflammation, distention, or ischemia

_____ 7. pain perceived in a location other than the one from which it originates

_____ 8. pain frequently characterized by the patient as sharp and well localized

_____ 9. condition caused by presence of free blood or GI contents within the abdominal cavity, which is typically perceived by the patient as somatic pain that is eased in a knee-chest position

_____ 10. pain frequently originating in the capsules of solid organs and typically perceived by the patient as sharp or tearing in character

_____ 11. pain between the shoulder blades that may be produced by a dissecting abdominal aorta

_____ 12. pain that an appendicitis patient may perceive when the inflamed appendix ruptures

_____ 13. pain that seems to the patient to move from one location to another

CHAPTER 26

*

Environmental Emergencies

Review of Chapter Objectives

After reading this chapter, you should be able to:

1. Define environmental emergency. pp. 1055–1056

An environmental emergency is a medical condition caused by or exacerbated by environmental factors such as weather, terrain, atmospheric pressure, or other local factors.

2. Identify risk factors most predisposing to environmental emergencies. pp. 1055–1056

General risk factors that place an individual at greater risk for an environmental emergency include age (very young and very old), poor general health, fatigue, predisposing medical conditions, and certain prescription or over-the-counter medications. Among drowning and near-drowning cases, alcohol use by an adult victim or the supervising adult is common.

3. Identify environmental factors that may cause illness or exacerbate a pre-existing illness or complicate treatment or transport decisions. pp. 1055–1056

Environments with certain characteristics are more likely to have emergencies: For instance, deserts may have tremendous variation in temperature between the hottest part of the day and overnight. Other such factors include current season, local weather patterns, atmospheric (high altitude) or hydrostatic (underwater) pressure, and the type of terrain. Rough or isolated terrain may significantly increase time for EMS response and for transport to the appropriate treating facility.

4. Identify normal, critically high, and critically low body temperatures. pp. 1058–1060

In the core of the body, temperature usually varies within 1° of 98.6°F (37°C). Heat exhaustion occurs at core temperatures above 100°F (37.8°C), and heatstroke can occur at 105°F (40.6°C) and higher. In contrast, mild hypothermia is associated with core temperatures of roughly 90–95°F (32–35°C). Severe hypothermia develops when core temperature drops below 90°F (32°C). The upper and lower core-body temperatures compatible with survival are roughly 114°F and 86°F, respectively.

5. Describe several methods of temperature monitoring. p. 1060

Core body temperature can be monitored with a tympanic or rectal thermometer. Peripheral body temperature, which is usually a little bit lower, can be measured with use of an oral thermometer or a thermometer placed under the armpit (an axillary temperature). Approximate peripheral temperature or change in peripheral temperature can often be discerned by touch.

Medical Emergencies

6. **Describe the body's compensatory processes for over-heating and for excess heat loss.** pp. 1056–1060, 1065

The human body does not generate "cold," it generates heat, and this process is called thermogenesis. There are three types of thermogenesis: The most basic and vital type is thermoregulatory thermogenesis, in which the nervous system and endocrine system work together to control the rate of cellular metabolism, which directly changes the rate of internal heat production. In work-induced thermogenesis, heat is produced through the work of skeletal muscles during exercise. In a cool or cold environment, muscles will produce some additional heat through shivering. The last type of heat generation is diet-induced thermogenesis, and it reflects the heat generated by cells as they process food and nutrients and eventually metabolize the breakdown products.

The body's thermal regulation is achieved through coordination of the nervous and endocrine systems. This is intuitively logical because these two systems are the control systems for all major body functions. Cells in the hypothalamus, a structure at the base of the brain, have the ability to act as a thermostat. As nerve cells, they sense the temperature of the core blood passing by them and they can receive messages from temperature sensors located in other parts of the body. Additional sensor cells for core temperature are located in the spinal cord, abdomen, and around the great veins in the chest. Peripheral sensors are in the skin and subcutaneous tissue.

On a cool day, peripheral temperature may drop. When the hypothalamic cells get the message, the cells act as endocrine cells, producing and secreting a hormone into the blood that acts to increase work-induced thermogenesis. Heat is produced through shivering. Also piloerection, or "goose bumps," the standing of small hairs, results in decreased air flow over the skin surface. If the environment is so cold that both peripheral and core temperature drop, the hypothalamic cells secrete hormones that increase heat production through all three means: thermoregulatory, work-induced, and diet-induced thermogenesis. (In the last, body cells burn fats and thus produce more heat.) In addition, core temperature, which is critical for survival, is maintained in part by reducing blood flow (and thus, heat) to the most peripheral tissues, the skin and subcutaneous tissues. In contrast, when the thermostat cells sense peripheral temperature is too high (as when you exercise vigorously), they stop releasing the hormone that stimulates thermogenesis. Not only is heat production slowed, but mechanisms to dissipate heat into the external environment are also activated. These include dilation of blood vessels in the skin and subcutaneous tissue (why people flush in the heat) and sweating.

This method of control, in which the production of a substance (in this case, heat) is turned off by the presence of that substance, is called negative feedback. Heat feeds back on the thermostat cells to turn off production of more heat. Think about the thermostat and furnace in a house. They work in a very similar fashion.

Thermogenesis consumes nutrient fuel for cells—fats, proteins, and carbohydrates—and it results in waste products such as carbon dioxide and water (from cellular respiration and fat breakdown) and urea (from protein breakdown). Extensive skeletal muscle use may also result in lactic acid accumulation. Heat dissipation through sweating consumes water, urea, and salts that are lost onto the skin surface.

7. **List the common forms of heat and cold disorders.** pp. 1060–1072

The common heat disorders are variants of hyperthermia, elevated core body temperature: In terms of increasing severity, these conditions are heat (muscle) cramps, heat exhaustion, and heatstroke. Cold disorders are frostbite, trench foot, and hypothermia.

8. **Define heat illness and hyperthermia and list the common predisposing factors and preventive measures.** pp. 1060–1061

Heat illness is increased core body temperature (CBT) due to inadequate thermolysis (heat dissipation). Hyperthermia is a state of unusually high core body temperature.

Important predisposing factors for hyperthermia include age, general health, and medications. Both the very young and the very old have less responsive heat regulating systems and can tolerate less variation in their core body temperature. Persons who have diabetes with autonomic neuropathy are at higher risk for hyperthermia because damage to the autonomic nervous system may interfere with proper messaging to the CNS about temperature and may interfere with the

©2004 Pearson Education, Inc.
Intermediate Emergency Care: Principles & Practice

heat-dissipating processes of vasodilation and sweating. Several groups of medications can affect body temperature. Diuretics predispose to dehydration, which impairs ability to sweat. Beta blockers interfere with vasodilation, impair ability to increase heart rate in response to volume loss, and may interfere with temperature messages to the CNS. Psychotropics and antihistamines interfere with thermoregulation within the CNS. Additional factors include acclimatization to local conditions, length and intensity of heat exposure, and environmental factors such as humidity and wind. Preventive measures for heat disorders include three major elements. First, maintenance of adequate fluid intake is vital, and remember that thirst alone is an inadequate indicator for dehydration. Second, you should allow yourself time for acclimatization to the hot environment, which results in more perspiration with lower salt concentration, thus conserving body-fluid volume. Last, it is important to limit exposure to hot environments.

9. Identify the signs, symptoms, and treatment for heat cramps, heat exhaustion, and heatstroke.
pp. 1061–1063

Heat cramps are caused by overexertion and dehydration in a hot environment. They occur when the temperature- and exercise-induced sweating (which consumes water and electrolytes including sodium) depletes the body of so much water and electrolytes that the actively exercising skeletal muscle fibers cramp. Signs and symptoms include cramping in fingers, arms, legs, or abdominal muscles. Patients are generally mentally alert with a feeling of weakness, but they may be dizzy or faint. Vital signs are stable, although temperature may be normal or slightly elevated. Skin is likely to be moist and warm. Note that heat cramps may be painful but they are NOT considered to be an actual heat illness. The general predisposing factors and preventive measures for all heat-related disorders are discussed with objective 8. Treatment for heat cramps is usually easily accomplished. First, remove the patient from the hot environment to a cooler one such as a shady area or an air-conditioned ambulance. For severe cramps, you can administer an oral saline solution (approximately 4 tsp salt/gallon water) or a sports electrolyte drink. Do NOT use salt tablets, which are not absorbed readily and can irritate the stomach causing ulceration or hypernatremia. If the patient cannot take liquids readily, an IV of normal saline may be needed. Palliative care may include muscle massage or moist towels over patient's head and the cramping muscles.

Heat exhaustion, which is considered a mild heat illness, is an acute reaction to heat exposure, and it is the most common heat-related illness seen by EMS providers. The loss of water and electrolytes (notably sodium) from working in a hot environment, combined with general vasodilation as a heat-dissipating mechanism, leads to a decreased circulating blood volume, venous pooling, and reduced cardiac output. The presenting symptoms are due to dehydration and sodium loss secondary to sweating. Because the symptoms are not unique to heat exhaustion, diagnosis requires presentation in the appropriate environmental setting. Remember that untreated heat exhaustion can progress to heatstroke. The signs and symptoms of heat exhaustion include increased body temperature (over 100°F, 37.8°C), cool clammy skin with heavy perspiration, rapid, shallow breathing, and a weak pulse. Signs of active thermolysis may include diarrhea and muscle cramps. The patient will feel weak and, in some cases, may lose consciousness. There also may be CNS symptoms such as headache, anxiety, paresthesia, and impaired judgment or even psychosis. The general predisposing factors and preventive measures for all heat-related disorders are discussed with objective 8. Treatment includes removal of the patient from the hot environment and placement in a supine position. For severe cramps, you can administer an oral saline solution (approximately 4 tsp salt/gallon water) or a sports electrolyte drink. Do NOT use salt tablets, as discussed above. If the patient cannot take liquids readily, an IV of normal saline may be needed. Remove some clothing and fan the patient to increase heat dissipation. Be careful not to cool the patient to the point of chilling him or her. Stop fanning if shivering develops, and consider covering the patient lightly. If shock is suspected, treat accordingly. If symptoms do not resolve, consider the possibility of increased core body temperature and evolution of heatstroke.

Heatstroke is a true environmental emergency, one in which the body's hypothalamic temperature regulation is lost and there is uncompensated hyperthermia resulting in cell death and damage to the brain, liver, and kidneys. Generally, heatstroke is characterized by body temperature above 105°F (40.6°C), CNS disturbances, and (usually) cessation of perspiration. It is thought that sweating stops either because of destruction of sweat glands or because of sensory overload resulting in their temporary dysfunction. Patients may present with signs and symptoms including cessation of sweating, hot skin that is either moist or dry (depending on whether sweat has dried), very high core temperatures, deep respirations that become shallow and rapid respirations that may later slow, a rapid, full pulse that may slow later, hypotension with low or absent diastolic reading, confusion or disorientation or unconsciousness, and possible seizures. Field management centers on immediate cooling of the patient's body and replacement of fluids. First, remove the patient from the environment; if this is not done, other measures will be only minimally useful. Initiate rapid active body cooling to a target temperature of 102°F (39°C). This can be accomplished en route to the hospital. Remove the patient's clothing and cover with sheets soaked in tepid water. If necessary, either fanning or misting may be used. Be sure you avoid overcooling because this can trigger reflex hypothermia. Tepid water avoids the risk of producing reflex peripheral vasoconstriction and shivering that can be produced by exposure to cold water. In addition, use high-flow oxygen and assist respirations if they are shallow. Use pulse oximetry if available. Administer fluid therapy orally (if possible) or IV. In many cases, orally will suffice. Remember in this setting that electrolyte replacement is not nearly as necessary as water/volume replacement. If IVs are needed, start one or two and make the initial infusion with the line(s) wide open. Be sure to monitor the ECG because dysrhythmias can develop at any time. Avoid vasopressors and anticholinergic drugs because they may inhibit sweating and can contribute to development of a hyperthermic state in high-humidity, high-temperature environments. Lastly, monitor body temperature for trends toward target temperature or for other shift. If you work in a hot climate, try to make sure your thermometers measure above 106°F and below 95°F.

10. Discuss the role of dehydration and the role of fluid therapy in heat disorders. p. 1064

Dehydration often accompanies heat disorders because it inhibits vasodilation and heat dissipation (thermolysis). Dehydration leads to orthostatic hypotension and the following symptoms: nausea, vomiting, abdominal distress, vision disturbances, decreased urine output, poor skin turgor, and signs of hypovolemic shock. These may present along with the signs and symptoms of heatstroke. When assessment suggests dehydration, rehydration is critical. IV fluids may be needed, especially when the patient has altered mental status or is nauseated. An adult with moderate to severe dehydration may require 2–3 liters of IV fluids or more.

Because dehydration plays an increasingly significant role in heat cramps, heat exhaustion, and heatstroke, rehydration becomes increasingly pivotal to treatment success. Remember in milder forms of heat disorders, such as heat cramps, that the patient's perception of thirst is a poor indication of the degree of dehydration present. Fluid, whether it is administered orally or IV, is important in restoring the body's thermolytic abilities. In heat exhaustion and heatstroke, replacement of fluid (often by IV due to patient nausea, inability to swallow, or inability to take in fluids orally fast enough to be successful) is critical. Remember that an adult with moderate to severe dehydration can require 2–3 liters or more of replacement fluid.

11. Discuss how to differentiate fever from heatstroke and treatment for fever. p. 1064

The fundamental difference is that the trigger for temperature disruption is endogenous (internal) in fever and exogenous (external) in heatstroke. In fever, the hypothalamic thermostat is actually reset to a high level by pyrogens, substances associated with infection and the body's responses to it. The thermostat resets to the normal level when pyrogens disappear from the body. In heatstroke, exposure to high ambient temperatures depletes the body of the materials necessary for compensation (such as water and electrolytes for perspiration) and then causes the hypothalamic thermoregulatory processes to be lost. The ensuing uncompensated hyperthermia, with very high core body temperatures, begins the process of organ damage (if untreated) with potential for death.

12. Define hypothermia and list its common predisposing and preventive measures. pp. 1065–1066

Hypothermia is a state of low body temperature, particularly low core body temperature. Important predisposing factors for hypothermia are the same: age, general health, and medications. Both the very young and the very old have less responsive heat generating systems to combat cold exposure and cannot tolerate cold environments. The elderly may become hypothermic in environments that are only somewhat cool to others. Persons with inadequately treated hypothyroidism have suppressed metabolisms, which prevents proper responsiveness to cold. In addition, malnutrition, hypoglycemia, Parkinson's disease, fatigue, and other medical conditions can interfere with the body's ability to combat cold exposure. Drugs that interfere with heat-generating mechanisms include narcotics, alcohol, phenothiazines, barbiturates, antiseizure medications, antihistamines and other allergy medications, antipsychotics, sedatives, antidepressants, and various analgesics such as aspirin, acetaminophen, and NSAIDs. Additional factors include prolonged or intense exposure, which directly affects both morbidity and mortality, and coexisting weather conditions (such as high humidity, brisk winds, or accompanying rain, all of which magnify the effect of cold). Preventive measures can decrease the morbidity of cold-related injury, and these include dressing warmly, being rested, which maximizes the ability of the heat-generating mechanisms to replenish energy reserves, appropriate eating at proper intervals to support metabolism, and limitation of exposure to cold environments.

13. Identify differences between mild, severe, chronic, and acute hypothermia.   **p. 1066**

Mild hypothermia is defined by a core temperature greater than 90°F (32°C) in the presence of signs/symptoms of hypothermia, whereas severe hypothermia is defined as core temperature less than 90°F in the presence of signs/symptoms of hypothermia. Acute hypothermia involves sudden exposure to a cold environment as can happen when someone falls through the ice on a frozen lake. Chronic hypothermia may occur in predisposed persons in ambient temperatures inadequately cold to produce hypothermia in a healthy, appropriately dressed individual. In the U.S., look for it among homeless persons who have endured frequent and prolonged cold stress outdoors.

14. Identify signs, symptoms, and treatment for hypothermia.   **pp. 1066–1071**

Signs and symptoms of hypothermia are given in Table 26-2 (text page 1067). Your assessment of an individual with mild hypothermia will likely reveal lethargy, shivering, lack of coordination, pale, cold, dry skin, and an early rise in blood pressure, heart rate, and respiratory rates. In severe hypothermia, you may find no shivering, loss of voluntary muscle control, hypotension, and an unpredictable pulse and respiration. On the ECG, you may find dysrhythmias. The most common presenting dysrhythmia is atrial fibrillation. With progressive cooling of the body core, a variety of dysrhythmias may appear, with eventual bradycardia or asystole. Note: The severely hypothermic patient requires assessment of pulse and respirations for at least 30 seconds every 1–2 minutes. Management includes: (1) removal of wet garments; (2) protection against further heat loss and wind chill (calling for passive external warming with blankets, moisture barriers, etc.); (3) maintenance of patient in horizontal position; (4) avoidance of rough handling, which can trigger dysrhythmias; (5) monitoring of core temperature; and (6) monitoring of cardiac rhythm. Persons with mild hypothermia may be rewarmed with active external techniques such as warmed blankets or heat packs. In contrast, active rewarming of the severely hypothermic patient is best carried out in the hospital because of the possibility of complications such as ventricular fibrillation. If transport to the hospital will require more than 15 minutes, you may need to begin active rewarming in the field. Beware of rewarming shock and cold diuresis, both of which are discussed on text pages 1068–1069. As a final aid in putting the pieces of hypothermia care together, review the algorithm on text page 1069.

15. Discuss the impact of severe hypothermia on standard BCLS and ACLS algorithms and transport considerations.   **pp. 1069, 1070–1071**

Severe hypothermia (core temperature less than 86°F or 30°C) mandates a switch from passive rewarming and some degree of active external rewarming to active internal rewarming, which may include use of warm IV fluids, warm, humid oxygen, peritoneal lavage, extracorporeal rewarming, and esophageal rewarming tubes. If pulse or breathing is absent, severe hypothermia mandates continuance of CPR but withholding of IV fluids and limitation of electrical conversion to three times maximum. There are also specific considerations for resuscitation when core temperature is 86°F or less (discussed on text pages 1069–1071). Drug metabolism in the severely

©2004 Pearson Education, Inc.
Intermediate Emergency Care: Principles & Practice

hypothermic patient is significantly decreased, and levels may accumulate that will become toxic when the patient is rewarmed. In addition, it may not be possible to electrically defibrillate a heart that is at a temperature less than 86°F.

16. Define frostbite and trench foot, and discuss the degree of frostbite and the treatment of frostbite and trench foot. pp. 1071–1072

Frostbite is an environmentally induced freezing of body tissues. As tissues freeze due to the excessive cold, ice crystals form within cells and water is drawn from cells into the extracellular space. As the ice crystals expand, cells are destroyed. Damage to blood vessels from ice-crystal formation causes loss of vascular integrity, which results in further tissue swelling and loss of distal blood flow. Peripheral tissues are more exposed to cold and thus more likely to be involved in frostbite. Thus, frostbite is largely seen in the extremities and in areas of the head and face.

Two types of frostbite are defined based on the extent of tissue freezing: superficial and deep frostbite. Superficial frostbite (also called frostnip) involves some freezing of epidermal tissue, resulting in initial redness followed by blanching and diminished sensation. Deep frostbite involves both the epidermal and subcutaneous layers; there is a white, hardened appearance. Sensation is lost. Subfreezing temperatures are necessary for frostbite (otherwise, cellular water wouldn't freeze) but are not necessary for hypothermia. You will find that many patients with frostbite also do have hypothermia. You will also find that there is tremendous variation in presentation of frostbite. Some patients will feel little pain at the outset, whereas other will complain of bitter pain. Physical exam is a better indicator of the extent of frostbite. In superficial frostbite, there will be some degree of compliance felt beneath the frozen layer upon palpation; in deep frostbite, the frozen part will be hard and noncompliant. Treatment involves the following steps. First, do not thaw the affected area if there is any possibility of refreezing and do not massage the frozen area or rub with snow. Both may result in more extensive damage. Do administer analgesia prior to thawing, and do transport to the hospital for rewarming by immersion. If transport will be delayed, thaw the frozen part in a 102–104°F water bath. Water will need to be changed frequently as it cools. Do cover the thawed part with loosely applied, dry, sterile dressings and elevate and immobilize the thawed part. Do not puncture or drain blisters, and do not rewarm frozen feet if they are required for walking out of a hazardous situation.

Trench foot, also knows as immersion foot, is similar to frostbite but occurs at temperatures above freezing and occurs when standing for prolonged periods of time in cold water. Symptoms are similar to frostbite though pain is usually present. Management includes warming, drying, elevating, and aerating the extremity.

17. Define near-drowning, list its signs and symptoms, and discuss its treatment. pp. 1072–1075

Near-drowning is defined as submersion that is survived for at least 24 hours. The pathophysiology parallels that of drowning. Following submersion, a conscious person will have complete apnea for up to three minutes as an involuntary reflex as he struggles to keep his head above water, and during this period blood is shunted to the heart and brain. During apnea, $PaCO_2$ will rise to greater than 50 mmHg while PaO_2 falls to less than 50 mmHg. The hypoxic stimulus eventually overrides the sedative effects of the hypercarbia, resulting in CNS stimulation. While conscious, the panicky victim typically swallows a lot of water into the stomach, stimulating severe laryngospasm and bronchospasm. Especially in near-drowning victims, this effect prevents significant influx of water into the lungs (and is thus termed a dry drowning or near-drowning). Another effect of laryngospasm is worsening hypoxia, which causes a deepening coma. Morbidity or delayed mortality in near-drowning is primarily due to asphyxia from airway obstruction secondary to water in the airways (if a wet event) or laryngospasm and bronchospasm (if a dry near-drowning). Water in the lungs of a near-drowning survivor may cause lower-airway disease. A number of factors affect survival, and these include the cleanliness of the water, the duration of submersion, and the age and general health of the victim. Children have a longer survival time and a greater probability of successful resuscitation. Most significant is water temperature. In general, the colder the water, the greater the chance for survival. Usually, you expect brain death after 4–6 minutes without oxygen. However, some patients in cold water (below 68°F) may be

©2004 Pearson Education, Inc.
Intermediate Emergency Care: Principles & Practice

resuscitated after 30 minutes or more in cardiac arrest. A possible physiologic factor in this phenomenon is the mammalian diving reflex. When a person dives into cold water, the submersion of the face inhibits breathing, drops heart rate, and causes vasoconstriction in tissues relatively resistant to asphyxia even as blood flow to the heart and brain continue. The colder the water, the greater the shunting of blood to brain and heart. This is the origin of the saying "the cold water drowning victim is not dead until he is warm and dead."

Field treatment for near-drownings in either saltwater or fresh water is similar: The first goal is to correct the profound hypoxia. Treatment includes the following steps: Remove the patient from the water. If possible, initiate ventilation while the victim is still in the water. Note that both steps require a trained, equipped rescue swimmer. Suspect head and neck injury if there was a fall or a dive involved; rapidly place victim on long backboard and use C-spine precautions. Then, protect from heat loss by removing wet clothing, laying the patient on a warm surface, and covering the body to the extent possible. The remaining steps are familiar to all resuscitations: Examine for airway patency, breathing, and pulse. If needed, begin CPR and defibrillation. Manage the airway as needed with suctioning and airway adjuncts. Administer 100% oxygen. Use respiratory rewarming, if available and if transport time will exceed 15 minutes. Establish an IV of lactated Ringer's or normal saline for venous access and run at 75 mL/hr. Follow ACLS protocols if the patient is normothermic. If hypothermic, the patient should be treated for hypothermia as discussed in the text. Note: Resuscitation is NOT indicated if immersion is known to have been extremely prolonged (unless hypothermia IS present) or if there is evidence of decomposition. All near-drowning victims should be admitted for observation for possible late complications including adult respiratory distress syndrome (ARDS).

18. Discuss the complications and protective role of hypothermia in the context of near-drowning. pp. 1072–1074

In general, the colder the water, the greater the patient's chance for survival. Usually, you expect brain death after 4–6 minutes without oxygen. However, some patients in cold water (below 68°F) may be resuscitated after 30 minutes or more in cardiac arrest. A possible physiologic factor in this phenomenon is the mammalian diving reflex. When a person dives into cold water, the submersion of the face inhibits breathing, drops heart rate, and causes vasoconstriction in tissues relatively resistant to asphyxia even as blood flow to the heart and brain continues. The colder the water, the greater the shunting of blood to brain and heart. This is the origin of the saying "the cold water drowning victim is not dead until he is warm and dead."

19. Discuss the pathophysiology, signs and symptoms, and management of diving emergencies. pp. 1075–1081

The underlying physiology of diving emergencies is based on dissolution of gases in water, specifically, oxygen, carbon dioxide, and other gases dissolved in a diver's blood and body tissues. Pressure increases during descent, causing more gas to dissolve. During ascent, decreasing pressure allows gases to come out of solution, and they are eliminated gradually through respiration. If ascent is too rapid, however, dissolved gases, primarily nitrogen, come out of solution and expand in volume quickly, forming bubbles in the blood, brain, spinal cord, inner ear, muscles, and joints. Scuba diving injuries are due to barotrauma (changes in pressure), pulmonary overpressure, arterial gas embolism, decompression illness, cold, panic, or a combination. Accidents generally occur at one of four phases of the dive: on the surface, during descent, at the bottom, or during ascent. Risk factors at the surface include presence of lines or kelp in which a diver can become entangled, cold water, which might induce shivering or even blackout, and boats or other large objects in the area. Barotrauma during descent is a factor in emergencies occurring during that period. If the diver cannot equilibrate the pressure between the nasopharynx and middle ear, he or she can experience severe pain, ringing in the ears, dizziness, and hearing loss, any of which can cause disorientation or panic, leading to an emergency. A similar problem of disequilibration can occur in the sinuses, producing frontal headache or pain below the eyes. Emergencies at the bottom often involve nitrogen narcosis, a state of stupor commonly called "rapture of the deep." Other emergencies occur when a diver begins to run out of oxygen and panics. Injury during ascent can involve barotrauma or decompression illness. The most serious form of barotrauma is

Medical Emergencies

pulmonary over-pressure, a condition in which expansion of air within the alveoli is greater than the tissue can handle and rupture of alveoli occur. If this occurs, the lung sustains structural damage and air entering the circulatory system can cause an arterial gas embolism. Pneumomediastinum (air in the mediastinum) and pneumothorax can also occur.

In a diving emergency, gather all evidence of air embolism and decompression illness together. Specific questions center on the timing and nature of the phases of the dive, as well as the diver's experience and state of equipment. Signs and symptoms of pulmonary over-pressure include substernal chest pain, respiratory distress, and diminished breath sounds. Treatment is the same as for pneumothorax of any other origin (see Chapter 19, "Respiratory Emergencies"). The signs and symptoms of arterial gas embolism (AGE) begin within 2–10 minutes of ascent with a rapid, dramatic onset of sharp tearing pain and other symptoms related to the specific organ system affected by lack of blood flow. The most common presentation resembles that of a stroke, with confusion, vertigo, visual disturbances, and loss of consciousness. Presentation may include hemiplegia as well as cardiopulmonary collapse. The key to diagnosis is the history of the dive. Treatment after assessment of ABCs includes use of 100% oxygen via nonrebreather mask, placement of patient in supine position, frequent monitoring of vitals, IV fluids at keep-vein-open rate, and use of a corticosteroid if ordered by medical direction. Transport to a recompression chamber as rapidly as possible under conditions that keep air pressure at that of sea level. Pneumomediastinum produces substernal chest pain, irregular pulse, abnormal heart sounds, reduced blood pressure and narrow pulse pressure, and change in voice. Cyanosis may or may not be present. Field management includes use of high-concentration oxygen via nonrebreather mask, IV with lactated Ringer's or normal saline per medical direction, and transport to an emergency department. Nitrogen narcosis causes the same concerns regarding mental and physical function as present with any other type of intoxication, with the addition of a person's functioning underwater during a dive. Altered level of consciousness and impaired judgment are key in assessment. Treatment involves return to shallow depth as this produces self-resolution.

Less frequent diving problems include oxygen toxicity due to prolonged exposure to high partial pressures of oxygen, hyperventilation, and hypercapnia due to inadequate clearance of carbon dioxide through the breathing equipment. Oxygen toxicity can lead to lung damage or even seizures. Hyperventilation due to excitement or panic may lead to muscle cramps or even decreased level of consciousness. Hypercapnia may also lead to unconsciousness. Finally, poorly prepared air tanks may be contaminated with other gases, which can increase the risk of hypoxia, narcosis, and accidental injury.

20. Discuss the pathophysiology, signs and symptoms, and management of high altitude illness. pp. 1081–1084

In contrast to diving emergencies, high altitude illnesses are due to decreased ambient pressure creating a low-oxygen environment. As barometric pressure decreases at higher altitudes, lower oxygen availability can both trigger related disorders and aggravate existing medical conditions such as angina, congestive heart failure, COPD, and hypertension. Even in very healthy individuals, rapid ascent to high altitudes without time for acclimatization can cause illness. It is difficult to predict who will be affected by altitude illness: The predictor is hypoxic ventilatory response. There are two medications that may act to prevent altitude illness: acetazolamide and nifedipine. High altitude illness begins to be manifest at approximately 8,000 ft (2,400 m) above sea level. Aspen, Colorado is located at 2,438 m, and it has 26% less oxygen per volume of air than at sea level. The range considered high altitude is 4,900–11,500 ft. Here, the hypoxic environment causes decreased exercise tolerance, although without major disruption of normal oxygen transport in the blood. The range for very high altitude is 11,500–18,000 ft, and this causes extreme hypoxia during exercise or sleep. Extreme altitude (greater than 18,000 ft) will cause severe illness in virtually everyone. Some signs and symptoms of altitude illness include malaise, anorexia, headache, sleep disturbance, and respiratory distress that worsens with exertion. Specific disorders include acute mountain sickness, high altitude pulmonary edema, and high altitude cerebral edema.

Acute mountain sickness (AMS) usually manifests in an unacclimatized person who ascends rapidly to an altitude of 2,000 m (6,600 ft) or higher. Signs and symptoms include lightheadedness, breathlessness, weakness, headache, and nausea and vomiting. More serious signs can

©2004 Pearson Education, Inc.
Intermediate Emergency Care: Principles & Practice

develop, especially if the person continues to ascend: weakness to the point of requiring assistance to dress and eat, severe vomiting, decreased urine output, shortness of breath, and altered level of consciousness. Mild AMS is self-limiting and often improves in 1–2 days if no further ascent occurs. Treatment for AMS consists of halting ascent or possibly lowering altitude, use of acetazolamide and anti-nauseants as needed. Supplemental oxygen will relieve symptoms but is typically used only in severe cases. Definitive treatment for all high altitude illnesses is descent.

High altitude pulmonary edema (HAPE) results from increased pulmonary pressure and hypertension caused by changed blood flow in higher altitude. Children are most susceptible, and men are more susceptible than women. Initial symptoms include dry cough, mild shortness of breath on exertion, and slight crackles in the lungs. Symptoms of progression include severe dyspnea and cyanosis, coughing productive of frothy sputum, and weakness that may progress to coma and death. In its early stages, HAPE is completely reversed by descent and use of oxygen. If immediate descent isn't possible, oxygen can completely reverse HAPE but requires 36–72 hours to do so. Such a supply is rarely available to mountain climbers. An alternative is a portable hyperbaric bag, the use of which simulates a descent of roughly 5,000 ft. Acetazolamide may decrease symptoms. Other medications such as morphine, nifedipine, and furosemide may be useful but carry risk for complications such as hypotension and dehydration.

The exact cause of high altitude cerebral edema (HACE) is unknown. It usually presents as deteriorating neurological status in a patient with AMS or HAPE. The increased fluid in the brain tissue causes increased intracranial pressure. Symptoms include altered mental status, ataxia, decreased level of consciousness, and coma. If descent isn't possible, oxygen and steroids and a hyperbaric bag may help. If coma develops, it may persist for days after descent to sea level, but it usually resolves, although it may leave residual disability.

21. Discuss the pathophysiology, signs and symptoms, and management of radiation injuries.
pp. 1084–1088

Ionizing radiation cannot be seen, felt, or heard. It may cause alterations in the body's cells, primarily it's genetic material (DNA). This cell damage is cumulative over a lifetime and may result in a decrease in white blood cells, defects in offspring, damage to to the bone marrow, and an increased incidence of cancer. As indicated earlier, there are no signs of ionizing radiation exposure (unless the exposure is extremely great).

Management for the patient exposed to radiation is directed at reducing the risk to you, your patient, and fellow rescuers. Maintain a safe distance upwind from the site and assure victims are properly decontaminated, then brought to you for care of other injuries. Care for those injuries as you would any other patient.

22. Given several preprogrammed simulated environmental emergency patients, provide the appropriate assessment, management, and transportation.
pp. 1056–1088

Attention to the ABCs is always important, and this doesn't change with environmental emergencies. The need to move the patient from the harmful environment to one conducive to recovery is special, although not unique (as with inhalation toxicological emergencies). Among the heat disorders, heatstroke is the most serious, and rapid transport is always required.

Hypothermia always requires transport to a hospital setting. The urgency in rewarming varies with the degree of hypothermia, as do some potential complications on rewarming such as cardiac dysrhythmias. Superficial and deep frostbite differ in the depth of tissue affected by freezing; care while en route to the hospital is similar. Early recognition is important to the EMS provider, but prevention is the most important of all steps.

Near-drownings require immediate care and rapid transport to the hospital. Although more than 90% of near-drowning patients survive without sequelae, ARDS can occur as a potentially deadly late complication. Emergencies related to air pressure (diving and altitude) can vary in severity and setting, but immediate care and removal to an appropriate environment as soon as possible are key to treatment. Again, these emergencies are better prevented than treated. Knowing what resources are available in the area is important to treating any of these types of emergencies.

CASE STUDY REVIEW

This case study demonstrates how EMT-Is react to a relatively common wintertime emergency: a patient with apparent hypothermia. The case study demonstrates how assessment findings reveal diagnosis, and, as presentation changes, how diagnosis and treatment change as well. The case study also demonstrates how contraindications to certain management steps appear at different stages of hypothermia.

The EMS team is en route to work on a winter day described as "bitterly cold" when they hear a priority call for an unconscious man found lying in snow. As they respond, they do not know any particulars regarding age, possible medical conditions, or even how long the man has been exposed to the snow and cold air.

They find a young man who is huddled and shivering on ice-covered ground. Breathing is shallow and irregular; the approximate number of respirations per minute is not given. The man is conscious, and, although confused, gives a brief, plausible history. He had been out celebrating and passed out. (The case study does not state whether the man admitted to use of alcohol or other drugs during the celebration, substances that may increase vulnerability to hypothermia.) The patient adds he may have been exposed to the elements for a "couple of hours." Important assessment findings include bradycardia, mild hypotension, and a core temperature of 86°F.

At this point, the assessment contains a few elements suggesting mild hypothermia and others pointing to severe hypothermia. Findings consistent with mild hypothermia include the presence of shivering, detectable although irregular respirations, and a level of consciousness sufficient to give a brief history. In contrast, there are also more ominous signs of severe hypothermia: bradycardia and hypotension. The core temperature of 86°F defines the case as severe hypothermia (core temp. less than 90°F).

The team knows that the man has severe hypothermia, and they know they must act quickly as they can expect his condition to continue to deteriorate, perhaps precipitously, as long as he is in the cold environment. Indeed, before they can intervene, the patient's presentation does decline: Shivering stops and speech becomes unintelligible.

The partners quickly move the man into the warm ambulance, remove his wet clothing, apply cardiac and core temperature monitors, and then begin active external rewarming with water bottles at the head, neck, chest, and groin. (The study does not note if the patient was covered with blankets or other insulating material, but you can assume that he was because the other initial actions taken by the team comply with management guidelines.) During this period core temperature does continue to drop, to 85°F. Findings from the cardiac monitor are not given but presumably are stable, as no action is taken against dysrhythmia.

The temperature drop below 86°F signals a new level of urgency. At this temperature, active internal rewarming is mandated with measures such as warm IV fluid, warm humid oxygen, as well as the possible steps of peritoneal lavage, extracorporeal rewarming, and esophageal rewarming tubes. In the prehospital setting, the measures most likely to be available are the warm IV fluid and warm, humid oxygen. The team also knows that they have reached a critical temperature in terms of cardiac instability: Dysrhythmias or asystole are now very real possibilities, and, indeed, the rough handling associated with road construction triggers ventricular fibrillation. Cardioversion is unsuccessful (an expected finding as hearts are generally considered to be incapable of response to defibrillation at temperatures below 86°F).

The providers respond with traditional support for the ABCs: intubation, ventilation with warmed oxygen, and chest compressions. The team makes another correct decision for treatment at this low temperature: They refrain from giving medications via the IV because they know drug metabolism is significantly decreased at this low core body temperature. The drugs may not be useful in the short term and may accumulate to a toxic level once the body core is rewarmed.

At the emergency department, more resources are available to rewarm the patient, and, after core temperature comes rises over 86°F, the usual ACLS protocols are used to stabilize the patient, who eventually recovers fully.

CONTENT SELF-EVALUATION

MULTIPLE CHOICE

_____ 1. General risk factors that predispose a person to developing an environmental illness include all of the following EXCEPT:
   A. predisposing medical conditions such as diabetes.
   B. fatigue.
   C. high levels of fluid intake.
   D. use of certain over-the-counter or prescription medications.
   E. age: either very young or old persons.

_____ 2. Homeostasis is the body's ability to maintain a steady, normal internal environment in the face of changing external conditions.
   A. True
   B. False

_____ 3. Which process is NOT one that results in body heat loss into the environment?
   A. evaporation
   B. convection
   C. respiration
   D. radiation
   E. diffusion

_____ 4. Which group of medications does NOT predispose a person to hyperthermia?
   A. psychotropics
   B. antiepileptics
   C. diuretics
   D. beta blockers
   E. antihistamines

_____ 5. Thirst is an adequate indicator of dehydration.
   A. True
   B. False

_____ 6. Dehydration is often intimately associated with heat disorders because it inhibits peripheral vasodilation and limits sweating.
   A. True
   B. False

_____ 7. In situations where it is unclear whether the diagnosis is fever or heatstroke, always treat for both conditions.
   A. True
   B. False

_____ 8. Medical conditions that may predispose to hypothermia include all of the following EXCEPT:
   A. hypothyroidism.
   B. malnutrition.
   C. Parkinson's disease.
   D. thin body build.
   E. hypoglycemia.

_____ 9. Rewarming is not the mirror image of the cooling process.
   A. True
   B. False

_____ 10. Which is NOT appropriate as a rewarming measure for mild to moderate hypothermia?
   A. warmed blankets
   B. warmed IV fluids
   C. peritoneal lavage
   D. heat packs
   E. heat lamp

_____ 11. Management guidelines for frostbite include all of the following negatives EXCEPT:
   A. Do not thaw affected area if possibility of refreezing exists.
   B. Do not massage the frozen area or rub with snow.
   C. Do not puncture or drain any blisters.
   D. Do not warm frozen feet if patient will need to walk out of hostile environment.
   E. Do not give analgesia prior to thawing.

Medical Emergencies

_____ 12. The physiology of fresh-water and saltwater drownings differs, and these differences contribute to differences in prognosis and field management.
A. True
B. False

_____ 13. Resuscitation of a drowning victim is not indicated when:
A. respirations have ceased.
B. cardiac asystole exists.
C. the patient has been pulled from freezing water and is very cold himself.
D. immersion is known to have been extremely long.
E. head or neck injury due to trauma is evident.

_____ 14. Which gas law is most applicable to decompression illness?
A. Boyle's law
B. Dalton's law
C. Henry's law
D. Ohm's law
E. Venturi's law

_____ 15. Which of the following might be administered IV to a near-drowning patient?
A. plasmanate
B. dextran
C. lactated Ringer's
D. D_5W
E. hetastarch

_____ 16. One of the most severe complications of near-downing is:
A. "the squeeze."
B. ARDS.
C. DAN.
D. barotrauma.
E. pneumomediastinum.

_____ 17. The condition whose chief signs and symptoms include altered levels of consciousness and impaired judgment is:
A. AGE.
B. "the squeeze."
C. "the bends."
D. pneumomediastinum.
E. nitrogen narcosis.

_____ 18. The condition whose signs and symptoms include substernal chest pain, irregular pulse, abnormal heart sounds, reduced blood pressure and narrow pulse pressure, and a change in voice is:
A. AGE.
B. "the squeeze."
C. "the bends."
D. pneumomediastinum.
E. nitrogen narcosis.

_____ 19. The condition whose signs and symptoms include altered mental status, ataxia, decreased level of consciousness, and coma is:
A. AGE.
B. DAN.
C. HACE.
D. HAPE.
E. AMS.

_____ 20. The unit of local tissue energy deposition in cases of radiation exposure is the:
A. Geiger.
B. RAD.
C. QF.
D. gamma.
E. radioisotope.

©2004 Pearson Education, Inc.
Intermediate Emergency Care: Principles & Practice

MATCHING

Write the letter of the clinical characteristics in the space provided next to the appropriate disorder.

_____ 21. heat exhaustion

_____ 22. deep frostbite

_____ 23. high altitude cerebral edema

_____ 24. severe hypothermia

_____ 25. acute mountain sickness (early phase)

_____ 26. pulmonary over-pressure

_____ 27. nitrogen narcosis

_____ 28. mild hypothermia

_____ 39. decompression illness

_____ 30. high altitude pulmonary edema

A. moderately decreased core temperature, shivering, lethargy, early rise in heart and respiratory rates

B. dry cough and dyspnea progressing to cough productive of frothy sputum and severe dyspnea

C. severe pain and CNS disturbances that develop during a rapid ascent from a dive to depth below 40 feet

D. environmentally induced freezing of skin and subcutaneous tissues with hardness on palpation, no sensation

E. altered mental status and decreasing level of consciousness, ataxia

F. substernal chest pain that develops during ascent, often from shallow depths, associated with respiratory distress and diminished breath sounds

G. lightheadedness, shortness of breath, nausea after rapid ascent to altitude of 6,600 feet or more

H. stuporous state that develops during deep dives rather than during descent or ascent

I. somewhat increased core temperature, rapid, shallow respirations, weak pulses

J. severely decreased core temperature, no shivering, hypotension, dysrhythmias, undetectable pulse and respirations

CHAPTER 27
✳
Behavioral Emergencies

Review of Chapter Objectives

After reading this chapter, you should be able to:

1. **Distinguish between normal and abnormal behavior.**　　　　　　**p. 1090**

   Behavior is a person's observable conduct and activity, while a behavioral emergency is a situation in which a patient's behavior becomes so unusual, bizarre, or threatening that it alarms the patient or another person and requires the intervention of EMS and/or mental health personnel. The differentiation between "normal" and "abnormal" behavior is largely subjective and widely variable based on culture, ethnic group, socioeconomic class, environment, and personal interpretation and opinion.

2. **Discuss the pathophysiology of behavioral and psychiatric disorders.**　　**pp. 1091–1092**

   The general causes of behavioral and psychiatric disorders are biological (organic), psychosocial, and sociocultural. Biological (organic) causes are related to disease processes or structural changes in the brain. Psychosocial causes are related to the patient's personality, dynamics of unresolved conflict, or crisis management methods. Sociocultural causes are related to the patient's actions and interactions within society. It should be noted that many psychiatric disorders are due to altered brain chemistry.

3. **Describe the medical legal considerations for management of emotionally disturbed patients.**　　　　　　**p. 1107**

   The laws of consent specify that any competent person has the right to refuse to consent to treatment. Further, no competent person may be transported against his/her will. Any person who is in imminent danger of harming him-/herself or others is not considered competent to refuse treatment and transport. Most states have laws that allow persons fitting this criterion to be transported against their will to a hospital or approved psychiatric facility for evaluation.

4. **Describe the overt behaviors associated with behavioral and psychiatric disorders.**　　　　　　**pp. 1095–1105**

   Overt behaviors that may be associated with behavioral emergencies include hand gestures (clenched fists, wringing hands, etc.) or postures (cowering, visible tension, etc.) that you may observe in your patient. The patient may display strange or threatening facial expressions. The patient's speech may reveal disorientation, fixations, unrealistic judgments, or unusual thought processes. Other behaviors you may observe include pacing, picking at one's skin, or appearing to pull things from the air. There are many different kinds of such overt behaviors, and they can differ or overlap depending on the specific disorder.

©2004 Pearson Education, Inc.
Intermediate Emergency Care: Principles & Practice

5. List the appropriate measures to ensure the safety of the EMT-Intermediate, the patient, and others. pp. 1092–1094, 1107–1110

As with any call, determining scene safety is critical. Many behavioral emergencies, for which you are dispatched, will also warrant mutual response by law enforcement personnel. Gain control of the scene. Remove anyone who agitates the patient or adds confusion to the scene. Examine the environment for signs of violence and potential weapons. Approach every situation cautiously and when feasible observe the patient from a distance first before approaching. Avoid invading the patient's personal space. Watch for signs of aggression. If a patient becomes violent, use of restraint may become necessary; in such cases, carefully follow your service's protocols for such circumstances and be sure to document your actions thoroughly.

6. Describe the circumstances when relatives, bystanders, and others should be removed from the scene. p. 1093

It is important to gain control of the scene as quickly as possible. Remove anyone who agitates the patient or adds to the confusion on the scene. Generally, it is a good idea to limit the number of people around the patient. You may even find it necessary to totally clear the room or to move the patient to a quiet area.

7. Describe techniques to systematically gather information from the disturbed patient. pp. 1093–1094, 1106–1107

Your interpersonal skills are crucial to your success as an EMS professional but never more so than when you are caring for a patient who is having a behavioral emergency. Limit environmental distractions at the scene. Introduce yourself and note how the patient responds to you, altering your approach if the patient becomes agitated. Establish eye contact. Place yourself at the patient's level. Listen carefully. Take your time. Do not physically threaten the patient. Ask open-ended questions. Be truthful with the patient and never play along with hallucinations or delusions. Focus your questioning and assessment on the immediate problem.

8. Identify techniques for physical assessment in a patient with behavioral problems. pp. 1093–1094

All of the interpersonal skills discussed above that allow you to effectively interview patients will need to be incorporated into your physical assessment activities. Generally, the examination of a behavioral emergency patient is largely conversational. If you need to perform hands-on assessment activities, defer their completion until you have had the opportunity to establish rapport and, even then, do not make any sudden moves that may startle the patient. If a patient is restrained, be sure to monitor him or her frequently and carefully to ensure that the airway is patent and that he or she is not experiencing positional asphyxia.

9. List situations in which you are expected to transport a patient forcibly and against his will. p. 1107

Any person who is in imminent danger of harming him-/herself or others is not considered competent to refuse treatment and transport. Patients who are suicidal or homicidal meet this criterion. Most states have laws that allow persons fitting this criterion to be transported against their will for evaluation. The authority to make this decision varies from state to state. Other situations are not so clear-cut and require you to use clinical judgment and follow your service's protocols.

10. Describe restraint methods necessary in managing the emotionally disturbed patient. pp. 1107–1110

The primary objective is to restrict the patient's movement to prevent him from harming himself or others. Your own agency's rules will dictate the appropriate technique and method for restraint. The following rules always apply: use minimum necessary force; use appropriate devices; remember that restraint is not punitive; and carefully monitor anyone who is restrained.

Medical Emergencies

Before initiating any restraint activities, make sure that you have sufficient help, as this minimizes the potential for injury to the patient or yourself.

11. List the risk factors and behaviors that indicate a patient is at risk for suicide. pp. 1103–1104

All of the following are considered to be risk factors for suicide: previously attempted suicide, depression, age (15 to 24 years of age or over 40), substance abuse, social isolation, major separation trauma, major physical stresses, loss of independence, suicide of a parent. Also significant is having possession of a mechanism for suicide and having a specific plan and/or expressing it.

12. Given several preprogrammed behavioral emergency patients, provide the appropriate scene size-up, initial assessment, focused assessment, and detailed assessment, then provide the appropriate care and patient transport. pp. 1090–1110

Throughout your training, you will encounter a variety of real and simulated patients with behavioral or psychiatric emergencies. Use the information in the text, as well as the application of this information as demonstrated by your instructors, preceptors, and mentors to enhance your ability to assess, manage, and transport patients with behavioral emergencies. Every emergency call has an element of behavioral emergency in it; your patience and professionalism will help minimize the emotional component for everyone involved.

CASE STUDY REVIEW

This case study draws attention to the assessment and management of a commonly encountered patient presentation, in which an individual is exhibiting bizarre behavior in a public setting.

The EMT-Is arrive on-scene and obtain information about the situation from the store manager who has placed the 911 call. When the patient notices their arrival and becomes more agitated, they retreat to the ambulance and request assistance from law enforcement personnel.

As is often the case, the police officers recognize the patient from previous interactions with him. Before approaching the patient, the EMT-Is and police officers coordinate their plans and anticipate the potential need for restraint. Using a team approach to subdue and restrain the patient minimizes the risk of injury for all involved. Once the patient is safely restrained, a thorough assessment is performed to rule out possible medical or traumatic causes for the patient's altered mental status and agitation. En route to the hospital the patient is carefully monitored to insure his well-being.

CONTENT SELF-EVALUATION

MULTIPLE CHOICE

_____ 1. Organic causes for behavioral emergencies include all of the following EXCEPT:
  A. tumor.
  B. depression.
  C. substance abuse.
  D. infection.
  E. hypoglycemia.

_____ 2. It is always safe to assume that a patient exhibiting bizarre behavior is suffering from a psychological problem or disease.
  A. True
  B. False

_____ 3. The term that describes the state of a patient's cerebral functioning is:
  A. affect.
  B. mood.
  C. mental status.
  D. orientation.
  E. sensorium.

©2004 Pearson Education, Inc.
Intermediate Emergency Care: Principles & Practice

_____ 4. The best approach for gaining information from a behavioral emergency patient is to:
   A. ask questions requiring yes or no answers.
   B. talk loudly to establish control.
   C. ask open-ended questions.
   D. physically restrain the patient before questioning.
   E. move quickly to expedite transport and then question.

_____ 5. The structured exam designed to quickly evaluate a patient's level of mental functioning is the:
   A. neurologic exam.
   B. mental status exam.
   C. psychiatric evaluation.
   D. Glasgow Coma Score.
   E. stroke assessment scale.

_____ 6. The most likely way to provoke violence or aggression in a behavioral emergency patient is to:
   A. listen carefully to his responses.
   B. appear patient and unhurried.
   C. ask open-ended questions.
   D. invade his personal space.
   E. avoid rapid or sudden movements.

_____ 7. Panic attack, phobias, and posttraumatic stress syndrome are classified as:
   A. types of schizophrenia.
   B. personality disorders.
   C. variants of depression.
   D. bipolar disorders.
   E. anxiety disorders.

_____ 8. The most prevalent form of psychiatric problem is:
   A. schizophrenia.
   B. personality disorder.
   C. depression.
   D. bipolar disorder.
   E. anxiety disorder.

_____ 9. Profound sadness, diminished ability to concentrate, and feelings of worthlessness are commonly associated with:
   A. schizophrenia.
   B. personality disorders.
   C. depression.
   D. bipolar disorders.
   E. anxiety disorders.

_____ 10. Medications commonly used in the management of schizophrenia are:
   A. antipsychotics.
   B. sedatives.
   C. antihistamines.
   D. antipsychotics and sedatives.
   E. sedatives and antihistamines.

_____ 11. Common causes of dementia include all of the following EXCEPT:
   A. Alzheimer's disease.
   B. head trauma.
   C. cardiac seizure.
   D. Parkinson's disease.
   E. AIDS.

_____ 12. Hallucinations, delusions, and disorganized thought, speech, and behavior are commonly associated with:
   A. schizophrenia.
   B. personality disorders.
   C. depression.
   D. bipolar disorders.
   E. anxiety disorders.

_____ 13. The compelling desire to use a substance, inability to reduce use of a substance, and repeated unsuccessful efforts to quit using that substance are indicators of:
   A. psychological dependence.
   B. physical dependence.
   C. substance tolerance.
   D. factitious disorder.
   E. somatoform disorder.

_____ 14. The primary objective in patient restraint is to:
   A. initiate punitive response.
   B. stop dangerous behaviors.
   C. limit patient strength.
   D. reduce legal liability.
   E. encourage patient cooperation.

Medical Emergencies

_____ **15.** When a EMT-I or geriatric patient is experiencing a behavioral emergency, the paramedic should always consider using chemical restraints.
   A. True
   B. False

MATCHING

Write the letter of the word or phrase in the space provided next to its definition.

A.	delirium	**F.**	catatonia
B.	dementia	**G.**	paranoid
C.	schizophrenia	**H.**	bipolar disorder
D.	delusions	**I.**	personality disorder
E.	hallucinations	**J.**	depersonalization

_____ **16.** Feeling detached from oneself

_____ **17.** Condition characterized by relatively rapid onset of widespread disorganized thought

_____ **18.** Fixed false beliefs

_____ **19.** Condition that results in persistently maladaptive behavior

_____ **20.** Sensory perceptions with no basis in reality

_____ **21.** Condition characterized by one or more manic episodes, with or without subsequent or alternating periods of depression

_____ **22.** Condition characterized by immobility, rigidity, and stupor

_____ **23.** Common disorder involving significant behavioral changes and disorganized thought

_____ **24.** Preoccupation with feelings of persecution

_____ **25.** Condition involving gradual development of memory impairment and cognitive disturbance

CHAPTER 28

*

Gynecological Emergencies

Review of Chapter Objectives

After reading this chapter, you should be able to:

1. **Review the anatomic structures and physiology of the female reproductive system.** (see Chapter 2)

   The most important female reproductive structures are located within the pelvic cavity. Essential to reproduction, these structures include the ovaries, fallopian tubes, uterus, and vagina. The external genitalia have accessory functions, in that they protect body openings and play an important role in sexual functioning.

2. **Describe how to assess a patient with a gynecological complaint.** pp. 1113–1115

   The most common gynecological complaints are abdominal pain and vaginal bleeding. Complete your initial assessment in the usual manner and then proceed with a focused history and physical exam. Specific questions will need to be asked that are pertinent to reproductive function and dysfunction. If pertinent, be sure to gather information about her obstetrical history, including pregnancies and deliveries. It is important to document the date of the patient's last menstrual period (LMP). You should also ask what form of birth control, if any, she uses and, if pertinent, whether she uses it regularly. Pay particular attention to the physical exam, which will be limited to assessment of the abdomen and potentially (in the presence of serious bleeding) inspection of the patient's perineum. Gently auscultate and palpate the abdomen. Be sure to note the color, character, and volume of any blood lost. An internal vaginal exam should never be performed in the prehospital setting.

3. **Explain how to recognize a gynecological emergency.** pp. 1113–1115

   As with any emergency situation, vital signs are useful clues as to your patient's status as well as its severity. Be alert for early signs of shock or a positive tilt test, both of which point to significant blood loss. If possible, estimate blood loss. The use of two sanitary pads per hour is considered significant bleeding.

4. **Describe the general care for any patient experiencing a gynecological emergency.** p. 1115

   Management of gynecological emergencies is focused on supportive care. Rely on your initial assessment guidance in your decision making about oxygen therapy, ventilatory support, and vascular access. In the presence of shock, follow your local protocols for fluid resuscitation and use of the PASG. In cases of heavy bleeding, do not pack dressings in the vagina. Continue to monitor the patient's status and bleeding en route to definitive care. Equally important is the psychological support that you give your patient. Protect her modesty and privacy.

5. **Describe the pathophysiology, assessment, and management of the following gynecological emergencies.**

a. Pelvic inflammatory disease pp. 1115–1116

Pelvic inflammatory disease (PID), the most common cause of nontraumatic abdominal pain in women in the childbearing years, is an infection of the female reproductive tract that is most commonly caused by gonorrhea or chlamydia. Predisposing factors include: multiple sexual partners, prior history of PID, recent gynecological procedure, or an IUD. The patient will look acutely ill and will often present with diffuse lower abdominal pain, and may also have fever, chills, nausea, vomiting, and possibly a foul-smelling vaginal discharge. The patient may also walk with a shuffling gait due to pain. Blood pressure may be normal, and fever may or may not be present. Palpation of the lower abdomen usually elicits moderate to severe pain. The primary management in the field is supportive care and a position of comfort during transport. If the patient appears septic, then administer oxygen and initiate IV therapy.

b. Ruptured ovarian cyst p. 1116

Cysts are fluid-filled pockets, and, when they develop in the ovary, they can rupture and be a source of abdominal pain. The rupture spills a small amount of blood into the abdomen, irritating the peritoneum and causing abdominal pain and rebound tenderness. Usually the patient complains of moderate to severe unilateral abdominal pain that may radiate to the back; it may be associated with vaginal bleeding. The patient may also report pain during intercourse or a delayed menstrual period. The primary management in the field is supportive care and a position of comfort during transport.

c. Cystitis p. 1116

A bacterial infection of the urinary bladder (cystitis) is a common cause of abdominal pain that may be accompanied by urinary frequency, dysuria, and a low-grade fever. The pain is generally located just above the symphysis pubis unless the infection has spread to the kidneys, in which case there is likely to be flank pain as well. The primary management in the field is supportive care and a position of comfort during transport.

d. Ectopic pregnancy p. 1117

Ectopic pregnancy is the implantation of a fetus outside of the uterus, most commonly in the fallopian tubes. Patients usually report severe unilateral abdominal pain that may radiate to the shoulder on the affected side, a late or missed menstrual period, and sometimes vaginal bleeding. As the fetus develops, the tube can rupture, triggering a massive, life-threatening hemorrhage. Absorb the bleeding but do not pack the vagina. Ectopic pregnancy is a surgical emergency, and the primary management in the field is supportive care and a position of comfort during transport, as well as oxygen administration and IV therapy for fluid resuscitation.

e. Vaginal hemorrhage pp. 1117–1118

Nontraumatic vaginal hemorrhage is rarely encountered in the prehospital setting unless it is severe. Do not presume that such bleeding is due to normal menstrual flow. Most commonly, it is due to a spontaneous abortion (miscarriage) and is associated with cramping abdominal pain and the passage of clots and tissue. Other possible causes include cancerous lesions, PID, or the onset of labor. Absorb bleeding but do not pack the vagina. The primary management in the field is supportive care and a position of comfort for the patient, as well as oxygen administration and IV therapy for fluid resuscitation. If the bleeding is due to miscarriage, this will likely be a significant emotional event for your patient, so your kind and considerate care is important.

Traumatic vaginal bleeding may result from sexual assault, blunt-force injuries to the lower abdomen, seat-belt injuries, objects inserted into the vagina, self-attempts at abortion, and lacerations following childbirth. Bleeding in such cases should be managed by direct pressure over a laceration or a cold pack applied to a hematoma. Never pack the vagina. Provide expedited transport to the hospital, with oxygen administration and IV access as necessary.

©2004 Pearson Education, Inc.
Intermediate Emergency Care: Principles & Practice

6. **Describe the assessment, care, and emotional support of the sexual assault patient.**   pp. 1118–1120

Sexual assault victims are unique patients with unique needs. The psychological care of these patients is as important, if not more so, than the physical care they may need. Confine your questions to the physical injuries that the patient may have received. Unless your patient is unconscious, do not touch the patient, even to take vital signs, without her permission. Explain what's going to be done before initiating any treatment. Avoid touching the patient other than to take vital signs or to examine other physical injuries. Do not examine the external genitalia of the sexual assault victim unless there is life-threatening hemorrhage. Consider the patient to be a crime scene and protect that scene; handle clothing as little as possible, collect all bloody articles as potential evidence, do not allow the patient to change clothes or bathe and do not clean wounds if possible. Be sure to document the treatment of the sexual assault victim carefully, thoroughly, and objectively.

7. **Given several preprogrammed gynecological patients, provide the appropriate assessment, management and transportation.**   pp. 1113–1120

Throughout your classroom, clinical, and field training, you will encounter a variety of real and simulated gynecologic patients. Use the information provided in this chapter of your text, as well as the application of this information as demonstrated by your instructors, preceptors, and mentors to enhance your ability to assess, manage, and transport these patients. Keep in mind that gynecological emergencies are likely to be a very stressful situations for your patients, and they will appreciate your gentle, considerate care and professionalism.

CASE STUDY REVIEW

This case study draws attention to the assessment and management of a sexual assault patient in the prehospital setting. Sexual assault continues to represent the most rapidly growing violent crime in the United States, so it is likely that you will encounter these patients in the course of your career.

In this scenario, the EMT-Is meet their patient in the care of the park police officer that found her. Stephanie has been allowed to cover herself and afforded privacy prior to the arrival of the EMT-Is. Being mindful of the psychological aspects of her care, the EMT-I explains every necessary procedure and asks her permission before any action is initiated. Recognizing the need to preserve potential evidence, the EMT-I keeps the blanket around Stephanie. The initial and rapid trauma assessments revealed no significant injuries or immediate life threats. The EMT-I consistently gave control to Stephanie and reassured her that she was safe now. She was transported to the hospital for evaluation by the Sexual Assault Nurse Examiner.

CONTENT SELF-EVALUATION

MULTIPLE CHOICE

_____ 1. Painful discomfort during menstrual periods is known as:
   A. menarche.
   B. dyspareunia.
   C. cystitis.
   D. dysmenorrhea.
   E. pelvic inflammatory disease.

_____ 2. The term used to describe the number of times a woman has been pregnant is parity.
   A. True
   B. False

3. Which of the following questions is LEAST likely to get an accurate response from a female who is complaining of abdominal pain?
   A. Are you currently menstruating?
   B. Are you sexually active?
   C. Could you be pregnant?
   D. Have you ever experienced this pain before when menstruating?
   E. Have you experienced dizziness?

4. The term used to describe the number of deliveries a woman has had is:
   A. gravida.   D. parita.
   B. gravity.   E. completa.
   C. parity.

5. A palpable abdominal mass found midway between the symphysis pubis and the umbilicus in the lower abdomen of a 25-year-old woman is most likely to be a(n):
   A. tumor.
   B. intrauterine pregnancy of 5 months gestation.
   C. intrauterine pregnancy of 4 months gestation.
   D. intrauterine pregnancy of 3 months gestation.
   E. ovarian cyst.

6. Pelvic inflammatory disease is most often caused by:
   A. gonorrhea and chlamydia.   D. chlamydia and streptococcus.
   B. streptococcus and staphylococcus.   E. HIV and staphylococcus.
   C. gonorrhea and HIV.

7. Mid-cycle abdominal pain associated with ovulation is known as:
   A. endometriosis.   D. cystitis.
   B. PID.   E. mittelschmerz.
   C. a miscarriage.

8. The most effective means to control vaginal hemorrhage is to apply direct pressure to the perineum.
   A. True
   B. False

9. All of the following signs and symptoms are associated with endometritis EXCEPT:
   A. history of gynecologic procedure.   D. bradycardia.
   B. severe abdominal pain.   E. bloody, foul-smelling discharge.
   C. fever.

10. All of the following signs and symptoms are associated with a ruptured ovarian cyst EXCEPT:
   A. dyspareunia.   D. delayed menstrual period.
   B. severe abdominal pain.   E. irregular bleeding.
   C. fever.

11. If a female patient presents with severe unilateral abdominal pain that radiates to the shoulder on one side, a missed menstrual period, and vaginal bleeding, you should suspect:
   A. mittelschmerz.   D. endometriosis.
   B. ectopic pregnancy.   E. cystitis.
   C. PID.

©2004 Pearson Education, Inc.
Intermediate Emergency Care: Principles & Practice

_____ 12. A female reports that during intercourse she felt a sudden and sharp tearing sensation. She is now bleeding from the external genitalia, although the bleeding is minimal. Management should include:
A. asking the woman to hold a dressing over the area and apply direct pressure.
B. establishing an IV and beginning fluid resuscitation regardless of blood loss.
C. packing the vagina with sterile dressings.
D. palpating the interior of the vagina to determine the extent of bleeding.
E. securing a hot pack over the vaginal opening with tape.

_____ 13. The prehospital priorities for care of the sexual assault victim include all of the following EXCEPT:
A. examining for perineal tears.
B. determining if life-threatening injuries exist.
C. providing emotional support.
D. preserving evidence.
E. protecting patient's privacy.

_____ 14. The BEST management for a victim of a sexual assault is:
A. aggressive questioning and internal examination.
B. discouraging the patient from dressing since this may taint evidence.
C. examining the genitalia.
D. psychological and emotional support.
E. prompt summoning of law enforcement officials.

LABEL THE DIAGRAM

In the spaces provided write the names of the organs of the female reproductive system marked A through E on the diagram below.

A. _____

B. _____

C. _____

D. _____

E. _____

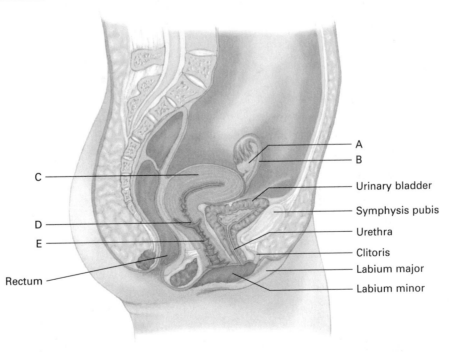

Medical Emergencies

SPECIAL PROJECT

Problem Solving—Abdominal Pain

You are dispatched for "woman with abdominal pain." Your patient is a 26-year-old female who looks acutely ill and complains of severe abdominal pain.

1. Given this information, what would you attempt to determine when gathering a focused history?

   _____

   _____

   _____

   _____

   _____

Having obtained the history, you perform a physical exam. Your findings include the following:

- tachypnea
- tachycardia
- pale, cool, diaphoretic skin
- narrowed pulse pressure
- vaginal bleeding or discharge
- abdominal exam: masses, distention, guarding, localized tenderness, rebound

2. Based on this information, provide a differential diagnosis for this patient.

   _____

   _____

   _____

©2004 Pearson Education, Inc.
Intermediate Emergency Care: Principles & Practice

Intermediate Emergency Care: Principles & Practice

Division 5
Special Considerations

CHAPTER 29

✳

Obstetrical Emergencies

Review of Chapter Objectives

After reading this chapter, you should be able to:

1. Describe the anatomic structures and physiology of the reproductive system during pregnancy. pp. 1122–1126

The primary "organ of pregnancy" is the placenta, which arises from the site on the uterine wall where the blastocyst (fertilized egg) implants itself. This temporary, blood-rich structure serves as a lifeline for the developing fetus via the umbilical cord. Its functions include the transfer of heat while exchanging oxygen and carbon dioxide, delivering nutrients, and removing waste. The placenta also serves as an endocrine gland throughout the pregnancy, secreting hormones necessary for fetal survival as well as the estrogen and progesterone required to maintain the pregnancy. The placenta is also a protective barrier against harmful substances that might cross the placental barrier to the fetus.

    The fetus develops within the amniotic sac, a thin-walled membranous covering containing amniotic fluid that surrounds and protects the fetus during intrauterine life.

2. Identify the normal events of pregnancy. p. 1126

Fetal development begins at the moment of conception (fertilization). Normally, the duration of pregnancy is 40 weeks after the date of the mother's last menstrual period or 280 days. This is comparable to 10 lunar months or 9 calendar months. This time period is divided into trimesters, each of 3 calendar months duration.

    Implantation of the fertilized egg into the uterine wall occurs during the pre-embryonic stage that lasts approximately 14 days. The embryonic stage begins at day 15 and ends at approximately 8 weeks, by which time all of the body systems have been formed. It is midway through this stage that the fetal heart begins to beat. The period from 8 weeks gestation until delivery is known as the fetal stage. The gender of the infant can usually be determined by 16 weeks, and by the 20th week, fetal heart tones are audible by stethoscope. The mother usually feels fetal movement (quickening) by the 24th week. By the 38th week, the baby is considered to be full term.

3. Describe how to assess an obstetrical patient. pp. 1128–1130

The initial assessment for an obstetric patient is the same as for any other patient. Utilization of the SAMPLE history will allow you to obtain specific information about the pregnancy. Ask about gravidity, parity, length of gestation, and EDC (estimated date of confinement or due date). You should also obtain information about past OB/GYN history (e.g., C-section) or complications as well as prenatal care. Determine current medications and any drug allergies as well. It is important to obtain the past medical history because pregnancy may aggravate pre-existing medical problems or trigger new ones such as gestational diabetes. It is possible to estimate the due date by measuring fundal height above the symphysis pubis. Continue the physical exam, which is essentially the same for any patient, while being mindful of the need for modesty and privacy.

4. Identify the stages of labor and the EMT-Intermediate's role in each stage. pp. 1140–1141

Labor is the physiologic and mechanical process by which the baby, placenta, and amniotic sac are expelled through the birth canal. The three stages of labor are dilatation, expulsion, and placental. The first stage (dilatation stage) begins with the onset of true labor and ends with the complete dilatation and effacement of the cervix. The second stage (expulsion stage) begins with the complete dilatation of the cervix and ends with the delivery of the baby. The third and final stage of labor (placental stage) begins immediately after the birth of the baby and ends with the delivery of the placenta. The role of the EMT-I during labor is to assist in the delivery and to recognize and treat life-threatening problems for the mother or baby.

5. Differentiate between normal and abnormal delivery. pp. 1147–1151

Normally, most infants present from the birth canal in a headfirst, face-down position (vertex presentation), which allows the infant to be delivered vaginally. Abnormal delivery situations generally preclude vaginal delivery and are likely to require caesarean section, so transport must be expedited. These situations include breech presentation (buttocks present first), prolapsed cord (umbilical cord protrudes from the birth canal), limb presentation (baby's arm or leg protrudes from the birth canal) or occiput posterior presentation (baby's brow is facing forward).

6. Identify and describe complications associated with pregnancy and delivery. pp. 1131–1140, 1147–1153

Medical complications of pregnancy include ectopic pregnancy, bleeding problems, supine hypotensive syndrome, gestational diabetes, and hypertensive disorders. Ectopic pregnancy refers to the implantation of the fertilized egg outside of the uterus. Abdominal pain and evidence of intra-abdominal and/or vaginal bleeding usually herald this event. Bleeding is generally differentiated as painful or painless. Vaginal bleeding, accompanied by cramping abdominal pain, prior to the 20th week of gestation is almost always associated with a spontaneous abortion. Painless bleeding is most commonly associated with *placenta previa* where, due to abnormal implantation of the placenta on the uterine wall, labor is accompanied by bleeding. Painful bleeding is the hallmark of *abruptio placenta* or the premature separation of the placenta from the uterine wall. It poses an immediate life threat to mother and child.

Supine hypotensive syndrome occurs most commonly in the third trimester as a result of compression of the inferior vena cava by the gravid uterus. Insulin resistance and decreased glucose tolerance characterize gestational diabetes, occurring in the last 20 weeks of pregnancy. Hypertensive disorders of pregnancy (formerly called toxemia) include preeclampsia or eclampsia and chronic and transient hypertension. Major motor seizures are the hallmark of eclampsia, which is the most serious of the hypertensive disorders, posing a life threat to the mother and child.

Some of complications associated with delivery are discussed in objective 5. Other problems can occur after delivery. One of these is postpartum hemorrhage, which is the loss of 500 cc or more of blood immediately following delivery. A common cause of the condition is lack of uterine muscle tone, and it occurs most frequently in the multigravida, with multiple births, and with the births of large infants. Uterine rupture is another complication of delivery. It can result from blunt abdominal trauma, prolonged uterine contractions, or a surgically scarred uterus. Uterine rupture presents with a patient in excruciating abdominal pain and often in shock. Uterine inversion occurs when the uterus turns inside out after delivery and extends through the cervix. Blood loss from 800 to 1,800 cc occurs, and the patient often experiences profound shock. Pulmonary embolism can also occur after pregnancy as a result of venous thromboembolism. It often presents with sudden dyspnea accompanied by sharp chest pain and a sense of impending doom.

7. Identify predelivery emergencies. pp. 1131–1140

Recognition of a predelivery emergency is based on information obtained from the focused history and physical exam that relates to the reported abnormality, such as pain, discomfort, or bleeding. While any of the complications listed above has potential to be an emergency, the most likely are *abruptio placenta* and eclampsia, both of which pose potential life threats to mother and child and require prompt and appropriate intervention.

8. State indications of an imminent delivery.   p. 1141

Increasing frequency and duration of contractions and the sensation of needing to move one's bowels (urge to push) are all signs of impending delivery. However, crowning is the definitive sign that birth is imminent.

9. Differentiate the management of a patient with predelivery emergencies from a normal delivery.   pp. 1131–1140

Management of predelivery emergencies requires that the EMT-I correctly recognize their presence based on information obtained from the focused history and physical exam and then expedite transport while anticipating the development of shock and maintaining adequate oxygenation, fluid resuscitation as necessary, and, if appropriate, pharmacological intervention. Most of the time, the mother will be transported in the left lateral recumbent position.

10. State the steps in the predelivery preparation of the mother.   pp. 1141, 1144

The first priority is to provide the mother with privacy. Then, time permitting, administer oxygen via a nasal cannula and establish vascular access. Position the mother on her back with knees and hips flexed and buttocks slightly elevated, or the mother may prefer squatting or to be in a semi-Fowler position with knees and hips flexed. Drape the mother's perineum to minimize contamination of the infant during delivery.

Normally, preparation for childbirth in the prehospital setting would entail thoroughly washing hands and forearms before donning a gown, in addition to sterile gloves and goggles. Body substance isolation for childbirth generally includes draping the mother to minimize contamination of the baby during delivery.

11. State the steps to assist in the delivery of a newborn, including cutting the umbilical cord and delivery of placenta.   pp. 1141–1145

Key EMS actions during a routine (normal) delivery are primarily supportive, but you should remain vigilant to signs of impending problems. Providing gentle support to the perineum as the delivery progresses decreases the likelihood of an explosive delivery causing vaginal tears and the potential for neonatal head trauma. While supporting the head, gently slide your finger along the head and neck to ensure that the cord is not wrapped around the baby's head and neck. As the head emerges from the vaginal opening, suction the airway (mouth first, then nose) to insure that the airway is clear prior to the neonate taking his first breath. It may be necessary to tear the amniotic sac to release the amniotic fluid and permit the baby to breathe.

Gently guide the baby's head downward to allow delivery of the upper shoulder. Do not pull! Then gently guide the baby's body upward to allow delivery of the lower shoulder. Once the shoulders are delivered, the rest of the body will be quickly delivered. Keep the baby at the level of the mother's hips until the cord has been clamped and cut. Once the body has fully emerged from the birth canal, the baby should again be suctioned until the airway is clear. After clamping the umbilical cord at 10 cm and 15 cm from the baby and cutting in between, carefully dry the baby and wrap in a warming blanket to prevent hypothermia.

Once the baby's body has been delivered, suction the airway until clear while keeping the baby at the level of the mother's hips until the cord has been clamped and cut. Do not "milk" the cord. Supporting the baby's body, place the first umbilical clamp approximately 10 cm from the baby and the second clamp at 15 cm and carefully cut in between.

Following delivery of the baby, the vaginal opening will continue to ooze blood. Do not pull on the umbilical cord! Eventually, the cord will appear to lengthen indicating separation of the placenta from the uterine wall. Once the placenta is expelled through the vaginal opening, it should be placed in a biohazard bag and be transported to the hospital for examination.

©2004 Pearson Education, Inc.
Intermediate Emergency Care: Principles & Practice

12. **Describe how to care for the newborn, including routine care and neonatal resuscitation.** pp. 1145–1147

The essential emergency care of the newborn includes the establishment and maintenance of adequate airway and breathing status and the prevention of heat loss. Support the infant's head and torso, using both hands. Maintain warmth, repeat suctioning of the mouth and nose as needed until the airway is clear, and then assess using the APGAR score. Do not delay resuscitation or transport to perform APGAR scoring.

If the infant's respirations are below 30 per minute and tactile stimulation does not increase the rate to a normal range (30–60), immediately assist ventilations using a pediatric bag-valve mask with high-flow oxygen. If the heart rate is below 80 and does not increase in response to ventilations, initiate chest compressions. Transport to a facility with neonatal intensive care capabilities.

13. **Describe the management of the mother post-delivery.** pp. 1151–1153

The mother should receive fundal massage to control postpartum bleeding and the perineum should be inspected for tears. Continuously monitor vital signs. If not accomplished prior to delivery, vascular access should be established should fluid resuscitation become necessary.

14. **Describe the procedures for handling abnormal deliveries, complications of pregnancy, and maternal complications of labor.** pp. 1131–1140, 1147–1153

Management of abnormal deliveries or complications of pregnancy and labor require that the EMT-I correctly recognize the problem and expedite transport while anticipating the development of shock and maintaining adequate oxygenation, fluid resuscitation as necessary and, if appropriate, pharmacological intervention. Most of the time, the mother will be transported in the left lateral recumbent position. When the baby's position (breech presentation, prolapsed cord, or limb presentation) dictates, the mother should be placed on oxygen and then assisted in assuming the knee-chest position. Additionally, in the management of prolapsed cord, two gloved fingers should be placed inside the vagina to prevent the baby's weight from compressing the cord and inhibiting oxygen delivery to the baby.

15. **Describe special considerations when meconium is present in amniotic fluid or during delivery.** p. 1151

The presence of meconium (fetal fecal matter) in the amniotic fluid is indicative of a fetal hypoxic incident. The thicker and darker the color of the meconium staining in the amniotic fluid, the higher the risk of fetal morbidity. Once the head has emerged from the birth canal, suction the mouth and nose thoroughly while still on the perineum. However, if the meconium is thick, visualize the glottis and use an endotracheal tube to suction the hypopharynx and trachea until clear. Failure to suction will cause the meconium to be pushed further down the trachea and into the lungs.

16. **Describe special considerations of a premature baby.** pp. 1139–1140

Premature infants are ill suited for extrauterine life, particularly with regard to their pulmonary function. All of the concerns about caring for a neonate are exaggerated when the neonate is less than 38 weeks gestation. Of greatest concern are airway maintenance, ventilatory support, and oxygen delivery. These critically ill neonates should be taken immediately to a facility with neonatal intensive care capabilities.

17. **Given several simulated delivery situations, provide the appropriate assessment, management, and transport for the mother and child.** pp. 1122–1153

Throughout your training, you will encounter a variety of real and simulated obstetric patients. Use the information provided in this chapter, as well as the application of this information as demonstrated by your instructors, preceptors, and mentors to enhance your ability to assess, manage, and transport these patients. Keep in mind that this is likely to be a stressful situation for your patient, and she will appreciate your kind, considerate care and professionalism.

©2004 Pearson Education, Inc.
Intermediate Emergency Care: Principles & Practice

CASE STUDY REVIEW

This case study draws attention to the management of childbirth in the prehospital setting. In most cases, the role of the EMS provider in a childbirth situation is merely supportive, as often no "emergency" care is needed.

As is often the case, a great deal of information about the imminence of delivery can be obtained prior to physically examining the patient. This patient reveals that she has had six pregnancies, a good indicator that this delivery may proceed very quickly. The urge to move the bowels is a sign that the cervix is fully effaced and the child is moving down the birth canal. Lastly, when exam of the perineum displays crowning this indicates that the cervix is fully dilated and that delivery is imminent.

Normally, preparation for delivery would entail thoroughly washing hands and forearms before donning a gown, in addition to the gloves and goggles that were used by the EMTs. Body substance isolation for childbirth generally includes draping the patient to minimize contamination of the baby during delivery. In this situation, there is no time to open the OB kit or provide for the mother's privacy.

Key EMS actions during a routine delivery are primarily supportive, but you should remain vigilant to signs of impending problems. Providing gentle support to the perineum as the delivery progresses decreases the likelihood of an explosive delivery causing vaginal tears and the potential for neonatal head trauma. As the head emerges from the vaginal opening, the EMT suctions the airway to insure that the airway is clear prior to the neonate taking her first breath. The EMT-Is arrive in time to assist the EMT in cutting the cord, after placing clamps at 10 cm and 15 cm from the baby and cutting in between, and then drying and wrapping the baby in a warming blanket to prevent hypothermia. The mother receives fundal massage to control postpartum bleeding. Vascular access is established should fluid resuscitation become necessary. The baby is assessed and APGAR scores are identified en route to the hospital.

Childbirth is one "emergency" which almost always has a positive outcome. It is common for EMS agencies to celebrate and acknowledge such calls. Rest assured that this delivery is one the EMT will remember for the balance of his career, even without a stork painted on his window.

CONTENT SELF-EVALUATION

MULTIPLE CHOICE

_____ 1. Thickening of the uterine lining in anticipation of implantation of the fertilized egg is stimulated by:
A. estrogen.
B. progesterone.
C. follicle-stimulating hormone.
D. luteinizing hormone.
E. oxytocin.

_____ 2. All of the following are placental functions EXCEPT:
A. acting as the "organ of pregnancy."
B. production of hormones.
C. serving as a protective barrier.
D. providing fertilization.
E. providing a means of heat transfer.

_____ 3. The normal duration of pregnancy is:
A. 40 weeks.
B. 280 days.
C. 10 lunar months.
D. 9 calendar months.
E. all of the above

_____ 4. Blood volume increases by what percentage during pregnancy?
A. 10%
B. 25%
C. 30%
D. 45%
E. 60%

_____ 5. The fetus receives its blood from the placenta by means of the:
A. umbilical vein.
B. umbilical artery.
C. inferior vena cava.
D. superior vena cava.
E. aorta.

_____ 6. Fetal circulation changes to normal circulation with the:
A. onset of labor.
B. expulsion from the birth canal.
C. baby's first breath.
D. clamping of the umbilical cord.
E. dilation and effacement of the cervix.

_____ 7. When performing a focused history on a pregnant patient, which of the following questions would be appropriate?
A. Are you experiencing any pain or discomfort?
B. Have you had any vaginal discharge or bleeding?
C. When is your due date?
D. Have you ever been pregnant before?
E. all of the above

_____ 8. All of the following are common signs or symptoms of a predelivery emergency EXCEPT:
A. abdominal pain or trauma.
B. vaginal bleeding or discharge.
C. painful deformed extremities.
D. altered mental status or seizures.
E. hypertension or hypotension.

_____ 9. All of the following are causes of bleeding during pregnancy EXCEPT:
A. abortion.
B. ovarian cyst.
C. ectopic pregnancy.
D. placenta previa.
E. abruptio placenta.

_____ 10. Treatment of a female patient who is 16 weeks pregnant, is complaining of cramping abdominal pain, and has bright red vaginal bleeding should include all of the following EXCEPT:
A. packing the vagina to control bleeding.
B. treating for shock if indicated.
C. maintaining oxygenation.
D. providing emotional support.
E. saving any tissue and clots for evaluation.

_____ 11. You suspect the patient in the situation described in question 10 is having a(n):
A. abortion.
B. ovarian cyst.
C. ectopic pregnancy.
D. placenta previa.
E. abruptio placenta.

_____ 12. Pelvic inflammatory disease, endometriosis, and tubal ligation are predisposing factors for:
A. abortion.
B. ovarian cyst.
C. ectopic pregnancy.
D. placenta previa.
E. abruptio placenta.

_____ 13. You find that your patient is 36 weeks pregnant, has an altered mental status, and is reported to have had a major motor seizure, which you suspect is due to:
A. placenta previa.
B. eclampsia.
C. epilepsy.
D. abruptio placenta.
E. supine hypotensive syndrome.

_____ 14. Care of the patient in question 13 should include all of the following EXCEPT:
A. administering high-flow oxygen via a nonrebreather mask.
B. protecting the patient from injury if seizures recur.
C. minimizing noise and light to prevent seizure activity.
D. administering magnesium sulfate per protocol.
E. transporting on right side to protect airway.

_____ 15. All of the following are signs and symptoms of an imminent delivery EXCEPT:
A. the presence of crowning.
B. contractions occurring every 1–2 minutes.
C. passage of "bloody show."
D. sensation of an urge for bowel movement.
E. rupture of membranes.

_____ 16. The stage of labor that begins with complete cervical dilatation and ends with the delivery of the fetus is called the dilatation stage.
A. True
B. False

_____ 17. Your patient has just delivered a healthy baby boy. Following the delivery of the placenta, her vaginal bleeding seems to increase. Which of the following best describes what you should do provide emergency care for this patient?
A. Massage the uterus and position your patient on her right side.
B. Administer oxygen and firmly massage the uterus.
C. Massage the uterus and pack the vagina to control bleeding
D. Administer oxygen and pack the vagina with sanitary napkins.
E. Provide fluid resuscitation and position patient on her right side.

_____ 18. Meconium-stained amniotic fluid should first be managed by:
A. immediate transport to the hospital for physician evaluation.
B. administration of oxygen to the mother to resolve fetal distress.
C. suctioning of the mouth and nose before the infant takes his first breath.
D. stimulation of the infant to encourage coughing to clear meconium from airway.
E. expediting completion of delivery to decrease fetal distress.

_____ 19. Management of a limb presentation should include all of the following EXCEPT:
A. administration of high-flow oxygen to the mother.
B. immediate transport to the hospital.
C. attempting to push the limb back into the vagina.
D. positioning the mother with her head down and pelvis elevated.
E. providing reassurance to the mother.

_____ 20. The administration of an IV fluid bolus to control premature labor is based on increasing intravascular volume and thus causing inhibition of:
A. antidiuretic hormone.   D. luteinizing hormone.
B. progesterone.   E. follicle-stimulating hormone.
C. estrogen.

_____ 21. Elements of the APGAR assessment include appearance, pulse, grimace, activity and respirations.
A. True
B. False

_____ 22. Acrocyanosis in the neonate is always a sign of inadequate oxygenation.
A. True
B. False

_____ 23. You have just assisted with the delivery of a baby girl. She has shallow, gasping respirations and a heart rate that is less than 100 beats per minute. Which of the following best describes your emergency care for this patient?
A. administering "blow by" oxygen and monitoring her pulse for 60 seconds
B. assisting ventilations with a BVM and reassessing in 30 seconds
C. administering high-flow, high-concentration oxygen with a nonrebreather mask
D. assisting ventilations with a BVM and beginning chest compressions
E. continuing to monitor and expedite transport

_____ 24. Shoulder dystocia is commonly associated with diabetic or obese mothers and:

    A. prematurity.   D. hormonal deficits.

    B. hormonal excesses.   E. fetal distress.

    C. post-term pregnancy.

_____ 25. If the uterus protrudes from the vaginal opening following the delivery of the placenta, you should:

    A. wrap it tightly in dry towels.

    B. wrap it in dextrose-soaked dressings.

    C. make no more than 3 attempts to replace it.

    D. make no more than 1 attempt to replace it.

    E. cover it with plastic wrap.

MATCHING

Write the letter of the definition in the space provided next to the term it describes.

_____ 26. amniotic sac   _____ 31. effacement

_____ 27. ovulation   _____ 32. Braxton-Hicks contractions

_____ 28. fetus   _____ 33. parity

_____ 29. placenta   _____ 34. tocolysis

_____ 30. umbilical cord   _____ 35. puerperium

  A. unborn infant from the third month of pregnancy to birth

  B. fetal lifeline, a placental extension through which the child is nourished

  C. organ of pregnancy for the exchange of oxygen and waste products

  D. transparent membrane forming the sac which holds the fetus

  E. release of an egg from the ovary

  F. the time period surrounding the birth of the fetus

  G. thinning and shortening of the cervix during labor

  H. number of pregnancies carried to term

  I. process of stopping labor

  J. painless, irregular uterine contractions

©2004 Pearson Education, Inc.
Intermediate Emergency Care: Principles & Practice

CHAPTER 30
✳
Neonatal Resuscitation

Review of Chapter Objectives

After reading this chapter, you should be able to:

1. Define newborn and neonate.   p. 1155

A newborn is a baby in the first few hours of its life, also called a *newly born infant*. A neonate is a baby less than one month old.

2. Identify important antepartum factors that can affect childbirth and high-risk newborns.   p. 1156

Antepartum factors are those that occur before the onset of labor. Examples of important antepartum factors that can adversely affect childbirth include multiple gestation, inadequate prenatal care, a mother who is younger than 16 years of age or older than 35, a history of perinatal morbidity or mortality, post-term gestation, drugs or medications, and a mother with a history of toxemia, hypertension, or diabetes.

Intrapartum factors are those that occur during childbirth. Examples of intrapartum factors that can help determine high-risk newborn patients include a mother with premature labor, meconium-stained amniotic fluid, rupture of membranes more than 24 hours prior to delivery, use of narcotics within four hours of delivery, an abnormal presentation, prolonged labor or precipitous delivery, and a prolapsed cord or bleeding.

3. Identify the primary signs utilized for evaluating a newborn during resuscitation.   p. 1158

The newborn should be assessed immediately after birth. The primary signs used for evaluating a newborn during resuscitation include respiratory rate, heart rate, and skin color. The newborn's respiratory rate should average 40–60 breaths per minute. The normal heart rate is between 150 and 180 beats per minute at birth, slowing to 130–140 beats per minute thereafter. A pulse less than 100 beats per minute indicates distress and requires emergency intervention. Some cyanosis of the extremities is common immediately after birth. However, if the newborn is cyanotic in the central part of the body or if peripheral cyanosis persists, the newborn must be treated with 100% oxygen.

4. Identify the appropriate use of the APGAR scale and calculate the APGAR score given various newborn situations.   pp. 1158–1159; see also Chapter 29

The APGAR scale—designed for use at 1 and 5 minutes after birth—helps distinguish between newborns who need only routine care and those who need greater assistance. The system also predicts long-term survival. A severely distressed newborn (one with an APGAR score of less than 4) requires immediate resuscitation.

To calculate the APGAR score, a value of 0, 1, or 2 is given for each of the following categories: pulse rate (heart rate), grimace (irritability), activity (muscle tone), and respiratory rate.

Special Considerations

5. **Formulate an appropriate treatment plan for providing initial care to a newborn.**　　p. 1159

Treatment of the newborn begins by preparing the environment and assembling the equipment needed for delivery and immediate care of the newborn. The initial care of the newborn follows the same priorities as for all patients. Complete the initial assessment first. Correct any problems detected in the initial assessment before proceeding to the next step. The majority of term newborns require no resuscitation beyond suctioning of the airway, mild stimulation, and maintenance of body temperature by drying and warming with blankets.

6. **Discuss the initial steps in resuscitation of a newborn.**　　pp. 1162–1170

Resuscitation of the newborn follows an inverted pyramid. In chronological order, initial steps include drying, warming, positioning, suctioning, and tactical stimulation; administration of supplemental oxygen; bag-valve ventilation; and chest compressions. If these steps fail, advanced measures include intubation and administration of medications.

7. **Describe the indications, equipment needed, application, and evaluation of the following management techniques for the newborn in distress:**

  a. **Blow-by oxygen**　　pp. 1167–1168

  Blow-by oxygen—the process of blowing oxygen across a newborn's face—is applied if central cyanosis is present or if the adequacy of ventilations is uncertain. If possible, the oxygen should be warmed and humidified.

  b. **Ventilatory assistance**　　p. 1168

  Positive-pressure ventilation should be applied to a newborn if any of the following conditions exist: heart rate less than 100 beats per minute, apnea, or persistence of central cyanosis after administration of supplemental oxygen. A bag-valve-mask unit is the device of choice. A self-inflating bag of appropriate size should be used (450 mL is optimal). If prolonged ventilation is required, it may be necessary to disable the pop-off valve.

  c. **Chest compressions**　　pp. 1168–1169

  Chest compressions should be applied to newborns with heart rates of less than 60 beats per minute or with heart rates between 60 and 80 beats per minute *that do not increase* with 30 seconds of positive-pressure ventilation and supplemental oxygen. Begin chest compressions by encircling the newborn's chest, placing both thumbs on the lower one-third of the sternum. Compress the sternum 1.5 to 2.0 cm (1/2 to 3/4 inch) at a rate of 120 times per minute. Maintain a ratio of 3 compressions to 1 ventilation. Reassess the newborn after 20 cycles of compressions (1-minute intervals). Discontinue compressions if the spontaneous heart rate exceeds 80 beats per minute.

8. **Discuss appropriate transport guidelines for a newborn.**　　p. 1172

EMT-I are frequently called upon to transport a high-risk newborn from a facility where stabilization has occurred to a neonatal intensive care unit. During transport you will help maintain the newborn's body temperature, control oxygen administration, and maintain ventilatory support. Often, a transport isolette with its own heat, light, and oxygen source is available. If a self-contained isolette is not available for transport, you might wrap the newborn in several blankets, keep the infant's head covered, and place hot-water bottles containing water heated to no more than 40°C (104°F) near, but not touching, the newborn. DO NOT use chemical packs to keep the newborn warm.

9. **Describe the epidemiology, including the incidence, morbidity/mortality, risk factors and prevention strategies, pathophysiology, assessment findings, and management for the following neonatal problems:**

  a. **Meconium aspiration**　　pp. 1159, 1164–1165, 1172–1173

  Meconium-stained amniotic fluid occurs in approximately 10–15 percent of deliveries, mostly in post-term or small-for-gestational-age newborns. Meconium aspiration accounts for a significant proportion of neonatal deaths. Fetal distress and hypoxia can cause meconium to be

©2004 Pearson Education, Inc.
Intermediate Emergency Care: Principles & Practice

passed into the amniotic fluid. Either *in utero* or more often with the first breath, thick meconium is aspirated into the lungs, resulting in small airway obstruction and aspiration pneumonia. The infant may have respiratory distress within the first hours, or even the first minutes, of life as evidenced by tachypnea, retraction, grunting, and cyanosis in severely affected newborns. The partial obstruction of some airways may lead to a pneumothorax.

An infant born through thin meconium may not require treatment, but depressed infants born through thick, particulate (pea-soup) meconium-stained fluid should be intubated immediately, prior to the first ventilation. Before stimulating such infants to breathe, apply suction with a meconium aspirator attached to an endotracheal tube. Connect to suction at 100 cc/H$_2$O or less to remove meconium from the airway. Withdraw the ET tube as suction is applied. It may be necessary to repeat this procedure to clear the airway. The patient should then be taken to a facility that can manage a high-risk neonate.

b. Bradycardia pp. 1174–1175

Bradycardia is most commonly caused by hypoxia in newborns. However, the bradycardia may also be due to several other factors, including increased intracranial pressure, hypothyroidism, or acidosis. In cases of hypoxia, the infant experiences minimal risk if the hypoxia is corrected quickly. In providing treatment, follow the procedures in the inverted pyramid. Resist the inclination to treat the bradycardia with pharmacological measures alone. Keep the newborn warm and transport to the nearest facility.

c. Respiratory distress/cyanosis p. 1176

Prematurity is the single most common factor causing respiratory distress and cyanosis in the newborn. The problem occurs most frequently in infants less than 1,200 grams (2 pounds, 10 ounces) and 30 weeks of gestation. Premature infants have an immature central respiratory control center and are easily affected by environmental or metabolic changes. There are many factors contributing to respiratory distress, including lung or heart disease, central nervous system disorders, meconium aspiration, metabolic problems, obstruction of the nasal passages, shock and sepsis, and diaphragmatic hernia. Expect the following assessment findings: tachypnea, paradoxical breathing, intercostal retractions, nasal flaring, and expiratory grunt.

In providing treatment, follow the inverted pyramid, paying particular attention to airway and ventilation. Suction as needed and provide a high concentration of oxygen. If prolonged ventilation will be required, consider placing an ET tube. Perform chest compressions, if indicated. Consider dextrose (D$_{10}$W or D$_{25}$W) if the newborn is hypoglycemic. Maintain body temperature and transport to the most appropriate facility.

d. Hypothermia p. 1178

Hypothermia presents a common and life-threatening condition for newborns. The increased surface-to-volume relationship in newborns makes them extremely sensitive to environmental temperatures, especially right after delivery when they are wet. In treating hypothermia—a body temperature below 35°C (95°F)—try to control the loss of heat through evaporation, conduction, convection, and radiation. Also remember that hypothermia can be an indicator of sepsis in the newborn. Regardless of the cause, the increase in the metabolic demands can produce a variety of related conditions including metabolic acidosis, pulmonary hypertension, and hypoxemia.

In assessing hypothermic newborns, remember that they do not shiver. Instead, expect the following findings: pale color, skin cool to the touch (especially in the extremities), acrocyanosis, respiratory distress, possible apnea, bradycardia, central cyanosis, initial irritability, and lethargy in later stages. Management focuses on ensuring adequate ventilations and oxygenation. Chest compressions may be necessary with bradycardia.

e. Cardiac arrest p. 1181

The incidence of neonatal cardiac arrest is related primarily to hypoxia. The condition can be caused by primary or secondary apnea, bradycardia, persistent fetal circulation, or pulmonary hypertension. Unless appropriate interventions are initiated immediately, the outcome is poor.

Risk factors for cardiac arrest in newborns include bradycardia, intrauterine asphyxia, prematurity, drugs administered to or taken by the mother, congenital neuromuscular diseases, congenital malformations, and intrapartum hypoxemia. Assessment findings may include peripheral cyanosis, inadequate respiratory effort, and ineffective or absent heart rate. In managing the neonatal cardiac arrest, follow the inverted pyramid for resuscitation and administer drugs or fluids according to medical direction.

10. Given several neonatal emergencies, provide the appropriate procedures for assessment, management, and transport. pp. 1151–1181

During your classroom, clinical, and field training, you will assess and develop a management plan for the real and simulated patients you attend. Use the information presented in this chapter, the information on neonatal emergencies in the field provided by your instructors, and the guidance given by your clinical and field preceptors to develop the skills needed to assess, manage, and transport the newborn and neonate patient. Continue to refine these skills once your training ends and you begin your career as a EMT-I.

CASE STUDY REVIEW

This case study draws attention to one of the complications that may occur at an out-of-hospital delivery of a newborn.

In this case, you arrive on scene to attend one patient, a woman who has just gone into labor, and quickly find yourself managing a second patient—a newly born infant who remains blue and limp, even after suctioning. The situation can be highly stressful, especially with the two parents nearby. You recall the steps in the inverted pyramid for resuscitating a distressed newborn. You quickly dry the infant and wrap her in a dry blanket, reducing the life-threatening risk of hypothermia. As you prepare to suction, you remember that you will also need to apply tactile stimulation, either by flicking the soles of the newborn's feet or by gently rubbing her back.

When the baby does not "pink up," many thoughts probably run through your mind. You know, for example, that a prolonged lack of oxygen can cause permanent brain damage—and death. Use of the APGAR score is out of the question. You must immediately provide the patient with oxygen. Again following the inverted pyramid, you administer supplemental oxygen (preferably warmed and humidified) using the "blow-by" method. When the patient's heart rate remains below 100 beats per minute, you begin positive-pressure ventilation with a bag-valve-mask unit, the device of choice. Perhaps you also depress the pop-off valve to deactivate it and ensure adequate ventilation.

Because the baby starts breathing spontaneously, you do not have to initiate endotracheal intubation or chest compressions. Nonetheless, you still use the pulse oximeter to ensure adequate oxygen saturation. In preparing the newborn for transport, you keep in mind the risk of hypothermia and cover the baby's head to prevent unnecessary heat loss. En route to the hospital, with the baby receiving blow-by oxygen, you finally compute the APGAR score. You come up with a 9—just one point below the maximum!

Your calm, professional conduct throughout the call helped reassure the parents—the two other people in your care—of their daughter's safety. In recognition of a job well done, they name her after you.

CONTENT SELF-EVALUATION

MULTIPLE CHOICE

_____ 1. Examples of antepartum factors indicating possible complications in newborns would include multiple gestation and:
  A. premature labor.
  B. inadequate prenatal care.
  C. abnormal presentation.
  D. prolapsed cord.
  E. prolonged labor.

_____ 2. Examples of intrapartum factors indicating possible complications in newborns would include the use of narcotics within four hours of delivery and:
   A. meconium-stained amniotic fluid.   D. toxemia or diabetes.
   B. post-term gestation.   E. a mother over 35 years old.
   C. a mother under 16 years old.

_____ 3. When the fetus is in the uterus, the respiratory system is:
   A. working at a very rapid speed.   D. essentially functional.
   B. working at a very slow speed.   E. flushed with meconium.
   C. essentially nonfunctional.

_____ 4. Factors that stimulate the baby's first breath include:
   A. mild acidosis.
   B. hypoxia.
   C. hypothermia.
   D. initiation of stretch reflexes in the lungs.
   E. all of the above

_____ 5. Persistent fetal circulation is a condition in which the:
   A. ductus arteriosus remains closed.   D. both A and C
   B. ductus arteriosus reopens.   E. both B and C
   C. pulmonary vascular bed dilates.

_____ 6. Always assume that apnea in the newborn is secondary apnea and rapidly treat it with ventilatory assistance.
   A. True
   B. False

_____ 7. Most of the fetal development that could lead to congenital problems occurs during the:
   A. first trimester.   D. onset of labor.
   B. second trimester.   E. intrapartum period.
   C. third trimester.

_____ 8. Some infants are born with a defect in their spinal cord. In some cases, the spinal cord and associated structures may be exposed. This abnormality is called diaphragmatic hernia.
   A. True
   B. False

_____ 9. A congenital hernia of the umbilicus found in the neonate is called a(n):
   A. choanal atresia.   D. meningomyelocele.
   B. Pierre Robin Syndrome.   E. omphalocele.
   C. spina bifida.

_____ 10. A congenital condition characterized by a small jaw combined with a cleft palate, downward displacement of the tongue, and an absent gag reflex is called a(n):
   A. cleft lip.   D. Pierre Robin Syndrome.
   B. omphalocele.   E. choanal atresia.
   C. cleft palate.

_____ 11. The APGAR score should be assigned at 1 and 10 minutes after the infant's birth.
   A. True
   B. False

_____ 12. The G in APGAR stands for:
   A. gravida.   D. gray tone.
   B. gestation.   E. none of the above
   C. grimace.

_____ 13. A dark green material found in the intestine of the full-term newborn is called:
   A. bile.   D. vomitus.
   B. meconium.   E. hyperbilirubinemia.
   C. mucus.

CHAPTER 30 *Neonatal Resuscitation* **403**

_____ 14. Loss of heat by the newborn can occur through:
  A. evaporation.   D. radiation.
  B. convection.   E. all of the above
  C. conduction.

_____ 15. Immediately after birth, the newborn's core temperature can drop 4 degrees or more from its birth temperature.
  A. True
  B. False

_____ 16. Prior to cutting the umbilical cord, it should not be "milked" as this can cause:
  A. polycythemia.   D. hemophilia.
  B. anemia.   E. both A and C
  C. hyperbilirubinemia.

_____ 17. An increase in the level of bilirubin in the blood can cause:
  A. jaundice.   D. flushing.
  B. pallor.   E. anemia.
  C. cyanosis.

_____ 18. The most important indicator of neonatal distress is the fetal respiratory rate.
  A. True
  B. False

_____ 19. EMS units should contain all of the following equipment in their neonatal resuscitation kit EXCEPT a(n):
  A. meconium aspirator.
  B. laryngoscope with size 3 and 4 blades.
  C. device to secure the endotracheal tube.
  D. umbilical catheter and 10 mL syringe.
  E. DeLee suction trap.

_____ 20. Following the inverted pyramid of neonatal resuscitation, which would be done first?
  A. intubation   D. drying and warming
  B. bag-valve-mask ventilations   E. administration of medications
  C. chest compressions

_____ 21. In distressed newborns, monitor the heart rate with external electronic monitors.
  A. True
  B. False

_____ 22. The danger of deep suctioning a newborn is that it can cause a(n):
  A. vagal response.   D. allergic reaction.
  B. increased heart rate.   E. tachypnea.
  C. decreased respiratory rate.

_____ 23. Suctioning of a newborn should last no longer than 10 seconds.
  A. True
  B. False

_____ 24. Normal newborn respirations are approximately _____ times a minute.
  A. 10–30   D. 40–70
  B. 20–50   E. 60–90
  C. 30–60

_____ 25. Insertion of an endotracheal tube is recommended when prolonged ventilation of a newborn will be required.
  A. True
  B. False

©2004 Pearson Education, Inc.
Intermediate Emergency Care: Principles & Practice

SPECIAL PROJECT

The APGAR Scale

The APGAR scoring system will help you distinguish between newborns who need only routine care and those who needed greater assistance. To gain practice in using this system, complete the following exercises.

Part I

You have just assisted in the delivery of a newborn. Your quick assessment reveals a blue baby with very slow movement of the extremities. Your initial vital signs indicate a slow respiratory rate and a heart rate around 80–90 beats per minute. The infant seems distressed but does not cry when touched. Complete the first 1-minute APGAR score for this infant using the following chart.

The APGAR Score				Score	
Sign	0	1	2	1 min	5 min
Appearance (Skin color)	Blue, pale	Body pink, extremities blue	Completely pink		
Pulse Rate (Heart rate)	Absent	Below 100	Above 100		
Grimace (Irritability)	No response	Grimace	Cries		
Activity (Muscle tone)	Limp	Some flexion of extremities	Active motion		
Respiratory Effort	Absent	Slow and irregular	Strong cry		
			TOTAL SCORE =		

Part II

You have begun to follow the inverted pyramid by drying, warming, positioning, suctioning, and providing tactile stimulation to the newborn. Based upon the inverted pyramid, what would be the next steps if the infant does not "perk up"? Indicate these steps, in the correct order, on the following incomplete diagram.

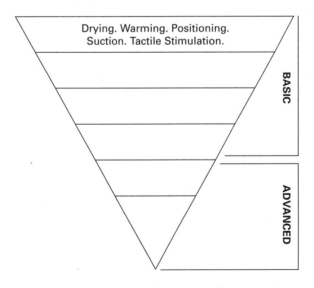

Part III

Fortunately, the stimulation that you provided has been helpful. At this time, both the family and your crew feel immense relief as the infant begins to cry and thrash about. A quick assessment of the vitals reveals a pulse rate well over 100 beats per minute. The infant's body is now pink, but the extremities are still a bit blue. Recalculate the APGAR score, using the chart in Part I, now that 5 minutes have quickly gone by.

CHAPTER 31

✳

Pediatric Emergencies

Review of Chapter Objectives

After reading this chapter, you should be able to:

1. Identify methods/mechanisms that prevent injuries to infants and children.   **p. 1186**

As a EMT-I, you can help reduce the rate of injury by taking advantage of opportunities to share "teaching points" in your daily life, both personally and professionally. Take part in, or offer to organize, school or community programs in injury prevention or health care. Engage student interest in the EMS profession by volunteering to speak at "career days," emphasizing those aspects of your job that relate to young people. Use nonurgent ambulance calls as a chance to educate family members or caregivers on the importance of "child-proofing" a home or neighborhood. Work with appropriate agencies in initiating or conducting safety inspections, block watches, and more.

2. Identify the common family responses to acute illness and injury of an infant or child.   **pp. 1187–1188**

As you might expect, the reaction of parents or caregivers to a pediatric emergency will vary. Initial responses by parents or caregivers might include shock, grief, denial, anger, guilt, fear, or complete loss of control. Their behavior may change during the course of the emergency.

3. Describe techniques for successful interaction with families of acutely ill or injured infants and children.   **pp. 1187–1188**

Communication is the key to successful interaction with families of acutely ill or injured pediatric patients. Preferably only one EMT-I will speak with adults at the scene. This will avoid any chance of conflicting information and allow a second EMT-I to focus on the child. If parents or caregivers sense your confidence and professionalism, they will regain control and trust your suggestions for care. As with the child, most parents and caregivers feel overwhelmed by fear.

If conditions permit, you should allow one of the parents or caregivers to remain with the child at all times. Some family members may be extremely emotional in emergency situations. The child will react more positively to a family member who appears calm and reassuring. If a parent or caregiver is "out of control," have another person take him or her away from the immediate area to settle down. Maintain a reasonable level of suspicion if a child shows a pattern of injuries, some old and some new. In such cases, the parent or caregiver may try to cover up what may be an abusive situation. They may also try to block examination and treatment.

4. Identify key anatomical, physiological, growth, and developmental characteristics of infants and children and their implications.   **pp. 1188–1191**

Children are broken into age groups because they differ in terms of anatomical, physiological, growth, and developmental characteristics. The following are some of the differences:

©2004 Pearson Education, Inc.
Intermediate Emergency Care: Principles & Practice

- **Newborns (first hours after birth).** The term "newborn" refers to a baby in the first hours of extrauterine life. These patients are assessed using the APGAR scoring system, which was described in Chapters 29 and 30. Resuscitation of the newborn generally follows the inverted pyramid and the guidelines established in the Neonatal Advanced Life Support (NALS) curriculum.

- **Neonates (ages birth to 1 month).** The neonate typically loses up to 10 percent of its birth weight as it adjusts to extrauterine life. This lost weight, however, is ordinarily recovered within 10 days. Gestational age affects early growth. Children born at term (40 weeks) should follow accepted developmental guidelines. Infants born prematurely will not be as developed, either neurologically or physically, as their term counterparts.

  The neonatal stage of development centers on reflexes. The neonate's personality also begins to form. Obviously, the history must be obtained from the parents or caregivers. However, it is also important to observe the child. Common illnesses in this age group include jaundice, vomiting, and respiratory distress. The approach to this age group should include several factors. First, the child should always be kept warm. Observe skin color, tone, and respiratory activity. The absence of tears when crying may indicate dehydration. The lungs should be auscultated early during this exam, while the infant is quiet.

- **Infants (ages 1 to 5 months).** Infants should have doubled their birth weight by 5 to 6 months of age and can follow the movement of others with their eyes. Muscle control develops in a cephalo-caudal ("head-to-tail") progression, with control spreading from the trunk toward the extremities. Although the infant's personality continues to form, it still centers strongly on the parents or caregivers. Concentrate on keeping these patients warm and comfortable, allowing them to remain the parent's or caregiver's lap, if possible. A pacifier or bottle can be used to help keep the baby quiet during the examination.

- **Infants (ages 6 to 12 months).** Patients in this age group are active and enjoy exploring the world with their mouths. In this stage of development, the risk of foreign body airway obstruction (FBAO) becomes a serious concern. Infants 6 months and older have more fully formed personalities and express themselves more readily than younger babies. They have a considerable anxiety toward strangers. They don't like lying on their backs, and they tend to cling to their mother, though the father "will do." Common illnesses and accidents include febrile seizures, vomiting, diarrhea, dehydration, bronchiolitis, car accidents, croup, child abuse, poisonings, falls, airway obstructions, and meningitis. These children should be examined while sitting in the lap of the parent or caregiver. The exam should progress in a toe-to-head order, since starting at the face may upset the child. If time and conditions permit, allow the child to become familiar with you before beginning the examination.

- **Toddlers (ages 1 to 3 years).** Great strides in gross motor development occur during this stage. Children tend to run underneath or stand on almost anything. As they grow older, toddlers become braver and more curious or stubborn. They begin to stray away from the parents or caregivers more frequently. Yet these remain the only people who can comfort them quickly, and most children will cling to a parent or caregiver if frightened. At ages 1 to 3, language development begins. Although the majority of the history comes from interaction with the parent or caregiver, it is possible to ask the toddler simple questions.

  Accidents of all types are the leading cause of injury deaths in pediatric patients ages 1 to 15. Common accidents in this age group include motor vehicle collisions, homicides, burn injuries, drownings, and pedestrian accidents. Common illnesses and injuries in the toddler age group include vomiting, diarrhea, febrile seizures, poisonings, falls, child abuse, croup, and meningitis. Keep in mind that FBAO is still a high risk for toddlers.

  Be cautious when treating toddlers. Approach toddlers slowly and try to gain their confidence. Conduct the exam in a toe-to-head order. The child may be difficult to examine and may resist being touched. Be sure to tell the child if something will hurt. If at all possible, avoid procedures on the dominant arm/hand, which the child will try to pull away.

- **Preschoolers (ages 3 to 5 years).** Children in this age group show a tremendous increase in fine and gross motor development. Language skills increase greatly. However, if frightened, these children often refuse to speak. They usually have vivid imaginations and may see monsters as part of their world. Preschoolers may have tempers and will express them. During this stage of development, children fear mutilation and may feel threatened by treatment. Avoid frightening or misleading comments. When evaluating a child in this age group, question the child first, keeping in mind that imagination may interfere with the facts. The child often has a distorted sense of time, and thus you must rely on the parents or caregivers to fill in the gaps. Common illnesses and accidents in this age group include croup, asthma, poisonings, auto accidents, burns, child abuse, ingestion of foreign bodies, drownings, epiglottitis, febrile seizures, and meningitis.

Start the examination with the chest and evaluate the head last. Do not lie or try to trick the patient. Avoid baby talk. If time and situation permit, give the preschooler health care choices.

- **School-age children (ages 6 to 12 years).** School-age children are active and carefree. Growth spurts sometimes lead to clumsiness. The personality continues to develop, and these children are proud and protective of their parents and caregivers. Common illnesses and injuries for this age group include drownings, auto accidents, bicycle accidents, falls, fractures, sports injuries, child abuse, and burns.

When examining school-age children, give them responsibility for providing the history. However, remember that children may be reluctant to provide information if they sustained an injury while doing something forbidden. The parents or caregivers can fill in the pertinent details. During assessment, respect the modesty of school-age children. Also, remember to be honest and tell the child what is wrong.

- **Adolescents (ages 13 to 18).** Adolescence covers the period from the end of childhood to the start of adulthood (age 18). It begins with puberty, roughly at age 13 for males and 11 for females. Puberty is highly child specific and can begin at various ages. Adolescents vary significantly in their development. Those over age 15 are physically nearer to adults in terms of their vital signs but emotionally may still be children. Regardless of physical maturity, remember that teenagers as a group are "body conscious." The slightest possibility of a lasting scar may be a tremendous issue to the adolescent patient. Common illnesses and injuries in this age group include mononucleosis, asthma, auto collisions, sports injuries, drug and alcohol problems, suicide gestures, and sexual abuse. Remember that pregnancy is also possible in female adolescents.

In examining an adolescent patient, it may be wise to conduct the interview away from the parents or caregivers. If you must perform a detailed physical exam, respect the teenager's sense of privacy. If the patient exhibits modesty or bodily shame, have an EMT-I of the same sex as the teenager conduct the exam. Although patients in this age group are not legally adults, keep in mind that most of them see themselves as grown up and will take offense at the use of the word "child."

5. **Outline differences in adult and childhood anatomy, physiology, and "normal" age-group-related vital signs.** pp. 1191–1194

Anatomical or physiological differences in infants and children as compared with adults include:

- A proportionally larger tongue
- Smaller airway structures
- Abundant secretions
- Deciduous (baby) teeth
- Flatter nose and face
- Head heavier relative to body and less-developed neck structures and muscles
- Fontanelle and open sutures (soft spots) palpable on top of a young infant's head
- Thinner, softer brain tissue
- Head larger in proportion to the body
- Shorter, narrower, more elastic (flexible) trachea
- Shorter neck
- Abdominal breathers with a faster respiratory rate
- In the case of newborns, breathe primarily through the nose (obligate nose breathers)

- Larger body surface relative to their body mass
- Softer bones
- More exposed spleen and liver
- More easily dehydrated
- Less blood and in greater danger of developing severe shock or bleeding to death from a relatively minor wound
- Immature temperature control mechanism (unstable in babies)

Age-related differences in vital signs include:

- Pulse rates (average) by age group:
  —Newborn: 100–180
  —Infant 0–5 months: 100–160
  —Infant 6–12 months: 100–160
  —Toddler 1–3 years: 80–110
  —Preschooler 3–5 years: 80–110
  —School-age child 6–10 years: 65–110
  —Early adolescent 11–14 years: 60–90

- Respiratory rates (average) by age group:
  —Newborn: 30–60
  —Infant 0–5 months: 30–60
  —Infant 6–12 months: 30–60
  —Preschooler 3–5 years: 22–34
  —School-age child 6–10 years: 18–30
  —Early adolescent 11–14 years: 12–26

- Blood pressure (average/mmHg at rest) by age group:

	Systolic *Approx. 90 plus 2 × age*	Diastolic *Approx. 2/3 systolic*
—Preschooler 3–5 years:	average 98 (78–116)	average 65
—School-age child 6–10 years:	average 105 (80–122)	average 69
—Early adolescent 11–14 years:	average 114 (88–140)	average 76

6. Describe techniques for successful assessment and treatment of infants and children. pp. 1195–1204

Many of the components of the initial patient assessment can be done during a visual examination of the scene ("assessment from the doorway"). Whenever possible, involve the parent or caregiver in efforts to calm or comfort the child. Depending on the situation, you may decide to allow the parent or caregiver to remain with the child during treatment and transport. The developmental stage of the patient and the coping skills of the parents or guardians will be key factors in making this decision.

When interacting with parents or other responsible adults, pay attention to the way in which parents or caregivers interact with the child. Are the interactions appropriate to the emergency? Are family members concerned? Are they angry? Are they overly emotional or entirely indifferent?

From the time of dispatch, you will continually acquire information relative to the patient's condition. As with all patients, personal safety must be your first priority. In treating pediatric patients, follow the same guidelines in approaching the scene as you would with any other patient. Observe for potentially hazardous situations, and make sure you take appropriate BSI precautions. Remember that infants and young children are at especially high risk of an infectious process.

7. Discuss normal age-group vital signs and the appropriate equipment used to obtain pediatric vital signs. pp. 1203–1204

Remember that poorly taken vital signs are of less value than no vital signs at all. Therefore, you must have the correct equipment to obtain pediatric vital signs. Items include appropriate-sized BP cuffs, a pediatric stethoscope, and so on. Modern noninvasive monitoring devices all have their application to emergency care. These devices may include pulse oximeter, automated blood pressure devices, self-registering thermometers, and ECGs. However, these devices may frighten a child. Before applying any monitoring device, explain what you are going to do and then demonstrate the device.

8. Determine appropriate airway adjuncts, ventilation devices, and endotracheal intubation equipment; their proper use; and complications of use for infants and children. pp. 1204–1213

As a general rule, use airway adjuncts in pediatric patients only if prolonged artificial ventilations are required. There are two reasons for this. First, infants and children often improve quickly through the administration of 100% oxygen. Second, airway adjuncts may create greater complications in children than in adults.

Keeping this in mind, be sure to have available the appropriate-sized airway adjuncts for each pediatric age group. Basic equipment includes oral and nasal airways, a pediatric BVM, smaller sized suction catheters, smaller sized masks for the BVM, age-appropriate nasogastric tubes, and a pediatric laryngoscope, blades, and endotracheal tubes. It is also a good idea to carry a Broselow® tape, which, after measuring the child's height, displays the appropriate sizes of tubes.

The biggest complication of airway management for the pediatric patient is the possibility of overinflation, which allows air to gather in the stomach. Gastric distention can cause pressure on the diaphragm, making full expansion of the lungs difficult. For specific techniques in airway management in the pediatric patient, review the steps and scans in the textbook, especially those dealing with advanced airway and ventilatory management.

9. List the indications and methods of gastric decompression for infants and children. pp. 1213, 1214

If gastric distention is present in a pediatric patient, you may consider placing a nasogastric tube (NG tube). In infants and children, gastric distention may result from overly aggressive artificial ventilations or from air swallowing. Placement of an NG tube will allow you to decompress the stomach and the proximal bowel of air. An NG tube can also be used to empty the stomach of blood or other substances. Indications for use of nasogastric intubation include an inability to achieve adequate tidal volumes during ventilation due to gastric distention and the presence of gastric distention in an unresponsive patient.

As with nasopharyngeal airways, an NG tube is contraindicated in pediatric patients who have sustained head or facial trauma. Because the NG tube might migrate into the cranial sinuses, consider the use of an orogastric tube instead. Other contraindications include possible soft-tissue damage in the nose and inducement of vomiting.

In determining the correct length of NG tube, measure the tube from the top of the nose, over the ear, to the tip of the xiphoid process. To insert an NG tube, you should:

- Oxygenate and continue to ventilate, if possible.
- Measure the NG tube from the tip of the nose, over the ear, to the tip of the xiphoid process.
- Lubricate the end of the tube. Then pass it gently downward along the nasal floor to the stomach.
- Auscultate over the epigastrium to confirm correct placement. Listen for bubbling while injecting 10–20 cc of air into the tube.
- Use suction to aspirate stomach contents.
- Secure the tube in place.

10. Define and discuss the pathophysiology and assessment findings associated with pediatric respiratory distress, failure, and arrest. pp. 1220–1221

The severity of respiratory compromise can be quickly classified into the following categories:

Respiratory distress. The mildest form of respiratory impairment is classified as respiratory distress. The most noticeable finding is the increased work of breathing. The signs and symptoms of respiratory distress include a normal mental status deteriorating to irritability or anxiety, tachypnea, retractions, nasal flaring (in infants), good muscle tone, head bobbing, grunting, and cyanosis that improves with supplemental oxygen. If not corrected immediately, respiratory distress will lead to respiratory failure.

Respiratory failure. Respiratory failure occurs when the respiratory system is not able to meet the demands of the body for oxygen intake and for carbon dioxide removal. It is characterized by inadequate ventilation and oxygenation. During respiratory failure, the carbon dioxide level begins to rise as the body is not able to remove it. This ultimately leads to respiratory acidosis. The signs and symptoms of respiratory failure include irritability or anxiety deteriorating to lethargy, marked tachypnea later deteriorating to bradypnea, marked retractions later deteriorating to agonal respirations, poor muscle tone, marked tachycardia later deteriorating to bradycardia, and central cyanosis. Respiratory failure is a very ominous sign. If immediate intervention is not provided, the child will deteriorate to full respiratory arrest.

Respiratory arrest. The end result of respiratory impairment, if untreated, is respiratory arrest. The cessation of breathing typically follows a period of bradypnea and agonal respirations. The signs and symptoms of respiratory arrest include unresponsiveness deteriorating to coma, bradypnea deteriorating to apnea, absent chest wall movement, bradycardia deteriorating to asystole, and profound cyanosis. Respiratory arrest will quickly deteriorate to full cardiopulmonary arrest if appropriate interventions are not made. The child's chances of survival markedly decrease when cardiopulmonary arrest occurs.

11. Differentiate between upper airway obstruction and lower airway disease.   pp. 1221–1227

Obstruction of the upper airway can be caused by many factors and may be partial or complete. Obstruction can result from inflamed or swollen tissues, which may be caused by infection or by aspirating a foreign body. Two medical conditions that can lead to upper airway obstruction in pediatric patients include croup and epiglottitis. Appropriate care depends on prompt and immediate identification of the disorder and its severity.

Suspect lower airway distress when the following conditions exist: an absence of stridor, presence of wheezing during exhalation, and increased work of breathing. Common causes of lower airway disease include respiratory diseases such as asthma, bronchiolitis, and pneumonia. Although infrequent, you may also encounter cases of foreign body lower airway aspiration, especially in toddlers and preschoolers.

12. Describe the general approach to the treatment of children with respiratory distress, failure, or arrest from upper airway obstruction or lower airway disease.   pp. 1221–1227

The general approach to the child with respiratory distress or failure from an upper or lower airway problem is to assess the child in the least stressful way possible and to administer oxygen. If the child has a complete upper airway obstruction, the appropriate FBAO maneuvers will need to be quickly done. If the child is in respiratory arrest, begin BVM resuscitation and consider the need for ET tube insertion. An NG tube may be useful to minimize gastric distention. If the child is in respiratory failure, assisted ventilations should also be considered.

In cases of upper airway obstruction, keep this precaution in mind: Because it is difficult to distinguish between croup from epiglottitis in the prehospital setting, never examine the oropharynx. If epiglottitis is present, examination of the oropharynx may result in laryngospasm and complete airway obstruction. In fact, if the patient is maintaining his or her airway, *do not put anything into the child's mouth,* including a thermometer. In the case of foreign body aspiration, do not attempt to look into the child's mouth if the obstruction is partial. Instead make the child comfortable and administer humidified oxygen. If the obstruction is complete, clear the airway with accepted basic life support techniques. However, DO NOT perform blind finger sweeps, as this can push a foreign body deeper into the airway.

When treating lower airway diseases, the primary goal is to support ventilations through the use of supplemental, humidified oxygen and appropriate pharmacological therapy such as bronchodilator medications (asthma and bronchiolitis). If prolonged ventilation will be required, perform endotracheal intubation.

13. **Describe the epidemiology, including the incidence, morbidity/mortality risk factors, preventive strategies, pathophysiology, assessment, and treatment of infants and children with:**

a. Croup
p. 1222

Croup (or laryngotracheobronchitis) is a viral infection of the upper airway affecting children of 6 months to 4 years of age, most commonly in the fall and winter months. The child will have a barking cough secondary to inflammation and swelling of the tissues just beneath the glottis and larynx. In the evening the child develops a harsh barking cough with inspiratory stridor, nasal flaring, and tracheal tugging. Management is supportive with calming and reassurance to both the child and parents. Administer oxygen, preferably with a cool water mist and racemic epinephrine or albuterol, as per physician order.

b. Epiglottitis
pp. 1222–1224

Epiglottitis presents similarly to croup and occurs usually at night. The child awakens with a high fever and brassy cough. There is often pain on swallowing, sore throat, dyspnea, inspiratory stridor and drooling. Do not attempt to visualize the airway as the procedure may result in complete airway obstruction. Management includes reduction of the child's anxiety and blow-by oxygen, humidified if possible. Do not attempt intubation unless absolutely necessary and then be prepared to use a tube somewhat smaller than otherwise indicated. The airway will be restricted by the glottic swelling.

c. Foreign body aspiration
pp. 1224–1225

Toddlers and preschoolers (ages 1 to 4) are likely to put objects in their mouths and are at increased risk for aspiration. This mechanism of injury is the number one cause of death in children under 6 years of age. The child will likely present with minimal air movement (complete obstruction) or severe respiratory distress, stridor, hoarse voice, drooling, throat pain, retractions, and cyanosis (partial obstruction). Management for partial obstruction is supportive with calming and reassurance, oxygen, and placement of the child in the sitting position. Attempts to remove the object may turn the partial obstruction into a complete obstruction. If the obstruction is complete, visualize the airway and sweep the obstruction from it or use the laryngoscope and try to remove the obstruction with the Magill forceps. If the object is very small, it may lodge in the lower airway. The child will present with cough and diminished breath sounds on one side. Care is directed to calming, reassurance, and oxygen administration.

d. Asthma
pp. 1225–1226

Asthma is a chronic inflammation of the lower respiratory tract and is usually associated with allergies. It is associated with bronchospasm and excessive mucus production that obstructs airflow. The lungs become progressively hyperinflated which reduces vital capacity and gas exchange in the alveoli. Asthma is often recognized by patient history, though it can be difficult to differentiate from other pediatric respiratory disease. The patient is often sitting bolt upright and using the accessory muscles of respiration. Wheezing is often present, though in a severe attack, air exchange may be so compromised that it and respiratory sounds may be absent. Management includes calming and reassurance, the administration of high-flow/high concentration oxygen, and an inhaled beta agonist. Status asthmaticus is a serious and prolonged asthma attack that cannot be broken by pharmacologic means. It is a serious event that often precedes respiratory arrest.

e. Bronchiolitis
pp. 1226–1227

Bronchiloitis is a contagious viral infection affecting the medium-sized airways and most often occurs in early childhood. It resembles asthma and presents with an expiratory wheeze in children under two years of age. Management is much the same as with asthma: reassurance, blow-by, humidified oxygen, and albuterol.

f. Pneumonia
p. 1227

Pneumonia is an infectious disease affecting the lower airways and lungs of pediatric patients between 1 and 5 years old. The child will often present with a history of respiratory infection, low grade fever, decreased breath sounds, crackles, and chest pain. Management is basically

©2004 Pearson Education, Inc.
Intermediate Emergency Care: Principles & Practice

supportive with emphasis on patient comfort and reassurance, oxygen, and bag-valve-masking as necessary.

g. Foreign Body Lower Airway Obstruction   p. 1227

Pediatric patients at risk for upper airway obstruction are also at risk for lower airway obstruction. A foreign object can enter the lower airway if it is too small to lodge in the upper airway. Think of foods like nuts, seeds, and candy, as well as small toys or parts of toys. Depending on the positioning, the foreign object can act like a one-way valve either trapping air in distal lung tissues or preventing aeration of distal lung tissues, causing a ventilation/perfusion mismatch.

Assessment usually reveals that the child had a foreign object in his/her mouth, and it then quickly disappeared. There is often considerable, often intractable, coughing. The child will be anxious and have diminished breath sounds in the part of the chest affected by the foreign body. You may hear crackles or rhonchi, usually unilateral. Unilateral wheezing should be considered a result of an aspirated foreign body until proven otherwise.

Management is supportive. Place the child in a position of comfort; avoid agitation. Provide supplemental oxygen. Transport the child to a facility that can perform pediatric fiberoptic bronchoscopy.

h. Shock (hypoperfusion)   pp. 1227–1231

The second major cause of pediatric cardiopulmonary arrest—after respiratory impairment—is shock. Shock can most simply be defined as inadequate perfusion of the tissues with oxygen and other essential nutrients and inadequate removal of metabolic waste products.

When compared with the incidence of shock in adults, shock is an unusual occurrence in children because their blood vessels constrict so efficiently. However, when the blood pressure does drop, it drops so far and so fast that the child may quickly develop cardiopulmonary arrest. A number of factors place infants and young children at risk for shock. Newborns and neonates will develop shock as a result of a loss of body heat. Other causes include dehydration (from vomiting and/or diarrhea), infection (particularly septicemia), trauma, and blood loss. Less common causes of shock in infants and children include allergic reactions, poisoning, and cardiac events.

As in adults, the severity of shock in a pediatric patient is classified as compensated shock, decompensated shock, and irreversible shock. It can also be categorized as *cardiogenic* or *noncardiogenic*. Cardiogenic shock results from an inability of the heart to maintain an adequate cardiac output to the circulatory tissues. Cardiogenic shock in a pediatric patient is ominous and often fatal. Noncardiogenic shock—types of shock that result from causes other than inadequate cardiac output—is more frequently encountered in pediatric patients, because they have a much lower incidence of cardiac problems that adults. Causes of noncardiogenic shock may include hemorrhage, abdominal trauma, systemic bacterial infection, spinal cord injury, and others.

The definitive care of shock takes place in the emergency department of a hospital. Because shock is a life-threatening condition in pediatric patients, it is important to recognize early signs and symptoms—or even the possibility of shock in a situation where the signs and symptoms may not have yet developed. In a situation in which you suspect a possibility of shock, provide oxygen to boost tissue perfusion and transport as quickly as possible. Also, keep the patient in a supine position and take steps to protect the child from hypothermia and agitation that might worsen the condition. In some cases (compensated shock), fluid therapy as ordered by medical direction can buy time until the patient arrives an appropriate treatment center.

i. Dysrhythmias including tachydysrhythmias, bradydysrhythmias, and arrest   pp. 1232–1234

Dysrhythmias in children are uncommon. When dysrhythmias occur, bradydysrhythmias are the most common. Supraventricular tachydysrhythmias are very uncommon. Dysrhythmias can cause pump failure, ultimately leading to cardiogenic shock. Children have a very limited capacity to increase stroke volume. The primary mechanism through which they increase cardiac output is through changes in the heart rate. The treatment of dysrhythmias is specific for the dysrhythmia in question.

Special Considerations

j. Seizures **pp. 1236–1237**

The etiology for seizures is often unknown. However, several risk factors have been identified. They include fever, hypoxia, infections, idiopathic epilepsy (epilepsy of unknown origin), electrolyte disturbances, head trauma, hypoglycemia, toxic ingestions or exposure, tumor, or CNS malformations. Management of pediatric seizure is essentially the same as for the seizing adult. Place patients on the floor or on the bed. Be sure to lay them on their side, away from furniture. Do not restrain patients, but take steps to protect them from injury. Maintain the airway, but do not force anything, such as a bite stick, between the teeth. Administer supplemental oxygen. Then take and record all vital signs. If the patient is febrile, remove excess layers of clothing, while avoiding extreme cooling. If status epilepticus is present, institute the following steps:

- Start an IV of normal saline or lactated Ringer's and perform a glucometer evaluation.
- Administer diazepam as follows:
  —*Children 1 month to 5 years:* 0.2–0.5 mg slow IV push every 2–5 minutes up to a maximum of 2.5 milligrams.
  —*Children 5 years and older:* 1 mg slow IV push every 2–5 minutes to a maximum of 5 milligrams.
- Contact medical direction for additional dosing. Diazepam can be administered rectally if an IV cannot be established.
- If the seizure appears to be due to a fever and a long transport time is anticipated, medical direction may request the administration of acetaminophen to lower the fever. Acetaminophen is supplied as an elixir or as suppositories. The dose should be 15 mg/kg body weight.

k. Hypoglycemia and hypoglycemia **pp. 1238–1240**

Hypoglycemia is an abnormally low blood sugar level and is a true and immediate emergency. It most frequently occurs in newborns and diabetic children. Suspect hypoglycemia when a patient exhibits weakness, dizziness, tachycardia, pallor, sweating, vomiting, or an altered mental status. Test the patient's blood sugar level and initiate treatment if the level falls below 70 mg/dl. Monitor the ABCs and the glucose level, administer oxygen and, if indicated, administer dextrose ($D_{25}W$) (you may dilute $D_{50}W$).

Hyperglycemia is an abnormally high blood sugar and is usually associated with Type I diabetes (insulin dependant). It may lead to dehydration and diabetic ketoacidosis. The patient may present with a progressive malaise and lethargy as well as a fruity (ketone) breath and other signs (see Table 31-13). Care for the hyperglycemia patient includes monitoring the ABCs and glucose level and administering fluids. If oral intake is not practical, consider administration of normal saline or lactate Ringer's solution in an IV bolus of 20 mL/kg, repeated if necessary. Intubation and overdrive ventilation may be necessary in cases of hyperventilation.

l. Trauma emergencies, including injuries to the head, neck, chest, abdomen, and extremities and burns **pp. 1242–1250**

Trauma is the number one cause of death in infants and children. Most pediatric injuries result from blunt trauma. Children have thinner body walls that allow forces to be more readily transmitted to body contents, increasing the possibility of injury to internal tissues and organs. If you serve in an urban area, you can expect to see a higher incidence of penetrating trauma, mostly intentional and mostly from gunfire or knife wounds. There is also a significant incidence of penetrating trauma outside the cities (mostly unintentional) from hunting accidents and agricultural accidents.

Although pediatric patients can be injured in the same way as adults, children tend to more susceptible to certain types of injuries than grownups. Falls, for example, are the single most common cause of injury in children. Other mechanisms of injury include motor vehicle collisions, car vs. pedestrian collisions, drownings and near drownings, penetrating injuries, burns, and physical abuse.

The treatment of trauma is injury specific. It involves management of the ABCS, management of the injury (e.g., spinal immobilization, splinting of fractures, control of bleeding), and treatment for possible shock.

Burn injuries are the leading cause of death in the home for children under 14 years of age. Burns in children are assessed as for adults except that the child's surface area to body weight is increased and the child's fluid reserves are decreased. Therefore, the burn injuries are more serious in children than adults due to this factor.

m. Abuse or neglect pp. 1251–1254

Child abuse is the second leading cause of death in infants less than 6 months of age. An estimated 2,000 to 5,000 children die each year as a result of abuse or neglect. There are several characteristics common among abused children. Often the child is seen as "special" and different from others. Premature infants and twins stand a higher risk of abuse than other children. Many abused children are less than 5 years of age. Physically and mentally handicapped children as well as those with special needs are at greater risk. So are uncommunicative children. Boys are more often abused than girls. A child who is not what the parents wanted (e.g., the "wrong" gender) is at increased risk of abuse, too.

Signs of abuse or neglect can be startling. As a guide, the following findings should trigger a high index of suspicion:

- Any obvious or suspected fractures in a child under 2 years of age
- Injuries in various stages of healing, especially burns and bruises
- More injuries than usually seen in children of the same age or size
- Injuries scattered on many areas of the body
- Bruises or burns in patterns that suggest intentional infliction
- Increased intracranial pressure in an infant
- Suspected intra-abdominal trauma in a young child
- Any injury that does not fit with the description of the cause given

Information in the medical history may also raise the index of suspicion. Examples include:

- A history that does not match the nature or severity of the injury
- Vague parental accounts or accounts that change during the interview
- Accusations that the child injured himself or herself intentionally
- Delay in seeking help
- Child dressed inappropriately for the situation
- Revealing comment by bystanders, especially siblings

Suspect child neglect if you spot any of the following conditions:

- Extreme malnutrition
- Multiple insect bites
- Long-standing skin infections
- Extreme lack of cleanliness
- Verbal or social skills far below those you would expect for a child of similar age and background
- Lack of appropriate medical care

In cases of child abuse or neglect, the goals of management include appropriate treatment of injuries, protection of the child from further abuse, and notification of proper authorities.

n. Sudden infant death syndrome (SIDS) including parent/caregiver responses pp. 1250–1251

The incidence of SIDS in the U.S. is approximately 2 deaths per 1,000 births. It is the leading cause of death between 2 weeks and 1 year of age, with peak incidence occurring at 2–4 months. SIDS occurs most frequently in the fall and winter months. It tends to be more common in males than in females. It is more prevalent in premature and low birth-weight infants, in infants of young mothers, and in infants whose mothers did not receive prenatal care. Infants of mothers who used cocaine, methadone, or heroin during pregnancy are at greater risk. Occasionally, a mild upper respiratory infection will be reported prior to the death. SIDS is not caused by external suffocation from blankets or pillows. Neither is it related to allergies to cow's milk or regurgitation and aspiration of stomach contents. It is not thought to be hereditary.

Current theories vary about the etiology of SIDS. Some authorities feel it may result from an immature respiratory center in the brain that leads the child to simply stop breathing. Others think there may be an airway obstruction in the posterior pharynx as a result of pharyngeal relaxation during sleep, a hypermobile mandible, or an enlarged tongue. Studies strongly link SIDS to a prone sleeping position. Soft bedding, waterbed mattresses, smoking in the home, and/or an overheated environment are other potential associations. A small percentage of SIDS may be abuse related.

Unless the infant is obviously dead, undertake active and aggressive care of the infant to assure the family or caregivers that everything possible is being done. A first responder or other personnel should be assigned to assist the parents or caregivers and to explain the procedure. At all points, use the baby's name.

The responses of the parent or caregiver to the death of a child include the normal grief reactions. Initially, there may be shock, disbelief, and denial. Other times, the parents or caregivers may express anger, rage, hostility, blame, or guilt. Often, there is a feeling or inadequacy as well as helplessness, confusion, and fear. The grief process is likely to last for years, as in the case of a SIDS death.

o. **Children with special needs, including children dependent on various technological devices** pp. 1255–1258

For most of human history, infants and children with devastating congenital conditions or diseases died or remained confined to a hospital. In recent decades, however, medical technology has lowered infant mortality rates and allowed a greater number of children with special needs to live at home.

In recent years medical technology has lowered infant mortality rates and allowed a greater number of children with special needs to live at home. Some of these infants and children include:

- Premature babies
- Infants and children with lung disease, heart disease, or neurological disorders
- Infants and children with chronic diseases, such as cystic fibrosis, asthma, childhood cancers, cerebral palsy, and others
- Infants and children with altered functions from birth (e.g., spina bifida, congenital birth defects, and cerebral palsy)

On some calls, you may be asked to treat technology-assisted children who depend, in varying degrees, upon special equipment. Commonly found devices include tracheostomy tubes, apnea monitors, home artificial ventilators, central intravenous lines, gastric feeding tubes, gastrostomy tubes, and shunts.

In treating pediatric patients with special needs, remember that they require the same assessment as other patients. (Recall that in the initial assessment, "disability" refers to a patient's neurological status—not to the child's special need.) Keep in mind that the child's special need is often an ongoing process, which may make the parent or caregiver an excellent source of information. In most cases, you should concentrate on the acute problem—the reason for the call. In managing patients with special needs, try to keep several thoughts in mind.

- Avoid using the term "disability" (in reference to the child's special need). Instead, think of the patient's many abilities.
- Never assume that the patient cannot understand what you are saying.
- Involve the parents, caregivers, or the patient, if appropriate, in treatment. They manage the illness or congenital condition on a daily basis.
- Treat the patient with a special need with the same respect as any other patient.

14. **Discuss the primary etiologies of cardiopulmonary arrest in infants and children.** pp. 1196, 1209–1221

The primary causes of cardiopulmonary arrest in infants and children include untreated respiratory failure, immaturity of the cardiac conductive system, bradycardia, hypoxia, vagal stimulation (rare), drug overdose, drowning, multiple system trauma, electrocution, pericardial tamponade, tension pneumothorax, acidosis, hypothermia, hypoglycemia, and FBAO.

©2004 Pearson Education, Inc.
Intermediate Emergency Care: Principles & Practice

15. Discuss basic cardiac life support (CPR) guidelines for infants and children. pp. 1204–1209

The CPR guidelines for infants and children were changed in August 2000 when the Guidelines 2000 were published. The Brady website at: www.bradybooks.com will provide a link to the most up-to-date information on these standards.

16. Discuss age-appropriate sites, equipment, techniques, and complications of vascular access and fluid therapy for infants and children. pp. 1215–1216

Intravenous techniques for children are basically the same as for adults. (See Chapter 4, "Venous Access and Medication Administration.") However, additional veins may be accessed in an infant. These include veins of the neck and scalp, as well as of the arms, hands, and feet. The external jugular vein, however, should only be used in life-threatening situations.

The use of intraosseous (IO) infusion has become popular in the pediatric patient. This is especially true when large volumes of fluid must be administered, as occurs in hypovolemic shock, and when other means of venous access are unavailable. The indications for IO include the existence of shock or cardiac arrest, an unresponsive patient, or an unsuccessful attempt at a peripheral IV insertion. The contraindications for IO infusion include the presence of a fracture in the bone chosen for infusion and a fracture of the pelvis or extremity fracture in the bone proximal to the chosen site.

In performing IO perfusion, you can use a standard 16- or 18-gauge needle (either hypodermic or spinal). However, an intraosseous needle is preferred and significantly better. Basic steps are as follows: Prep the anterior surface of the leg below the knee with antiseptic solution (povidone iodine), and insert the needle in twisting fashion 1–3 centimeters below the tuberosity. Insertion should be slightly inferior in direction (to avoid the growth plate) and perpendicular to the skin. Signs of correct placement of the needle into the marrow cavity include a lack of resistance as the needle passes through the bony cortex, the ability of the needle to stand upright without support, the ability to aspirate bone marrow into a syringe, or free flow of the infusion without infiltration into the subcutaneous tissues.

17. Identify common lethal mechanisms of injury in infants and children. pp. 1243–1245

The most common pediatric mechanisms of injury (MOI) include falls, motor vehicle crashes, car vs. pedestrian collisions, drownings and near drownings, penetrating injuries, burns, and physical abuse.

18. Discuss anatomical features of children that predispose or protect them from certain injuries. pp. 1248–1250

Head. Small children have larger heads in proportion to the rest of their bodies. For this reason, when they fall or are thrown through the air, they often land head first, predisposing them to serious head injury. The larger relative mass of the head and lack of neck muscle strength also provide increased momentum in acceleration-deceleration injuries and a greater stress on the cervical spine. Because the skull is softer and more compliant in infants and young children than in adults, brain injuries occur more readily.

Chest and abdomen. Infants and young children lack the rigid rib cages of adults. Therefore, they suffer fewer rib fractures and more intrathoracic injuries. Remember that chest injuries are the second most common cause of pediatric trauma death. Because of the compliance of the chest wall, severe intrathoracic injury can be present without signs of external injury. Likewise, their relatively underdeveloped abdominal musculature affords minimal protection to the viscera, particularly the spleen.

Extremities. Because children have more flexible bones than adults, they tend to have incomplete fractures such as bend fractures, buckle fractures, and greenstick fractures. Therefore, you should treat "sprains" and "strains" as fractures and immobilize accordingly. In younger children, the bone growth plates have not yet closed. Some growth plate fractures can lead to permanent disability if not managed correctly.

Body surface area. There are three distinguishing features of the pediatric patient's skin and BSA. First, the skin of an infant or child is thinner than that of an adult. Second, infants and children generally have less subcutaneous fat. Finally, they have a larger body-surface-area-to-weight ratio. As a result of these features, children risk greater injury from extremes in temperature or thermal exposure. They lose fluids and heat more quickly than adults and have a greater likelihood of dehydration and hypothermia. They also burn more easily and deeper than adults, which explains why burns are one of the leading causes of death among pediatric trauma patients.

19. **Describe aspects of infant and child airway management that are affected by potential cervical spine injury.**   pp. 1245–1246

An infant's open airway is in the neutral or extended position but not in the hyperextended position. This needs to be kept in mind when positioning the infant who may have sustained a neck injury where there can be little to no movement of the neck for fear of worsening the potential neck injury. Children under the age of 6 usually have large heads in proportion to the rest of their bodies. Therefore, it is often necessary to pad behind the shoulders when a cervical collar is applied as a part of the spinal immobilization. Keep infants, toddlers, and preschoolers with the cervical spine in a neutral in-line position by placing padding from the shoulders to the hips.

Always make sure that you use appropriate-sized pediatric immobilization equipment. These supplies may include rigid cervical collars, towel or blanket rolls, foam head blocks, commercial pediatric immobilization devices, vest-type or short wooden backboards, and long boards with the appropriate padding.

20. **Identify infant and child trauma patients who require spinal immobilization.**   pp. 1217–1218

Children are not small adults. Although spinal injuries are not as common as in adults, they do occur, especially because of a child's disproportionately larger and heavier head. Any time an infant or child sustains a significant head injury, assume that a neck injury may be present. Children can suffer a spinal cord injury with no noticeable damage to the vertebral column as seen on cervical spine X-rays. Thus, negative cervical spine X-rays do not necessary assure that a spinal cord injury does not exist. As a result, children should remain immobilized until a spinal cord injury has been ruled out by hospital personnel.

Remember that many children, especially those under age 5, will protest or fight restraints. Try to minimize the emotional stress by having a parent or caregiver stand near or touch the child.

21. **Given several pre-programmed simulated pediatric patients, provide the appropriate assessment, treatment, and transport.**   pp. 1185–1258

During your classroom, clinical, and field training, you will be presented with real and simulated pediatric patients and assess and treat them. Use the information provided in this chapter and the information and skills you gain from your instructors and clinical and field preceptors to develop your skill on caring for these patients. Continue to refine newly learned skills once your training ends and you begin your EMT-I career.

CASE STUDY REVIEW

This case study examines the treatment of a severely dehydrated pediatric patient—a common condition encountered on calls involving infants and young children.

This case involves an infant who has been unable to hold down any food for three days. In just a short time, she has developed signs and symptoms that point to possible shock, which the EMT-Is immediately notice. Their initial assessment starts as soon they observe the quality of the baby's skin (pale, cool, clammy) and the noticeably sunken anterior fontanelle. As the EMT-Is take vital signs and assess the level of consciousness, they note that the baby cries but does not produce tears. After taking appropriate BSI precautions, they wisely check the infant's diaper to see if it is dry or wet. (If it had been wet, they would have checked the quality of the urine. Dehydrated patients, when they do uri-

©2004 Pearson Education, Inc.
Intermediate Emergency Care: Principles & Practice

nate, have very dark yellow urine because it is a concentrated solute with less solvent [water] than usual.) The dry diaper and the mother's comment confirms a suspicion of dehydration, giving the crew enough information to develop a treatment plan.

The EMT-Is take this patient very seriously and begin transport before starting fluid therapy. En route to the hospital, they start an IV, which is not always an easy task in a patient this small. They probably keep in mind the use of an intraosseous needle in case an IV cannot be placed. For a patient this dehydrated, it would not be surprising that she might have needed a second bolus of 20 mL/kg of the normal saline. Of course, as is always the case, a parent should be nearby to assist in comforting the patient.

During your EMT-I career, you can expect to take part in a call similar to this one. Dehydration in infants and small children is a common condition, and you should be prepared to respond, assess, and manage the patient accordingly. Remember that dehydration is one of the causes of hypoperfusion (shock) in pediatric patients.

CONTENT SELF-EVALUATION

MULTIPLE CHOICE

_C_ 1. The leading cause of death in pediatric patients in the United States is:
A. AIDS.
B. asthma.
C. trauma.
D. neglect.
E. cardiac arrest.

_D_ 2. Factors that account for high rates of pediatric injury include all of the following EXCEPT:
A. weather.
B. geography.
C. dangers in the home.
D. HMOs.
E. motor vehicle accidents.

_A_ 3. The federally funded program aimed at improving the health of pediatric patients who suffer from life-threatening illnesses and injuries is called:
A. EMSC.
B. PBTLS.
C. PALS.
D. APLS.
E. TRIPP.

_B_ 4. The most common response of children to illness or injury is:
A. denial.
B. fear.
C. excitement.
D. indifference.
E. grief.

_E_ 5. Treatment of a pediatric patient begins with:
A. obtaining vital signs.
B. placement of an ET tube.
C. administration of oxygen.
D. focused head-to-toe exam.
E. communications and psychological support.

_C_ 6. While caring for the pediatric patient, whenever possible, the EMT-I should:
A. avoid discussing painful procedures.
B. administer high-flow oxygen.
C. allow a parent or caregiver to stay with the child.
D. use correct medical and anatomical terms.
E. stand in an authoritative posture.

_C_ 7. The term neonate describes a baby that is:
A. newly born.
B. 10 days or less in age.
C. up to 1 month in age.
D. 1 to 5 months in age.
E. 6 months or more in age.

_B_   8. The age group for which foreign body airway obstruction (FBAO) becomes a concern is:
- A. infants ages 1–5 months.
- B. infants ages 6–12 months.
- C. toddlers.
- D. preschoolers.
- E. school-age children.

_____ 9. An infant's airway differs from that of an adult in all of the following ways EXCEPT that it:
- A. is narrower at all levels.
- B. has a softer and more flexible trachea.
- C. is less likely to be blocked by secretions.
- D. has a greater likelihood of soft-tissue injury.
- E. is more prone to obstruction by the tongue.

_____ 10. In comparing pediatric heart and respiratory rates with those of an adult, infants and young children have:
- A. about the same heart and respiratory rates as an adult.
- B. slower heart rates and slower respiratory rates.
- C. slower heart rates and faster respiratory rates.
- D. faster heart rates and slower respiratory rates.
- E. faster heart rates and faster respiratory rates.

_____ 11. Unlike an adult, the trachea of a child can collapse if the neck and head are hyperextended because:
- A. the trachea is softer and more flexible.
- B. a child's tongue takes up more space proportionately.
- C. the cricoid rings are firmer.
- D. a child's larynx is higher.
- E. the airway is wider at all levels.

_____ 12. The two abdominal organs that are most likely to suffer traumatic injury in a pediatric patient are the:
- A. kidney and gallbladder.
- B. liver and spleen.
- C. stomach and small intestine.
- D. colon and appendix.
- E. bladder and pancreas.

_____ 13. A child's larger body-surface-area-to-weight ratio causes a pediatric patient to be:
- A. resilient to temperature changes.
- B. prone to hypothermia.
- C. difficult to assess.
- D. prone to excess subcutaneous fat.
- E. less likely to lose fluids quickly.

_____ 14. Although infants and children have a circulating blood volume proportionately larger than adults, their absolute blood volume is:
- A. about the same.
- B. smaller.
- C. even larger.
- D. rate dependent.
- E. variable.

_____ 15. The pediatric assessment triangle focuses on airway, breathing, and circulation.
- A. True
- B. False

_____ 16. In an infant or small child, tachypnea, an abnormally rapid rate of breathing, may indicate:
- A. fear.
- B. pain.
- C. inadequate oxygenation.
- D. exposure to cold.
- E. all of the above

_____ 17. A respiratory rate of 18–30 breaths per minute would be considered normal for a(n):
- A. newborn.
- B. 6-month old infant.
- C. toddler.
- D. preschooler.
- E. school-age child.

©2004 Pearson Education, Inc.
Intermediate Emergency Care: Principles & Practice

18. Which of the following approaches is the correct method for conducting the physical examination of an infant or a very young child?
    A. toe-to-head
    B. head-to-chest
    C. head-to-toe
    D. chest-to-head
    E. both A and B

19. To obtain the blood pressure of a pediatric patient, the cuff should be _____ the width of the patient's arm.
    A. one-fourth
    B. one-third
    C. one-half
    D. two-thirds
    E. three-fourths

20. Poorly taken vital signs are of less value than no vital signs at all.
    A. True
    B. False

21. Medication administration in the pediatric patient is modified to the patient's:
    A. age.
    B. height.
    C. weight.
    E. level of distress.
    D. level of consciousness.

22. The hallmark of pediatric management is:
    A. frequent pulse checks.
    B. prompt transport.
    C. administration of fluids.
    D. adequate oxygenation.
    E. diagnosis of medical conditions.

23. As a rule, an oropharyngeal airway should only be used on pediatric patients who:
    A. have sustained head or facial trauma.
    B. are known to suffer from seizures.
    C. show signs of cardiac arrest.
    D. exhibit a vagal response.
    E. lack a gag reflex.

24. An indication to perform abdominal thrusts in the pediatric patient is:
    A. failure to obtain an airway by any other method.
    B. desire to suction the airway.
    C. a foreign body airway obstruction.
    D. desire to ventilate by a BVM.
    E. both A and C

25. Indications for performing an endotracheal intubation in a pediatric patient include all of the following EXCEPT the:
    A. need to gain access for suctioning.
    B. necessity of providing a route for drug administration.
    C. need for prolonged artificial ventilations.
    D. failure to provide adequate ventilations with a BVM.
    E. all of the above

26. The optimal positioning of the head for pediatric intubation in the absence of a spinal injury is:
    A. neutral.
    B. hyperextended.
    C. sniffing.
    D. head-tilt.
    E. spine.

27. If gastric distention is present in a pediatric patient, an EMT-I might consider placing a(n):
    A. oropharyngeal airway.
    B. nasopharyngeal airway.
    C. needle cricothyrotomy.
    D. nasogastric tube.
    E. endotracheal tube.

Special Considerations

_____ 28. In obtaining vascular access in a pediatric patient, the external jugular vein should only be used in life-threatening situations.
    A. True
    B. False

_____ 29. The indications for use of intraosseous infusion include all of the following EXCEPT:
    A. a patient less than 6 years old.
    B. existence of shock or cardiac arrest.
    C. presence of a facture in the pelvis.
    D. an unresponsive patient.
    E. failure to place a peripheral IV.

_____ 30. You are more likely to use electrical therapy on pediatric patients than adult patients.
    A. True
    B. False

_____ 31. All of the following are symptoms of epiglottitis EXCEPT:
    A. a rapid onset.   **D.** drooling.
    B. occasional stridor.   **E.** a fever of approximately 102–104°F.
    C. a barking cough.

_____ 32. In treating a patient with epiglottitis, an EMT-I should:
    A. take blood pressure regularly.
    B. attempt to visualize the oropharynx.
    C. take the child's temperature orally.
    D. place the child in a supine position.
    E. none of the above

_____ 33. Common causes of lower airway distress include all of the following EXCEPT:
    A. pneumonia.   **D.** bronchiolitis.
    B. asthma.   **E.** status asthmaticus.
    C. croup.

_____ 34. When a child experiences a severe asthma attack without wheezing, this is:
    A. an ominous sign.
    B. because of a lack of expectorant.
    C. a sign of improvement.
    D. because of an inability to cough.
    E. common, and should not alarm the EMT-I.

_____ 35. All of the following are signs and symptoms of shock in a child EXCEPT:
    A. pale, cool, clammy skin.   **D.** increased urination.
    B. impaired mental status.   **E.** a rapid respiratory rate.
    C. absence of tears when crying.

_____ 36. Cardiogenic shock is more frequently encountered in prehospital pediatric care than noncardiogenic shock.
    A. True
    B. False

_____ 37. When dysrhythmias do occur in children, the most common form is a(n):
    A. bradydysrhythmia.   **D.** asystole.
    B. supraventricular tachydysrhythmia.   **E.** ventricular fibrillation.
    C. ventricular tachydysrhythmia.

_____ 38. A pediatric patient is seen by an EMT-I for a seizure. Assessment and history reveal that the child has a fever of 101°F, was very sleepy and irritable before the seizure, and has had no similar episodes. The child complained of a stiff neck and headache earlier in the day. You suspect that the episode may have been caused by:
    A. febrile convulsions.   **D.** hypoxia.
    B. meningitis.   **E.** hyperglycemia.
    C. hypoglycemia.

©2004 Pearson Education, Inc.
Intermediate Emergency Care: Principles & Practice

_____ 39. Whenever a glucometer reading reveals a blood sugar of less than 70 mg/dL, an EMT-I might suspect:
  A. hypoxia.
  B. hyperglycemia.
  C. hypoglycemia.
  D. ketoacidosis.
  E. dehydration.

_____ 40. The single most common cause of trauma-related injuries in children is:
  A. motor-vehicle collisions.
  B. burns.
  C. falls.
  D. physical abuse.
  E. drownings.

_____ 41. Appropriate-sized pediatric immobilization equipment includes all of the following EXCEPT:
  A. towel or blanket roll.
  B. vest-type device (KED).
  C. sandbag.
  D. straps and cravats.
  E. padding.

_____ 42. All of the following are true statements about sudden infant death syndrome EXCEPT that it:
  A. occurs most frequently in the fall and winter.
  B. is not caused by external suffocation by blankets.
  C. tends to be more common in females than in males.
  D. is not thought to be hereditary.
  E. is possibly linked to a prone sleeping position.

_____ 43. Child abuse can take the form of:
  A. psychological abuse.
  B. physical abuse.
  C. sexual abuse.
  D. neglect.
  E. all of the above

_____ 44. In cases of suspected child abuse, management goals include all of the following EXCEPT:
  A. protection of the child from further injury.
  B. notification of proper authorities.
  C. appropriate treatment of injuries.
  D. cross-examination of the parents or caregivers.
  E. documentation of all findings and statements.

_____ 45. A surgical connection that runs from the brain to the abdomen in a pediatric patient is called a(n):
  A. central IV.
  B. tracheostomy.
  C. shunt.
  D. inner cannula.
  E. epigastric tube.

SPECIAL PROJECT

Burn Injuries

Burn injuries are the leading cause of accidental death in the home for children under 14 years of age. As with other assessment tools, you must modify the "rule of nines" to estimate the extent of a burn in a pediatric patient. Read the following short patient description and complete the diagram on the following page. Then answer the questions that follow.

You have been called to the scene of a fire at a single-family residence. The dispatcher tells you that a two-year-old female patient has been critically burned. Upon arrival at the scene, first responders with the fire department lead you to the little girl. They report that the patient has full-thickness burns on the right arm, right leg, and the anterior trunk.

Special Considerations

THE RULE OF NINES

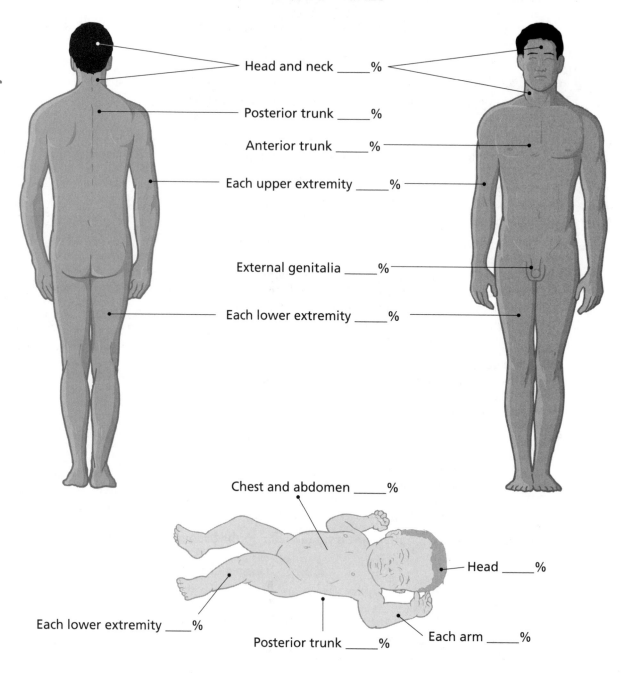

Head and neck _____%

Posterior trunk _____%

Anterior trunk _____%

Each upper extremity _____%

External genitalia _____%

Each lower extremity _____%

Chest and abdomen _____%

Head _____%

Each lower extremity _____%

Posterior trunk _____%

Each arm _____%

1. If the patient had been an adult, what would the rule of nines add up to? _____

2. What does the rule of nines add up to for this toddler? _____

3. Why do the percentages differ? _____

4. Suppose the burns had been less extensive. What alternative method for calculating the burn area might be used? _____

©2004 Pearson Education, Inc.
Intermediate Emergency Care: Principles & Practice

CHAPTER 32
✳
Geriatric Emergencies

Review of Chapter Objectives

After reading this chapter, you should be able to:

1. Discuss dependent and independent living environments of the elderly patients.

pp. 1262–1263

The elderly live in both independent and dependent living environments. Many continue to live alone or with their partner until well into their 80s or 90s. The "oldest" old are the most likely to live alone, and, in fact, nearly half of those age 85 and older live by themselves. The great majority of these people—an estimated 78 percent—are women. This is because married men tend to die before their wives, and widowed men tend to remarry more often than widowed women. Elderly persons living alone represent one of the most impoverished and vulnerable parts of society.

Usually the elderly own their own homes or apartments. In addition to these traditional residences, they may choose among a variety of options for assisted living. Among the elderly who receive help, more than 43 percent rely on paid assistance. Another 54 percent use unpaid assistance, and 3 percent use both types of help. Those elderly who turn to dependent care arrangements select live-in nursing, life-care communities, congregate care, or personal-care homes. Approximately 5 percent of the elderly live in nursing homes.

2. Discuss common emotional and psychological reactions to aging, including causes and manifestations.

pp. 1261–1263, 1229–1301

When behavioral or psychological problems develop later in life, they are often dismissed as normal age-related changes. This attitude denies an elderly person the opportunity to correct a treatable condition and/or overlooks an underlying physical disorder. Studies have shown that the elderly retain their basic personalities and their adaptive cognitive abilities. Intellectual decline and regressive behavior are not normal age-related changes and could in fact have a physiological cause, such as head trauma.

It is important to keep in mind the emotionally stressful situations facing many elderly people such as isolation, loneliness, loss of independence, loss of strength, fear of the future, and more. The elderly are at risk for alcoholism as well as facing a higher incidence of secondary depression as a result of neuroleptic medications such as Haldol or Thorazine.

The emotional well-being of the elderly impacts upon their overall physical health. Therefore, it is important that you note evidence of altered behavior in any elderly patient that you assess and examine. Also, keep in mind that many emotional conditions, such as depression, are normal reactions to stressful situations and can be resolved with appropriate counseling and treatment. Finally, remember that medical disorders in the elderly often present as functional impairment and should be treated as an early warning of a possibly undetected medical problem.

Special Considerations

3. Discuss pathophysiology changes associated with the elderly in regard to drug distribution, metabolism, and elimination—including polypharmacy, dosing errors, increased drug sensitivity, and medication non-compliance. pp. 1264–1265

In general, a person's sensitivity to drugs increases with age. When compared with younger patients, the elderly experience more adverse drug reactions, more drug–drug interactions, and more drug–disease interactions. Because of age-related pharmacokinetic changes such as a loss of body fluids and atrophy of organs, drugs concentrate more readily in the plasma and tissues of elderly patients. As a result, drug dosages often must be adjusted to prevent toxicity. Additionally, due to differences in the GI tract, medications are metabolized and excreted at a slower rate in the elderly patient.

If medications are not correctly monitored, polypharmacy can cause a number of problems among the elderly. In taking a medical history of an elderly patient, remember to ask questions to determine if the patient is taking a prescribed medication as directed. Noncompliance with drug therapy, usually underadherence, is common among the elderly. Up to 40 percent do not take medications as prescribed. Of these individuals, 35 percent experience some type of medical problem.

Factors that can decrease compliance in the elderly include limited income, memory loss (due to decreased or diseased neural activity), limited mobility, sensory impairment (cannot hear/read/understand directions), multiple or complicated drug therapies, fear of toxicity, child-proof containers (especially difficult for arthritic patients), and lengthy drug therapy plans.

4. Discuss the use and effects of commonly prescribed drugs for the elderly patient. pp. 1264–1265, 1296–1298

Functional changes in the kidneys, liver, and gastrointestinal system slow the absorption and elimination of many medications in the elderly. In addition, the various compensatory mechanisms that help buffer against medication side effects are less effective in the elderly than in younger patients.

Approximately 30 percent of all hospital admissions are related to drug-induced illness. About 50 percent of all drug-related deaths occur in people over the age of 60. Accidental overdoses may occur more frequently in the aged due to confusion, vision impairment, self-selection of medications, forgetfulness, and concurrent drug use. Intentional drug overdose also occurs in attempts at self-destruction. Another complicating factor is the abuse of alcohol among the elderly.

5. Discuss the problem of mobility in the elderly, and develop strategies to prevent falls. pp. 1265–1266

Regular exercise and a good diet are two of the most effective prevention measures for ensuring mobility among the elderly. Some elderly may suffer from a severe medical problem, such as crippling arthritis. They may fear for their personal safety, either from accidental injury or intentional injury, such as robbery. Certain medications also may increase their lethargy. Whatever the cause, a lack of mobility can have detrimental physical and emotional effects. Some of these include poor nutrition, difficulty with elimination, poor skin integrity, a greater predisposition for falls, loss of independence and/or confidence, depression from "feeling old," and isolation.

Falls present an especially serious problem for the elderly. Fall-related injuries represent the leading cause of accidental death among the elderly and the seventh highest cause of death overall. As a result, the EMT-I should consider strategies for making a home safe for the elderly and point these out to the elderly patient or family of the elderly patient, whichever may be appropriate. Examples of hazards that can easily be corrected include torn or slippery rugs, chairs without armrests, chairs with low backs, chairs with wheels, obstructing furniture, slippery bathtubs, dim lighting, high cabinet shelves, missing handrails on stairways, and high steps on stairways.

6. **Discuss age-related changes in sensations in the elderly, and describe the implications of these changes for communication and patient assessment.** pp. 1266, 1269–1270

Most elderly patients suffer from some form of age-related sensory changes. Normal physiological changes may include impaired vision or blindness, impaired or loss of hearing, an altered sense of taste or smell, and/or a lower sensitivity to pain or touch. Any of these conditions can affect your ability to communicate with the patient. In general, be prepared to spend more time obtaining histories from elderly patients.

7. **Discuss the problems with continence and elimination in the elderly patient.** pp. 1266–1267

The elderly often find it embarrassing to talk about problems with continence and elimination. They may feel stigmatized, isolated, and/or helpless. When confronted with these problems, DO NOT make a big deal out of them. Respect the patient's dignity, and assure the person that, in many cases, the problem is treatable.

Remember, too, that problems with continence and elimination are not necessarily caused by aging. They may be the result of drug therapy or medical conditions such as diabetes. As a result, in assessing a patient with incontinence or constipation, inquire about their medications and any chronic medical disorders. Also keep in mind the variety of other conditions that can result from problems with continence or elimination. In the case of incontinence, for example, a patient may experience rashes, skin infections, skin breakdown (ulcers), urinary tract infections, sepsis, and falls or fractures (caused by a frequent need to eliminate). In elderly people with cerebrovascular disease or impaired baroreceptor reflexes, efforts to force a bowel movement can lead to a transient ischemic attack (TIA) or syncope.

8. **Discuss factors that may complicate the assessment of the elderly patient.** pp. 1267–1272

In assessing an elderly patient, keep in mind the variety of causes of functional impairment. If identified early, an environmental or disease-related condition can often be reversed. Your success depends upon a thorough understanding of age-related changes and the implications of these changes for patient assessment and management. You will need to recall at all times the complications that can arise from comorbidity (having more than one disease at a time) and polypharmacy (concurrent use of a number of drugs).

Communications challenges may also complicate the assessment. Patients may be blind, have speech difficulties, or have some kind of hearing loss that can make assessment more difficult. They also often have a lower sensitivity to pain or touch.

In general, assessment of the elderly patient follows the same basic approach used with any other patient. However, you should keep in mind these points:

- Set a context for illness, taking into account the patient's living situation, level of activity, network of social support, level of dependence, medication history (both prescriptive and non-prescriptive), and sleep patterns.
- Pay close attention to an elderly person's nutrition, noting conditions that may complicate or discourage eating.
- Keep in mind that elderly patients may minimize or fail to report important symptoms. Therefore, try to distinguish the patient's chief complaint from the patient's primary problem.
- Because of presence of multiple chronic diseases, treat the patient on a "threat-to-life" basis.
- Recall at all times that alterations in the temperature-regulating mechanism can result in a lack of fever, or a minimal fever, even in the presence of a severe infection.
- When confronted with a confused patient, try to determine whether the patient's mental status represents a significant change from normal for them. DO NOT assume that a confused, disoriented patient is "just senile," thus failing to assess for a serious underlying problem.
- Remember that some patients are often easily fatigued and cannot tolerate a long physical examination. Also, because of problems with temperature regulation, the patient may be wearing several layers of clothing.

Special Considerations

- Be aware that the elderly patient may minimize or deny symptoms because of a fear of institutionalization or a loss of self-sufficiency.
- Try to distinguish signs of chronic disease from acute problems. For example:
  —Peripheral pulses may be difficult to evaluate because of peripheral vascular disease and arthritis.
  —The elderly may have nonpathological crackles (rales) upon lung auscultation.
  —The elderly often exhibit an increase in mouth breathing and a loss of skin elasticity, which may be confused with dehydration.
  —Dependent edema may be caused by inactivity, not congestive heart failure.

9. Discuss common complaints of elderly patients.   pp. 1278–1301

Common complaints of elderly patients include fatigue and weakness, dizziness, vertigo or syncope, falls, headaches, insomnia, dysphagia, loss of appetite, inability to void, and constipation or diarrhea. Many of these complaints in and of themselves would not be too serious. However, given the context of complicated medical histories of the elderly, each of these complaints are important and should be followed up and taken very seriously.

10. Discuss the normal and abnormal changes of age in relation to the:

a. Pulmonary system   p. 1273

The effects of aging on the respiratory system begin as early as age 30. Without regular exercise and/or training, the lungs start to lose their ability to defend themselves and to carry out their prime function of ventilation. Age-related changes in the respiratory system include decreased chest wall compliance, loss of lung elasticity, increased air trapping due to collapse of the smaller airways, and reduced strength and endurance of the respiratory muscles. In addition, there is a decrease in an effective cough reflex and the activity of the cilia. The decline of these two defense mechanisms leave the lungs more susceptible to recurring infection. Other factors that may affect pulmonary function in the elderly are kyphosis (exaggeration of the normal posterior curvature of the spine), chronic exposure to pollutants, and long-term cigarette smoking.

b. Cardiovascular system   pp. 1273–1275

A number of variables unrelated to aging influence cardiovascular functions—diet, smoking and alcohol use, education, socioeconomic status, and even personality traits. Of particular importance is the level of physical activity.

This said, the cardiovascular system still experiences, in varying degrees, age-related deterioration. Changes include a loss of elasticity and hardening of the arteries, an increase in the size and bulk of the left ventricle (hypertrophy), development of fibrosis (formation of fiber-like connective/scar tissue), and changes in the rate, rhythm, and overall efficiency of the heart.

c. Nervous system   pp. 1275–1276

Unlike cells in other organ systems, cells in the central nervous system cannot reproduce. The brain can lose as much as 45 percent of its cells in certain areas of the cortex. Overall, there is an average 10 percent reduction in brain weight from age 20 to age 90. Keep in mind, however, that reductions in brain weight and ventricular size are not well correlated with intelligence, and elderly people may still be capable of highly creative and productive thought. In addition to shrinkage of brain tissue, the elderly may experience some memory loss, clinical depression, altered mental status, and impaired balance. Keep in mind that these changes vary greatly and may not be seen in all elderly patients, even at the close of very long lives.

d. Endocrine system   p. 1276

The elderly experience a variety of age-related hormonal changes. Women, for example, experience menopause, the result of reductions in estrogen production. Men also experience a decline in levels of testosterone. In addition, the elderly commonly experience a decline in insulin sensitivity and/or an increase in insulin resistance. Finally, thyroid disorders, especially hypothyroidism and thyroid nodules, increase with age as well.

©2004 Pearson Education, Inc.
Intermediate Emergency Care: Principles & Practice

e. Gastrointestinal system p. 1276

Age affects the gastrointestinal system in various ways. The volume of saliva may decrease by as much as 33 percent, leading to complaints of dry mouth, nutritional deficiencies, and a predisposition to choking. Gastric secretions may decrease to as little as 20 percent of the quantity present in younger people. Esophageal and intestinal motility also decrease, making swallowing more difficult and delaying digestive processes. The production of hydrochloric acid also declines, further disrupting digestion and, in some adults, contributing to nutritional anemia. Gums atrophy and the number of taste buds decrease, reducing even further the desire to eat.

Other conditions may also develop. Hiatal hernias are not age-related per se, but can have serious consequences for the elderly. The hernias may incarcerate, strangulate, or, in the most severe cases, result in massive GI hemorrhage. A diminished liver function, which is associated with aging, can delay or impede detoxification. It also can reduce the production of clotting proteins, which in turn leads to bleeding abnormalities.

f. Thermoregulatory system pp. 1276–1277

As people age, the thermoregulatory system becomes altered or impaired. Aging seems to reduce the effectiveness of sweating in cooling the body. Older people tend to sweat at higher core temperatures and have less sweat output per gland than younger people. As people age, they also experience deterioration of the autonomic nervous system, including a decrease in shivering and lower resting peripheral blood flow. In addition, the elderly may have a diminished perception of the cold. Drugs and disease can further alter an elderly patient's response to temperature extremes, resulting in hyperthermia or accidental hypothermia.

g. Integumentary system p. 1277

As people age, the skin loses collagen, a connective tissue that gives elasticity and support to the skin. Without this support, the skin is subject to a great number of injuries from bumping or tearing. In addition, the skin thins as people age. Because cells reproduce more slowly, older patients often suffer more severe skin injuries than younger patients and healing takes a longer time. As a rule, the elderly are at a higher risk of secondary infections, skin tumors, drug-induced eruptions, and fungal or viral infections. Decades of exposure to the sun also makes the elderly vulnerable to melanoma and other sun-related carcinomas.

h. Musculoskeletal system p. 1277

An aging person may lose as much as 2–3 inches of height from narrowing of the intervertebral disks and osteoporosis (softening of bone tissue due to the loss of essential minerals). This is especially evident in the vertebral bodies, thus causing a change in posture. The posture of the aged individual often reveals an increase in the curvature of the thoracic spine (kyphosis) and slight flexion of the knee and hip joints. The demineralization of bone makes the elderly patient much more susceptible to hip and other fractures.

In addition to skeletal changes, a decrease in skeletal muscle weight commonly occurs with age—especially with sedentary individuals. To compensate, elderly women develop a narrow, short gait, while older men develop a wide gait. These changes make the elderly more susceptible to falls.

i. Renal system p. 1277

Aging affects the renal system through a reduction in the number of functioning nephrons by 30% to 40%. Renal blood flow may also be reduced by up to 45% increasing waste products in the blood and upsetting the fluid and electrolyte balance. A decrease in renal function may result in anemia or hypertension in older patients. Pay close attention to the airway as nausea and vomiting are complications of pain secondary to renal obstruction.

j. Genitourinary system pp. 1277–1278

Aging produces a loss of bladder sensation and tone causing incomplete emptying. This causes frequent urges to urinate and increases the chances of falling when walking to the bathroom half asleep at night. It also increases the chance of UTI and bladder infections as well as sepsis. In the male the prostrate often becomes enlarged (benign prostatic hypertrophy) causing difficulty in urination or urinary retention. Incontinence is also a problem.

Special Considerations

k. Immune system

The function of the T cells declines making the elderly person's body less able to notify the immune system of invasion by antigens. This diminished response, called immune senescence, increases susceptibility to infections and increases the duration and severity of the infection. The elderly should receive vaccinations suggested by the Health Department. Always consider infectious diseases to be potentially life threatening to the fragile elderly patient.

l. Hematology system
p. 1278

The hematology system is affected by a failure of the renal system to stimulate the production of red blood cells. Nutritional abnormalities may also produce abnormal RBCs. Since there is less body water present in the elderly, blood volume similarly decreases. This makes it difficult for an elderly patient to bounce back from an illness or injury. Intervention must be started early in order to make a lasting difference.

11. Discuss the assessment and management of the elderly patient with complaints related to the following body systems:

a. Respiratory
pp. 1278–1281

Respiratory emergencies are some of the most common reasons elderly persons summon EMS or seek emergency care. Most elderly patients with a respiratory disorder present with a chief complaint of dyspnea. However, coughing, congestion, and wheezing are also common chief complaints

- *Pneumonia* occurs more frequently in the elderly than younger patients due to the following reasons found in an elderly population: decreased immune response, reduced pulmonary function, increased colonization of the pharynx by gram-negative bacteria, abnormal or ineffective cough reflex, and decreased effectiveness of mucociliary cells of the upper respiratory system. Common signs and symptoms of pneumonia include increasing dyspnea, congestion, fever, chills, tachypnea, sputum production, and altered mental status. Occasionally, abdominal pain may be the only symptom, and a fever may be absent in the elderly patient. In treating an elderly patient with pneumonia, manage the life-threats, maintain ABCs, and transport to the hospital for diagnosis.
- *Chronic obstructive pulmonary disease (COPD)* is a collection of diseases characterized by chronic airflow obstruction with reversible and/or irreversible components. COPD patients often have a combination of emphysema, chronic bronchitis, and asthma. The usual signs and symptoms include cough, increased sputum production, dyspnea, accessory muscle use, pursed-lip breathing, tripod positioning, exercise intolerance, wheezing, pleuritic chest pain, and tachypnea. When confronted by an elderly patient with COPD, treatment is essentially the same as for all age groups. Administer supplemental oxygen and drug therapy, most frequently bronchodilators, according to your local medical direction to reduce the patient's dyspnea.
- *Pulmonary embolism* (PE) should always be considered as a possible cause of respiratory distress in the elderly patient. Blood clots are the most frequent cause of PE, yet they may also be caused by fat, air, bone marrow, tumor cells, or foreign bodies. Risk factors for developing a PE include deep venous thrombosis, prolonged immobility, malignancy, paralysis, fractures of the pelvis, hip, or leg, obesity, trauma to the leg vessels, major surgery, presence of a venous catheter, use of estrogen (in women), and atrial fibrillation. Treatment goals involve delivery of high-flow, high-concentration oxygen via mask, maintaining oxygen levels above SaO_2 or 90%. An IV should be established but vigorous fluid therapy avoided. Pain medications should be discussed with medical direction.
- *Pulmonary edema* is an escape of serous fluids into the alveoli and interstitial tissues of the lungs. Pulmonary edema can develop very rapidly in the elderly patient having an acute myocardial infarction. It can also be caused by pulmonary factors such as infections, inhaled toxins, narcotic overdose, pulmonary embolism, and decreased atmospheric pressure. The treatment is directed at altering the cause of the condition through actively positioning the patient in the Fowler's position, administering high-flow, high-concentration oxygen, assessing the need for ventilatory assistance, obtaining IV access, ECG monitoring,

430 DIVISION 5 *Special Considerations*

©2004 Pearson Education, Inc.
Intermediate Emergency Care: Principles & Practice

and providing appropriate drug therapy including morphine, nitrates, Lasix, or other medications as ordered by medical direction.

b. Cardiovascular pp. 1281–1285

The leading cause of death in the elderly is cardiovascular disease. When conducting a patient history, determine the patient's level of cardiovascular fitness, changes in exercise tolerance, recent diet history, use of medications, and use of cigarettes and/or alcohol. Ask questions about breathing difficulty, especially at night, and evidence of palpitations, flutter, or skipped beats. In performing the physical exam watch for hypertension, orthostatic hypotension, and consider checking both arms for BP differences from side-to-side. Look for signs of dehydration or dependent edema. In evaluating the problem, recall the cardiovascular disorders commonly found in elderly patients. They include angina pectoris, myocardial infarction, heart failure, dysrhythmias, aortic dissection, aneurysm, hypertension, and syncope.

- *Angina pectoris* literally means "pain in the chest." However, the pain of angina is actually felt in only about 10% to 20% of elderly patients. The changes in sensory nerves, combined with the myocardial changes of aging, make dyspnea a more likely symptom of angina than pain. In the elderly patient, exercise intolerance is a key symptom of angina. In obtaining a history, you should ask the patient about sudden changes in routine. In addition, inquire about any increased stresses on the heart, such as anemia, infection, dysrhythmias, and thyroid changes.

- *Myocardial infarction* (MI) involves actual death of muscle tissue due to a partial or complete occlusion of one or more of the coronary arteries. The greatest number of patients hospitalized for acute MI are older than 65. The elderly patient with MI is less likely to present with the classic symptoms such as chest pain that a younger patient would have. These "atypical" presentations seen in the elderly may also include absence of pain, exercise intolerance, confusion and dizziness, syncope, dyspnea (especially >85 years old), neck, dental, and/or epigastric pain, fatigue, and weakness. The mortality rate associated with MI and/or resulting complications doubles after age 70. Unlike younger patients, the elderly are more likely to suffer a silent MI. They also tend to have larger MIs. The majority of the deaths that occur in the first few hours following a MI are due to dysrhythmias.

- *Heart failure* takes place when cardiac output cannot meet the body's metabolic demands. The incidence rises exponentially after age 60. The causes of heart failure fall in one of four categories: impairment to flow, inadequate cardiac filling, volume overload, and myocardial failure. Typical age-related factors, such as prolonged myocardial contractions, make the elderly vulnerable to heart failure. Assessment findings specific to the elderly include fatigue from left heart failure; two-pillow orthopnea; dyspnea on exertion; dry, hacking cough progressing to a productive cough; dependent edema from right heart failure; nocturia; anorexia; hepatomegaly; and ascites.

- *Dysrhythmias* usually develop with age, and atrial fibrillation is the most common of the rhythms. Dysrhythmias occur primarily as a result of degeneration of the patient's conductive system. Anything that decreases myocardial blood flow can produce a dysrhythmia. They may also be caused by electrolyte abnormalities. To complicate matters further, the elderly do not tolerate extremes in heart rate as well as a younger person would. Treatment considerations depend upon the type of dysrhythmia. Patients who may already have a pacemaker have a low but significant rate of complications such as a failed battery, fibrosis around the catheter site, lead fracture, or electrode dislodgement. Drug therapy may be indicated. Whenever you discover a dysrhythmia remember the irregular heart rhythm may be the only clinical finding in an elderly patient suffering an acute MI.

- *Aortic dissection* is the degeneration of the wall of the aorta, either in the thoracic or abdominal cavity. It can result in an aneurysm or in the rupture of the vessel. Approximately 80% of thoracic aneurysms are due to atherosclerosis combined with hypertension. The remaining cases occur secondary to other factors like Marfan's syndrome or blunt trauma to the chest. These patients often present with tearing chest pain radiating to the back or if ruptured, cardiac arrest. The distal portion of the aorta is the most common site for abdominal aneurysms. The aneurysm may appear as a pulsatile mass in a patient with a normal girth, but lack of identifiable mass does not eliminate this condition. The patient may have

Special Considerations

a tearing abdominal pain or unexplained low back pain. Pulses in the legs are diminished or absent and the lower extremities feel cold to the touch. The treatment of an aneurysm depends on its size, location, and the severity of the condition. Rapid transportation is in order, and many of these patients will need a surgical procedure.

- Today over 50% of the people in the U.S. over the age of 65 have clinically diagnosed *hypertension*—defined as blood pressure greater than 140/90 mmHg. Prolonged elevated blood pressure will eventually damage the heart, brain, or kidneys. As a result of hypertension, the elderly are at greater risk for heart failure, stroke, blindness, renal failure, coronary heart disease, and peripheral vascular disease. Management of hypertension depends upon its severity and the existence of other conditions. Hypertension is often treated chronically with beta blockers which are contraindicated in patients who have COPD, asthma, or heart blocks greater than a first degree. Diuretics are another common drug used to treat hypertension but should be used cautiously in patients who are also taking digitalis.

- *Syncope* is a common presenting complaint in the elderly. The condition results when blood flow to the brain is temporarily interrupted or decreased. It is usually caused by problems with either the nervous system or the cardiovascular system. Common presentations of syncope would include the following:
  —Vasodepressor syncope or common fainting may occur following an emotional distress, pain, prolonged bed rest, mild blood loss, prolonged standing in warm crowded rooms, anemia, or fever.
  —Orthostatic syncope occurs when a person rises from a seated or supine position. This is due to pooling of the blood in the legs reducing the flow of blood to the brain. This is common in hypovolemia, venous varicosities, prolonged bed rest, and autonomic dysfunction. It can also be drug induced by blood pressure medications.
  —Vasavagal syncope occurs as a result of a valsalva maneuver during defecation, coughing, or similar maneuvers. This slows the heart rate and cardiac output, thus decreasing the blood flow to the brain.
  —Cardiac syncope results from transient reduction in cerebral blood flow due to a sudden decrease in cardiac output. It can result from a silent MI or a dysrhythmia, such as a bradycardia, Stokes-Adam syndrome, heart block, tachydysrhythmia, and sick sinus syndrome.
  —Seizures may result from a seizure disorder or syncope may cause seizure activity. Syncope due to seizures tends to occur without warning. It is associated with muscular jerking or convulsions, incontinence, and tongue-biting.
  —Transient ischemic attacks occur more frequently in the elderly and may cause syncope.

c. Nervous pp. 1285–1289

Elderly patients are at risk for several neurological emergencies. Many of these disorders involve an altered mental status and are discussed below:

- *Cerebrovascular disease (stroke/brain attack).* Strokes are the third leading cause of death in the U.S. Older patients are at higher risk than younger patients because of atherosclerosis, hypertension, immobility, limb paralysis, congestive heart failure, and atrial fibrillation. Transient ischemic attacks (TIAs) are also more common in older patients. Strokes usually fall in one of two major categories: (1) brain ischemia injuries caused by inadequate supply of oxygen and nutrients, which accounts for 80% of the strokes, and (2) subarachnoid hemorrhage or intracerebral hemorrhages which account for the rest. Due to the different types of strokes, signs and symptoms can present in many ways including: altered mental status, coma, paralysis, slurred speech, a change in mood, and seizures. When assessing a stroke, complete a GCS for later comparison in the ED. Many EMS systems also use the Cincinnati Prehospital Stroke Scale which assesses the smile, pronator drift, and speech to predict the potential for a stroke. Stroke patients need to be assessed and removed to the most appropriate facility quickly so that fibrinolytics (thrombolytics) can be utilized if the patient is an appropriate candidate and it is within three hours of the onset of the symptoms. By far the most preferred treatment for a stroke is prevention. Strategies for stroke prevention include control of hypertension, treatment of cardiac disorders and blood disorders, cessation of smoking, cessation of recreational drug use, moderate use of alcohol, regular exercise, improving eating habits.

- *Seizures* may be mistaken for stroke in the elderly patient. Some seizures are subtle in the elderly, and the common causes include seizure disorders (epilepsy), syncope, recent or past head trauma, mass lesion (tumor or bleed), alcohol withdrawal, hypoglycemia, or stroke. If the patient has fallen during a seizure, always remember to check for evidence of trauma and treat accordingly.
- *Dizziness* is a frequent complaint of the elderly. It may indicate the patient has suffered syncope, pre-syncope, lightheadedness, or true vertigo. Vertigo is a specific sensation of motion perceived by the patient as spinning or whirling. Vertigo is often accompanied by sweating, pallor, nausea, and vomiting. Meniere's disease can cause severe, intractable vertigo as well as a "roaring" sound in the ears. Any factor that impairs visual input, inner-ear function, peripheral sensory input, or the central nervous system can cause dizziness, including alcohol and many prescription drugs. Therefore, it is virtually impossible to distinguish dizziness, syncope, and pre-syncope in the prehospital setting.
- *Delirium* can be caused by organic brain disease or disorders that occur elsewhere in the body. Delirium in the elderly is a serious condition leading to death in approximately 18% of hospitalized patients. Delirium is a global mental impairment of sudden onset and self-limited duration. Common signs and symptoms include the acute onset of anxiety, an inability to focus, disordered thinking, irritability, inappropriate behavior, fearfulness, excessive energy, or psychotic behavior such as hallucinations or paranoia. Aphasic or speaking errors and/or prominent slurring may be present. In distinguishing between delirium and dementia, err on the side of delirium.
- *Dementia* is more prevalent in the elderly than delirium. Over 50% of all nursing home patients have some form of dementia. Dementia is a chronic global cognitive impairment, often progressive or irreversible. This mental deterioration is often called "organic brain syndrome," "senile dementia," or "senility." Causes of dementia include small strokes, atherosclerosis, age-related neurological changes, neurological diseases, certain hereditary diseases (e.g., Huntington's disease), and Alzheimer's disease. The signs and symptoms of dementia include progressive disorientation, shortened attention span, aphasia or nonsense talking, and hallucinations. Stay alert for signs of abuse or neglect which occurs in a disproportionate number of elderly suffering from dementia.
- *Alzheimer's disease* is a specific type of dementia that affects 4 million people in the United States. It is a chronic degenerative disorder that attacks the brain and results in impaired memory, thinking, and behavior. The disease generally occurs in three stages: early, intermediate and terminal stages. The early stage is characterized by loss of recent memory, inability to learn new material, mood swings, and personality changes. Patients may believe someone is plotting against them when they lose items or forget things. Aggression or hostility is common and poor judgment is evident. In the intermediate stage, the patient has a complete inability to learn new material. They wander, particularly at night, have increased falls, lose the ability for self-care, including bathing and use of the toilet. In the terminal stage, the patient is unable to walk and regresses to an infant stage including the loss of bowel and bladder function. Eventually the patient loses the ability to eat and swallow. Remember that the families of these patients also have need for support. If they show signs of stress, you may want to alert the emergency department so additional assistance in caring for their loved ones can be provided.
- *Parkinson's disease* is a degenerative disorder characterized by changes in muscle response, including tremors, loss of facial expression, and gait disturbances. It mainly appears in people over age 50 and peaks at age 70. Primary Parkinson's disease still has an unknown cause. Secondary Parkinson's disease has one of a number of potential causes such as viral encephalitis, atherosclerosis of cerebral vessels, reaction to certain drugs or toxins (such as antipsychotic or carbon monoxide), metabolic disorders (such as anoxia), tumors, head trauma, and degenerative disorders (such as Shy-Drager syndrome). Patients have a resting tremor and a pill rolling motion. As the disease progresses, muscles become more rigid and movements become slower and/or jerkier. Their feet may feel "frozen to the ground." Gaits become shuffled with short steps and unexpected bursts of speed, often used to avoid falling. Kyphotic deformity is a hallmark of the disease. They also develop a mask-like face devoid of all expression and speak in a slow, monotone voice. Difficulties in communication,

Special Considerations

coupled with a loss of mobility, often lead to anxiety and depression. In treating the patient with Parkinson's, observe for conditions that may indicate a fall or the inability to move. Manage treatable conditions and transport as needed.

d. Endocrine

The endocrine system undergoes a number of age-related changes, which affect hormone levels. The most common endocrine disorders include diabetes mellitus and thyroid gland disorders.

- *Diabetes mellitus* (primarily Type II) is estimated to be present in 20% of older adults, and almost 40% of the elderly have a form of glucose intolerance. The reasons the elderly develop these disorders include poor diet, decreased physical activity, loss of lean body mass, impaired insulin production, and resistance by body cells to the actions of insulin. Left unchecked, over time vague constitutional symptoms like fatigue or weakness may actually be indications of diabetes and ultimately lead to high glucose levels, neuropathy, and visual impairment. The acute management of an elderly diabetic and/or hypoglycemic patient is generally the same as for any other patient. Do not rule out alcohol as a complicating factor, especially in cases of hypoglycemia. In addition, remember that diabetes places the elderly at increased risk of other complications, including atherosclerosis delayed healing, retinopathy, blindness, altered renal function, and severe peripheral vascular disease, leading to foot ulcers and even amputations.
- *Thyroid disorders* occur due to the moderate atrophy and changes in hormone production that come with aging of the thyroid gland. Often when an elderly patient presents with complaints of typical signs and symptoms of hypothyroidism, they are attributed to aging. Common nonspecific complaints in the elderly include mental confusion, anorexia, falls, incontinence, and decreased mobility. Some patients may also experience an increase in muscle or joint pain. Hyperthyroidism is less common among the elderly but may result from medication errors such as an overdose of thyroid hormone replacement. The typical symptom of heat intolerance is often present in the elderly patient. Common nonspecific features or complaints include atrial fibrillation, failure to thrive, abdominal distress, diarrhea, exhaustion, and depression. Since thyroid disorders are not diagnosed in the field, these patients should always be encouraged to go to the hospital for further evaluation.

e. Gastrointestinal

The most frequent GI emergency is bleeding; however, the elderly will describe a variety of other GI complaints such as nausea, poor appetite, diarrhea, and constipation. Remember these conditions may be symptomatic of more serious diseases and should not be downplayed. Keep in mind that older patients are far more intolerant of hypotension and anoxia than younger patients. Treatment should include airway management, support of breathing and circulation, high-flow, high-concentration oxygen therapy, IV fluid replacement with a crystalloid solution, PASG placement (if indicated), and rapid transport. The following are the most serious of the GI problems found in the elderly patient in the field:

- *GI hemorrhage* falls into two general categories of upper GI and lower GI bleeds. The upper GI bleeds include peptic ulcer disease, gastritis, esophageal varices, and Mallory-Weiss tears. Lower GI bleeds include diverticulosis, tumors, ischemic colitis, and arterio-venous malformations. Signs of significant GI blood loss include the presence of "coffee ground" emesis, black tar-like stool (melena), obvious blood in the emesis or stool, orthostatic hypotension, pulse greater than 100 (unless the patient is on beta blockers), and confusion. GI bleeding in the elderly may result in such complications as a recent increase in angina symptoms, congestive heart failure, weakness, or dyspnea.
- *Bowel obstruction* in the elderly typically involves the small bowel. Causes include tumors, prior abdominal surgery, use of certain medications, and occasionally the presence of vertebral compression fractures. The patient will typically complain of diffuse abdominal pain, bloating, nausea, and vomiting. The abdomen may feel distended when palpated and the bowel sounds may be hypoactive or absent. If the obstruction has been present for a prolonged period of time, the patient may have a fever, weakness, shock, and various electrolyte disturbances.

©2004 Pearson Education, Inc.
Intermediate Emergency Care: Principles & Practice

434 DIVISION 5 *Special Considerations*

- *Mesenteric infarct* involves the vessels arising from the superior or inferior mesenteric arteries which serve the bowel. An infarct occurs when a portion of the bowel does not receive enough blood to survive. The primary symptom of a bowel infarct is pain out of proportion to the physical exam. Signs include bloody diarrhea (but usually not a massive hemorrhage), some tachycardia (although there may be a vagal effect masking the sign), and abdominal distention. The patient is at great risk for shock as the dead bowel attracts interstitial and intravascular fluids, thus removing them from use. Necrotic products are released to the peritoneal cavity, leading to a massive infection.

f. Integumentary   pp. 1291–1292

Age-related changes in the immune system make the elderly more prone to certain chronic skin diseases and infections. They are also likely to develop pressure ulcers or bedsores more than any other age group.

- *Skin diseases* elderly patients commonly complain about include pruritus, or itching. This condition can be caused by dermatitis (eczema) or environmental conditions, such as dry air in the home and cold windy air outside. Keep in mind that generalized itching can also be a sign of systemic diseases, particularly liver and renal disorders. When itching is strong and unrelenting, suspect an underlying disease and encourage the patient to seek medical evaluation. Slower healing and compromised tissue perfusion in the elderly makes them more susceptible to bacterial infection of wounds, appearing as cellutitis; impetigo; and, in the case of immunocompromised adults, staphylococcal scalded skin. The elderly also experience a higher incidence of fungal infections, due in part to decreases in the cutaneous immunologic response. In addition, they suffer higher rates of herpes zoster (shingles), which peaks between ages 50 and 70. Most skin disorders are managed in the ED and not in the field setting.
- *Pressure ulcers* (decubitus ulcers) occur commonly in patients over the age of 70. As many as 25% of the patients in nursing homes develop pressure ulcers. Typically the ulcers develop from the waist down, usually over bony prominences, in bedridden patients. They usually result from tissue hypoxia and affect the skin, subcutaneous tissues, and muscle. Factors that can increase the risk of this condition include external compression of tissues, altered sensory perception, maceration caused by excessive moisture, decreased activity, decreased mobility, poor nutrition, friction, or shear. Pressure ulcers are generally not managed in the prehospital setting.

g. Musculoskeletal   pp. 1293–1294

Musculoskeletal diseases are the leading cause of functional impairment in the elderly. Although usually not fatal, musculoskeletal disorders often produce chronic disability, which in turn creates a context for illness. Two of the most widespread disorders are osteoarthritis and osteoporosis.

- *Osteoarthritis* is the leading cause of disability among people age 65 and older. Contributing causes to the disease include loss of muscle mass, obesity, inflammatory arthritis, trauma, and congenital abnormalities such as hip dysplasia. The disease initially presents as joint pain, worsened by exercise and improved by rest. As the disease progresses, pain may be accompanied by diminished mobility, joint deformity, and crepitus or grating sensations. Late signs include tenderness upon palpation or during passive motion. Immobilization, even for short periods, can accelerate the condition.
- *Osteoporosis* affects an estimated 20 million people in the U.S. and is largely responsible for fractures of the hip, wrist, and vertebral bones following a fall or other injury. The risk factors include age (peak bone mass occurs in 3rd and 4th decades of life), gender (women are at a higher risk especially if they experience an early menopause), race (whites and Asians are more likely to have), body weight (thin, light people), family history, genetic factors, use of caffeine, alcohol, and cigarettes. The condition may go unnoticed until the first fracture occurs or a bone density test is done.

h. Renal and Urinary   pp. 1294–1295

The most common renal and urinary disorders in the elderly are discussed below.

Special Considerations

- *Renal diseases* in the elderly include renal failure, glomerulonephritis, and renal blood clots. These problems may be traced to two age-related factors: loss in kidney size and changes in the walls of the renal arteries and in the arterioles serving the glomeruli. In general, the kidney loses approximately one-third of its weight between the ages of 30 and 80. Most of this loss occurs in the tissues that filter blood. When filtering tissue is gone, blood is shunted from the precapillary side directly to venules on the postcapillary side, thus bypassing any tissue still capable of filtering. The result is a reduction in kidney efficiency. This condition is complicated by changes in renal arteries, which promote the development of renal emboli and thrombi. With renal changes, elderly patients are more likely to accumulate toxins and medications within the bloodstream. Occasionally this will be obvious to the patient as he or she experiences a substantial decrease in urine output. More often, however, the elderly are prone to a type of renal failure in which urine output remains normal to high while kidneys remain ineffective in clearing wastes. Processes that precipitate acute renal failure include hypotension, heart failure, major surgery, sepsis, angiographic procedures (the dye is nephrotoxic), and use of nephrotoxic antibiotics. Ongoing hypertension also can contribute to the development of chronic renal failure.
- *Urinary tract infections (UTI)* affect as many as 10% of the elderly each year. Factors that contribute to these infections in the elderly include bladder outlet obstruction from benign prostatic hyperplasia (in men), atrophic vaginitis (in women), stroke, immobilization, use of indwelling bladder catheters, diabetes, upper urinary tract stone, dementia with resulting poor hygiene. The signs or symptoms of a UTI range from cloudy, foul smelling urine to the typical complications of bladder pain and frequent urination. Urosepsis presents as an acute process, including fever, chills, abdominal discomfort, and other signs of septic shock. The septicemia generally begins within 24–72 hours after catheterization or cystoscopy. Treatment of urosepsis commonly includes placement of a large-bore IV catheter for administration of fluids and parenteral antibiotics. Diagnosis of urosepsis is based on history and other physical findings. Prompt transport is critical. The prognosis for elderly patients with urosepsis is poor, with a mortality rate of approximately 30%. Maintenance of fluid balance as well as adequate BP is essential.

12. **Describe the assessment and management of the elderly patient with an environmental emergency.** pp. 1295–1296

Hypothermia. Thermoregulatory emergencies represent some of the most common EMS calls involving the elderly. As a group, the elderly are vulnerable to low temperatures, suffering about 750,000 winter deaths annually, primarily from hypothermia and "winter risks" such as pneumonia and influenza. Factors that predispose the elderly to hypothermia include accidental exposure to cold, CNS disorders, head trauma, stroke, endocrine disorders (particularly hypoglycemia and diabetes), drugs that interfere with heat production, malnutrition or starvation, chronic illness, forced inactivity as a result of a medical condition, low or fixed income (which discourages use of home heating), inflammatory dermatitis, and A-V shunts.

Hypothermic patients may exhibit slow speech, cold skin, confusion, and sleepiness. In early stages, vitals may reveal hypertension and an increased heart rate. As hypothermia progresses, however, blood pressure drops and the heart rate slows, sometimes to a barely detectable level. Keep in mind that the elderly patient with hypothermia often does not shiver. Check the abdomen and back to see if the skin is cool to the touch or, if your unit has a low-temperature thermometer, check the patient's core temperature.

Treatment is focused on rewarming the patient and rapid transport. Once the elderly develop hypothermia, they become progressively impaired, with their condition worsening other chronic medical problems. Remain alert for complications, most commonly cardiac arrest or ventricular fibrillation.

Hyperthermia. Age-related changes in the sweat glands and increased incidence of heart disease place the elderly at risk of heat stress. They may develop heat cramps, heat exhaustion, or heat stroke. Risk factors for severe hyperthermia include altered sensory output, inadequate liquid intake, decreased functioning of the thermoregulatory center, commonly prescribed medications that inhibit sweating (such as antihistamines and tricyclic antidepressants), low or fixed incomes (which may result in a lack of fans or air conditioning), alcoholism, concomitant medical disorders, and use of diuretics (which increase fluid loss).

Early heatstroke may present with nonspecific signs and symptoms such as nausea, light-headedness, dizziness, headache, and high fever. Prevention strategies include adequate fluid intake, reduced activity, shelter in an air conditioned environment, and use of light clothing. If hyperthermia develops, however, rapid treatment and transport are necessary.

13. Describe the assessment and management of the elderly patient with a toxicological or substance abuse problem. pp. 1296–1299

Toxicological problems. Aging alters pharmacokinetics and pharmacodynamics in the elderly. Functional changes in the kidneys, liver, and GI system slow the absorption and elimination of many medications. In addition, the various compensatory mechanisms that help buffer against medication side effects are less effective in the elderly than in younger patients.

Approximately 30 percent of all hospital admissions are related to drug-induced illnesses. About 50 percent of all drug-related deaths occur in people over age 60. Accidental overdoses may occur more frequently in the aged due to confusion, vision impairment, self-selection of medications, forgetfulness, and concurrent drug use. Intentional drug overdose also occurs in attempts at self-destruction. Another complicating factor is the abuse of alcohol in the elderly.

In assessing the elderly patient, always take these steps:
- Obtain a full list of medications currently taken by the patient.
- Elicit any medications that are newly prescribed.
- Obtain a good past medical history, including prior renal or hepatic depression.
- Know your medications, their routes of elimination, and their potential side effects.
- If possible, always take all medications to the hospital along with the patient.

Some of the drugs or substances that have been identified as commonly causing toxicity in the elderly include:

- *Lidocaine.* Lidocaine is recommended for the treatment of ventricular dysrhythmias in the acute setting, especially in acute myocardial infarction and in dysrhythmias that arise from cardiac surgery or catheterization. Patients with liver or kidney problems will have problems metabolizing this drug. Lidocaine toxicity is characterized by vision disturbances, GI effects, tinnitus, trembling, breathing difficulties, dizziness or syncope, seizures, and bradycardic dysrhythmias. Since the cardiac antidysrhythmics in general can cause a decrease in cardiac function and output, observe for shortness of breath, lightheadedness, loss of consciousness, fatigue, chest discomfort, and palpitations.
- *Beta blockers.* Beta blockers are widely used to treat hypertension, angina pectoris, and cardiac dysrhythmias. Elderly patients, however, are susceptible to CNS side effects such as depression, lethargy, and sleep disorders. Because geriatric patients often have pre-existing cardiovascular problems that can cause decreased cardiac function and output, beta blockers will limit the heart's ability to respond to postural changes, causing orthostatic hypotension. Beta blockers also limit the heart's ability to increase contractile force and cardiac output whenever a sympathetic response is necessary in situations such as exercise or hypovolemia. This can be detrimental to the trauma patient who is hemorrhaging and cannot mount the sympathetic response necessary to maintain perfusion of vital organs.

    Treatment of beta-blocker overdoses includes general supportive measures, the removal of gastric contents, support of the ABCs, fluids, and administration of nonadrenergic inotropic agents such as glucagons for hypotension. Excessive bradycardia can be countered with atropine.
- *Antihypertensives/diuretics.* These medications act on the kidneys to increase urine flow and the excretion of water and sodium. They are used primarily in the treatment of hypertension and congestive heart failure. Of these drugs, furosemide is the most widely used diuretic in the elderly. The elimination half-life of furosemide is markedly prolonged in the patient with acute pulmonary edema and renal and hepatic failure. As a result, the geriatric patient is at risk for a drug buildup. Excessive urination caused by the drug may put the elderly at risk for postural hypotension, circulatory collapse, potassium depletion, and renal function impairment. To

reduce this risk, a smaller dose is often prescribed and the patient usually takes a daily potassium supplement.

- *Angiotensin-converting enzyme (ACE) inhibitors.* ACE inhibitors are used for the management of hypertension and congestive heart failure. Geriatric patients generally respond well to treatment with ACE inhibitors. However, these drugs can cause chronic hypotension in patients with severe heart failure who are also taking high-dose loop diuretics. ACE inhibitors can also cause plasma volume reduction and hypotension with prolonged vomiting and diarrhea in the elderly patient. Some hemodialysis patients can experience anaphylactic reactions if treated with ACE inhibitors. Other side effects of ACE inhibitors include dizziness or lightheadedness upon standing, presence of a rash, muscle cramps, swelling of the hands, face, or eyes, cough, headache, stomach upset, and fatigue.

- *Digitalis (digoxin, lanoxin).* Digoxin is the most widely used cardiac glycoside for the management of congestive heart failure, atrial fibrillation, atrial flutter, paroxysmal atrial tachycardia, and cardiogenic shock. The drug is unique in that it has a positive inotropic effect and a negative chronotropic effect. Because digoxin has a low margin of safety and a narrow therapeutic index, the amount of drug required to produce a desired effect is very close to the toxic range. Digoxin toxicity in the elderly can result from accidental or intentional ingestion. In the renally impaired elderly patient, any change in kidney function usually warrants an alteration in the dosing of digoxin. Diuretics, which are often given to patients with congestive heart failure, cause the loss of large amounts of potassium in the urine. If potassium is not adequately replenished in the patient taking digoxin, toxicity will develop.

  Signs and symptoms of digoxin toxicity include visual disturbances, fatigue, weakness, nausea, loss of appetite, abdominal discomfort, dizziness, abnormal dreams, headache, and vomiting. Low potassium (hypokalemia) is also common with chronic digoxin toxicity due to concurrent diuretic therapy. Dysrhythmias commonly associated with digoxin toxicity include sinoatrial (SA) exit block, SA arrest, second- or third-degree AV block, atrial fibrillation with a slow ventricular response, accelerated AV junctional rhythms, patterns of premature ventricular contractions, ventricular tachycardia, and atrial tachycardia with AV block.

  The management of digoxin toxicity includes gastric lavage with activated charcoal, correction of confirmed hypokalemia with K+ supplements, treatment of bradycardias with atropine or pacing, and the treatment of rapid ventricular rhythms with lidocaine. Digoxin-specific FAB fragment antibodies (Digibind), an antidote for digoxin toxicity, is used in the treatment of potentially life-threatening situations.

- *Antipsychotics/antidepressants.* Psychotropic medications comprise a variety of agents that affect mood, behavior, and other aspects of mental function. The elderly often experience a high incidence of psychiatric disorders and may take any number of medications, including antidepressants, anti-anxiety agents, sedative-hypnotic agents, and antipsychotics.

  Antidepressant use in the elderly may result in side effects such as sedation, lethargy, and muscle weakness. Some antidepressants tend to produce anticholinergic effects, including dry mouth, constipation, urinary retention, and confusion. Newly prescribed tricyclic antidepressants can also cause orthostatic hypotension, which can be compounded if the geriatric patient is taking diuretics or other antihypertensive medications. Side effects such as sedation and confusion may also impair the patient's cognitive abilities and possibly endanger the elderly patient who lives alone.

  Antipsychotic medications produce a number of minor side effects such as sedation and anticholinergic effects. Extrapyramidal side effects can also occur, including restlessness and involuntary muscle movements, particularly in the face, jaw, and extremities.

  Field treatment for overdose of antipsychotics and antidepressants is aimed primarily at the ABCs, with special emphasis on airway management.

- *Medications for Parkinson's disease.* Drug treatment for Parkinson's disease is aimed at restoring the balance of neurotransmitters in the basal ganglia. Toxicity of Parkinson's drugs commonly presents as dyskinesia (the inability to execute voluntary movements) and psychological disturbances such as visual hallucinations and nightmares. When these medications are first taken, orthostatic hypotension may also occur. The goal of field management is aimed at decreasing the patient's anxiety and providing a supportive environment. Remember that patients with gross involuntary motor movements are at risk for aspiration and choking.

- *Anti-seizure medications.* Seizure disorders are not uncommon in the elderly, and the selection of anti-seizure medication depends upon the type of seizure present in the patient. The most common side effect of anti-seizure medications is sedation. Other side effects include GI distress, headache, dizziness, lack of coordination, and dermatological reactions (rashes). Recommended treatment involves airway management and supportive therapy.
- *Analgesics and anti-inflammatory agents.* Treatment of pain and inflammation for chronic conditions such as rheumatoid arthritis and osteoarthritis includes narcotics and non-narcotic analgesics and corticosteroids. Adverse side effects of these drugs include sedation, mood changes, nausea, vomiting, and constipation. Orthostatic hypotension and respiratory depression may also occur. Over long periods of time, patients may develop drug tolerance and physical dependence on narcotic agents. In the case of corticosteroids, side effects may include hypertension, peptic ulcer, aggravation of diabetes mellitus, glaucoma, increased risk of infection, and suppression of normally produced corticosteroids.

Substance abuse, drug abuse, alcohol abuse. In general, the factors that contribute to substance abuse among the elderly are different than those of younger people. They include age-related changes, loss of employment, loss of spouse or partner, malnutrition, loneliness, moving from a long-loved home, and multiple prescriptions.

The elderly who become physically and/or psychologically dependent upon drugs or alcohol are more likely to hide their dependence and less likely to seek help than other age groups. Common signs and symptoms of drug abuse include memory changes, drowsiness, decreased vision/hearing, orthostatic hypotension, poor dexterity, mood changes, falling, restlessness, and weight loss. Pertinent findings for alcohol abuse include mood swings, denial and hostility (when questioned about alcohol), confusion, history of falls, anorexia, insomnia, visible anxiety, and nausea.

Treatment follows many of the same steps as for any other patient with a pattern of substance abuse. DO NOT judge the patient. Manage the ABCs and evaluate the need for fluid therapy or medications to accommodate withdrawal. Transport the patient to the hospital for further evaluation and referral.

14. **Describe the assessment and management of the elderly patient with a behavioral or psychological problem.** pp. 1299–1301

Psychological disorders. When behavioral or psychological problems develop later in life, they are often dismissed as normal age-related changes. This attitude denies an elderly person the opportunity to correct a treatable condition and may overlook an underlying physical disorder. It is important to keep in mind the emotionally stressful situations facing many elderly people—isolation, loneliness, loss of self-dependence, loss of strength, and fear of the future. The elderly also face a higher incidence of secondary depression as a result of neuroleptic medications such as Haldol and Thorazine. Some of the common classifications of psychological disorders related to age include organic brain syndrome, affective disorders, neurotic disorders, and paranoid disorders.

Depression and suicide. Up to 15 percent of the non-institutionalized elderly experience depression. Within institutions, that figures rises to about 30 percent. In general, depressed patients should receive supportive care, with caregivers delicately raising questions about suicidal thoughts. Keep in mind that the elderly account for 20 percent of all suicides even though they only represent 12 percent of the total population. In fact, suicide is the third leading cause of death among the elderly, following falls and car accidents.

In cases of seriously depressed patients, elicit behavior patterns from family, friends, or caregivers. Warning signs may include curtailing activities and self-care, breaking from medical or exercise regimens, grieving a personal loss, expressing feelings of uselessness, putting affairs in order, and stock-piling medications. Be particularly alert to suicide among the acutely ill, especially those in a home-care setting.

Your first priorities in the management of a suicidal elderly patient are to protect yourself and then to protect the patient from self-harm. Conduct a brief interview with the patient, if possible, to determine the need for further action. DO NOT leave the suicidal patient alone. Administer medications with caution, keeping in mind polypharmacy and drug interactions in the elderly. (Consult with medical direction.) *All suicidal elderly patients should be transported to the hospital.*

Special Considerations

15. Describe the incidence, morbidity/mortality, risk factors, prevention strategies, pathophysiology, assessment, need for intervention and transport, and management of the elderly trauma patient. pp. 1301–1303

Trauma is the leading cause of death among the elderly. Older patients who sustain moderate to severe injuries are more likely to die than their younger counterparts. Post-injury disability is also more common in the elderly than in the young. Contributing factors to the high incidence and severity of trauma among the elderly include slower reflexes, arthritis, diminished eyesight and hearing predisposing them to accidents (especially falls), high risk for criminal assault (due to physical state and vulnerability), osteoporosis (muscle weakness increases the chance of fractures), reduced cardiac reserve (decreases the ability to compensate for blood loss), decreased respiratory function (increases the likelihood of acute respiratory distress syndrome (ARDS), impaired renal function (decreased ability to adapt to fluid shifts), and decreased elasticity in the peripheral blood vessels (greater susceptibility to tearing).

General assessment of an elderly patient should include determining the MOI. Leading mechanisms include falls, motor-vehicle crashes, burns, assault or abuse, and underlying medical problems such as syncope. In assessing the elderly patient remember that the BP may be deceptive since older patients usually have higher BPs compared to younger patients. Elderly trauma patients also may not exhibit an elevated pulse, which is common in shock because they are on a beta blocker. Fractures may also be obscured or concealed because of a diminished sense of pain among the elderly. One of the best indicators of shock in the elderly is an altered mental status or changes in consciousness during assessment. Elderly trauma patients who exhibit confusion or agitation are candidates for rapid transport.

Whenever assessing the elderly patient observe the scene for signs of abuse and neglect. Abuse of the elderly is as big a problem in our society as child abuse and neglect. Geriatric abuse is defined as a syndrome in which an elderly person has received serious physical or psychological injury from family members or other caregivers. Abuse of the elderly knows no socioeconomic bounds. It often occurs when an older person is no longer able to be totally independent, and the family has difficulty upholding their commitment to care for the patient. It can occur in nursing homes and other health facilities. Signs and symptoms of geriatric abuse and neglect are often obvious. Unexplained trauma is usually the primary presentation. The average abused patient is older than 80 and has multiple medical problems, such as cancer, congestive heart failure, heart disease, and incontinence. Senile dementia is often present. In these cases, it can be hard to determine whether the dementia is chronic or acute, especially if there is an increased likelihood of head trauma from the abuse. Follow your local procedures for reporting and documenting suspected abuse.

General management of trauma to the elderly patient is similar to that of all trauma patients. However, you must keep in mind age-related systemic changes and the presence of chronic diseases. This is especially true of the cardiovascular system, respiratory system, renal system, transport considerations, and the specific injuries discussed below.

- *Cardiovascular considerations*—Recent or past MI may contribute to the risk of dysrhythmia or congestive heart failure in the trauma patient. It may also decrease the response of the heart in adjusting its rate and stroke volume to the stress of hypovolemia. The elderly trauma patient may require higher than usual arterial pressures for perfusion of vital organs, due to increased peripheral vascular resistance and hypertension. Hypotension, hypovolemia, and hypervolemia are poorly tolerated in the elderly patient.
- *Respiratory considerations*—In managing the airway and ventilation in an elderly trauma patient, you must consider the physical changes that may affect treatment. Check for dentures that may need to be removed. Keep in mind age-related changes can decrease chest wall movement and vital capacity. Age also reduces the tolerance of all organs for anoxia. Also, COPD is a widespread problem of the elderly.
- *Renal considerations*—The decreased ability of the kidneys to maintain normal acid/base balance, and to compensate for fluid changes, can further complicate the management of the elderly trauma patient. Any preexisting renal disease can decrease the kidneys' ability to compensate. A decrease in renal function, along with a decreased cardiac reserve, places the elderly injured patient at risk for fluid overload and pulmonary edema.

©2004 Pearson Education, Inc.
Intermediate Emergency Care: Principles & Practice

- *Transport considerations*—You may have to modify positioning, immobilization, and packaging of the elderly trauma patient before transport. Be attentive to physical deformities such as arthritis, spinal abnormalities, or frozen limbs that may cause pain or require special care. Recall the frailty of an elderly person's skin and avoid creating skin tears or pressure sores.

16. Describe the assessment and management of the elderly patient with:

a. Orthopedic injuries   pp. 1304–1305

The elderly suffer the greatest mortality and greatest incidence of disability from falls. Approximately 33 percent of the falls in the elderly result in at least one fractured bone. The most common fall-related fracture is a fracture of the hip or pelvis. Falls also result in a variety of stress fractures in the elderly, including fractures of the proximal humerus, distal radius, proximal tibia, and thoracic and lumbar bodies. In treating orthopedic injuries, remember to ask questions aimed at detecting an underlying medical condition.

b. Burns   pp. 1305–1306

People age 60 and older are more likely to suffer death from burns than any other age group except neonates and infants. Factors that help explain the high mortality rate among the elderly include age-related changes that slow reaction time, pre-existing diseases that increase the risk of medical complications, age-related skin changes (thinning) that increase the severity of burns, immunological and metabolic changes that increase the risk of infection, and reductions in physiologic function and the reduced reserves of several organ systems that make the elderly more vulnerable to systemic stress.

Management of the elderly burn patient follows the same general procedures as other patients. However, remember that the elderly are at increased risk of shock. Administration of fluids is important to prevent renal tubular damage. Assess hydration in the initial hours after the burn injury by blood pressure, pulse, and urine output. Keep in mind that complications in the elderly may manifest themselves in the days and weeks following the incident. For serious burns to heal, the body may use up to 20,000 calories a day. Elderly patients, with altered metabolisms and complications such as diabetes, may not be able to meet this demand, increasing the chances for infection and systemic failure. Part of your job may be to prepare the family for such a delayed response.

c. Head and spinal injuries   p. 1306

As people age, the brain decreases in size and weight. The skull, however, remains constant in size, allowing the brain more room to move, thus increasing the likelihood of brain injury. Because of this, the signs and symptoms of brain injury may develop more slowly in the elderly patient, sometimes over days or weeks. In fact, the patient may often have forgotten the offending incident.

The cervical spine is also more susceptible to injury due to osteoporosis and spondylosis—a degeneration of the vertebral body. In addition, arthritic changes can gradually compress the nerve rootlets or spinal cord. Thus, injury to the spine in the elderly makes them much more susceptible to spinal cord injury. Therefore, it is important to provide older patients with suspected spinal-cord injury, especially those involved in motor vehicle collisions, with immediate manual cervical stabilization at the time of initial assessment.

17. Given several pre-programmed simulated geriatric patients with various complaints, provide the appropriate assessment, management, and transport.   pp. 1261–1306

During your classroom, clinical, and field training, you will assess real and simulated geriatric patients and develop a management plan for them. Use the information presented in this text chapter, the information on assessment of geriatric patients in the field presented by your instructors, and the guidance given by your clinical and field preceptors to develop good patient assessment skills. Continue to refine these skills once your training ends and you begin your career as an EMT-I.

©2004 Pearson Education, Inc.
Intermediate Emergency Care: Principles & Practice

Special Considerations

CASE STUDY REVIEW

This case study draws attention to the importance of recognizing the vital lives led by elderly people and the need to take their complaints seriously, rather than dismissing them as normal age-related changes.

The case study puts you in the position of an EMT-I who decides to teach a student intern about the treatment of elderly patients. At the end of the call, the intern is asked: "So Andy, do you want to talk about what went right with this call and what we could have done better while we restock the ambulance?"

So let's discuss it! The complaint of abdominal pain can be caused by many different factors, most of which cannot not be resolved in an out-of-hospital setting. Even so, after reading the text, you now know that the most frequent gastrointestinal emergency in the elderly is GI bleeding, a condition that can place the elderly at a significant risk of hemorrhage and shock. The elderly are also far more intolerant of hypotension and anoxia than younger patients. Any GI emergency should be aggressively managed.

In this case, the initial assessment ruled out an immediate life threat. The general impression was that of an elderly woman with severe abdominal pain. As noted, the pain was out of proportion to the physical exam—a symptom suggestive of mesenteric infarct. Care steps included administration of high-flow oxygen, IV fluid replacement therapy with a crystalloid solution, and, most importantly, rapid transport.

It was correct to place the patient on a cardiac monitor. An ECG of atrial fibrillation is common in elderly patients. Based on the patient's vital signs, Mrs. Hildegaard seemed to be tolerating the dysrhythmias. The monitor helped show that the pain was not cardiac-related, though complications could result, depending upon pre-existing medical conditions.

It might have been helpful to inquire in more detail about any other GI distress experienced by the patient, such as diarrhea, vomiting, and nausea. Also, a pulse oximeter might have been useful to measure the patient's oxygen saturation en route to the hospital. However, considering the patient's presentation, she was managed appropriately.

Andy's quip about a beer and taco provided a "teachable moment" in that it corrected a mistaken attitude about the aging process—the idea that an elderly patient might not live like a younger counterpart. In fact, it would have been relevant to ask just what the patient ate—and drank—at dinner. It also highlighted the problem of alcohol abuse among the elderly. They are not only exposed to the stresses of aging, but age-related systemic changes and medical problems make it more difficult for them to metabolize alcohol or many other drugs. So it would have also been relevant to ask whether Mrs. Hildegaard consumed alcohol on a regular basis.

CONTENT SELF-EVALUATION

MULTIPLE CHOICE

_____ 1. All of the following are responsible for the growing number of elderly people in the United States—and the projected increase in the number of elderly patients treated by EMS services—EXCEPT a(n):
   A. increase in the mean survival rate of older persons.
   B. increase in the birth rate.
   C. absence of major wars.
   D. improved health care.
   E. higher standard of living.

_____ 2. The scientific study of the effects of aging and of age-related diseases on humans is known as:
   A. geriatrics.   D. eldercare.
   B. ageism.   E. gerontotherapeutics.
   C. gerontology.

3. The existence of multiple diseases in the elderly is known as:
   A. functional impairment.   D. polypharmacy.
   B. dysphagia.   E. senility.
   C. comorbidity.

4. Common complaints in the elderly include:
   A. falls, weakness, syncope.   D. MVC, meningitis, poisoning.
   B. fractures, drowning, diabetes. E. fever, epiglottitis, febrile seizures.
   C. GSW, croup, nausea.

5. When compared to younger patients, the elderly experience fewer adverse drug reactions.
   A. True
   B. False

6. Drugs concentrate more readily in the plasma and tissues of elderly patients because of:
   A. diminished neurologic function.
   B. increased body fluid.
   C. atrophy of organs.
   D. more efficient compensatory mechanisms.
   E. increased renal function.

7. Factors that can decrease medication compliance in the elderly include all of the following EXCEPT:
   A. limited mobility.   D. multiple-compartment pill boxes.
   B. fear of toxicity.   E. sensory impairment.
   C. child-proof containers.

8. Factors that can increase medication compliance in the elderly include:
   A. compliance counseling.   D. blister-pack packaging.
   B. a belief that an illness is serious. E. all of the above
   C. clear, simple directions.

9. A lack of mobility can have detrimental physical and emotional effects on the elderly.
   A. True
   B. False

10. Which of the following is the leading cause of accidental deaths among the elderly?
    A. drownings   D. gunshot wounds
    B. fall-related injuries   E. poisonings
    C. motor vehicle collisions

11. Intrinsic factors that can cause an elderly person to fall include all of the following EXCEPT:
    A. dizziness.   D. impaired vision.
    B. slippery floors.   E. CNS problems.
    C. decreased mental status.

12. Extrinsic factors that can cause an elderly person to fall include:
    A. an altered gait.   D. use of certain medications.
    B. a sense of weakness.   E. a history of repeated falls.
    C. a lack of hand rails.

13. The inability to retain urine or feces because of loss of sphincter control or because of cerebral or spinal lesions is called:
    A. diarrhea.   D. incontinence.
    B. involuntary elimination.   E. uremia.
    C. diuresis.

_____ 14. In elderly people with cerebrovascular disease or impaired baroreceptor reflexes, efforts to force a bowel movement can lead to a transient ischemic attack.
   A. True
   B. False

_____ 15. Possible causes of elimination problems in the elderly include:
   A. diverticular disease.
   B. constipation.
   C. colorectal cancer.
   D. use of opioids.
   E. all of the above

_____ 16. One of the most common reasons that elderly patients underestimate the severity of a primary medical problem is that they have a(n):
   A. shrinkage of structures in the ear.
   B. clouding and thickening of lenses in the eyes.
   C. lowered sensitivity to pain.
   D. deterioration of the teeth and gums.
   E. altered sense of taste.

_____ 17. All of the following factors play a part in forming a general assessment of the elderly patient EXCEPT:
   A. average cost of rent.
   B. medication history.
   C. living situations.
   D. sleep patterns.
   E. level of nutrition.

_____ 18. Conditions that may discourage eating among the elderly include:
   A. breathing or respiratory problems.
   B. nausea or vomiting.
   C. poor dental care.
   D. alcohol or drug abuse.
   E. all of the above

_____ 19. Which of the following is a byproduct of malnutrition?
   A. electrolyte abnormalities
   B. dehydration
   C. vitamin deficiencies
   D. hypoglycemia
   E. all of the above

_____ 20. The elderly are more prone to environmental thermal problems due to changes in the sweat glands.
   A. True
   B. False

_____ 21. A medical condition in which eye pressure increases and ultimately diminishes sight is known as:
   A. Meniere's disease.
   B. tinnitus.
   C. cataracts.
   D. glaucoma.
   E. retinitis.

_____ 22. A disease of the inner ear characterized by vertigo, nerve deafness, and a roar or buzzing in the ear is called:
   A. Meniere's disease.
   B. tinnitus.
   C. cataracts.
   D. glaucoma.
   E. cerumen.

_____ 23. To improve communication with an elderly patient, you should try to:
   A. display verbal and nonverbal signs of concern.
   B. dim the room lights.
   C. avoid looking directly into the patient's eyes.
   D. first talk to family members, then the patient.
   E. remain as quiet as possible.

_____ 24. Both senility and organic brain syndrome may manifest themselves as:
   A. distractibility.
   B. excitability.
   C. hostility.
   D. restlessness.
   E. all of the above

©2004 Pearson Education, Inc.
Intermediate Emergency Care: Principles & Practice

_____ 25. When assessing an elderly person, if they are confused or disoriented, you can conclude that the patient is senile.
  A. True
  B. False

_____ 26. Changes in mental status in the elderly patient may be due to which of the following?
  A. traumatic head injury
  B. dementia
  C. decreased sugar level
  D. infection
  E. all of the above

_____ 27. To help reduce an elderly patient's fears, you should:
  A. downplay the patient's fears.
  B. ignore nonverbal messages.
  C. discourage the expression of feelings.
  D. confirm what the patient has said.
  E. instruct the patient to calm down.

_____ 28. Compared to younger people, the skin of elderly people:
  A. is thicker and oilier.
  B. heals more quickly.
  C. tears less easily.
  D. is less subject to fungal infections.
  E. perspires less.

_____ 29. The elderly have a greater risk of trauma-related complications due a decrease in blood volume.
  A. True
  B. False

_____ 30. Age-related changes to the respiratory system include all of the following EXCEPT:
  A. increased chest wall compliance.
  B. diminished breathing capacity.
  C. reduced strength and endurance.
  D. increased air trapping.
  E. reduced gag reflex.

_____ 31. The decrease of an effective cough reflex and the activity of the _____ make the elderly more prone to respiratory infection.
  A. gag reflex
  B. alveoli
  C. cilia
  D. bronchioles
  E. vagal response

_____ 32. In treating respiratory disorders in the elderly patient, do not fluid overload.
  A. True
  B. False

_____ 33. An exaggeration of the normal posterior curvature of the spine is called:
  A. scoliosis.
  B. kyphosis.
  C. fibrosis.
  D. hypertrophy.
  E. spondylosis.

_____ 34. An increase in the size and bulk of the left ventricle wall in some elderly patients is an example of:
  A. kyphosis.
  B. anoxia hypoxemia.
  C. hypertrophy.
  D. fibrosis.
  E. Marfan's syndrome.

_____ 35. In managing elderly patients with complaints related to the cardiovascular system, take all of the following steps EXCEPT:
  A. inquire about age-related dosages.
  B. provide high-concentration supplemental oxygen.
  C. walk the patient slowly to the rig.
  D. remain empathetic to the patient's fears.
  E. start an IV for medication administration.

Special Considerations

_____ 36. All of the following are age-related changes to the nervous system EXCEPT:
  A. decreased reaction time.
  B. increased brain weight.
  C. impaired balance.
  D. shrinkage of brain tissue.
  E. recent memory loss.

_____ 37. The elderly are less susceptible to subdural hematomas than younger people.
  A. True
  B. False

_____ 38. Age-related changes in the gastrointestinal system include all of the following EXCEPT:
  A. impaired swallowing.
  B. diminished digestive functions.
  C. decreased liver efficiency.
  D. a predisposition to choking.
  E. increased gastric secretions.

_____ 39. A protrusion of the stomach upward into the mediastinal cavity through the diaphragm is known as:
  A. a hiatal hernia.
  B. Marfan's syndrome.
  C. a diaphragmatic hernia.
  D. an inguinal hernia.
  E. an epigastric hernia.

_____ 40. Reasons that the elderly develop pneumonia more frequently than younger people include all of the following EXCEPT a(n):
  A. decreased immune response.
  B. increased pulmonary function.
  C. abnormal or ineffective cough reflex.
  D. decreased activity of mucociliary cells.
  E. decreased colonization of the pharynx by gram-negative bacteria.

_____ 41. An elderly patient in an institutional setting is up to 50 times more likely to contract pneumonia that an elderly patient receiving home care.
  A. True
  B. False

_____ 42. The usual signs and symptoms of COPD include:
  A. cough and wheezing.
  B. dyspnea and tachypnea.
  C. exercise intolerance.
  D. pleuritic chest pain.
  E. all of the above

_____ 43. The most effective prevention of COPD involves:
  A. elimination of smoking.
  B. lowering blood sugar.
  C. reducing physical activity.
  D. lowering blood pressure.
  E. use of supplemental oxygen.

_____ 44. Your elderly patient is complaining of acute onset of sharp chest pain and shortness of breath. The patient was recently released from the hospital for a leg fracture. What is the most likely suspected disorder?
  A. pneumonia
  B. pulmonary embolism
  C. heart attack
  D. COPD
  E. pulmonary edema

_____ 45. Although all of the following can contribute to a pulmonary embolism, the condition is most frequently caused by:
  A. fat.
  B. bone marrow.
  C. blood clots.
  D. tumor cells.
  E. air.

_____ 46. The leading cause of death in the elderly is:
  A. pneumonia.
  B. stroke.
  C. cardiovascular disease.
  D. Alzheimer's disease.
  E. COPD.

©2004 Pearson Education, Inc.
Intermediate Emergency Care: Principles & Practice

_____ 47. The heart sounds in an elderly patient are generally louder than those in a young patient.
   A. True
   B. False

_____ 48. All of the following are atypical presentations of a myocardial infarction in the elderly EXCEPT:
   A. syncope.
   B. tearing chest pain.
   C. dyspnea.
   D. neck or dental pain.
   E. exercise intolerance.

_____ 49. Assessment findings specific to the elderly such as anorexia, nocturia, dependent edema, and hepatomegaly may be found in a patient with:
   A. a pulmonary embolism.
   B. heart failure.
   C. hypertension.
   D. an aneurysm.
   E. syncope.

_____ 50. An abnormal dilation of a blood vessel, usually an artery, due to a congenital defect or weakness in the wall of the vessel is called:
   A. an aneurysm.
   B. an infarct.
   C. thrombosis.
   D. an embolism.
   E. a hernia.

_____ 51. A series of symptoms resulting from decreased blood flow to the brain that are caused by a sudden decrease in cardiac output from a heart block are known as:
   A. autonomic dysfunction.
   B. Stokes-Adams syndrome.
   C. sick sinus syndrome.
   D. dying heart muscle.
   E. Marfan's syndrome.

_____ 52. Injury to or death of brain tissue resulting from interruption of cerebral blood flow and oxygenation is called a(n):
   A. subarachnoid hemorrhage.
   B. autonomic dysfunction.
   C. TIA.
   D. stroke.
   E. intracerebral hemorrhage.

_____ 53. Common causes of seizures in the elderly include all of the following EXCEPT:
   A. head trauma.
   B. alcohol withdrawal.
   C. spinal injury.
   D. stroke.
   E. hypoglycemia.

_____ 54. A progressive, degenerative disease that attacks the brain and results in impaired memory, thinking, and behavior is called:
   A. dementia.
   B. Parkinson's disease.
   C. delirium.
   D. Alzheimer's disease.
   E. aphasia.

_____ 55. A chronic, degenerative nervous disease characterized by tremors, muscular weakness and rigidity, and loss of postural reflexes is called:
   A. Parkinson's disease.
   B. Shy-Drager syndrome.
   C. Alzheimer's disease.
   D. sick sinus syndrome.
   E. grand mal seizure.

_____ 56. All of the following are forms of upper GI bleed EXCEPT:
   A. peptic ulcer disease.
   B. ischemic colitis.
   C. esophageal varices.
   D. gastritis.
   E. peptic ulcer disease.

_____ 57. An example of a lower GI bleed is:
   A. a Mallory-Weiss tear.
   B. diverticulosis.
   C. peptic ulcer disease.
   D. a bowel obstruction.
   E. a mesenteric infarct.

_____ 58. An inflammation of the colon due to impaired or decreased blood supply is called:
   A. diverticulosis.   D. colostomy.
   B. ischemic colitis.   E. gastritis.
   C. arterio-venous malformation.

_____ 59. An abnormal dilation of veins in the lower esophagus common in patients with cirrhosis of the liver is called esophageal varices.
   A. True
   B. False

_____ 60. The acute skin eruption caused by a reactivation of latent varicella virus that peaks between ages 50 and 70 is known as:
   A. shingles.   D. herpes zoster.
   B. pruritus.   E. both A and D
   C. maceration.

_____ 61. When transporting an elderly patient with pressure ulcers, you should encourage the patient to remain still.
   A. True
   B. False

_____ 62. Risk factors for osteoporosis include all of the following EXCEPT:
   A. African or Latino ancestry.   D. family history of fractures.
   B. low body weight.   E. use of caffeine, alcohol, and cigarettes.
   C. early menopause.

_____ 63. In general, the kidney loses approximately one-third of its weight between the ages of 30 and 80.
   A. True
   B. False

_____ 64. All of the following are signs and symptoms of hypothermia in an elderly patient EXCEPT:
   A. confusion.   D. skin cool to the touch.
   B. slow speech.   E. sleepiness.
   C. shivering.

_____ 65. Elderly patients with hepatic impairment and decreased renal function should receive the normal dose of lidocaine.
   A. True
   B. False

MATCHING

Write the letter of the term in the space provided next to the appropriate description.

   A. epistaxis   I. polycythemia
   B. varicosities   J. delirium
   C. sick sinus syndrome   K. senile dementia
   D. autonomic dysfunction   L. vertigo
   E. transient ischemic attack   M. mesenteric infarct
   F. brain ischemia   N. spondylosis
   G. urosepsis   O. dysphoria
   H. nocturia

_____ 66. acute alteration in mental functioning that is often reversible

_____ 67. septicemia originating from the urinary tract

_____ 68. medical term for a nosebleed

_____ 69. excessive urination, usually at night

©2004 Pearson Education, Inc.
Intermediate Emergency Care: Principles & Practice

_____ 70. death of tissue in the peritoneal fold that encircles the small intestine

_____ 71. exaggerated feeling of depression or unrest

_____ 72. excess of red blood cells

_____ 73. abnormal dilation of a vein

_____ 74. group of disorders characterized by dysfunction of the SA node

_____ 75. sensation of faintness or dizziness causing loss of balance

_____ 76. general term used to describe an abnormal decline in mental function in the elderly

_____ 77. degeneration of the vertebral body

_____ 78. abnormality of the involuntary aspect of the nervous system

_____ 79. injury to the brain tissues caused by an inadequate supply of oxygen and nutrients

_____ 80. medical condition like a stroke but reversible and commonly involving syncope

Chapter 33

Assessment-Based Management

Review of Chapter Objectives

After reading this chapter, you should be able to:

1. Explain how effective assessment is critical to clinical decision making.   pp. 1310–1311

Assessment forms the foundation for patient care. You can't treat or report a problem that is not found or identified. To find a problem, you must gather, evaluate, and synthesize information. Based on this process, you can then make a decision and take the appropriate actions to formulate a management plan and determine the priorities for patient care.

An EMT-I is entrusted with a great deal of independent judgment and responsibility for performing correct actions for each individual patient, including such advanced skills as ECG interpretation, rapid sequence intubation, and medication administration. Additionally, the medical director and hospital staff must rely on your experience and expertise as you describe the patient's condition and your conclusions about it. Consequently, the ability to reason and to reach a field diagnosis is critical to EMT-I practice.

2. Explain how the EMT-Intermediate's attitude and uncooperative patients affect assessment and decision making.   pp. 1311–1313

Attitude

Your attitude is one of the most critical factors in performing an effective assessment. You must be as nonjudgmental as possible to avoid "short-circuiting" accurate data collection and pattern recognition by leaping to conclusions before completing a thorough assessment. Remember the popular computer mnemonic GIGO—garbage in/garbage out. You can't reach valid conclusions about your patient based on hasty or incomplete assessment. Seek to identify any preconceived notions that you may have about a group and then work to eliminate them.

Uncooperative patients

Admittedly, uncooperative patients make it difficult to perform good assessments. However, you must remember that there are many possible causes for patient belligerence. Whenever you assess an uncooperative or a restless patient, consider medical causes for the behavior—hypoxia, hypovolemia, hypoglycemia, or a head injury. Be careful not to jump to the conclusion that the patient is "just another drunk" or a "frequent flyer." The frequent flier that you have transported for alcoholic behavior in the past may, this time, be suffering from trauma or a medical emergency.

In addition, cultural and ethnic barriers—as well as prior negative experiences—may cause a patient to lack confidence in the rescuers. Such situations make it difficult for you to be effective at the scene, and the patient in fact may refuse to provide express consent for treatment or transport. However, it is your job to increase patient confidence. Become familiar with the cultural customs of any large ethnic populations in your area. Find out about available translation services. Above all, don't permit yourself to make snap judgments about the patient.

©2004 Pearson Education, Inc.
Intermediate Emergency Care: Principles & Practice

3. Explain strategies to prevent labeling, tunnel vision, and to decrease environmental distractions.

pp. 1310–1313

A number of factors—both internal (for example, your personal attitudes) and external (for example, the patient's attitude, distracting injuries, or environmental factors at the scene)—can affect your assessment of the patient and ultimately your decisions on how to manage treatment.

Labeling and tunnel vision

The dangers of labeling have been discussed in objective 2. However, another internal factor that can negatively affect your assessment is tunnel vision. Do not focus on distracting injuries, such as a scalp laceration, that look worse than they really are. Instead, resist the temptation to form a field diagnosis too early. Always take a systematic approach to patient assessment to avoid distractions and to find and prioritize care for all of the patient's injuries and conditions. In general, follow an inverted pyramid format that progresses from a differential diagnosis to a narrowing process to your field diagnosis. (For more information on the inverted pyramid format, see the diagram on page 1309 of your textbook.)

Environmental distractions

You've probably already experienced some of the environmental factors that can affect patient assessment and care—scene chaos, violent or dangerous situations, high noise levels, crowds of bystanders, or even crowds of responders. Limit these distractions through the careful staging of personnel (see objectives 4 and 5). In the case of a large number of rescuers, you might assign crowd control tasks to some of them or stage them nearby. They can then be brought to the scene when and if necessary. Finally, you might change environments completely. Sometimes the best way to deal with excessive environmental noise and distractions is to rapidly load the patient into the ambulance and leave the scene. You can always pull over for further assessment in a quieter environment.

4. Describe how personnel considerations and staffing configurations affect assessment and decision making.

pp. 1313–1314

As a rule, assessment is best achieved by one rescuer. A single EMT-I can gather information and provide treatment sequentially. In the case of two EMT-Is, one EMT-I can assess the patient, while the other provides simultaneous treatment. With multiple responders, however, assessment and history may take place entirely by "committee," which often leads to disorganized management. It can also be difficult to manage a patient if the responders are all at the same professional level and have no clear direction. Therefore, it is important to plan for these events so that personnel can have pre-designated roles. These roles may be rotated among team members so no one is left out, but there must be a plan to avoid "freelancing." If there is only one EMT-I, then that person must assume all ALS roles.

5. Synthesize and apply concepts of scene management and choreography to simulated emergency calls.

pp. 1313–1314

Points in the textbook and direction by your instructors and clinical or field preceptors will help you to manage and choreograph simulated emergency calls. When approaching these practice sessions, remember the importance of an effective preplan. In the case of a two-person team, the roles of team care leader and patient care provider can be assigned on an alternating basis. EMT-Is who work together regularly may develop their own plan, but a universally understood plan allows for other rescuers to participate in a rescue without interrupting the flow. While the dynamics of field situations may necessitate changes in plans, a general "game plan" can go a long way toward preventing chaos. If field dynamics dictate a change in the preplanned roles, you are still working from a solid base.

6. Explain the roles of the team leader and the patient care person.

p. 1314

In setting up a two-person team, keep in mind the general tasks performed by the team leader and patient care provider as outlined below.

Roles of Team Leader	Roles of Patient Care Provider
Establishes patient contact	Provides "scene cover"
Obtains history	Gathers scene information
Performs physical exam	Talks to relatives/bystanders
Presents patient	Obtains vital signs
Handles documentation	Performs interventions
Acts as EMS commander	Acts as triage group leader

7. List and explain the rationale for bringing the essential care items to the patient. pp. 1314–1315

Having the right equipment at the patient's side is essential. As an EMT-I, you must be prepared to manage many conditions and injuries or changes in the patient's condition. Assessment and management must usually be done simultaneously. If you do not have the right equipment readily available, then you have compromised patient care and, in fact, the patient may die.

8. When given a simulated call, list the appropriate equipment to be taken to the patient. pp. 1314–1315

Think of your equipment as items in a backpack. Just like backpacking, you must downsize your equipment to minimum weight and bulk to facilitate rapid movement. At the same time, you need certain essential items to ensure survival—in this case, patient survival. The following is a list of the essential equipment for EMT-I management of life-threatening conditions. You must bring these items to the side of every patient, regardless of what you initially think you may need.

- Infection Control
    —Infection control supplies—e.g., gloves, eye shields
- Airway Control
    —Oral airways
    —Nasal airways
    —Suction (electric or manual)
    —Rigid tonsil-tip and flexible suction catheters
    —Laryngoscope and blades
    —Endotracheal tubes, stylettes, syringes, tape
- Breathing
    —Pocket mask
    —Manual ventilation bag-valve mask
    —Spare masks in various sizes
    —Oxygen masks, cannulas, and extension tubing
    —Occlusive dressings
    —Large-bore IV catheter for thoracic decompression
- Circulation
    —Dressings
    —Bandages and tape
    —Sphygmomanometer, stethoscope
    —Note pad and pen or pencil
- Disability
    —Rigid collars
    —Flashlights
- Dysrhythmia
    —Cardiac monitor/defibrillator
- Exposure and Protection
    —Scissors
    —Space blankets or something to cover the patient

You may also pack some optional "take in" equipment, such as drug therapy and venous access supplies. The method by which these supplies are carried may depend upon how your system is designed—e.g., EMT-I ambulances versus EMT-Is in non-transporting vehicles. It may also

©2004 Pearson Education, Inc.
Intermediate Emergency Care: Principles & Practice

depend upon local protocols, flexibility of standing orders, the number of EMT-I responders in your area, and the difficulty of accessing patients because of terrain or some other problem.

9. Explain the general approach to the emergency patient. pp. 1315–1319

In addition to having the right equipment, you need to have the essential demeanor to calm or reassure the patient. You must look and act the professional, while exhibiting the compassion and understanding associated with an effective "bedside manner." While patients may not have the ability to rate your medical performance, they can certainly rate your people skills and service. Be aware of your body language and the messages it sends, either intentionally or unintentionally. Think carefully about what you say and how you say it—this includes your conversations with other members of the ALS team and anyone else on the scene.

Once again, it helps to preplan your general approach to the patient. This will prevent confusion and improve the accuracy of your assessment. One team member should engage in an active, concerned dialogue with the patient. This same person should also demonstrate the listening skills needed to collect information and to convey a caring attitude. Taking notes may prevent asking the same question repeatedly as well as ensuring that you acquire and pass on accurate data.

10. Explain the general approach, patient assessment differentials, and management priorities for patients with various types of emergencies that may be experienced in prehospital care. pp. 1310–1319

Scene size-up
Before approaching the patient (see objective 9), you must carefully size up the scene. The scene size-up has the following components: body substance isolation, ensuring scene safety, locating all patients, and identifying the mechanism of injury or the nature of the illness.

Initial assessment
After you size up the scene, you quickly begin the initial assessment for the purpose of detecting and treating immediate life threats. The components of the initial assessment are:

- Forming a general impression
- Determining mental status (AVPU)
- Assessing airway, breathing, and circulation
- Determining the patient's priority for further on-scene care or immediate transport

Depending upon your findings during initial assessment, you might take either the contemplative or the resuscitative approach to patient care. You might also decide to immediately transport the patient.

Contemplative approach. In general, use the contemplative approach when immediate intervention is not necessary. In such situations, the focused history and physical exam, followed by any required interventions can be performed at the scene, before transport to the hospital.

Resuscitative approach. Use the resuscitative approach whenever you suspect a life-threatening problem, including:

- Cardiac or respiratory arrest
- Respiratory distress or failure
- Unstable dysrhythmias
- Status epilepticus
- Coma or altered mental status
- Shock or hypotension
- Major trauma
- Possible C-spine injury

In these cases, you must take immediate resuscitative action (such as CPR, defibrillation, or ventilation) or other critical action (such as supplemental oxygen, control of major bleeding, or C-spine immobilization). Additional assessment and care can be performed after resuscitation and the rapid trauma assessment and/or en route to the hospital.

Immediate evacuation. In some cases, you will need to immediately evacuate the patient to the ambulance. For example, a patient with severe internal bleeding requires life-saving interventions beyond an EMT-I's skills. You might also resort to immediate evacuation if the scene is too chaotic for rational assessment or if it is too unsafe or unstable.

Focused history and physical exam

Following the initial assessment, you will perform the focused history and physical exam. Based on the patient's chief complaint and the information gathered during the initial assessment, you should consider your patient to belong to one of the following four categories:

- Trauma patient with a significant mechanism of injury or altered mental status
- Trauma patient with an isolated injury
- Medical patient who is unresponsive
- Medical patient who is responsive

For a trauma patient with a significant MOI or altered mental status or for an unresponsive medical patient, perform a complete head-to-toe physical examination (rapid trauma assessment for the trauma patient, rapid medical assessment for the medical patient). For a trauma patient with an isolated injury or for a responsive medical patient, perform a physical exam focused on body systems related to the chief complaint.

Ongoing assessment and detailed physical exam

The ongoing assessment must be performed on all patients to monitor and to observe trends in the person's condition—every 5 minutes if the patient is unstable, every 15 minutes if the patient is stable. Ongoing assessments must be performed until the patient is transferred to the care of hospital personnel. The ongoing assessment includes evaluation of the following:

- Mental status
- Airway, breathing, and circulation
- Transport priorities
- Vital signs
- Focused assessment of any problem areas or conditions
- Effectiveness of interventions
- Management plans

The detailed physical exam is similar to but more thorough than the rapid trauma assessment. It is generally performed only on trauma patients and only if time and the patient's condition permit.

Identification of life-threatening problems

At all stages of the assessment, from initial assessment through ongoing assessments, from the scene to the ambulance to arrival at the hospital, you must actively and continuously look for and manage any life-threatening problems. Basically your role as an EMT-I is to rapidly and accurately assess the patient and then to treat for the worst-case scenario. This is the underlying principle of assessment-based management—your guide to providing effective medical care.

---

11. **Describe how to effectively communicate patient information face to face, over the telephone, by radio, and in writing.** pp. 1319–1320

The ability to communicate effectively is the key to transferring patient information, whether in an out-of-hospital setting or within the hospital itself. Although neither basic nor advanced life-support interventions may be required for every patient, a skill that will be used on every single patient is that of presentation, whether it is over the radio or telephone, in writing, or in face-to-face transfers at the receiving facility.

Effective presentation and communication skills help establish an EMT-I's credibility. They also inspire trust and confidence in patients. If you present your assessment, your findings, and your treatment in a clear, concise manner, you give the impression of a job well done. A poor presentation, on the other hand, implies poor assessment and poor patient care.

©2004 Pearson Education, Inc.
Intermediate Emergency Care: Principles & Practice

The most effective oral presentations usually meet these guidelines:
- Last less than one minute
- Are very concise and clear
- Avoid excessive use of medical jargon
- Follow a basic format, usually the SOAP format or some variation
- Include both pertinent findings and pertinent negatives
- Conclude with specific actions, requests, or questions related to the plan

An ideal presentation should include the following:
- Patient identification, age, sex, and degree of distress
- Chief complaint
- Present illness/injury
  —Pertinent details about the present problem
  —Pertinent negatives
- Past medical history
  —Allergies
  —Medications
  —Pertinent medical history
- Physical signs
  —Vital signs
  —Pertinent positive findings
  —Pertinent negative findings
- Assessment
  — EMT-I impression
- Plan
  —What has been done
  —Orders requested

12. **Given various preprogrammed and moulaged patients, provide the appropriate scene size-up, initial assessment, focused assessment, and detailed assessment, then provide the appropriate care, ongoing assessments, and patient transport.** pp. 1310–1320

In order to develop as an entry-level practitioner at the EMT-I level, it is important to participate in scenario-based reviews of commonly encountered complaints. Laboratory-based simulations require you to assess a preprogrammed patient or mannequin. Use the information presented in the textbook, the information on assessment-based management provided by your instructors, and the guidance given by your clinical and field preceptors to develop good assessment-based management skills. Remember—the chance to practice does not stop at the classroom. While an EMT-I student or the new member of a team, take advantage of every opportunity to practice your new skills.

CASE STUDY REVIEW

This case study leads you through the thought process of an EMT-I who uses "inverted reasoning"— the foundation of assessment-based management—to choreograph a call involving a patient injured in a single-vehicle crash.

The EMT-I starts planning the call from the moment of dispatch, listing possible medical conditions and injuries that might be found upon arrival and reviewing the equipment that should be taken to the patient's side. Upon arrival, the EMT-I determines scene safety—the most important concern on any run—before determining the approach. Paramount on the EMT-I's mind is quick identification and treatment of any life-threatening injuries. Before even reaching the patient, the EMT-I has formed a general impression of a seriously injured patient—one who will in all likelihood require a resuscitative approach.

The importance of having the right equipment becomes clear as the EMT-I conducts the initial assessment. The EMT-I also illustrates the role of a team leader, quickly assigning additional personnel as they arrive on the scene. Ignoring distracting injuries, the EMT-I identifies immediate life threats, prioritizes care, and prepares the patient for immediate transport.

Despite obvious trauma, the EMT-I does not forget to rule out medical complications that may have led to the crash. Because of the seriousness of the injury, the ALS team stays with the patient in the back of the ambulance, while an EMT from another crew volunteers to drive.

In the end, it is all those little things—the right equipment at the patient's side, good scene choreography, use of inverted reasoning, good presentation skills, and more—that can save a life.

CONTENT SELF-EVALUATION

MULTIPLE CHOICE

_____ 1. Which of the following gives the correct order of steps in the clinical decision making of the inverted pyramid?
  A. field diagnosis, differential diagnosis, narrowing process
  B. differential diagnosis, narrowing process, field diagnosis
  C. narrowing process, field diagnosis, differential diagnosis
  D. differential diagnosis, field diagnosis, narrowing process
  E. field diagnosis, narrowing process, differential diagnosis

_____ 2. The foundation of patient care is:
  A. the detailed physical exam.   D. medication administration.
  B. BLS protocols.   E. ALS protocols.
  C. assessment.

_____ 3. In a medical patient, the physical exam takes precedence over the history.
  A. True
  B. False

_____ 4. All of the following are examples of external factors that can affect assessment EXCEPT:
  A. the attitude of family members.   D. scene chaos.
  B. an uncooperative patient.   E. personal attitudes.
  C. distracting injuries.

_____ 5. Protocols and standing orders do not replace:
  A. good history taking.   D. the team approach.
  B. a good attitude.   E. pattern recognition.
  C. good judgment.

_____ 6. An EMT-I can do something to correct or lessen obstacles to performing a good assessment such as:
  A. tunnel vision.   D. preconceived notions.
  B. labeling.   E. all of the above
  C. cultural and ethnic barriers.

_____ 7. You should treat a "frequent flier" just like you would any other patient.
  A. True
  B. False

_____ 8. A team leader's roles include all of the following EXCEPT:
  A. obtains a history.   D. triages patients.
  B. performs the physical exam.   E. performs a detailed exam.
  C. handles documentation.

©2004 Pearson Education, Inc.
Intermediate Emergency Care: Principles & Practice

_____ 9. Roles of a patient care provider include:
   A. talking to bystanders.
   B. obtaining vital signs.
   C. gathering scene information.
   D. providing scene cover.
   E. all of the above

_____ 10. Patient assessment is best performed by two EMT-Is rather than just one.
   A. True
   B. False

_____ 11. Which of the following is probably optional "take in" equipment carried by EMT-Is?
   A. rigid collars
   B. infection control supplies
   C. drug therapy
   D. space blankets
   E. sphygmomanometer

_____ 12. Components of the initial assessment include all of the following EXCEPT:
   A. forming a general impression.
   B. assessing ABCs.
   C. assessing the scene.
   D. determining the patient's priority.
   E. assessing mental status.

_____ 13. A patient with severe internal bleeding is a candidate for:
   A. the resuscitative approach.
   B. the contemplative approach.
   C. immediate evacuation.
   D. detailed physical exam.
   E. both B and D

_____ 14. In critical patients, a detailed physical exam is more important than continuing ongoing assessments.
   A. True
   B. False

_____ 15. The most effective patient presentations will:
   A. use medical jargon.
   B. follow the SOAP format.
   C. be done in writing.
   D. last 5 to 10 minutes.
   E. exclude subjective findings.

CHAPTER 34

*

Responding to Terrorist Acts

Review of Chapter Objectives

After reading this chapter, you should be able to:

1. Identify the typical weapons of mass destruction likely to be used by terrorists. **pp. 1323–1324**

The most likely weapon of mass destruction used by the terrorist, either foreign or domestic, is the conventional explosive. As terrorists gain greater funding and sophistication, however, the risk of terrorists using nuclear, biological, and chemical weapons is increasing. Terrorist may also use agents and mechanisms not yet mentioned as they search for new ways to terrify the public and bring attention to their cause. An example of this was crashing commercial airliners, laden with fuel, into large buildings.

2. Explain the mechanisms of injury associated with conventional and nuclear weapons of mass destruction. **pp. 1324–1325, 1327, 1332**

Chemical reactions in the conventional explosion release tremendous amounts of heat energy in milliseconds. This energy instantaneously creates super-heated gases and results in extreme pressure at the detonation site. This pressure moves outward rapidly, first creating a pressure wave traveling at sonic speeds and then becomes forceful blast wind. The pressure wave (called over-pressure) rapidly compresses and then decompresses all with which it comes in contact. Serious injury may result to any hollow and air-filled spaces, such as those in the middle ear, the bowel, and the lungs. The blast wind can propel the explosive container parts or other debris, such as glass or wood splinters, inducing injury in those it strikes. The blast wind may also throw victims resulting in blunt trauma as they strike objects or the ground. The pressure wave and blast wind may also cause structural collapse, resulting in crushing injury and/or entrapment. Finally, the blast heat may cause serious burn injury directly or burns from combustion of material it ignites.

The nuclear weapon releases energy as atoms are broken apart and reassembled. The energy released from a relatively small bomb is thousands of times greater than a conventional explosive of equal size. The nuclear detonation injures through the same mechanisms as the conventional explosion. The resulting injuries, however, are more extensive and serious. Additionally, the nuclear detonation releases exceptional amounts of heat energy that kills most individuals in the detonation area and causes serious burns at some distance from the blast epicenter. Lastly, the detonation emits great amounts of nuclear radiation causing direct radiation exposure and energizes dust and debris causing radioactive fallout. The fallout may travel with upper air currents and fall to earth many miles from the detonation site.

3. Identify and describe the major sub-classifications of chemical and biological weapons of mass destruction. **pp. 1327–1330, 1332–1333**

Chemical weapons
—*Nerve agents.* Nerve agents attack the central nervous system by causing an impulse transmission overload. This results in muscle spasms, convulsions, unconsciousness, and respiratory failure.

©2004 Pearson Education, Inc.
Intermediate Emergency Care: Principles & Practice

—*Vesicants.* Vesicants are chemical agents that damage exposed skin and cause blistering. They may also damage the eyes, respiratory tract, and lung tissue and may induce general illness as well.

—*Pulmonary agents.* Pulmonary agents attack the airway and lungs, producing inflammation and pulmonary edema. Their use frequently results in nasal and throat irritation, wheezing, cough, dyspnea, and hypoxia.

—*Bio-toxins.* Bio-toxins are chemicals produced by living organisms and behave more like chemical agents. Botulinum is the most toxic, 15,000 times more potent than the worst of the nerve agents (VX).

Biological weapons

—*Pulmonary or pneumonia-like agents.* Pulmonary agents are the most likely biologic agents to be used by terrorists. These agents are transmitted via the respiratory system and induce cough, dyspnea, fever, and malaise.

—*Encephalitis-like agents.* Encephalitis-like agents affect the central nervous system and present with flu-like signs and symptoms. However, these biological agents usually carry a much higher mortality rate than the flu or similar diseases.

Other biological agents

Cholera and *viral hemorrhagic fever* are other biologic agents terrorists may use. Cholera causes profuse diarrhea, and viral hemorrhagic fever attacks the blood's ability to coagulate.

4. List the scene evidence that might alert the EMS provider to a terrorist attack that involves a weapon of mass destruction. p. 1334

Terrorists are likely to target public places where the effects of their actions are the greatest on structures that symbolize an institution they oppose. The results of a conventional or nuclear explosion make them easy to recognize but chemical and biological releases may be insidious. Whenever a large number of people appear to be complaining of similar signs and symptoms, suspect the deployment of chemical or biological weapons. In a chemical release, the effects are likely to occur immediately or shortly after exposure. Confined spaces, such as within a building or in a subway terminal, are likely targets though terrorists may release an agent upwind of a large public gathering. A biological release is even more difficult to detect. You, or more likely, Emergency Medical Service personnel, may recognize many patients with similar generalized signs and symptoms. Only after extensive diagnostic tests and investigation may someone confirm that a weapon of mass destruction was deployed.

5. Describe the special safety precautions and safety equipment appropriate for an incident involving nuclear, biological, or chemical weapons. pp. 1333–1334, 1326–1327; also see Chapters 8, 13, and 16

The first step in responding to a possible weapon of mass destruction incident is to maintain the proper index of suspicion and to assure that you, fellow rescuers, and the public are not exposed to danger. Approach the scene from upwind and when in doubt about scene safety, request that a properly trained response team assess and enter the scene before you. Only after the response team determines the scene is safe should you enter (if at all).

Affected patients must be properly decontaminated before you offer care, both for your protection and theirs. This occurs whether they are brought to you or you enter the scene to treat them.

When responding to a nuclear incident, act at the direction of persons trained in radiation detection. Wear a dosimeter when appropriate and have your exposure level checked periodically. When off duty, properly decontaminate and move a good distance from the scene to limit cumulative exposure.

For biological agents, employ body substance isolation precautions as appropriate. In this case BSI usually means a properly fitted HEPA-filter mask and gloves. While it is unlikely that you will recognize the release of an agent, you may be called on to treat victims days after the initial exposure.

Chemical agent releases may present with a recognizable and immediate danger. Remain at a distance and upwind from the scene and call for the victims to self-evacuate. Only properly trained personnel wearing the appropriate protective gear (a properly trained and equipped haz-mat team) should enter the scene. Patients must be properly decontaminated before it is safe for you to care for them.

6. **Identify the assessment and management concerns for victims of conventional, nuclear, biological, and chemical weapons.** pp. 1326–1327, 1330, 1331, 1333; also see Chapters 13 and 16

Conventional. Victims of a conventional weapon detonation suffer compression injuries from the blast wave. The most serious injury is to the lungs. Any sign of compression injury such as mid-dle ear or bowel injury signs or any dyspnea should suggest lung injury. Blast victims may also suffer penetrating and blunt injuries due to debris propelled by the blast wind or from being thrown by the wind. Finally, the victim may be injured during structural collapse.

Focus management of the blast victim on care for the respiratory injury. Administer high-flow, high concentration oxygen. Provide intermittent positive pressure ventilation as needed, but conservatively, as the blast may have injured the alveolar walls. Care for other blunt and pene-trating injuries as indicated.

Nuclear. Victims of a nuclear blast are most likely to receive burns as their most serious injuries. Radiation exposure may come from the initial blast or from radioactive fallout at or downwind from the explosion. There will be limited signs and symptoms unless the radiation exposure was very high. With high radiation exposure, the patient will display nausea, vomiting, and malaise. The greater the radiation exposure, the faster these signs will appear following exposure.

Patient care includes decontamination and then care for thermal burns. Protection from fall-out is an additional concern and best addressed by moving the victims away from the expected fallout path. Care for the patient exposed to radioactivity is mostly supportive.

If there is a recognized release of radiation through a conventional explosion or other mech-anism, direct your first efforts to reduce further exposure. Then assure that the patients are prop-erly decontaminated. Only then, concentrate your efforts on specific injury care.

Biological. It is unlikely that anyone will immediately detect the release of a biologic agent. It is more likely that you or other health care workers will notice a group of people complaining of similar symptoms. These symptoms will most likely be fever, nausea, body aches, and malaise (symptoms similar to the flu).

Care for the victims of a biological agent release is first directed at reducing transmission. At the first sign of a possible biological agent (or any potentially contagious disease), don a mask and gloves and isolate the patient (or patients). Provide supportive care as for any other serious contagious disease.

Chemical. A chemical release is likely to affect its victims very quickly. They will complain of res-piratory symptoms such as chest tightness or burning or possibly skin irritation. If you receive reports of several or many individuals complaining of similar symptoms, suspect a chemical release and approach the scene with great caution. Alert the fire department or the designated hazardous materials team and position your vehicle upwind from the scene. Assure the evacua-tion of persons downwind and decontamination of those victims brought to you for care.

Care for the victims of a chemical release includes high-flow, high-concentration oxygen, respiratory support as needed (including bag-valve masking and intubation), and antidote admin-istration as indicated.

7. **Given a narrative description of a conventional, nuclear, biological, or chemical terrorist attack, identify the elements of scene size-up that suggest terrorism, and identify the likely injuries and any special patient management considerations necessary.** pp. 1324–1334

During your classroom training and practical skills session you will learn and practice the skills associated with recognizing, taking the proper protective precautions for you and the public, and caring for patients subject to illness or injury from weapons of mass destruction. Use this train-ing and practice to perfect your skills of WMD care.

CASE STUDY REVIEW

This case study illustrates how the events of September 11, 2001 have affected EMS professionals and their responsibilities. It highlights the need to include the possibility of terrorist acts in all aspects of emergency care decision making.

Adam and Sean have a heightened index of suspicion for a weapon of mass destruction incident that comes following the events of September 11, 2001. When presented with several patients with similar symptoms, they suspect a chemical agent release and request activation of the county's WMD plan. They also approach the scene with care, arriving upwind of the building and directing dispatch to request evacuation (thereby evacuating the building without risk to rescuers). Sean and Adam also request the fire department (their local hazmat team) to respond as well. Finally, by using a cell phone rather than using the EMS radio, they assure their suspicion of a WMD incident is not made public.

Adam and Sean direct the potential patients to their care station using the public address system, again reducing any risk to the rescuers. They establish incident command and effectively communicate pertinent information regarding the numbers and types of patients they are encountering. This helps the emergency department prepare for arrival of numerous patients with the same complaints. Before stepping from their rig, Sean and Adam don HEPA-filter masks and gloves to further protect themselves from any biologic threat.

Adam relinquishes incident command as soon as someone from the fire department arrives. He communicates his knowledge of the scene and then joins Sean in administering to the patients. Since the number of patients outnumbers the resources available, Sean and Adam provide oxygen only to the most seriously affected patients. Thankfully, the symptoms are only minor and other ambulances arrive quickly. As more information is gathered about the scene, the initial information suggest a simple furnace or chimney malfunction. However, further investigation suggests that this was truly a WMD incident involving the intentional production of carbon monoxide. The scene then becomes a crime scene and is investigated thoroughly by the police department.

CONTENT SELF-EVALUATION

MULTIPLE CHOICE

_____ 1. Which of the following is the most likely weapon of choice for terrorist groups?
- A. conventional explosives
- B. nuclear weapons
- C. biological agents
- D. chemical agents
- E. incendiary devices

_____ 2. Terrorists are likely to target which of the following?
- A. an embassy
- B. a symbol of government
- C. their employer
- D. corporations
- E. all of the above

_____ 3. The blast pressure wave is likely to injure all of the following EXCEPT:
- A. the lungs.
- B. the ears.
- C. the bowel.
- D. the heart.
- E. the sinuses.

_____ 4. Incendiary agents differ from conventional explosives in that they:
- A. have greater explosive energy.
- B. cause more burn injuries.
- C. consume more oxygen.
- D. are dropped from a high altitude.
- E. combine both explosive and nuclear damage.

©2004 Pearson Education, Inc.
Intermediate Emergency Care: Principles & Practice

_____ 5. Which of the following is the mechanism of injury associated with most deaths from a nuclear blast?
   A. radiation burns
   B. radiation illness
   C. cancer
   D. thermal burns
   E. pressure injuries

_____ 6. The best way to detect radiation in the absence of a Geiger counter is:
   A. by a strange taste in your mouth.
   B. a warm sensation in your muscles.
   C. immediate nausea.
   D. a tingling sensation from the exposed surface.
   E. none of the above

_____ 7. Fallout associated with the nuclear detonation is not likely to be a factor until how long after the detonation?
   A. 10 minutes
   B. 30 minutes
   C. 1 hour
   D. 4 hours
   E. 2 days

_____ 8. Once a victim is exposed to nuclear radiation and debris has been properly decontaminated, he poses no danger to himself or others.
   A. True
   B. False

_____ 9. Which of the following is a symptom associated with radiation exposure?
   A. nausea
   B. fatigue
   C. malaise
   D. hypertension
   E. all of the above except D

_____ 10. Which of the following influence the delivery of a chemical weapon?
   A. wind strength
   B. the agent's specific gravity
   C. the agent's volatility
   D. precipitation
   E. all of the above

_____ 11. Which of the following is NOT a common sign or symptom of a nerve agent?
   A. dry mouth
   B. tearing eyes
   C. urination
   D. defecation
   E. vomiting

_____ 12. Blistering agents are also known as:
   A. organophosphates.
   B. vesicants.
   C. carbamates.
   D. chambering agents.
   E. none of the above

_____ 13. Which of the following is NOT a blistering agent?
   A. lewisite
   B. phosgene oxime
   C. botulinum
   D. sulfur mustard
   E. nitrogen mustard

_____ 14. One of the most toxic agents known to man is:
   A. sulfur mustard.
   B. Ricin.
   C. VX gas.
   D. botulinum.
   E. none of the above

_____ 15. Which of the following suggests a chemical agent release?
   A. a strange smell
   B. numerous patients complaining of the same symptoms
   C. a cloud of dust or gas
   D. incapacitated or dead birds and insects
   E. all of the above

©2004 Pearson Education, Inc.
Intermediate Emergency Care: Principles & Practice

_____ **16.** Which of the following is NOT a biologic agent capable of spreading from person to person?
   A. Ebola
   B. smallpox
   C. plague
   D. anthrax
   E. cholera

_____ **17.** A biological release can be recognized by which of the following?
   A. a distinctive cloud of gas
   B. a distinctive odor
   C. immediate signs and symptoms
   D. very distinct signs and symptoms
   E. none of the above

_____ **18.** The most likely biologic agents to be used by terrorists are:
   A. pulmonary agents.
   B. flu-like agents.
   C. encephalitis-like agents.
   D. Ebola.
   E. all of the above

_____ **19.** Almost all bioterrorist weapons are transmitted via the respiratory route; therefore, the HEPA respirator is very effective at reducing transmission.
   A. True
   B. False

_____ **20.** Dangers of a conventional explosion used by terrorists include all of the following EXCEPT:
   A. the danger of a secondary explosion.
   B. inability to recognize the incident.
   C. radioactive contamination.
   D. structural collapse.
   E. all of the above

WORKBOOK ANSWER KEY

Note: Throughout Answer Key, textbook page references are shown in italic.

Division 1: Preparatory Information

CHAPTER 1: Foundations of the EMT-Intermediate

Part 1

MULTIPLE CHOICE

1. C	*p. 5*	6. C	*p. 6*	
2. A	*pp. 5–6*	7. B	*p. 6*	
3. E	*p. 6*	8. A	*p. 6*	
4. E	*p. 6*	9. C	*p. 6*	
5. D	*p. 6*	10. A	*p. 6*	

Part 2

MULTIPLE CHOICE

1. A	*p. 7*	19. A	*p. 14*	
2. A	*p. 8*	20. E	*p. 15*	
3. E	*p. 7*	21. B	*p. 15*	
4. B	*p. 9*	22. A	*p. 15*	
5. A	*p. 10*	23. D	*p. 16*	
6. D	*p. 11*	24. C	*p. 16*	
7. A	*p. 11*	25. B	*p. 16*	
8. E	*p. 11*	26. C	*pp. 16–17*	
9. C	*pp. 11–12*	27. E	*p. 17*	
10. C	*p. 12*	28. B	*p. 17*	
11. B	*p. 12*	29. C	*p. 18*	
12. C	*p. 13*	30. E	*p. 18*	
13. A	*p. 13*	31. B	*p. 18*	
14. D	*p. 14*	32. B	*p. 19*	
15. B	*p. 15*	33. A	*p. 19*	
16. A	*p. 14*	34. C	*p. 20*	
17. D	*p. 14*	35. A	*p. 20*	
18. D	*pp. 14–15*			

LISTING

36. U.S. DOT (National Highway Traffic Safety Administration) *p. 14*
37. U.S. General Services Administration *p. 16*
38. American College of Surgeons Committee on Trauma *p. 16*
39. American College of Emergency Physicians *p. 16*
40. National Registry of EMTs *p. 15*
    Joint Review Committee on Educational Programs for the EMT-Paramedic

Part 3

MULTIPLE CHOICE

1. A	*p. 21*
2. E	*p. 21*
3. E	*pp. 21–22*
4. A	*p. 22*
5. B	*p. 22*
6. C	*p. 23*
7. C	*p. 23*
8. E	*p. 23*
9. B	*pp. 23–24*
10. B	*p. 24*
11. B	*p. 25*
12. A	*p. 27*
13. D	*p. 26*
14. B	*p. 26*
15. C	*p. 27*

MATCHING

16. G	*p. 23*
17. C	*p. 22*
18. D	*pp. 22–23*
19. C	*p. 22*
20. F	*p. 23*
21. A	*p. 21*
22. C	*p. 22*
23. C	*p. 22*
24. E	*p. 23*
25. B	*p. 22*
26. D	*pp. 22–23*
27. A	*pp. 21–22*
28. G	*p. 23*
29. C	*p. 22*
30. C	*p. 22*

Part 4

MULTIPLE CHOICE

1. C	*p. 28*	19. E	*p. 35*	
2. A	*p. 28*	20. C	*p. 36*	
3. A	*p. 29*	21. C	*p. 37*	
4. B	*p. 29*	22. B	*p. 37*	
5. C	*p. 29*	23. B	*p. 38*	
6. E	*p. 29*	24. A	*p. 38*	
7. C	*p. 29*	25. A	*p. 39*	
8. C	*p. 30*	26. D	*p. 39*	
9. E	*pp. 30, 32*	27. D	*p. 40*	
10. C	*p. 32*	28. B	*p. 40*	
11. A	*p. 33*	29. B	*p. 41*	
12. A	*p. 33*	30. A	*p. 41*	
13. D	*pp. 33–34*	31. E	*p. 42*	
14. E	*pp. 33–34*	32. B	*pp. 41–43*	
15. B	*pp. 33–34*	33. E	*p. 43*	
16. E	*p. 34*	34. A	*p. 44*	
17. E	*p. 34*	35. B	*p. 45*	
18. A	*p. 35*			

MATCHING

36. A, B	*pp. 33–34*	
37. A, B, D	*pp. 33–34*	
38. A, B	*pp. 33–34*	
39. A, C	*pp. 33–34*	
40. A, B, D	*pp. 33–34*	

Part 5

MULTIPLE CHOICE

1.	C	p. 46	9.	C	p. 49
2.	A	p. 46	10.	A	p. 46
3.	A	p. 46	11.	C	p. 49
4.	B	p. 46	12.	A	p. 50
5.	A	p. 47	13.	E	pp. 50–51
6.	B	p. 48	14.	B	p. 51
7.	A	p. 49	15.	E	p. 51
8.	B	p. 49			

Part 6

MULTIPLE CHOICE

1.	B	p. 52	19.	C	p. 62
2.	C	p. 52	20.	E	pp. 61–62
3.	C	p. 53	21.	B	p. 62
4.	A	p. 53	22.	B	p. 62
5.	E	pp. 54–55	23.	E	p. 62
6.	D	p. 55	24.	B	pp. 62–63
7.	B	p. 55	25.	B	p. 63
8.	A	p. 56	26.	A	p. 64
9.	D	p. 56	27.	D	p. 64
10.	E	p. 56	28.	C	p. 65
11.	C	p. 57	29.	D	p. 65
12.	C	p. 57	30.	A	p. 65
13.	E	p. 58	31.	E	p. 66
14.	A	p. 58	32.	A	p. 67
15.	A	p. 59	33.	A	p. 67
16.	D	p. 60	34.	C	pp. 67–68
17.	E	p. 61	35.	C	pp. 68–69
18.	B	p. 62			

Part 7

MULTIPLE CHOICE

1.	A	p. 69	6.	B	p. 73
2.	B	p. 70	7.	A	p. 74
3.	D	p. 70	8.	B	p. 75
4.	A	p. 71	9.	A	p. 77
5.	D	p. 71	10.	E	pp. 77–78

SPECIAL PROJECT: Crossword Puzzle

CHAPTER 2: Overview of Human Systems

Part 1

MULTIPLE CHOICE

1.	A	p. 83	21.	E	p. 91
2.	A	p. 84	22.	B	p. 92
3.	C	p. 84	23.	A	p. 92
4.	E	p. 84	24.	B	p. 93
5.	C	p. 84	25.	E	p. 94
6.	D	p. 84	26.	D	p. 94
7.	A	p. 85	27.	A	p. 94
8.	E	p. 86	28.	B	p. 94
9.	D	p. 86	29.	A	pp. 94–95
10.	A	p. 86	30.	B	p. 95
11.	E	p. 86	31.	A	pp. 96–97
12.	E	p. 87	32.	D	p. 97
13.	A	p. 87	33.	E	p. 97
14.	B	p. 87	34.	A	p. 97
15.	A	p. 87	35.	B	p. 97
16.	B	p. 88	36.	C	p. 97
17.	B	p. 88	37.	B	p. 97
18.	C	pp. 89–90	38.	B	p. 97
19.	B	pp. 89–90	39.	D	p. 97
20.	D	p. 91	40.	B	p. 100

Part 2

MULTIPLE CHOICE

1.	A	p. 101	36.	E	p. 136
2.	A	p. 102	37.	D	p. 136
3.	E	p. 102	38.	B	p. 137
4.	A	p. 102	39.	B	p. 137
5.	D	p. 102	40.	A	pp. 137–138
6.	C	p. 103	41.	C	p. 138
7.	B	p. 103	42.	A	p. 138
8.	C	p. 104	43.	A	p. 139
9.	A	pp. 104–105	44.	E	p. 139
10.	D	p. 105	45.	C	p. 139
11.	A	p. 106	46.	E	p. 141
12.	E	p. 107	47.	B	p. 140
13.	B	p. 108	48.	C	p. 140
14.	A	p. 109	49.	C	p. 141
15.	B	p. 109	50.	D	p. 142
16.	E	p. 110	51.	A	p. 142
17.	D	p. 110	52.	A	p. 142
18.	B	p. 110	53.	C	p. 142
19.	C	p. 113	54.	B	p. 147
20.	B	p. 113	55.	C	p. 147
21.	A	p. 113	56.	B	p. 148
22.	C	p. 114	57.	A	p. 149
23.	D	p. 113	58.	C	p. 150
24.	A	p. 114	59.	A	p. 150
25.	B	p. 115	60.	E	p. 150
26.	A	p. 115	61.	B	p. 150
27.	C	p. 115	62.	E	p. 151
28.	A	p. 116	63.	B	p. 151
29.	C	p. 128	64.	E	p. 151
30.	E	p. 130	65.	C	p. 152
31.	D	p. 130	66.	A	p. 152
32.	A	p. 133	67.	D	p. 152
33.	E	pp. 134–135	68.	B	p. 153
34.	B	p. 135	69.	E	p. 154
35.	C	p. 136	70.	B	p. 154

71. A p. 154
72. C pp. 154–155
73. D p. 155
74. C p. 156
75. C p. 158
76. C p. 158
77. A p. 159
78. E pp. 159–160
79. D p. 160
80. D p. 161
81. A pp. 162–163, 166
82. D p. 170
83. C p. 172
84. B p. 174
85. A p. 178
86. B p. 179
87. B p. 180
88. D pp. 180–181
89. B p. 180
90. B p. 181
91. E p. 181
92. C p. 181
93. B p. 181
94. C p. 181
95. A p. 181
96. A p. 181
97. A p. 181
98. C p. 183
99. B p. 185
100. E p. 186
101. A p. 187
102. A pp. 187–188
103. D p. 188
104. A p. 190
105. D p. 191
106. D p. 192
107. B p. 193
108. C p. 195
109. C p. 196
110. E pp. 197–198
111. D p. 199
112. D p. 199
113. A p. 200

114. B p. 201
115. A p. 202
116. C p. 202
117. C pp. 201–203
118. D p. 204
119. A p. 204
120. E p. 205
121. D pp. 205–206
122. A p. 206
123. B p. 208
124. C p. 208
125. A p. 209
126. E pp. 209–210
127. C p. 210
128. C p. 210
129. B p. 210
130. A p. 211
131. E p. 211
132. C p. 212
133. C p. 212
134. A p. 213
135. C p. 213
136. E p. 213
137. E p. 216
138. B p. 216
139. A p. 216
140. E p. 218
141. A p. 218
142. B p. 221
143. A p. 223
144. D p. 223
145. B p. 224
146. B p. 224
147. C p. 225
148. E p. 227
149. A p. 227
150. B p. 228
151. A p. 228
152. C p. 228
153. D p. 228
154. C p. 229
155. C pp. 230–231

33. D p. 248
34. B p. 248
35. C pp. 248–249
36. A p. 248
37. A p. 249
38. D p. 250
39. E p. 250
40. C p. 250

Part 2

MULTIPLE CHOICE

1. E p. 252
2. A p. 252
3. D p. 252
4. B p. 252
5. B p. 253
6. A p. 253
7. A p. 253
8. D p. 253
9. D p. 253
10. C p. 253
11. B p. 253
12. D p. 254
13. B p. 255
14. A p. 257
15. E p. 256
16. B p. 257
17. D p. 258
18. D p. 258
19. A p. 256
20. A p. 258

Part 3

SPECIAL PROJECT: Crossword Puzzle

Crossword puzzle grid with answers including: SYNTHETIC, ACTIVE, FILTRATION, SYRUP, BIOASSAY, ION, MINERAL, ORAL, NASAL, SPIRIT, EFFICACY, AGONIST, BIOEQUIVALENT, ANIMAL, EXTRACT, TABLET, RECEPTOR.

CHAPTER 3: Emergency Pharmacology

Part 1

MULTIPLE CHOICE

1. D p. 234
2. A p. 235
3. B p. 235
4. A p. 235
5. B p. 235
6. B p. 235
7. C p. 236
8. C p. 236
9. E p. 237
10. B p. 238
11. E p. 238
12. E p. 238
13. A p. 239
14. B p. 240
15. D p. 240
16. E p. 240
17. D p. 241
18. A p. 241
19. C p. 242
20. B p. 242
21. D p. 242
22. A p. 243
23. D p. 245
24. B pp. 245–246
25. D p. 246
26. A p. 246
27. C p. 246
28. C p. 247
29. E p. 247
30. C p. 247
31. C p. 247
32. B p. 248

CHAPTER 4: Venous Access and Medication Administration

Part 1

MULTIPLE CHOICE

1.	A	*p. 273*	24.	B	*p. 283*
2.	B	*p. 274*	25.	A	*p. 284*
3.	D	*p. 274*	26.	B	*p. 285*
4.	E	*p. 274*	27.	C	*p. 285*
5.	A	*p. 275*	28.	B	*p. 288*
6.	A	*p. 275*	29.	D	*p. 288*
7.	C	*p. 275*	30.	B	*p. 290*
8.	D	*p. 275*	31.	B	*p. 290*
9.	A	*p. 276*	32.	B	*p. 291*
10.	C	*p. 276*	33.	A	*p. 293*
11.	E	*p. 277*	34.	A	*p. 293*
12.	D	*p. 277*	35.	E	*p. 293*
13.	C	*p. 277*	36.	A	*p. 297*
14.	C	*p. 278*	37.	C	*p. 298*
15.	E	*p. 278*	38.	D	*pp. 297–298*
16.	D	*p. 278*	39.	B	*pp. 298–299*
17.	B	*p. 279*	40.	A	*p. 301*
18.	B	*p. 280*	41.	D	*pp. 299, 303*
19.	B	*p. 281*	42.	C	*p. 303*
20.	C	*p. 282*	43.	D	*pp. 297–298, 303*
21.	A	*p. 283*	44.	D	*p. 303*
22.	E	*p. 283*	45.	B	*p. 303*
23.	A	*p. 283*			

Part 2

MULTIPLE CHOICE

1.	E	*p. 305*	26.	C	*p. 315*
2.	B	*p. 305*	27.	C	*p. 315*
3.	E	*p. 305*	28.	E	*p. 317*
4.	D	*p. 305*	29.	E	*pp. 317, 319*
5.	A	*p. 306*	30.	D	*p. 320*
6.	C	*p. 306*	31.	D	*p. 320*
7.	E	*p. 307*	32.	B	*p. 320*
8.	D	*p. 307*	33.	D	*p. 321*
9.	E	*p. 307*	34.	C	*p. 321*
10.	E	*p. 307*	35.	A	*p. 323*
11.	B	*p. 309*	36.	B	*pp. 329–330*
12.	A	*p. 309*	37.	A	*p. 330*
13.	D	*p. 309*	38.	B	*p. 331*
14.	C	*p. 310*	39.	B	*pp. 330–331*
15.	A	*p. 310*	40.	A	*p. 330*
16.	A	*p. 310*	41.	C	*p. 331*
17.	A	*p. 307*	42.	B	*p. 332*
18.	E	*p. 311*	43.	C	*p. 332*
19.	B	*p. 312*	44.	C	*p. 333*
20.	B	*p. 312*	45.	A	*p. 333*
21.	D	*p. 312*	46.	A	*p. 333*
22.	B	*p. 314*	47.	C	*p. 334*
23.	B	*p. 314*	48.	A	*p. 335*
24.	B	*p. 314*	49.	C	*p. 336*
25.	A	*p. 315*	50.	D	*p. 339*

Part 3

SPECIAL PROJECT: Drip Math Worksheet 1

1. R = 15 gtts/min
   V = ?
   T = 25 min
   D = 60 gtts/ml

   $V = R \times T = 15$ gtts/min $\times 25$ min

   $V = \dfrac{15 \text{ gtts} \times 25 \text{ min}}{\text{min}}$

   $V = 375 \text{ gtts}/D = \dfrac{375 \text{ gtts} \times \text{ml}}{60 \text{ gtts}} = \dfrac{375 \text{ ml}}{60} = \mathbf{6.25}$

2. R= V/T = 250 ml/60 min
   V = 250 ml
   T = 60 min
   D_1 = 60 gtts/ml
   D_2 = 10 gtts/ml

   A. $R = V/T = \dfrac{250 \text{ ml}}{60 \text{ min}} = \dfrac{4.17 \text{ ml}}{\text{min}} = \dfrac{4.17 \text{ ml} \times 60 \text{ gtts}}{\text{min} \times \text{ml}} = \mathbf{\dfrac{250 \text{ gtts}}{\text{min}}}$

   B. $R = V/T = \dfrac{250 \text{ ml}}{60 \text{ min}} = \dfrac{4.17 \text{ ml}}{\text{min}} = \dfrac{4.17 \text{ ml} \times 10 \text{ gtts}}{\text{min} \times \text{ml}} = \mathbf{\dfrac{41.7 \text{ gtts}}{\text{min}}}$

©2004 Pearson Education, Inc.
Intermediate Emergency Care: Principles & Practice

3. R = 32 gtts/min
    V = 50 ml
    T = ?
    D = 45 gtts/ml

$R(ml) = R(min) \times D$

$R(ml) = 32 \text{ gtts/min} \times 45 \text{ gtts/ml}$

$R(ml) = \dfrac{32 \text{ gtts} \times ml}{45 \text{ gtts} \times min} = \dfrac{32 \text{ ml}}{45 \text{ min}} = 0.71 \text{ ml/min}$

$T = V/R = \dfrac{50 \text{ ml}/0.71 \text{ ml/min}}{0.71 \text{ ml}} = \dfrac{50 \text{ ml} \times min}{0.71} = 50 \text{ min} = \mathbf{0.70 \text{ min}}$

4. $R = 4 \text{ gtts/sec} \times 60 \text{ sec/min} = \dfrac{4 \text{ gtts} \times 60 \text{ sec}}{\text{sec} \times min} = 240 \text{ gtts/min}$

    V = ?
    T = 45 min
    D = 10 gtts/ml

$V = R \times T = 240 \text{ gtts/min} \times 45 \text{ min} = \dfrac{240 \text{ gtts} \times 45 \text{ min}}{min} = 10{,}800 \text{ gtts}$

$V = 10{,}800 \text{ gtts}/D = \dfrac{10{,}800 \text{ gtts}/10 \text{ gtts/ml}}{10 \text{ gtts}} = \dfrac{10{,}800 \text{ ml} \times ml}{10} = \mathbf{1{,}080 \text{ ml}}$

5. R = ?
    V = 1.5 ml/min
    T = 1 min
    D_1 = 60 gtts/min
    D_2 = 45 gtts/min
    D_3 = 10 gtts/min

A. $R = V/T = \dfrac{1.5 \text{ ml}}{1 \text{ min}} = \dfrac{1.5 \text{ ml} \times D}{1 \text{ min}} = \dfrac{1.5 \text{ ml} \times 60 \text{ gtts}}{min \times ml} = \mathbf{90 \text{ gtts/min}}$

B. $R = V/T = \dfrac{1.5 \text{ ml}}{1 \text{ min}} = \dfrac{1.5 \text{ ml} \times D}{1 \text{ min}} = \dfrac{1.5 \text{ ml} \times 45 \text{ gtts}}{min \times ml} = \mathbf{67.5 \text{ gtts/min}}$

C. $R = V/T = \dfrac{1.5 \text{ ml}}{1 \text{ min}} = \dfrac{1.5 \text{ ml} \times D}{1 \text{ min}} = \dfrac{1.5 \text{ ml} \times 10 \text{ gtts}}{min \times ml} = \mathbf{15 \text{ gtts/min}}$

Drug Math Worksheet 1

1. Dh = 1 mg
    Vh = 5 ml
    Dd = 0.5 mg
    Va = ?

$Va = \dfrac{Vh \times Dd}{Dh} = \dfrac{5 \text{ ml} \times 0.5 \text{ mg}}{1 \text{ mg}} = \dfrac{2.5 \text{ ml}}{1} = \mathbf{2.5 \text{ ml}}$

2. Dh = 80 mg
    Vh = 4 ml
    Dd = 40 mg
    Va = ?

$Va = \dfrac{Vh \times Dd}{Dh} = \dfrac{4 \text{ ml} \times 40 \text{ mg}}{80 \text{ mg}} = \dfrac{160 \text{ ml}}{80} = \mathbf{2 \text{ ml}}$

3. A. Dh = 1 g (1,000 mg)
        Vh = 1,000 ml
        Dd = 1 mg
        Va = ?

$Va = \dfrac{Vh \times Dd}{Dh} = \dfrac{1{,}000 \text{ ml} \times 1 \text{ mg}}{1 \text{ g}} = \dfrac{1{,}000 \text{ ml} \times 1 \text{ mg}}{1{,}000 \text{ mg}} = \dfrac{1 \text{ ml}}{1} = \mathbf{1 \text{ ml}}$

(continued next page)

(Drug Math Worksheet 1 continued)

B. Dh = 1 g (1,000 mg)
   Vh = 10,000 ml
   Dd = 1 mg
   Va = ?

$$Va = \frac{Vh \times Dd}{Dh} = \frac{10,000 \text{ ml} \times 1 \text{ mg}}{1 \text{ g}} = \frac{10,000 \text{ ml} \times 1 \text{ mg}}{1,000 \text{ mg}} = \frac{10 \text{ ml}}{1} = 10 \text{ ml}$$

4. Desired dose = patient weight × 0.2 mg/kg = $\dfrac{6 \text{ kg} \times 0.2 \text{ mg}}{\text{kg}}$ = 1.2 mg

   Dh = 6 mg
   Vh = 2 ml
   Dd = 1.2 mg
   Va = ?

$$Va = \frac{Vh \times Dd}{Dh} = \frac{2 \text{ ml} \times 1.2 \text{ mg}}{6 \text{ mg}} = \frac{2.4 \text{ ml}}{6} = 0.4 \text{ ml}$$

CHAPTER 5: Airway Management and Ventilation

MULTIPLE CHOICE

1. A	p. 351	10. C	p. 361	19. B	p. 368	33. B	p. 381
2. C	p. 352	11. D	p. 361	20. C	p. 369	34. D	p. 381
3. B	pp. 352–353	12. D	p. 363	21. D	p. 370	35. E	p. 381
4. B	p. 353	13. D	p. 363	22. B	p. 370	36. A	p. 382
5. B	p. 354	14. A	pp. 364–365	23. A	p. 372	37. C	p. 367
6. E	p. 354	15. D	p. 365	24. A	p. 374	38. C	p. 376
7. D	p. 355	16. E	p. 367	25. C	p. 374	39. E	pp. 385–386
8. A	p. 356	17. B	p. 366	26. B	p. 375	40. A	p. 386
9. C	p. 358	18. C	p. 367	27. C	p. 375	41. B	p. 388
				28. C	p. 376	42. B	p. 390
				29. B	p. 377	43. A	pp. 390–391
				30. A	pp. 377–378	44. A	pp. 392–393
				31. E	p. 379	45. E	pp. 393–394
				32. B	p. 380		

Division 2: Patient Assessment

CHAPTER 6: History Taking

MULTIPLE CHOICE

1. D	p. 400	14. A	p. 413
2. A	p. 401	15. A	p. 414
3. A	p. 404		
4. B	p. 404	MATCHING	
5. C	p. 404	16. S	pp. 406–407
6. B	p. 406	17. P	pp. 406–407
7. A	p. 406	18. R	pp. 406–407
8. B	p. 407	19. Q	pp. 406–407
9. C	p. 408	20. P	pp. 406–407
10. E	p. 409	21. O	pp. 406–407
11. C	p. 409	22. R	pp. 406–407
12. D	p. 409	23. T	pp. 406–407
13. B	pp. 411–413	24. Q	pp. 406–407
		25. O	pp. 406–407

CHAPTER 7: Techniques of Physical Examination

MULTIPLE CHOICE

1. A	p. 420	5. B	p. 421
2. B	p. 423	6. C	p. 421
3. A	p. 422	7. A	p. 422
4. C	p. 420	8. A	p. 422
		9. C	p. 423

10. B	p. 424	36. D	p. 435
11. C	p. 424	37. E	p. 436
12. A	p. 424	38. A	p. 436
13. E	p. 425	39. B	p. 437
14. A	p. 425	40. D	p. 438
15. D	p. 425	41. A	p. 439
16. C	p. 426	42. A	p. 439
17. A	p. 426	43. B	p. 439
18. E	p. 426	44. E	p. 441
19. B	p. 426	45. A	p. 441
20. C	p. 426	46. D	p. 445
21. E	p. 427	47. B	pp. 445–446
22. C	p. 427	48. E	p. 446
23. D	p. 428	49. B	p. 449
24. D	p. 428	50. D	pp. 431, 437
25. B	p. 428	51. C	p. 446
26. B	p. 429	52. C	p. 448
27. D	p. 433	53. A	p. 448
28. B	p. 433	54. E	p. 449
29. A	p. 433	55. D	p. 450
30. E	p. 433	56. E	p. 452
31. C	p. 433	57. B	p. 455
32. A	p. 433	58. B	p. 455
33. E	p. 434	59. B	p. 462
34. D	p. 434	60. D	p. 462
35. B	p. 435	61. C	p. 465

©2004 Pearson Education, Inc.
Intermediate Emergency Care: Principles & Practice

62. A	p. 465	74. E	p. 472
63. D	p. 467	75. E	p. 472
64. E	p. 467	76. A	p. 472
65. A	p. 468	77. C	p. 473
66. E	p. 468	78. E	p. 473
67. B	p. 468	79. B	p. 473
68. C	p. 468	80. A	p. 474
69. D	p. 469	81. B	p. 474
70. E	p. 469	82. B	p. 475
71. A	p. 471	83. A	p. 475
72. D	p. 472	84. D	p. 475
73. C	p. 471	85. E	pp. 476–477

SPECIAL PROJECT: Vital Signs

Pulse: Evaluate pulse rate, quality (or strength), and rhythm. Pulses should be strong, regular, and have a rate of 60 to 100 beats per minute.

Respirations: Evaluate rate, effort, and quality (depth and pattern). The respiratory rate should be between 12 to 20 breaths per minute with minimal effort involved in using the diaphragm and intercostal muscles. Breathing should show a regular rhythm and move about 500 mL with each breath.

Blood Pressure: Evaluate the diastolic, systolic, and pulse pressure. The normal systolic blood pressure is 100 to 135 mmHg; the normal diastolic pressure is 60 to 80 mmHg; and the pulse pressure is between 30 and 40 mmHg. Blood pressures in premenopausal women are slightly lower.

Temperature: Evaluate the core body temperature. The normal core body temperature is 98.6°F or 37°C.

CHAPTER 8: Patient Assessment in the Field

MULTIPLE CHOICE

1. A	p. 480	31. C	p. 501
2. E	p. 480	32. D	p. 502
3. E	p. 481	33. B	p. 502
4. B	p. 481	34. A	p. 503
5. A	p. 482	35. E	p. 503
6. C	pp. 482–483	36. A	p. 503
7. A	p. 483	37. D	p. 503
8. E	p. 484	38. A	p. 503
9. E	p. 484	39. B	p. 505
10. C	pp. 484–485	40. C	p. 505
11. A	p. 485	41. B	p. 507
12. D	p. 488	42. D	p. 509
13. B	p. 488	43. B	p. 509
14. A	p. 488	44. D	p. 510
15. B	p. 488	45. C	p. 510
16. D	pp. 448–489	46. E	p. 511
17. E	p. 489	47. D	p. 512
18. C	p. 489	48. B	p. 512
19. E	p. 491	49. C	p. 513
20. C	p. 491	50. A	pp. 513–514
21. A	pp. 491–492	51. D	p. 514
22. E	p. 492	52. B	p. 514
23. C	p. 492	53. E	p. 514
24. A	p. 493	54. B	pp. 514–515
25. C	p. 494	55. E	p. 516
26. A	p. 494	56. A	p. 516
27. B	p. 495	57. E	p. 517
28. D	p. 495	58. A	p. 519
29. A	p. 496	59. A	p. 524
30. C	p. 497	60. E	p. 525

CHAPTER 9: Clinical Decision Making

MULTIPLE CHOICE

1. A	p. 530	14. D	p. 538
2. D	p. 532	15. B	p. 540
3. A	p. 531		

MATCHING

4. C	p. 532	16. B	pp. 538–539
5. D	p. 532	17. D	p. 539
6. C	pp. 532–533	18. A	p. 538
7. A	p. 532	19. A	p. 538
8. B	p. 532	20. C	p. 539
9. B	p. 533	21. B	pp. 538–539
10. A	p. 534	22. A	p. 538
11. D	p. 536	23. C	p. 539
12. B	p. 536	24. A	p. 538
13. A	p. 537	25. D	p. 539

CHAPTER 10: Communications

MULTIPLE CHOICE

1. E	p. 543	11. B	p. 551
2. B	pp. 543–544	12. D	p. 551
3. C	p. 544	13. C	p. 552
4. E	pp. 545–546	14. A	p. 554
5. D	p. 546	15. D	p. 554
6. B	p. 546	16. E	p. 555
7. A	p. 547	17. A	p. 555
8. E	pp. 547–549	18. D	p. 555
9. E	p. 548	19. A	p. 556
10. A	p. 550	20. C	p. 557

SPECIAL PROJECT: Documentation: Radio Report/Prehospital Care Report

Your report should include most of the following elements:

Radio message from the scene to medical direction:

Unit 89 to receiving hospital. We are at the ball field treating a 13-year-old male who collapsed while playing baseball. He is currently unresponsive to all but painful stimuli, is cool to the touch, and is sweating profusely. Vitals are BP 136/98, pulse 92 and strong, respirations 24 and regular, and pupils equal and slow to react. ECG is showing a normal sinus rhythm. No physical signs of trauma noted, and past medical history is unknown. Oxygen is applied at 12 liters via nonrebreather. Expected ETA, 20 minutes.

Follow-up radio message to Receiving Hospital:

One IV in left forearm is running TKO with NS. Patient now responding to verbal stimuli. Vitals are BP 134/96, pulse 90 and strong, respirations 24. ECG shows normal sinus rhythm. ETA, 10 minutes.

Ambulance run report form:

Please review the accompanying form (on the next page) and check to be sure the form you completed

(continued on p. 473)

Date **Today's Date**	Emergency Medical Services Run Report	Run # **911**

Patient Information	Service Information	Times

Name: **Thompson, Jim**	Agency: **Unit 89**	Rcvd	**15:15**
Address: **Unknown**	Location: **Ballfield**	Enrt	**15:16**
City: St: Zip:	Call Origin: **Dispatch**	Scne	**15:22**
Age: **13** Birth: / / Sex: [**M**][F]	Type: Emrg[**X**] Non[ ] Trnsfr[ ]	LvSn	**15:38**
Nature of Call: **Unconscious person**		ArHsp	**15:57**
Chief Complaint: **Unconsciousness—possible heat exhaustion**		InSv	**16:15**

Description of Current Problem:

The patient collapsed while playing baseball on a very hot, sunny

day. Pt. was found to be cool & diaphoretic, unresponsive to

verbal stimuli, and responsive to painful stimuli. Pupils were

normal in size but slow to react. Physical assessment reveals no

apparent signs of trauma or other medical problem.

Medical Problems

Past		Present
[ ]	Cardiac	[ ]
[ ]	Stroke	[ ]
[ ]	Acute Abdomen	[ ]
[ ]	Diabetes	[ ]
[ ]	Psychiatric	[ ]
[ ]	Epilepsy	[ ]
[ ]	Drug/Alcohol	[ ]
[ ]	Poisoning	[ ]
[ ]	Allergy/Asthma	[ ]
[ ]	Syncope	[ ]
[ ]	Obstetrical	[ ]
[ ]	GYN	[ ]

Other: **Unknown**

Trauma Scr: **n/a**   Glasgow: **6**

On Scene Care: **provided oxygen, removed**	First Aid: **pillow was placed under head**
patient from sun and heat. Attempted IV in right	
forearm (unsuccessful) started IV in left	
forearm w/ 16 ga NS – TKO	By Whom? **bystanders**

02 @ **12** L **15:27** Via **NRB**	C-Collar **n/a** :	S-Immob. **n/a**	Stretcher **15:37**

Allergies/Meds: **Unknown**	Past Med Hx: **Unknown**

Time	Pulse	Resp.	BP S/D	LOC	ECG
15:27	R: **92** [**X**][i]	R: **24** [s][l]	**136**/**98**	[a][v][**X**][u]	**Normal Sinus Rhythm**
Care/Comments: **Pt. unresponsive to all but painful stimuli**					
15:37	R: **90** [**X**][i]	R: **24** [s][l]	**134**/**96**	[a][**X**][p][u]	**Normal Sinus Rhythm**
Care/Comments: **Pt. became responsive to verbal stimuli**					
15:45	R: **88** [**X**][i]	R: **24** [s][l]	**132**/**90**	[**X**][v][p][u]	**Normal Sinus Rhythm**
Care/Comments: **Pt. became fully concious, alert, and oriented**					
:	R: [r][i]	R: [s][l]	/	[a][v][p][u]	
Care/Comments:					

Destination: **Receiving Hospital**	Personnel:	Certification
Reason:[ ]pt [**X**]Closest [ ]M.D. [ ]Other	1. **Your Name**	[**X**][E][O]
Contacted: [**X**]Radio [ ]Tele [ ]Direct	2. **Steve Phillips**	[P][**X**][O]
Ar Status: [**X**]Better [ ]UnC [ ]Worse	3. **n/a**	[P][E][O]

includes the appropriate information. Note that you should include most, if not all, of the information listed on the accompanying sample form. If you have not done this, please review the narrative in the Workbook and determine what is missing from your version. Assure that no important details are left out of the report.

CHAPTER 11: Documentation

MULTIPLE CHOICE			MATCHING		
1.	E	p. 560	31.	P	p. 564
2.	B	p. 560	32.	Y	p. 564
3.	A	p. 560	33.	L	p. 564
4.	B	p. 561	34.	T	p. 564
5.	B	p. 563	35.	A	p. 564
6.	C	p. 563	36.	E	p. 564
7.	A	p. 567	37.	B	p. 564
8.	D	p. 567	38.	O	p. 564
9.	C	p. 568	39.	U	p. 564
10.	B	p. 568	40.	X	p. 564
11.	B	p. 568	41.	M	p. 564
12.	A	p. 568	42.	J	p. 565
13.	E	p. 570	43.	Q	p. 565
14.	A	p. 570	44.	G	p. 565
15.	C	p. 571	45.	R	p. 565
16.	B	p. 571	46.	V	p. 565
17.	D	p. 571	47.	I	p. 566
18.	E	p. 571	48.	N	p. 566
19.	B	p. 572	49.	F	p. 566
20.	A	p. 572	50.	C	p. 566
21.	E	p. 572	51.	W	p. 566
22.	D	p. 573	52.	K	p. 566
23.	E	p. 573	53.	S	p. 566
24.	A	p. 574	54.	D	p. 567
25.	E	p. 574	55.	H	p. 567
26.	B	p. 574			
27.	A	p. 575			
28.	D	p. 575			
29.	E	p. 577			
30.	C	p. 577			

SPECIAL PROJECTS: Documentation: Radio Report/Prehospital Care Report

Radio message from the scene to medical direction:

Unit 21 to medical direction. We are attending a male victim of a one-car crash. He was initially unconscious but is now conscious, alert, and oriented. He has a small contusion on his forehead and a small welt on his neck. He was stung by a bee and has had a previous allergic reaction. Vitals are BP 110/76, pulse 90 and strong, respirations 30, and O_2 saturation of 94 percent. There are audible wheezes, and he is complaining of "a lump in the throat." He is on 12 L of O_2 via nonrebreather and has one IV of LR running TKO. A cervical collar has been applied and spinal immobilization is underway.

Follow-up radio message to Community Hospital:

0.3 mg epinephrine SQ and 50 mg Benadryl IM have been administered. Current vitals are BP 122/78, pulse 68 and strong, respirations 22 and regular, O_2 saturation 98%. Breath sounds are now clear. ETA is 10 minutes.

Ambulance run report form:

Please review the accompanying form (on the next page) and check to be sure the form you completed includes the appropriate information. Note that you should include most, if not all, of the information listed on the accompanying sample form. If you have not done this, please review the narrative in the Workbook and determine what is missing from your version. Assure that no important details are left out of the report.

Crossword Puzzle

Date **Today's Date**	Emergency Medical Services Run Report		Run # **912**

Patient Information		Service Information		Times

Patient Information

Name: **William Sobeski**

Address: **2145 E. Brookline Drive**

City: **Rochester**   St: Zip:

Age: **28**   Birth: /   /   Sex: [**M**][F]

Nature of Call: **One-car auto accident**

Chief Complaint: **Head injury—allergic reaction/bee sting**

Service Information

Agency: **Medic Rescue Unit 21**

Location: **Wildwood & Elm**

Call Origin: **Dispatch**

Type: Emrg[**X**] Non[ ] Trnsfr[ ]

Times

Rcvd	**18:32**
Enrt	**18:32**
Scne	**18:45**
LvSn	**19:02**
ArHsp	**19:25**
InSv	**19:55**

Description of Current Problem:

    Pt. was apparently stung by a bee, then struck a tree with his auto.

    Found unconscious, then awoke. Contusion on his forehead where

    it hit the windshield and a small welt on his neck. Pt. complains

    of a lump in his throat and mild dyspnea. Mild wheezes on

    auscultation. Pt. reports previous life-threatening allergic reaction,

    has a prescribed kit but it is at home. Assessment otherwise

    unremarkable.

Medical Problems

Past		Present
[ ]	Cardiac	[ ]
[ ]	Stroke	[ ]
[ ]	Acute Abdomen	[ ]
[ ]	Diabetes	[ ]
[ ]	Psychiatric	[ ]
[ ]	Epilepsy	[ ]
[ ]	Drug/Alcohol	[ ]
[ ]	Poisoning	[ ]
[**X**]	Allergy/Asthma	[**X**]
[ ]	Syncope	[ ]
[ ]	Obstetrical	[ ]
[ ]	GYN	[ ]

Other:

Trauma Scr: **16**   Glasgow: **15**

On Scene Care: **0_2, C-Collar, Spinal Imm.**	First Aid: **None**
IV – TKO LR w/ 16 ga R forearm	
0.3 mg Epi SQ, 50 mg Benadryl IM	
	By Whom?

02 @ **12** L **18:52** Via **NRB**	C-Collar **18:50**	S-Immob. **18:52**	Stretcher **18:55**

Allergies/Meds: **Bee sting, no other** **allergies known**	Past Med Hx: **Bee sting and reaction 2 yrs ago** **no other history noted.**

Time	Pulse	Resp.	BP S/D	LOC	ECG
18:52	R: **90** [**X**][i]	R: **30** [s][l]	**110/76**	[**X**][v][p][u]	**Normal Sinus Rhythm**
Care/Comments: **IV initiated via protocol – 16 ga R forearm, audible wheezes, SaO_2 94%**					
18:59	R: **78** [**X**][i]	R: **24** [s][l]	**118/88**	[**X**][v][p][u]	**Normal Sinus Rhythm**
Care/Comments: **Epi & Benadryl administered, SaO_2 98%, wheezes gone**					
19:02	R: **68** [**X**][i]	R: **22** [s][l]	**122/78**	[**X**][v][p][u]	**Normal Sinus Rhythm**
Care/Comments: **SaO_2 98%**					
19:20	R: **86** [**X**][i]	R: **24** [s][l]	**122/80**	[**X**][v][p][u]	**Normal Sinus Rhythm**
Care/Comments: **Wheezes reduced, SaO_2 98%**					

Destination: **Community Hospital**	Personnel:	Certification
Reason:[**X**]pt [ ]Closest [ ]M.D. [ ]Other	1. **Your Name**	[**R**][E][O]
Contacted: [**X**]Radio [ ]Tele [ ]Direct	2. **Mike Grailing**	[**R**][E][O]
Ar Status: [**X**]Better [ ]UnC [ ]Worse	3. **n/a**	[P][E][O]

©2004 Pearson Education, Inc.
Intermediate Emergency Care: Principles & Practice

Division 3: Trauma Emergencies

CHAPTER 12: Trauma and Trauma Systems

MULTIPLE CHOICE

1. C	*p. 583*	9. E	*p. 586*
2. A	*p. 583*	10. B	*p. 588*
3. A	*p. 584*	11. A	*p. 588*
4. A	*p. 584*	12. A	*p. 589*
5. C	*p. 584*	13. E	*pp. 589–590*
6. D	*p. 584*	14. C	*p. 590*
7. B	*p. 584*	15. A	*p. 590*
8. D	*p. 584*		

CHAPTER 13: Blunt Trauma

MULTIPLE CHOICE

1. A	*p. 593*	21. E	*p. 605*
2. B	*p. 593*	22. E	*p. 606*
3. B	*p. 593*	23. B	*p. 606*
4. D	*p. 594*	24. D	*pp. 608–609*
5. C	*p. 594*	25. A	*p. 609*
6. E	*p. 594*	26. B	*p. 610*
7. B	*p. 594*	27. C	*p. 611*
8. E	*p. 595*	28. A	*p. 611*
9. E	*p. 597*	29. A	*p. 613*
10. D	*p. 597*	30. E	*p. 614*
11. A	*p. 599*	31. D	*p. 615*
12. B	*p. 600*	32. B	*p. 615*
13. C	*p. 600*	33. C	*p. 615*
14. B	*p. 601*	34. A	*p. 616*
15. C	*p. 601*	35. C	*p. 616*
16. B	*p. 602*	36. A	*p. 617*
17. C	*p. 602*	37. D	*p. 618*
18. A	*p. 604*	38. B	*p. 618*
19. E	*p. 604*	39. A	*p. 620*
20. A	*p. 605*	40. E	*p. 621*

SPECIAL PROJECT: Injury Mechanism Analysis

A. Mechanism of Injury: sports injury, blunt trauma
   Anticipated Injuries: head (but well protected); neck/spine, skeletal—fractures/dislocations; muscular—sprains, strains *pp. 620–622*

B. Mechanism of Injury: frontal impact auto crash
   Anticipated Injuries: head injury; cervical spine injury; chest injury; abdominal injury; foot, leg and thigh injuries *pp. 602–604*

C. Mechanism of Injury: explosion, pressure wave, projectiles, structural collapse
   Anticipated Injuries: pressure wave—lung, bowel, ear injuries; penetrating trauma from projectiles; burns; inhalation injuries; blunt trauma; crush injuries *pp. 614–617*

CHAPTER 14: Penetrating Trauma

MULTIPLE CHOICE

1. B	*p. 624*	14. A	*p. 632*
2. C	*p. 625*	15. C	*p. 634*
3. A	*p. 626*	16. B	*p. 634*
4. C	*p. 626*	17. A	*pp. 635–636*
5. B	*p. 626*	18. A	*p. 636*
6. E	*p. 627*	19. A	*p. 636*
7. A	*p. 627*	20. D	*p. 636*
8. A	*p. 627*	21. C	*p. 637*
9. E	*p. 629*	22. B	*p. 637*
10. A	*p. 630*	23. E	*p. 638*
11. A	*p. 632*	24. D	*p. 638*
12. C	*p. 632*	25. C	*p. 639*
13. E	*p. 633*		

CHAPTER 15: Hemorrhage and Shock

MULTIPLE CHOICE

1. D	*p. 644*	21. E	*p. 655*
2. B	*p. 644*	22. E	*pp. 655–656*
3. A	*p. 644*	23. E	*p. 647*
4. D	*p. 644*	24. D	*p. 658*
5. D	*p. 644*	25. B	*p. 657*
6. B	*p. 644*	26. B	*p. 660*
7. E	*pp. 645–646*	27. B	*p. 661*
8. A	*p. 646*	28. A	*p. 661*
9. B	*p. 647*	29. C	*p. 661*
10. B	*p. 650*	30. B	*p. 662*
11. A	*p. 650*	31. E	*p. 663*
12. B	*p. 650*	32. D	*p. 663*
13. C	*p. 651*	33. A	*p. 663*
14. E	*p. 651*	34. B	*p. 664*
15. D	*p. 651*	35. E	*p. 665*
16. A	*p. 651*	36. C	*p. 665*
17. A	*p. 652*	37. E	*p. 666*
18. A	*p. 653*	38. B	*p. 666*
19. C	*p. 654*	39. E	*p. 667*
20. B	*p. 649*	40. A	*p. 668*

SPECIAL PROJECT: Drip Math Worksheet 2

(see next page for answers)

Drip Math Worksheet 2

1. R = 120 gtts/min
   V = ?
   T = 35 min
   D = 10 gtts/mL

   $V = R \times T = 120$ gtts/min $\times 35$ min

   $V = \dfrac{120 \text{ gtts} \times 35 \text{ min}}{\text{min}} = 4200$ gtts

   $V = \dfrac{4200 \text{ gtts/D}}{10 \text{ gtts}} = 4200 \text{ gtts} \times \text{mL}$ = 420 mL

2. R = 45 gtts/min
   D = 60 gtts/mL
   D´ = 45 gtts/mL

   $R(mL) = R(min)/D = 45$ gtts/min/60 gtts/mL

   $R(mL) = \dfrac{45 \text{ gtts} \times \text{mL}}{60 \text{ gtts} \times \text{min}} = \dfrac{45 \text{ mL}}{60 \text{ min}} = 0.75$ mL/min

   $R(min) = R(mL) \times D´ = 0.75$ mL/min $\times 45$ gtts/mL

   $R(min) = \dfrac{0.75 \text{ mL} \times 45 \text{ gtts}}{\text{mL} \times \text{min}} = 33.75$ gtts/min

   $R(sec) = 33.75$ gtts/60 sec   = 0.56 gtts/sec

3. R = ?
   V = 100 mL
   T = 115 min
   D = 60 gtts/mL

   $R = V/T = 100$ mL/115 min $= 0.87$ mL/min

   $R(min) = R(mL) \times D = 0.87$ mL/min $\times 60$ gtts/min

   $R(min) = \dfrac{0.87 \text{ mL} \times 60 \text{ gtts}}{\text{min} \times \text{mL}}$ = 52 gtts/min

4. R = ?
   V = 45 > 100 mL
   T = 60 min
   D = 60 – 45 – 10 gtts/mL
   R(min) = R(mL) × D

   $R = V/T = 45$ mL/60 min $= 0.75$ mL/min

   $R´ = V/T = 100$ mL/60 min $= 1.67$ mL/min

   $R(60) = \dfrac{0.75 \text{ mL/min} \times 60 \text{ gtts/mL}}{\text{min} \times \text{mL}} = 0.75 \text{ mL} \times 60 \text{ gtts}$ = 45 gtts/min

   $R´(60) = \dfrac{1.67 \text{ mL/min} \times 60 \text{ gtts/mL}}{\text{min} \times \text{mL}} = 1.67 \text{ mL} \times 60 \text{ gtts}$ = 100.2 gtts/mL

   $R(45) = \dfrac{0.75 \text{ mL/min} \times 45 \text{ gtts/mL}}{\text{min} \times \text{mL}} = 0.75 \text{ mL} \times 45 \text{ gtts}$ = 33.75 gtts/min

   $R´(45) = \dfrac{1.67 \text{ mL/min} \times 45 \text{ gtts/mL}}{\text{min} \times \text{mL}} = 1.67 \text{ mL} \times 45 \text{ gtts}$ = 75 gtts/mL

   $R(10) = \dfrac{0.75 \text{ mL/min} \times 10 \text{ gtts/mL}}{\text{min} \times \text{mL}} = 0.75 \text{ mL} \times 10 \text{ gtts}$ = 7.5 gtts/min

   $R´(10) = \dfrac{1.67 \text{ mL/min} \times 10 \text{ gtts/mL}}{\text{min} \times \text{mL}} = 1.67 \text{ mL} \times 10 \text{ gtts}$ = 16.7 gtts/mL

5. R = ?
   V = 150 mL
   T = 65 min

   $R = V/T = 150$ mL/65 min $= \dfrac{150 \text{ mL}}{65 \text{ min}}$ = 2.3 mL/min

©2004 Pearson Education, Inc.
Intermediate Emergency Care: Principles & Practice

CHAPTER 16: Burns

MULTIPLE CHOICE

1. A	p. 672	14. A	p. 679	27. E	p. 684	44. A	p. 693
2. D	p. 673	15. E	p. 679	28. E	p. 685	45. B	p. 693
3. A	p. 673	16. D	p. 679	29. B	p. 687	46. B	p. 693
4. D	p. 674	17. B	p. 679	30. A	p. 688	47. B	p. 694
5. B	p. 674	18. E	pp. 380–381	31. A	p. 688	48. A	p. 694
6. A	p. 674	19. C	p. 681	32. B	p. 694	49. E	p. 695
7. C	p. 676	20. D	p. 681	33. B	p. 681	50. D	p. 695
8. E	p. 676	21. B	p. 681	34. E	pp. 681–683	51. B	p. 695
9. A	p. 676	22. C	p. 682	35. A	p. 690	52. D	p. 697
10. B	p. 677	23. B	p. 683	36. D	p. 690	53. E	p. 697
11. B	p. 677	24. C	p. 683	37. D	p. 690	54. C	p. 697
12. B	p. 677	25. D	p. 683	38. D	p. 690	55. B	p. 697
13. C	p. 678	26. E	p. 683	39. A	p. 692	56. D	p. 698
				40. A	p. 693	57. A	p. 698
				41. B	p. 692	58. A	p. 699
				42. B	p. 692	59. E	p. 699
				43. B	p. 693	60. B	p. 699

SPECIAL PROJECT: Drip Math Worksheet 3

1. R = ?
   T = 2 hour (120 min)
   V = 250 mL

   $$\text{Rate} = \frac{\text{Volume}}{\text{Time}} = \frac{250 \text{ mL}}{120 \text{ min}} = \frac{2.08 \text{ mL}}{\text{min}} = 2.08 \text{ mL/min}$$

   A. D = 10 gtts/mL

   $$R = V \times D = \frac{2.08 \text{ mL} \times 10 \text{ gtts}}{\text{min} \times \text{mL}} = \frac{20.8 \text{ gtts}}{\text{min}} = 20.8 \text{ gtts/min}$$

   B. D = 15 gtts/mL

   $$R = V \times D = \frac{2.08 \text{ mL} \times 15 \text{ gtts}}{\text{min} \times \text{mL}} = \frac{31.2 \text{ gtts}}{\text{min}} = 31.2 \text{ gtts/min}$$

   C. D = 60 gtts/mL

   $$R = V \times D = \frac{2.08 \text{ mL} \times 60 \text{ gtts}}{\text{min} \times \text{mL}} = \frac{144 \text{ gtts}}{\text{min}} = 144 \text{ gtts/min}$$

2. R = 30 gtts/min
   T = ?
   D = 60 gtts/mL

   $$R = R/D = \frac{30 \text{ gtts} \times \text{mL}}{60 \text{ gtts} \times \text{min}} = \frac{0.5 \text{ mL}}{\text{min}} = 0.5 \text{ mL/min}$$

   A. V = 200

   $$T = \frac{V}{R} = \frac{200 \text{ mL} \times \text{min}}{0.5 \text{ mL}} = 400 \text{ min} \quad \frac{400 \text{ min} \times \text{hr}}{60 \text{ min}} = 6.67 \text{ hrs (6 hrs, 40 min)}$$

   B. V = 350

   $$T = \frac{V}{R} = \frac{350 \text{ mL} \times \text{min}}{0.5 \text{ mL}} = 700 \text{ min} \quad \frac{700 \text{ min} \times \text{hr}}{60 \text{ min}} = 11.67 \text{ hrs (11 hrs, 40 min)}$$

3. R = 1 gtts/sec = 60 gtts/min
   T = 15 min
   V = ?
   D = 15 gtts/mL

   $$R = \frac{60 \text{ gtts} \times \text{mL}}{15 \text{ gtts} \times \text{min}} = \frac{4 \text{ mL}}{\text{min}} = 4 \text{ mL/min}$$

   $$V = R \times T = \frac{4 \text{ mL} \times 15 \text{ min}}{\text{min}} = 60 \text{ mL}$$

4. Note: You must determine the volume (per minute) administered with the 60 gtts/ml set running at 15 gtts. Then determine the gtts (/min) with the 45 gtts/mL set necessary to administer the same volume.

   $$R = 15 \text{ gtts/min (60 gtts/mL)} = \frac{15 \text{ gtts} \times \text{mL}}{60 \text{ gtts} \times \text{min}} = \frac{0.25 \text{ mL}}{\text{min}} = 0.25 \text{ mL/min}$$

   T = 1 min
   V = ?
   D = 45 gtts/mL

   $$V = R \times T = \frac{0.25 \text{ mL} \times 1 \text{ min}}{\text{min}} = 0.25 \text{ mL}$$

   $$R = \frac{0.25 \text{ mL} \times 45 \text{ gtts}}{\text{min} \times \text{mL}} = \frac{11.25 \text{ gtts}}{\text{min}} = 11.25 \text{ gtts/min}$$

CHAPTER 17: Thoracic Trauma

MULTIPLE CHOICE

1.	A	pp. 704–705	26.	B	p. 718
2.	C	p. 707	27.	D	p. 718
3.	D	p. 708	28.	A	p. 719
4.	B	p. 708	29.	C	pp. 719–720
5.	A	p. 708	30.	B	p. 719
6.	A	p. 708	31.	E	p. 720
7.	E	pp. 708–709	32.	C	p. 720
8.	B	p. 709	33.	B	p. 720
9.	D	p. 709	34.	A	p. 720
10.	B	p. 710	35.	B	p. 721
11.	B	p. 711	36.	E	p. 721
12.	E	p. 709	37.	E	p. 722
13.	D	p. 713	38.	A	p. 723
14.	B	p. 712	39.	D	p. 724
15.	D	p. 713	40.	E	p. 724
16.	D	p. 713	41.	B	p. 725
17.	D	p. 714	42.	B	p. 725
18.	E	p. 714	43.	A	p. 728
19.	C	p. 714	44.	D	p. 728
20.	A	p. 716	45.	A	p. 728
21.	A	p. 716	46.	B	p. 729
22.	A	p. 716	47.	C	p. 729
23.	D	p. 717	48.	A	p. 729
24.	A	p. 717	49.	A	p. 730
25.	E	p. 717	50.	E	p. 732

SPECIAL PROJECT: Label the Diagram

A. sternum *p. 731*
B. lung *p. 731*
C. heart *p. 731*
D. trachea *p. 731*
E. pleura *p. 731*
F. ribs *p. 731*
G. diaphragm *p. 731*
H. pleural space *p. 731*

CHAPTER 18: Trauma Management Skills

MULTIPLE CHOICE

1.	D	p. 736	14.	E	p. 764
2.	E	p. 739	15.	B	p. 767
3.	C	p. 739	16.	C	p. 768
4.	E	p. 741	17.	B	p. 769
5.	E	p. 744	18.	E	p. 770
6.	C	p. 748	19.	A	p. 770
7.	E	p. 750	20.	E	p. 771
8.	A	p. 754	21.	B	p. 777
9.	C	p. 756	22.	A	p. 780
10.	E	p. 760	23.	E	p. 782
11.	A	p. 761	24.	C	p. 786
12.	A	p. 761	25.	B	p. 795
13.	B	p. 763			

Division 4: Medical Emergencies

CHAPTER 19: Respiratory Emergencies

MULTIPLE CHOICE

1.	C	p. 801	29.	C	p. 813
2.	A	p. 802	30.	C	p. 814
3.	A	p. 802	31.	E	p. 823
4.	D	p. 802	32.	C	p. 817
5.	E	p. 803	33.	A	p. 819
6.	C	p. 804	34.	A	p. 821
7.	D	p. 805	35.	B	p. 822
8.	B	p. 805	36.	B	p. 823
9.	B	p. 807	37.	B	p. 824
10.	E	p. 807	38.	D	p. 825
11.	B	p. 807	39.	D	p. 825
12.	A	p. 807	40.	B	p. 825
13.	C	pp. 808–809	41.	B	p. 827
14.	B	p. 809	42.	A	p. 827
15.	A	p. 808	43.	B	p. 829
16.	B	p. 810	44.	A	pp. 830–831
17.	A	p. 810	45.	B	p. 831
18.	C	p. 810	46.	A	p. 831
19.	A	p. 811	47.	A	p. 831
20.	E	p. 811	48.	B	p. 831
21.	D	p. 811	49.	C	p. 832
22.	D	p. 811	50.	A	p. 833
23.	D	p. 811	51.	A	p. 834
24.	B	p. 812	52.	A	p. 834
25.	E	p. 802	53.	C	p. 831
26.	B	p. 812	54.	B	p. 830
27.	E	p. 813	55.	D	p. 827
28.	D	p. 813			

MATCHING

56.	C	pp. 818–819
57.	F	p. 823
58.	A	p. 825
59.	E	p. 826
60.	G	p. 829
61.	B	p. 830
62.	D	pp. 831–832

LABEL THE DIAGRAMS

1.	J	p. 201
2.	H	p. 201
3.	G	p. 201
4.	C	p. 201
5.	E	p. 201
6.	F	p. 201
7.	B	p. 201
8.	A	p. 201
9.	D	p. 201
10.	I	p. 201
11.	M	p. 201
12.	N	p. 201
13.	O	p. 201
14.	K	p. 201
15.	L	p. 201
16.	B	p. 204
17.	E	p. 204
18.	D	p. 204
19.	C	p. 204
20.	A	p. 204

SPECIAL PROJECT: Evaluating Abnormal Breathing Patterns

A. Apneustic respirations *p. 806*
B. Cheyne-Stokes respirations *p. 806*
C. Central neurogenic hyperventilation *p. 806*
D. Kussmaul's respirations *p. 806*
E. Ataxic (Biot's) respirations *p. 806*

Suggested Responses to Scenarios:

Scenario 1: Breathing Pattern: Cheyne-Stokes
Probable Cause: terminal illness *p. 805*

Scenario 2: Breathing Pattern: Ataxic (Biot's)
Probable Cause: hemorrhagic stroke. (The ataxic breathing is a clue that the stroke is hemorrhagic

rather than obstructive because ataxic breathing typically results from a build-up of intracranial pressure as would be caused by bleeding into the brain.) Other possibilities include intracranial bleeding caused by a blow to the head when the patient fell. A brain infection or tumor could also cause increased intracranial pressure and ataxic breathing, but the sudden onset and severe headache are more indicative of a stroke. *p. 805*

Scenario 3: Breathing Pattern: Kussmaul's
Probable Cause: diabetic ketoacidosis (A variety of medical emergencies can result from diabetes.) The clue to acidosis is the deep, rapid breathing, which is a compensatory mechanism that rids the body of excess CO_2 to alleviate the acidic condition. The cause in this case is that the patient has not been taking her insulin. Insulin is necessary to help glucose enter the body cells. When insulin is absent, the cells tun to metabolism of fats instead of the normal glucose metabolism. A byproduct of fat metabolism is ketones, which result in acidosis. *p. 805*

CHAPTER 20: Cardiovascular Emergencies

Part 1

MULTIPLE CHOICE

1. C	*p. 839*
2. A	*p. 839*
3. D	*p. 840*
4. E	*p. 842*
5. B	*pp. 843–844*
6. B	*p. 851*
7. E	*p. 855*
8. C	*p. 858*
9. D	*p. 863*
10. B	*p. 873*
11. A	*p. 873*
12. E	*p. 876*
13. A	*p. 876*
14. C	*p. 877*
15. D	*p. 878*
16. B	*p. 883*
17. E	*p. 888*
18. C	*p. 886*
19. D	*p. 889*
20. A	*p. 893*

MATCHING

21. B	*p. 840*
22. G	*p. 840*
23. D	*p. 840*
24. A	*p. 840*
25. H	*p. 840*
26. C	*p. 840*
27. F	*p. 840*
28. E	*p. 840*
29. B	*p. 843*
30. C	*p. 843*
31. A	*p. 843*

LABEL THE DIAGRAMS

Figure 1

32. D	*p. 840*
33. A	*p. 840*
34. B	*p. 840*
35. C	*p. 840*
36. F	*p. 840*
37. E	*p. 840*

Figure 2

38. C	*p. 843*
39. D	*p. 843*
40. F	*p. 843*
41. G	*p. 843*
42. E	*p. 843*
43. B	*p. 843*
44. A	*p. 843*

Figure 3
pp. 847, 852

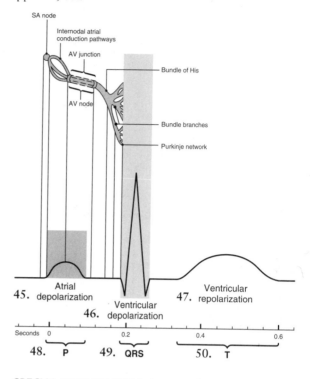

45. Atrial depolarization
46. Ventricular depolarization
47. Ventricular repolarization
48. P
49. QRS
50. T

SPECIAL PROJECT: ECG Interpretation

ECG #1 *p. 859*
Rate: roughly 150 bpm
Rhythm: regular
P waves: always present, upright, normal shape
P-R interval: approx. 0.10–0.12 sec
QRS complexes: normal appearance, approx. 0.08–0.10 sec
Overall rhythm (or dysrhythmia): Sinus tachycardia

ECG #2 *pp. 870–871*
Rate: roughly 100 bpm
Rhythm: irregularly regular
P waves: none detected, fibrillation (f) waves are visible
P-R interval: none (because of absence of P waves)
QRS complexes: normal appearance, approx. 0.10–0.12 sec
Overall rhythm (or dysrhythmia): Atrial fibrillation

ECG #3 *pp. 873–874*
Rate: roughly 90 bpm
Rhythm: ventricular rhythm is roughly regularly irregular
P waves: normal in appearance, two are not followed by a QRS complex
P-R interval: widens over five beats, then comes apparent missed beat
QRS complexes: inverted, approx. 0.10 sec
Overall rhythm (or dysrhythmia): Type I second-degree AV block

ECG #4 *pp. 857; 884–886*
Rate: roughly 60 bpm or less
Rhythm: slow, roughly regular except for premature beat (last shown on strip)
P waves: normal in appearance, precede all but last beat on strip

P-R Interval: none
QRS complexes: abnormal shape, S-T segment abnormal and lengthened, T waves peaked, somewhat tall
Overall rhythm (or dysrhythmia): Sinus bradycardia, one premature ventricular contraction (PVC). Possible hyperkalemia.

ECG #5 *p. 889*
Rate: impossible to determine
Rhythm: irregular, disorganized rhythm
P waves: not clearly discernible
P-R interval: not discernible
QRS complexes: Ventricular fibrillation
Overall rhythm (or dysrhythmia): Ventricular fibrillation

Part 2

MULTIPLE CHOICE

1.	A	*p. 898*	17.	A	*p. 943*
2.	D	*p. 911*	18.	E	*p. 910*
3.	E	*p. 911*	19.	D	*p. 916*
4.	B	*p. 911*	20.	A	*p. 910*
5.	B	*p. 915*	21.	B	*p. 915*
6.	A	*p. 923*	22.	C	*p. 916*
7.	E	*p. 933*	23.	A	*p. 852*
8.	B	*p. 935*	24.	C	*p. 852*
9.	A	*p. 938*	25.	B	*p. 852*
10.	D	*p. 941*	26.	B	*p. 852*
			27.	C	*p. 926*
			28.	D	*p. 930*
			29.	B	*p. 930*

MATCHING

11.	B	*p. 899*	30.	F	*p. 938*
12.	F	*p. 867*	31.	E	*p. 930*
13.	E	*p. 931*	32.	A	*p. 932*
14.	G	*p. 932*	33.	G	*p. 933*
15.	C	*p. 932*	34.	H	*p. 934*
16.	D	*p. 942*			

CHAPTER 21: Diabetic Emergencies

MULTIPLE CHOICE

1.	C	*p. 948*	9.	A	*p. 954*
2.	C	*p. 949*	10.	A	*p. 954*
3.	C	*p. 950*	11.	C	*p. 956*
4.	E	*p. 949*	12.	E	*p. 955*
5.	B	*p. 952*	13.	A	*p. 957*
6.	D	*p. 953*	14.	B	*p. 954*
7.	E	*p. 953*	15.	C	*p. 956*
8.	A	*p. 954*			

CHAPTER 22: Allergic Reactions

MULTIPLE CHOICE

1.	B	*p. 960*	9.	C	*p. 963*
2.	D	*p. 960*	10.	B	*p. 963*
3.	B	*p. 960*	11.	A	*p. 963*
4.	C	*p. 961*	12.	B	*p. 964*
5.	D	*p. 961*	13.	C	*p. 965*
6.	A	*p. 962*	14.	D	*p. 965*
7.	C	*p. 962*	15.	D	*p. 964*
8.	C	*p. 963*			

CHAPTER 23: Poisoning and Overdose Emergencies

MULTIPLE CHOICE

1.	C	*p. 971*	27.	E	*p. 985*
2.	A	*p. 971*	28.	A	*p. 991*
3.	D	*p. 972*	29.	A	*pp. 992–993*
4.	B	*p. 973*	30.	C	*p. 1000*
5.	A	*p. 973*	31.	A	*p. 1003*
6.	B	*p. 975*	32.	A	*p. 1002*
7.	E	*p. 974*	33.	A	*p. 1002*
8.	B	*p. 974*	34.	B	*pp. 1004–1005*
9.	B	*p. 975*			
10.	B	*p. 975*			

MATCHING

11.	C	*p. 976*	35.	B	*p. 972*
12.	A	*p. 976*	36.	H	*p. 999*
13.	D	*p. 977*	37.	N	*p. 970*
14.	B	*p. 978*	38.	M	*p. 972*
15.	A	*p. 977*	39.	A	*p. 970*
16.	E	*p. 982*	40.	O	*p. 999*
17.	A	*p. 980*	41.	G	*p. 985*
18.	B	*p. 983*	42.	P	*p. 971*
19.	A	*p. 983*	43.	F	*p. 1004*
20.	A	*p. 983*	44.	L	*p. 990*
21.	E	*p. 983*	45.	I	*p. 974*
22.	C	*p. 987*	46.	J	*p. 972*
23.	E	*p. 988*	47.	K	*p. 1000*
24.	A	*p. 985*	48.	D	*p. 978*
25.	B	*p. 986*	49.	C	*p. 999*
26.	D	*p. 990*	50.	E	*p. 999*

SPECIAL PROJECT: Analyzing an Emergency Scene

pp. 975–977

1. This probably represents an accidental ingestion overdose involving multiple medications of unknown type(s). This is not an uncommon call; you will see this kind of situation.

2. As in all other cases involving a potentially unstable patient, the first priority is support of the ABCs: After checking that the airway is clear, high-flow oxygen should be started and attention paid on an ongoing basis that the airway remains clear (suspect possible vomiting and aspiration; intubate if necessary). Ventilation does not appear to need support at the moment, but you are aware that ventilation can decompensate quickly. Circulation clearly is impaired based on the peripheral pulses. Prepare for ECG monitoring and for pulse oximetry. If it looks like IV access can be established easily, it may be done at this point.

3. Transport of this unstable, elderly man with unclear toxic ingestion and underlying medical conditions is the first priority. Contact with medical direction can be made en route as the focused physical is done and evaluation of vitals and patient condition continues. Poison Control is not useful until you have some idea of the medications involved in the ingestion.

4. Take the pill case. If there are any empty or partially full glasses/cups around, check for signs of alcohol or coffee or tea (which might contain caffeine). Look for opened bottles of over-the-counter medications such as aspirin. If one team partner has time while en route, he/she can inspect the medications to see if any are definitively recognizable.

CHAPTER 24: Neurological Emergencies

MULTIPLE CHOICE

1. C   *p. 1009*
2. C   *p. 1012*
3. E   *p. 1015*
4. C   *p. 1019*
5. B   *p. 1019*
6. D   *p. 1021*
7. C   *p. 1025*
8. B   *pp. 1025–1026*
9. B   *p. 1025*
10. C   *pp. 1026–1027*

MATCHING

11. B, G   *p. 1013*
12. E, H   *p. 1013*
13. A, D   *p. 1013*
14. C, I   *p. 1013*
15. F, J   *p. 1013*
16. A, D   *p. 1021*
17. C, E   *p. 1021*
18. C, F   *p. 1021*
19. B, C   *p. 1021*

CHAPTER 25: Non-Traumatic Abdominal Emergencies

MULTIPLE CHOICE

1. D   *p. 1036*
2. A   *p. 1036*
3. B   *p. 1052*
4. E   *pp. 1036–1037*
5. A   *p. 1053*

6. C   *pp. 1036–1037*
7. E   *p. 1037*
8. A   *p. 1037*
9. B   *p. 1037*
10. A   *p. 1037*
11. E   *p. 1037*
12. A   *p. 1037*
13. D   *p. 1051*

CHAPTER 26: Environmental Emergencies

MULTIPLE CHOICE

1. C   *pp. 1055–1056*
2. A   *p. 1056*
3. E   *pp. 1057–1058*
4. B   *p. 1060*
5. B   *p. 1061*
6. A   *p. 1064*
7. B   *p. 1064*
8. D   *p. 1065*
9. A   *p. 1068*
10. C   *p. 1068*
11. E   *p. 1071*
12. B   *p. 1073*
13. D   *p. 1075*
14. C   *p. 1076*
15. C   *p. 1079*
16. B   *p. 1075*

17. E   *p. 1081*
18. D   *p. 1080*
19. C   *p. 1084*
20. B   *p. 1086*

MATCHING

21. I   *p. 1062*
22. D   *p. 1071*
23. E   *p. 1084*
24. J   *p. 1067*
25. G   *p. 1083*
26. F   *p. 1080*
27. H   *p. 1081*
28. A   *p. 1067*
29. C   *p. 1078*
30. B   *p. 1084*

CHAPTER 27: Behavioral Emergencies

MULTIPLE CHOICE

1. B   *p. 1091*
2. B   *p. 1093*
3. C   *p. 1093*
4. C   *p. 1093*
5. B   *p. 1094*
6. D   *p. 1094*
7. E   *p. 1097*
8. C   *p. 1099*
9. C   *p. 1099*
10. A   *p. 1095*
11. C   *p. 1096*
12. A   *p. 1096*
13. A   *p. 1100*

14. B   *pp. 1107–1108*
15. B   *p. 1109*

MATCHING

16. J   *p. 1102*
17. A   *p. 1096*
18. D   *p. 1097*
19. I   *p. 1102*
20. E   *p. 1097*
21. H   *p. 1099*
22. F   *p. 1097*
23. C   *p. 1096*
24. G   *p. 1102*
25. B   *p. 1096*

CHAPTER 28: Gynecological Emergencies

MULTIPLE CHOICE

1. D   *p. 1113*
2. B   *p. 1113*
3. C   *pp. 1113–1114*
4. C   *p. 1113*
5. C   *p. 1115*
6. A   *p. 1116*
7. E   *p. 1116*
8. B   *p. 1118*
9. D   *p. 1117*
10. C   *p. 1116*
11. B   *p. 1117*

12. A   *p. 1118*
13. A   *pp. 1119–1120*
14. D   *p. 1119*

LABEL THE DIAGRAM

p. 226
  A. Ovary
  B. Fallopian tube
  C. Uterus
  D. Cervix
  E. Vagina

SPECIAL PROJECT: Problem-Solving: Abdominal Pain

1. Focused history elements: *pp. 1113–1114*
   • SAMPLE and OPQRST
   • Obstetric history: gravida, parity, abortion
   • Gynecologic history: past ectopic pregnancies, surgical procedures
   • History of trauma
   • Last menstrual period (LMP)
   • Form of birth control and regularity of use
2. Differential diagnosis possibilities: *pp. 1115–1117*
   • PID
   • Ruptured ovarian cyst
   • Endometritis
   • Ectopic pregnancy

Division 5: Special Considerations

CHAPTER 29: Obstetrical Emergencies

MULTIPLE CHOICE

1. A *p. 1122*	20. A *pp. 1139–1140*
2. D *p. 1123*	21. A *p. 1145*
3. E *p. 1126*	22. B *p. 1145*
4. D *p. 1124*	23. B *p. 1147*
5. A *p. 1126*	24. C *p. 1151*
6. C *p. 1126*	25. D *pp. 1152–1153*
7. E *p. 1128*	
8. C *pp. 1128–1132*	**MATCHING**
9. B *p. 1132*	26. D *p. 1123*
10. A *p. 1133*	27. E *p. 1122*
11. A *p. 1132*	28. A *p. 1127*
12. C *p. 1133*	29. C *p. 1123*
13. B *p. 1136*	30. B *p. 1123*
14. E *p. 1137*	31. G *p. 1138*
15. C *p. 1141*	32. J *p. 1138*
16. B *p. 1141*	33. H *p. 1127*
17. B *p. 1152*	34. I *p. 1139*
18. C *p. 1151*	35. F *p. 1140*
19. C *pp. 1148, 1150*	

CHAPTER 30: Neonatal Resuscitation

MULTIPLE CHOICE

1. B *p. 1156*	14. E *p. 1159*
2. A *p. 1156*	15. B *p. 1159*
3. C *p. 1156*	16. E *p. 1161*
4. E *p. 1156*	17. A *p. 1161*
5. B *p. 1157*	18. B *p. 1162*
6. A *p. 1157*	19. B *p. 1162*
7. A *pp. 1157–1158*	20. D *p. 1162*
8. B *p. 1158*	21. B *p. 1167*
9. E *p. 1158*	22. A *p. 1165*
10. D *p. 1158*	23. A *p. 1165*
11. B *p. 1158*	24. C *p. 1167*
12. C *p. 1158*	25. A *p. 1168*
13. B *p. 1159*	

SPECIAL PROJECT: APGAR Score

Part I: Total score = 5 *pp. 1145–1146, 1158–1159*

Part II: From top to bottom, items should read—
oxygen, bag-mask ventilation, chest compressions,
intubation, medications *p. 1163*

Part III: Total score = 9 *pp. 1145–1146, 1158–1159*

CHAPTER 31: Pediatric Emergencies

MULTIPLE CHOICE

1. C *p. 1185*	24. C *p. 1205*
2. D *p. 1185*	25. E *p. 1210*
3. A *p. 1186*	26. C *p. 1212*
4. B *p. 1187*	27. D *p. 1213*
5. E *p. 1187*	28. A *p. 1215*
6. C *p. 1188*	29. C *p. 1215*
7. C *p. 1188*	30. B *p. 1216*
8. B *p. 1189*	31. C *p. 1222*
9. C *p. 1191*	32. E *pp. 1223–1224*
10. E *p. 1198*	33. C *p. 1225*
11. A *p. 1192*	34. A *p. 1226*
12. B *p. 1193*	35. D *pp. 1228–1229*
13. B *p. 1193*	36. B *p. 1229*
14. B *p. 1194*	37. A *p. 1232*
15. B *p. 1196*	38. B *p. 1237*
16. E *p. 1198*	39. C *p. 1239*
17. E *p. 1198*	40. C *p. 1243*
18. E *p. 1201*	41. C *pp. 1245–1246*
19. D *p. 1203*	42. C *pp. 1250–1251*
20. A *p. 1203*	43. E *p. 1252*
21. C *p. 1217*	44. D *p. 1254*
22. D *p. 1206*	45. C *p. 1257*
23. E *p. 1206*	

SPECIAL PROJECT: Burn Injuries

pp. 1249–1250

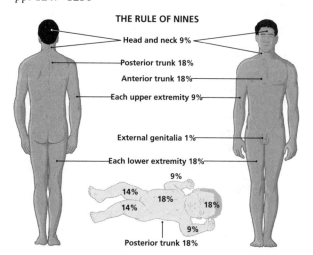

THE RULE OF NINES

Head and neck 9%
Posterior trunk 18%
Anterior trunk 18%
Each upper extremity 9%
External genitalia 1%
Each lower extremity 18%

9%
14%
18%
14%
18%
9%
Posterior trunk 18%

1. 49%
2. 41%
3. Sample answer: The modified rule of nines for the
   pediatric patient gives less body surface area to
   the legs and more to the head of a toddler.
4. "rule of palm"

©2004 Pearson Education, Inc.
Intermediate Emergency Care: Principles & Practice

CHAPTER 32: Geriatric Emergencies

MULTIPLE CHOICE

1.	B	*p. 1262*	42.	E	*p. 1280*
2.	C	*p. 1262*	43.	A	*p. 1280*
3.	C	*p. 1264*	44.	B	*pp. 1280–1281*
4.	A	*p. 1265*	45.	C	*p. 1280*
5.	B	*p. 1265*	46.	C	*p. 1281*
6.	C	*p. 1265*	47.	B	*p. 1282*
7.	D	*p. 1265*	48.	B	*p. 1282*
8.	E	*p. 1265*	49.	B	*p. 1283*
9.	A	*p. 1265*	50.	A	*p. 1284*
10.	B	*p. 1265*	51.	B	*p. 1285*
11.	B	*p. 1265*	52.	D	*p. 1285*
12.	C	*p. 1265*	53.	C	*p. 1286*
13.	D	*p. 1266*	54.	D	*p. 1287*
14.	A	*p. 1267*	55.	A	*p. 1288*
15.	E	*p. 1267*	56.	B	*pp. 1290–1291*
16.	C	*p. 1266*	57.	B	*p. 1291*
17.	A	*p. 1267*	58.	B	*p. 1291*
18.	E	*p. 1268*	59.	A	*p. 1291*
19.	E	*p. 1268*	60.	E	*p. 1292*
20.	A	*p. 1269*	61.	B	*p. 1292*
21.	D	*p. 1269*	62.	A	*pp. 1293–1294*
22.	A	*p. 1270*	63.	A	*p. 1294*
23.	A	*p. 1270*	64.	C	*p. 1295*
24.	E	*pp. 1270–1271*	65.	B	*p. 1297*
25.	B	*p. 1271*			
26.	E	*p. 1271*			

MATCHING

27.	D	*pp. 1272–1273*	66.	J	*p. 1287*
28.	E	*p. 1272*	67.	G	*p. 1294*
29.	A	*p. 1274*	68.	A	*p. 1284*
30.	A	*p. 1273*	69.	H	*p. 1283*
31.	C	*p. 1273*	70.	M	*p. 1290*
32.	A	*p. 1273*	71.	O	*p. 1300*
33.	B	*p. 1273*	72.	I	*p. 1286*
34.	C	*p. 1274*	73.	B	*p. 1285*
35.	C	*p. 1275*	74.	C	*p. 1285*
36.	B	*p. 1275*	75.	L	*p. 1287*
37.	B	*p. 1275*	76.	K	*p. 1288*
38.	E	*p. 1276*	77.	N	*p. 1306*
39.	A	*p. 1276*	78.	D	*p. 1285*
40.	B	*pp. 1278–1279*	79.	F	*p. 1286*
41.	A	*p. 1279*	80.	E	*p. 1267*

CHAPTER 33: Assessment-Based Management

MULTIPLE CHOICE

1.	B	*p. 1309*	9.	E	*p. 1314*
2.	C	*p. 1310*	10.	B	*p. 1314*
3.	B	*p. 1310*	11.	C	*p. 1315*
4.	E	*p. 1311*	12.	C	*p. 1316*
5.	C	*p. 1311*	13.	C	*p. 1317*
6.	E	*pp. 1311–1312*	14.	B	*p. 1318*
7.	A	*p. 1312*	15.	B	*p. 1319*
8.	D	*p. 1314*			

CHAPTER 34: Responding to Terrorist Acts

MULTIPLE CHOICE

1.	A	*p. 1323*	11.	A	*p. 1328*
2.	E	*p. 1323*	12.	B	*p. 1328*
3.	C	*p. 1324*	13.	C	*p. 1328*
4.	B	*p. 1324*	14.	D	*p. 1329*
5.	D	*p. 1325*	15.	E	*p. 1330*
6.	E	*p. 1325*	16.	D	*p. 1332*
7.	C	*pp. 1325–1326*	17.	E	*p. 1332*
8.	A	*p. 1326*	18.	A	*p. 1333*
9.	E	*p. 1327*	19.	A	*p. 1333*
10.	E	*pp. 1327–1328*	20.	B	*p. 1334*

National Registry of Emergency Medical Technicians

PRACTICAL EVALUATION FORMS

The forms on the next pages are provided to help you identify common criteria by which you will be evaluated. It may be valuable to review your practical skills by using these sheets during your class practice sessions and as you review those skills before class, state, and any national testing. Evaluation forms will vary; however, many of the important elements of EMT-Intermediate practice are common to all forms.

EMT-INTERMEDIATE FORMS

The following skill instruments for the EMT-Intermediate level were developed by the National Registry of EMTs and have been approved for use in advanced level National Registry examinations.

- Bleeding Control/Shock Management
- Dual Lumen Airway Device
- Dynamic Cardiology
- Intravenous Therapy
- Patient Assessment—Medical
- Patient Assessment—Trauma
- Pediatric Intraosseous Infusion
- Pediatric (less than 2 years) Ventilatory Management
- Spinal Immobilization (Seated Patient)
- Spinal Immobilization (Supine Patient)
- Static Cardiology
- Ventilatory Management—Adult

Candidate: _____ Examiner: _____

Date: _____ Signature: _____

Time Start:_____	Possible Points	Points Awarded
Takes or verbalizes body substance isolation precautions	1	
Applies direct pressure to the wound	1	
Elevates the extremity	1	
NOTE: The examiner must now inform the candidate that the wound continues to bleed.		
Applies an additional dressing to the wound	1	
NOTE: The examiner must now inform the candidate that the wound still continues to bleed. The second dressing does not control the bleeding.		
Locates and applies pressure to appropriate arterial pressure point	1	
NOTE: The examiner must now inform the candidate that the bleeding is controlled.		
Bandages the wound	1	
NOTE: The examiner must now inform the candidate that the patient is exhibiting signs and symptoms of hypoperfusion.		
Properly positions the patient	1	
Administers high concentration oxygen	1	
Initiates steps to prevent heat loss from the patient	1	
Indicates the need for immediate transportation	1	
Time End: _____	**TOTAL** 10	

CRITICAL CRITERIA

_____ Did not take or verbalize body substance isolation precautions
_____ Did not apply high concentration of oxygen
_____ Applied a tourniquet before attempting other methods of bleeding control
_____ Did not control hemorrhage in a timely manner
_____ Did not indicate the need for immediate transportation

You must factually document your rationale for checking any of the above critical items on the reverse side of this form.

p313/8-003k

DUAL LUMEN AIRWAY DEVICE (COMBITUBE® OR PTL®)

Candidate: _____ Examiner: _____

Date: _____ Signature: _____

NOTE: If candidate elects to initially ventilate with BVM attached to reservoir and oxygen, full credit must be awarded for steps denoted by "**" so long as first ventilation is delivered within 30 seconds.

	Possible Points	Points Awarded
Takes or verbalizes body substance isolation precautions	1	
Opens the airway manually	1	
Elevates tongue, inserts simple adjunct [oropharyngeal or nasopharyngeal airway]	1	
NOTE: Examiner now informs candidate no gag reflex is present and patient accepts adjunct		
**Ventilates patient immediately with bag-valve-mask device unattached to oxygen	1	
**Hyperventilates patient with room air	1	
NOTE: Examiner now informs candidate that ventilation is being performed without difficulty		
Attaches oxygen reservoir to bag-valve-mask device and connects to high flow oxygen regulator [12-15 L/minute]	1	
Ventilates patient at a rate of 10-20/minute with appropriate volumes	1	
NOTE: After 30 seconds, examiner auscultates and reports breath sounds are present and equal bilaterally and medical control has ordered insertion of a dual lumen airway. The examiner must now take over ventilation.		
Directs assistant to pre-oxygenate patient	1	
Checks/prepares airway device	1	
Lubricates distal tip of the device [may be verbalized]	1	
NOTE: Examiner to remove OPA and move out of the way when candidate is prepared to insert device		
Positions head properly	1	
Performs a tongue-jaw lift	1	

☐ USES COMBITUBE®	☐ USES PTL®		
Inserts device in mid-line and to depth so printed ring is at level of teeth	Inserts device in mid-line until bite block flange is at level of teeth	1	
Inflates pharyngeal cuff with proper volume and removes syringe	Secures strap	1	
Inflates distal cuff with proper volume and removes syringe	Blows into tube #1 to adequately inflate both cuffs	1	
Attaches/directs attachment of BVM to the first [esophageal placement] lumen and ventilates		1	
Confirms placement and ventilation through correct lumen by observing chest rise, auscultation over the epigastrium, and bilaterally over each lung		1	
NOTE: The examiner states, "You do not see rise and fall of the chest and you only hear sounds over the epigastrium."			
Attaches/directs attachment of BVM to the second [endotracheal placement] lumen and ventilates		1	
Confirms placement and ventilation through correct lumen by observing chest rise, auscultation over the epigastrium, and bilaterally over each lung		1	
NOTE: The examiner confirms adequate chest rise, absent sounds over the epigastrium, and equal bilateral breath sounds.			
Secures device or confirms that the device remains properly secured		1	
	TOTAL	20	

CRITICAL CRITERIA

_____ Failure to initiate ventilations within 30 seconds after taking body substance isolation precautions or interrupts ventilations for greater than 30 seconds at any time
_____ Failure to take or verbalize body substance isolation precautions
_____ Failure to voice and ultimately provide high oxygen concentrations [at least 85%]
_____ Failure to ventilate patient at a rate of at least 10/minute
_____ Failure to provide adequate volumes per breath [maximum 2 errors/minute permissible]
_____ Failure to pre-oxygenate patient prior to insertion of the dual lumen airway device
_____ Failure to insert the dual lumen airway device at a proper depth or at either proper place within 3 attempts
_____ Failure to inflate both cuffs properly
_____ **Combitube** - failure to remove the syringe immediately after inflation of each cuff
      PTL - failure to secure the strap prior to cuff inflation
_____ Failure to confirm that the proper lumen of the device is being ventilated by observing chest rise, auscultation over the epigastrium, and bilaterally over each lung
_____ Inserts any adjunct in a manner dangerous to patient

You must factually document your rationale for checking any of the above critical items on the reverse side of this form.

p304/8-003k

National Registry of Emergency Medical Technicians
Advanced Level Practical Examination

DYNAMIC CARDIOLOGY

Candidate: _____Examiner: _____

Date: _____Signature: _____

SET #_____

Level of Testing:　　□ NREMT-Intermediate/99　　　□ NREMT-Paramedic

Time Start:_____	Possible Points	Points Awarded
Takes or verbalizes infection control precautions	1	
Checks level of responsiveness	1	
Checks ABCs	1	
Initiates CPR if appropriate [verbally]	1	
Attaches ECG monitor in a timely fashion or applies paddles for "Quick Look"	1	
Correctly interprets initial rhythm	1	
Appropriately manages initial rhythm	2	
Notes change in rhythm	1	
Checks patient condition to include pulse and, if appropriate, BP	1	
Correctly interprets second rhythm	1	
Appropriately manages second rhythm	2	
Notes change in rhythm	1	
Checks patient condition to include pulse and, if appropriate, BP	1	
Correctly interprets third rhythm	1	
Appropriately manages third rhythm	2	
Notes change in rhythm	1	
Checks patient condition to include pulse and, if appropriate, BP	1	
Correctly interprets fourth rhythm	1	
Appropriately manages fourth rhythm	2	
Orders high percentages of supplemental oxygen at proper times	1	
Time End: _____　　　　　　　　　　　　　　　　**TOTAL**	24	

CRITICAL CRITERIA

_____ Failure to deliver first shock in a timely manner due to operator delay in machine use or providing treatments other than CPR with simple adjuncts

_____ Failure to deliver second or third shocks without delay other than the time required to reassess rhythm and recharge paddles

_____ Failure to verify rhythm before delivering each shock

_____ Failure to ensure the safety of self and others [verbalizes "All clear" and observes]

_____ Inability to deliver DC shock [does not use machine properly]

_____ Failure to demonstrate acceptable shock sequence

_____ Failure to order initiation or resumption of CPR when appropriate

_____ Failure to order correct management of airway [ET when appropriate]

_____ Failure to order administration of appropriate oxygen at proper time

_____ Failure to diagnose or treat 2 or more rhythms correctly

_____ Orders administration of an inappropriate drug or lethal dosage

_____ Failure to correctly diagnose or adequately treat v-fib, v-tach, or asystole

You must factually document your rationale for checking any of the above critical items on the reverse side of this form.

p306/8-003k

INTRAVENOUS THERAPY

Candidate: _____ Examiner: _____

Date: _____ Signature: _____

Level of Testing: ☐ NREMT-Intermediate/85   ☐ NREMT-Intermediate/99   ☐ NREMT-Paramedic

Time Start: _____

	Possible Points	Points Awarded

Checks selected IV fluid for:
     -Proper fluid (1 point)
     -Clarity (1 point)
	2	

Selects appropriate catheter	1	
Selects proper administration set	1	
Connects IV tubing to the IV bag	1	
Prepares administration set [fills drip chamber and flushes tubing]	1	
Cuts or tears tape [at any time before venipuncture]	1	
Takes/verbalizes body substance isolation precautions [prior to venipuncture]	1	
Applies tourniquet	1	
Palpates suitable vein	1	
Cleanses site appropriately	1	

Performs venipuncture
     -Inserts stylette (1 point)
     -Notes or verbalizes flashback (1 point)
     -Occludes vein proximal to catheter (1 point)
     -Removes stylette (1 point)
     -Connects IV tubing to catheter (1 point)
	5	

Disposes/verbalizes disposal of needle in proper container	1	
Releases tourniquet	1	
Runs IV for a brief period to assure patent line	1	
Secures catheter [tapes securely or verbalizes]	1	
Adjusts flow rate as appropriate	1	

Time End: _____   **TOTAL**   21

CRITICAL CRITERIA

_____ Failure to establish a patent and properly adjusted IV within 6 minute time limit
_____ Failure to take or verbalize body substance isolation precautions prior to performing venipuncture
_____ Contaminates equipment or site without appropriately correcting situation
_____ Performs any improper technique resulting in the potential for uncontrolled hemorrhage, catheter shear, or air embolism
_____ Failure to successfully establish IV within 3 attempts during 6 minute time limit
_____ Failure to dispose/verbalize disposal of needle in proper container

NOTE: Check here (_____) if candidate did not establish a patent IV and do not evaluate IV Bolus Medications.

INTRAVENOUS BOLUS MEDICATIONS

Time Start: _____

Asks patient for known allergies	1	
Selects correct medication	1	
Assures correct concentration of drug	1	
Assembles prefilled syringe correctly and dispels air	1	
Continues body substance isolation precautions	1	
Cleanses injection site [Y-port or hub]	1	
Reaffirms medication	1	
Stops IV flow [pinches tubing or shuts off]	1	
Administers correct dose at proper push rate	1	
Disposes/verbalizes proper disposal of syringe and needle in proper container	1	
Flushes tubing [runs wide open for a brief period]	1	
Adjusts drip rate to TKO/KVO	1	
Verbalizes need to observe patient for desired effect/adverse side effects	1	

Time End: _____   **TOTAL**   13

CRITICAL CRITERIA

_____ Failure to begin administration of medication within 3 minute time limit
_____ Contaminates equipment or site without appropriately correcting situation
_____ Failure to adequately dispel air resulting in potential for air embolism
_____ Injects improper drug or dosage [wrong drug, incorrect amount, or pushes at inappropriate rate]
_____ Failure to flush IV tubing after injecting medication
_____ Recaps needle or failure to dispose/verbalize disposal of syringe and needle in proper container

You must factually document your rationale for checking any of the above critical items on the reverse side of this form.

p309/8-003k

PATIENT ASSESSMENT - MEDICAL

Candidate: _____ Examiner: _____

Date: _____ Signature: _____

Scenario: _____

Time Start: _____

	Possible Points	Points Awarded
Takes or verbalizes body substance isolation precautions	1	
SCENE SIZE-UP		
Determines the scene/situation is safe	1	
Determines the mechanism of injury/nature of illness	1	
Determines the number of patients	1	
Requests additional help if necessary	1	
Considers stabilization of spine	1	
INITIAL ASSESSMENT		
Verbalizes general impression of the patient	1	
Determines responsiveness/level of consciousness	1	
Determines chief complaint/apparent life-threats	1	
Assesses airway and breathing -Assessment (1 point) -Assures adequate ventilation (1 point) -Initiates appropriate oxygen therapy (1 point)	3	
Assesses circulation -Assesses/controls major bleeding (1 point)　-Assesses skin [either skin color, temperature, or condition] (1 point) -Assesses pulse (1 point)	3	
Identifies priority patients/makes transport decision	1	
FOCUSED HISTORY AND PHYSICAL EXAMINATION/RAPID ASSESSMENT		
History of present illness -Onset (1 point)　　　　-Severity (1 point) -Provocation (1 point)　-Time (1 point) -Quality (1 point)　　　-Clarifying questions of associated signs and symptoms as related to OPQRST (2 points) -Radiation (1 point)	8	
Past medical history -Allergies (1 point)　　-Past pertinent history (1 point)　　-Events leading to present illness (1 point) -Medications (1 point)　-Last oral intake (1 point)	5	
Performs focused physical examination [assess affected body part/system or, if indicated, completes rapid assessment] -Cardiovascular　-Neurological　　-Integumentary　-Reproductive -Pulmonary　　　-Musculoskeletal　-GI/GU　　　　-Psychological/Social	5	
Vital signs -Pulse (1 point)　　　　　-Respiratory rate and quality (1 point each) -Blood pressure (1 point)　-AVPU (1 point)	5	
Diagnostics [must include application of ECG monitor for dyspnea and chest pain]	2	
States field impression of patient	1	
Verbalizes treatment plan for patient and calls for appropriate intervention(s)	1	
Transport decision re-evaluated	1	
ON-GOING ASSESSMENT		
Repeats initial assessment	1	
Repeats vital signs	1	
Evaluates response to treatments	1	
Repeats focused assessment regarding patient complaint or injuries	1	

Time End: _____

CRITICAL CRITERIA　　　　　　　　　　　　　　　　　　　　　　**TOTAL**　48

_____ Failure to initiate or call for transport of the patient within 15 minute time limit

_____ Failure to take or verbalize body substance isolation precautions

_____ Failure to determine scene safety before approaching patient

_____ Failure to voice and ultimately provide appropriate oxygen therapy

_____ Failure to assess/provide adequate ventilation

_____ Failure to find or appropriately manage problems associated with airway, breathing, hemorrhage or shock [hypoperfusion]

_____ Failure to differentiate patient's need for immediate transportation versus continued assessment and treatment at the scene

_____ Does other detailed or focused history or physical examination before assessing and treating threats to airway, breathing, and circulation

_____ Failure to determine the patient's primary problem

_____ Orders a dangerous or inappropriate intervention

_____ Failure to provide for spinal protection when indicated

You must factually document your rationale for checking any of the above critical items on the reverse side of this form.

p302/8-003k

PATIENT ASSESSMENT - TRAUMA

Candidate: _____ Examiner: _____

Date: _____ Signature: _____

Scenario # _____

Time Start: _____   NOTE: Areas denoted by "**" may be integrated within sequence of Initial Assessment

	Possible Points	Points Awarded
Takes or verbalizes body substance isolation precautions	1	
SCENE SIZE-UP		
Determines the scene/situation is safe	1	
Determines the mechanism of injury/nature of illness	1	
Determines the number of patients	1	
Requests additional help if necessary	1	
Considers stabilization of spine	1	
INITIAL ASSESSMENT/RESUSCITATION		
Verbalizes general impression of the patient	1	
Determines responsiveness/level of consciousness	1	
Determines chief complaint/apparent life-threats	1	
Airway -Opens and assesses airway (1 point) -Inserts adjunct as indicated (1 point)	2	

Breathing
  -Assess breathing (1 point)
  -Assures adequate ventilation (1 point)
  -Initiates appropriate oxygen therapy (1 point)
  -Manages any injury which may compromise breathing/ventilation (1 point)
	4	

Circulation
  -Checks pulse (1point)
  -Assess skin [either skin color, temperature, or condition] (1 point)
  -Assesses for and controls major bleeding if present (1 point)
  -Initiates shock management (1 point)
	4	

Identifies priority patients/makes transport decision	1	
FOCUSED HISTORY AND PHYSICAL EXAMINATION/RAPID TRAUMA ASSESSMENT		
Selects appropriate assessment	1	
Obtains, or directs assistant to obtain, baseline vital signs	1	
Obtains SAMPLE history	1	
DETAILED PHYSICAL EXAMINATION		

Head
  -Inspects mouth**, nose**, and assesses facial area (1 point)
  -Inspects and palpates scalp and ears (1 point)
  -Assesses eyes for PERRL** (1 point)
	3	

Neck**
  -Checks position of trachea (1 point)
  -Checks jugular veins (1 point)
  -Palpates cervical spine (1 point)
	3	

Chest**
  -Inspects chest (1 point)
  -Palpates chest (1 point)
  -Auscultates chest (1 point)
	3	

Abdomen/pelvis**
  -Inspects and palpates abdomen (1 point)
  -Assesses pelvis (1 point)
  -Verbalizes assessment of genitalia/perineum as needed (1 point)
	3	

Lower extremities** -Inspects, palpates, and assesses motor, sensory, and distal circulatory functions (1 point/leg)	2	
Upper extremities -Inspects, palpates, and assesses motor, sensory, and distal circulatory functions (1 point/arm)	2	

Posterior thorax, lumbar, and buttocks**
  -Inspects and palpates posterior thorax (1 point)
  -Inspects and palpates lumbar and buttocks area (1 point)
	2	

Manages secondary injuries and wounds appropriately	1	
Performs ongoing assessment	1	

Time End: _____   **TOTAL**   43

CRITICAL CRITERIA

_____ Failure to initiate or call for transport of the patient within 10 minute time limit
_____ Failure to take or verbalize body substance isolation precautions
_____ Failure to determine scene safety
_____ Failure to assess for and provide spinal protection when indicated
_____ Failure to voice and ultimately provide high concentration of oxygen
_____ Failure to assess/provide adequate ventilation
_____ Failure to find or appropriately manage problems associated with airway, breathing, hemorrhage or shock [hypoperfusion]
_____ Failure to differentiate patient's need for immediate transportation versus continued assessment/treatment at the scene
_____ Does other detailed/focused history or physical exam before assessing/treating threats to airway, breathing, and circulation
_____ Orders a dangerous or inappropriate intervention

You must factually document your rationale for checking any of the above critical items on the reverse side of this form.

p301/8-003k

PEDIATRIC INTRAOSSEOUS INFUSION

Candidate: _____ Examiner: _____

Date: _____ Signature: _____

Time Start:_____	Possible Points	Points Awarded

Checks selected IV fluid for:
   -Proper fluid (1 point)
   -Clarity (1 point)
	2	

Selects appropriate equipment to include:
   -IO needle (1 point)
   -Syringe (1 point)
   -Saline (1 point)
   -Extension set (1 point)
	4	

Selects proper administration set	1	
Connects administration set to bag	1	
Prepares administration set [fills drip chamber and flushes tubing]	1	
Prepares syringe and extension tubing	1	
Cuts or tears tape [at any time before IO puncture]	1	
Takes or verbalizes body substance isolation precautions [prior to IO puncture]	1	
Identifies proper anatomical site for IO puncture	1	
Cleanses site appropriately	1	

Performs IO puncture:
   -Stabilizes tibia (1 point)
   -Inserts needle at proper angle (1 point)
   -Advances needle with twisting motion until "pop" is felt (1 point)
   -Unscrews cap and removes stylette from needle (1 point)
	4	

Disposes of needle in proper container	1	
Attaches syringe and extension set to IO needle and aspirates	1	
Slowly injects saline to assure proper placement of needle	1	
Connects administration set and adjusts flow rate as appropriate	1	
Secures needle with tape and supports with bulky dressing	1	

Time End: _____   **TOTAL**   23

CRITICAL CRITERIA
_____ Failure to establish a patent and properly adjusted IO line within the 6 minute time limit
_____ Failure to take or verbalize body substance isolation precautions prior to performing IO puncture
_____ Contaminates equipment or site without appropriately correcting situation
_____ Performs any improper technique resulting in the potential for air embolism
_____ Failure to assure correct needle placement before attaching administration set
_____ Failure to successfully establish IO infusion within 2 attempts during 6 minute time limit
_____ Performing IO puncture in an unacceptable manner [improper site, incorrect needle angle, etc.]
_____ Failure to dispose of needle in proper container
_____ Orders or performs any dangerous or potentially harmful procedure

You must factually document your rationale for checking any of the above critical items on the reverse side of this form.

p310/8-003▶

PEDIATRIC (<2 yrs.) VENTILATORY MANAGEMENT

Candidate: _____ Examiner _____

Date: _____ Signature: _____

NOTE: If candidate elects to ventilate initially with BVM attached to reservoir and oxygen, full credit must be awarded for steps denoted by "**" so long as first ventilation is delivered within 30 seconds.

	Possible Points	Points Awarded
Takes or verbalizes body substance isolation precautions	1	
Opens the airway manually	1	
Elevates tongue, inserts simple adjunct [oropharyngeal or nasopharyngeal airway]	1	
NOTE: Examiner now informs candidate no gag reflex is present and patient accepts adjunct		
**Ventilates patient immediately with bag-valve-mask device unattached to oxygen	1	
**Hyperventilates patient with room air	1	
NOTE: Examiner now informs candidate that ventilation is being performed without difficulty and that pulse oximetry indicates the patient's blood oxygen saturation is 85%		
Attaches oxygen reservoir to bag-valve-mask device and connects to high flow oxygen regulator [12-15 L/minute]	1	
Ventilates patient at a rate of 20-30/minute and assures adequate chest expansion	1	
NOTE: After 30 seconds, examiner auscultates and reports breath sounds are present, equal bilaterally and medical direction has ordered intubation. The examiner must now take over ventilation.		
Directs assistant to pre-oxygenate patient	1	
Identifies/selects proper equipment for intubation	1	
Checks laryngoscope to assure operational with bulb tight	1	
NOTE: Examiner to remove OPA and move out of the way when candidate is prepared to intubate		
Places patient in neutral or sniffing position	1	
Inserts blade while displacing tongue	1	
Elevates mandible with laryngoscope	1	
Introduces ET tube and advances to proper depth	1	
Directs ventilation of patient	1	
Confirms proper placement by auscultation bilaterally over each lung and over epigastrium	1	
NOTE: Examiner to ask, "If you had proper placement, what should you expect to hear?"		
Secures ET tube [may be verbalized]	1	
TOTAL	17	

CRITICAL CRITERIA

_____ Failure to initiate ventilations within 30 seconds after applying gloves or interrupts ventilations for greater than 30 seconds at any time
_____ Failure to take or verbalize body substance isolation precautions
_____ Failure to pad under the torso to allow neutral head position or sniffing position
_____ Failure to voice and ultimately provide high oxygen concentrations [at least 85%]
_____ Failure to ventilate patient at a rate of at least 20/minute
_____ Failure to provide adequate volumes per breath [maximum 2 errors/minute permissible]
_____ Failure to pre-oxygenate patient prior to intubation
_____ Failure to successfully intubate within 3 attempts
_____ Uses gums as a fulcrum
_____ Failure to assure proper tube placement by auscultation bilaterally **and** over the epigastrium
_____ Inserts any adjunct in a manner dangerous to the patient
_____ Attempts to use any equipment not appropriate for the pediatric patient

You must factually document your rationale for checking any of the above critical items on the reverse side of this form.

SPINAL IMMOBILIZATION (SEATED PATIENT)

Candidate:_____Examiner:_____

Date: _____Signature:_____

	Possible Points	Points Awarded
Time Start: _____		
Takes or verbalizes body substance isolation precautions	1	
Directs assistant to place/maintain head in the neutral, in-line position	1	
Directs assistant to maintain manual immobilization of the head	1	
Reassesses motor, sensory, and circulatory function in each extremity	1	
Applies appropriately sized extrication collar	1	
Positions the immobilization device behind the patient	1	
Secures the device to the patient's torso	1	
Evaluates torso fixation and adjusts as necessary	1	
Evaluates and pads behind the patient's head as necessary	1	
Secures the patient's head to the device	1	
Verbalizes moving the patient to a long backboard	1	
Reassesses motor, sensory, and circulatory function in each extremity	1	
Time End: _____ **TOTAL**	12	

CRITICAL CRITERIA

_____ Did not immediately direct or take manual immobilization of the head
_____ Did not properly apply appropriately sized cervical collar before ordering release of manual immobilization
_____ Released or ordered release of manual immobilization before it was maintained mechanically
_____ Manipulated or moved patient excessively causing potential spinal compromise
_____ Head immobilized to the device **before** device sufficiently secured to torso
_____ Device moves excessively up, down, left, or right on the patient's torso
_____ Head immobilization allows for excessive movement
_____ Torso fixation inhibits chest rise, resulting in respiratory compromise
_____ Upon completion of immobilization, head is not in a neutral, in-line position
_____ Did not reassess motor, sensory, and circulatory functions in each extremity after voicing immobilization to the long backboard

You must factually document your rationale for checking any of the above critical items on the reverse side of this form.

SPINAL IMMOBILIZATION (SUPINE PATIENT)

Candidate:_____Examiner:_____

Date: _____Signature:_____

Time Start: _____	Possible Points	Points Awarded
Takes or verbalizes body substance isolation precautions	1	
Directs assistant to place/maintain head in the neutral, in-line position	1	
Directs assistant to maintain manual immobilization of the head	1	
Reassesses motor, sensory, and circulatory function in each extremity	1	
Applies appropriately sized extrication collar	1	
Positions the immobilization device appropriately	1	
Directs movement of the patient onto the device without compromising the integrity of the spine	1	
Applies padding to voids between the torso and the device as necessary	1	
Immobilizes the patient's torso to the device	1	
Evaluates and pads behind the patient's head as necessary	1	
Immobilizes the patient's head to the device	1	
Secures the patient's legs to the device	1	
Secures the patient's arms to the device	1	
Reassesses motor, sensory, and circulatory function in each extremity	1	

Time End: _____   **TOTAL**   14

CRITICAL CRITERIA

_____ Did not immediately direct or take manual immobilization of the head
_____ Did not properly apply appropriately sized cervical collar before ordering release of manual immobilization
_____ Released or ordered release of manual immobilization before it was maintained mechanically
_____ Manipulated or moved patient excessively causing potential spinal compromise
_____ Head immobilized to the device **before** device sufficiently secured to torso
_____ Patient moves excessively up, down, left, or right on the device
_____ Head immobilization allows for excessive movement
_____ Upon completion of immobilization, head is not in a neutral, in-line position
_____ Did not reassess motor, sensory, and circulatory functions in each extremity after voicing immobilization to the device

You must factually document your rationale for checking any of the above critical items on the reverse side of this form.

STATIC CARDIOLOGY

Candidate: _____ Examiner: _____

Date: _____ Signature: _____

SET #_____

Level of Testing: ☐ NREMT-Intermediate/99   ☐ NREMT-Paramedic

Note: No points for treatment may be awarded if the diagnosis is incorrect.
Only document incorrect responses in spaces provided.

Time Start:_____

	Possible Points	Points Awarded
STRIP #1		
Diagnosis:	1	
Treatment:	2	
STRIP #2		
Diagnosis:	1	
Treatment:	2	
STRIP #3		
Diagnosis:	1	
Treatment:	2	
STRIP #4		
Diagnosis:	1	
Treatment:	2	

Time End: _____   TOTAL   12

p307/8-003k

Candidate:_____ Examiner:_____

Date: _____ Signature: _____

NOTE: If candidate elects to ventilate initially with BVM attached to reservoir and oxygen, full credit must be awarded for steps denoted by "**" so long as first ventilation is delivered within 30 seconds.

	Possible Points	Points Awarded
Takes or verbalizes body substance isolation precautions	1	
Opens the airway manually	1	
Elevates tongue, inserts simple adjunct [oropharyngeal or nasopharyngeal airway]	1	
NOTE: Examiner now informs candidate no gag reflex is present and patient accepts adjunct		
**Ventilates patient immediately with bag-valve-mask device unattached to oxygen	1	
**Hyperventilates patient with room air	1	
NOTE: Examiner now informs candidate that ventilation is being performed without difficulty and that pulse oximetry indicates the patient's blood oxygen saturation is 85%		
Attaches oxygen reservoir to bag-valve-mask device and connects to high flow oxygen regulator [12-15 L/minute]	1	
Ventilates patient at a rate of 10-20/minute with appropriate volumes	1	
NOTE: After 30 seconds, examiner auscultates and reports breath sounds are present, equal bilaterally and medical direction has ordered intubation. The examiner must now take over ventilation.		
Directs assistant to pre-oxygenate patient	1	
Identifies/selects proper equipment for intubation	1	
Checks equipment for: -Cuff leaks (1 point) -Laryngoscope operational with bulb tight (1 point)	2	
NOTE: Examiner to remove OPA and move out of the way when candidate is prepared to intubate		
Positions head properly	1	
Inserts blade while displacing tongue	1	
Elevates mandible with laryngoscope	1	
Introduces ET tube and advances to proper depth	1	
Inflates cuff to proper pressure and disconnects syringe	1	
Directs ventilation of patient	1	
Confirms proper placement by auscultation bilaterally over each lung and over epigastrium	1	
NOTE: Examiner to ask, "If you had proper placement, what should you expect to hear?"		
Secures ET tube [may be verbalized]	1	
NOTE: Examiner now asks candidate, "Please demonstrate one additional method of verifying proper tube placement in this patient."		
Identifies/selects proper equipment	1	
Verbalizes findings and interpretations [compares indicator color to the colorimetric scale and states reading to examiner]	1	
NOTE: Examiner now states, "You see secretions in the tube and hear gurgling sounds with the patient's exhalation."		
Identifies/selects a flexible suction catheter	1	
Pre-oxygenates patient	1	
Marks maximum insertion length with thumb and forefinger	1	
Inserts catheter into the ET tube leaving catheter port open	1	
At proper insertion depth, covers catheter port and applies suction while withdrawing catheter	1	
Ventilates/directs ventilation of patient as catheter is flushed with sterile water	1	
TOTAL	**27**	

CRITICAL CRITERIA

_____ Failure to initiate ventilations within 30 seconds after applying gloves or interrupts ventilations for greater than 30 seconds at any time
_____ Failure to take or verbalize body substance isolation precautions
_____ Failure to voice and ultimately provide high oxygen concentrations [at least 85%]
_____ Failure to ventilate patient at a rate of at least 10/minute
_____ Failure to provide adequate volumes per breath [maximum 2 errors/minute permissible]
_____ Failure to pre-oxygenate patient prior to intubation and suctioning
_____ Failure to successfully intubate within 3 attempts
_____ Failure to disconnect syringe **immediately** after inflating cuff of ET tube
_____ Uses teeth as a fulcrum
_____ Failure to assure proper tube placement by auscultation bilaterally **and** over the epigastrium
_____ If used, stylette extends beyond end of ET tube
_____ Inserts any adjunct in a manner dangerous to the patient
_____ Suctions the patient for more than 15 seconds
_____ Does not suction the patient

You must factually document your rationale for checking any of the above critical items on the reverse side of this form.

p303/8-003k